KW-044-449

pathology

JOIN US ON THE INTERNET VIA WWW, GOPHER, FTP OR EMAIL:

WWW: http://www.thomson.com
GOPHER: gopher.thomson.com
FTP: ftp.thomson.com   A service of I(T)P ®
EMAIL: findit@kiosk.thomson.com

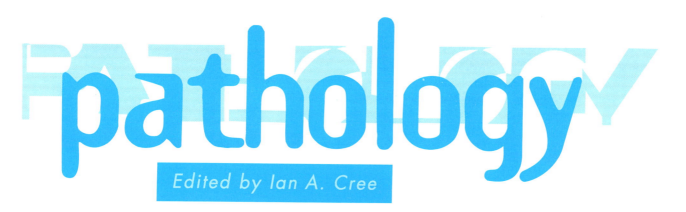

pathology

Edited by Ian A. Cree

MB, PhD, MRCPath

Clinical Senior Lecturer
Department of Pathology, Institute of Ophthalmology,
University College London
and
Honorary Consultant Pathologist,
Moorfields Eye Hospital, London, UK

CHAPMAN & HALL MEDICAL
London • Weinheim • New York • Tokyo • Melbourne • Madras

Published by Chapman & Hall, 2–6 Boundary Row,
London SE1 8HN, UK

Chapman & Hall, 2–6 Boundary Row, London SE1 8HN, UK

Chapman & Hall GmbH, Pappelallee 3, 69469 Weinheim, Germany

Chapman & Hall USA, 115 Fifth Avenue, New York, NY 10003, USA

Chapman & Hall Japan, ITP-Japan, Kyowa Building,
3F, 2-2-1 Hirakawacho, Chiyoda-ku, Tokyo 102, Japan

Chapman & Hall Australia, 102 Dodds Street, South Melbourne,
Victoria 3205, Australia

Chapman & Hall India, R. Seshadri, 32 Second Main Road, CIT East,
Madras 600 035, India

First edition 1997

© 1997 Ian A. Cree

Typeset in 10/13 Palatino by Newnorth Print Ltd, UK

Printed in Spain

ISBN 0 412 47200 7

Apart from any fair dealing for the purposes of research or private study,
or criticism or review, as permitted under the UK Copyright Designs and
Patents Act, 1988, this publication may not be reproduced, stored, or
transmitted, in any form or by any means, without the prior permission
in writing of the publishers, or in the case of reprographic reproduction
only in accordance with the terms of the licences issued by the Copyright
Licensing Agency in the UK, or in accordance with the terms of licences
issued by the appropriate Reproduction Rights Organization outside the
UK. Enquiries concerning reproduction outside the terms stated here
should be sent to the publishers at the London address printed on this
page.

The publisher makes no representation, express or implied, with
regard to the accuracy of the information contained in this book and
cannot accept any legal responsibility or liability for any errors or
omissions that may be made.

A catalogue record for this book is available from the British Library

Library of Congress Catalog Card Number: 96-85896

List of contributors

Suhail I.A. Baithun, FRCPath
Senior Lecturer/Honorary Consultant in Histopathology
St Bartholomew's and the Royal London School of Medicine and Dentistry,
London, UK

Nathaniel R.B. Carey, MA, MD, MRCPath, DMJ(Path)
Consultant Cardiac Histopathologist
Department of Histopathology, Papworth Hospital, Cambridge, UK

Derrick M. Chisholm, MDSc, BDS, PhD, FDSRCPS(Glas), FDSRCS(Ed)
Boyd Professor of Dental Surgery; Honorary Consultant in Oral Medicine and
Pathology
Department of Dental Surgery and Periodontology, University of Dundee,
Scotland, UK

Ian A. Cree, PhD, MRCPath
Clinical Senior Lecturer
Department of Pathology, Institute of Ophthalmology, University College
London; Honorary Consultant Pathologist, Moorfields Eye Hospital, London, UK

David J. Harrison, MRCPath
Senior Lecturer
University of Edinburgh; Honorary Consultant, Royal Infirmary NHS Trust,
Edinburgh, Scotland, UK

Steven Humphreys, FRCPath
Consultant Histopathologist
King's Healthcare and King's College Hospital School of Medicine and Dentistry,
London, UK

D. James Ironside, MRCPath
Senior Lecturer in Pathology
University of Edinburgh; Honorary Consultant in Neuropathology, Western
General Hospitals Trust, Edinburgh, Scotland, UK

Iona J.M. Jeffrey, MRCPath
Consultant and Honorary Senior Lecturer in Perinatal and Paediatric Pathology
Department of Histopathology, St George's Hospital Medical School, London,
UK

Klaus Kayser, MD, PhD
Associate Professor
University of Heidelberg; Chief, Department of Pathology, Thoraxklinik,
Heidelberg, Germany

Stephen Lang, MRCPath
Consultant Pathologist
Ninewells Hospital and Medical School, Dundee; Honorary Senior Lecturer,
University of Dundee, Scotland, UK

David G. Lowe, MD, FRCS, FIBiol, FRCPath
Reader and Consultant Histopathologist
Department of Histopathology, St Bartholomew's Hospital Medical School,
London, UK

Sebastian B. Lucas, FRCP, FRCPath
Professor of Pathology
UMDS Department of Histopathology, St Thomas' Hospital, London, UK

Anne-Marie McNicol, MD, FRCP(Glas), FRCPath
Reader in Pathology and Head of NHS Department
University Department of Pathology, Glasgow Royal Infirmary University NHS
Trust, Glasgow, Scotland, UK

Indira Nath, MD, FRCPath, FAMS, FNA, FASc, FNASc
Professor of Biotechnology
All India Institute of Medical Sciences, New Delhi, India

Graham R. Ogden, BDS, MDSc, PhD, FDSRCPS(Glas)
Senior Lecturer in Oral Surgery; Honorary Consultant in Oral and Maxillofacial
Surgery
Department of Dental Surgery and Periodontology, University of Dundee,
Scotland, UK

David M. Parham, MD, MRCPath
Consultant Pathologist
Royal Bournemouth Hospital, Dorset, UK

Robin P. Reid, MRCPath
Senior Lecturer in Osteoarticular Pathology
University Department of Pathology, Western Infirmary, Glasgow, Scotland, UK

Neil A. Shepherd, MRCPath
Consultant Pathologist
Department of Histopathology, Gloucester Royal Hospital, Gloucester, UK

Josef Smolle, MD
Associate Professor
Department of Dermatology, University of Graz, Graz, Austria

C. Michael Steel, PhD, DSc, FRCP(Edin), FRCSE(Edin), FRCPath, FRCE
Professor of Medical Science
University of St Andrews, Scotland, UK

Jon D. van der Walt, FRCPath
Senior Lecturer
Department of Histopathology, UMDS of Guy's and St Thomas' Hospitals;
Honorary Consultant, Guy's and St Thomas' Hospitals, London, UK

Preface

There is often a large difference between what a student wants from a textbook and what the tutor thinks the student needs from a textbook. In trying to bridge this gap with a new pathology textbook, I have been made very aware of the problems of trying to please both parties.

The rate of accumulation of medical knowledge continues to increase, and in most medical schools, the curriculum has been stretched to bursting point. The UK General Medical Council sought to reform the medical curriculum by addressing three major problems:

- Excessive factual load on students
- Passive acquisition of knowledge to the detriment of imagination and curiosity
- Lack of training for future self-education.

The primary aim of the undergraduate course is to acquire 'an understanding of health and disease, and of the prevention and management of the latter'. Understanding of the scientific basis of medicine and of disease in terms of processes is stressed as the basis for a sound medical training. Development of scientific skills of evaluation and experimentation should feature prominently.

Pathology is the study of disease and as such, it is essential to the study of medicine. Understanding the mechanisms of disease must be gained by the undergraduate at an early stage in the medical course to prepare him or her for instruction in other disciplines, to interpret their possible impact on patient care, and to give a basis for future postgraduate training. Systematic pathology can be studied later, and may be integrated with clinical teaching. There is no need to turn all medical students into pathologists – even for a year or two! There is, however, a core of knowledge in pathology which will be important whatever the student's chosen career.

Pathology is about disease – its aetiology, pathogenesis and possible opportunities for therapeutic intervention. Histopathology is primarily a matter of pattern recognition, either of cells or of tissue appearances. It is important for students to understand what diagnostic histopathology is and how it contributes to patient care; however, overemphasis on histopathology skills can put students off the more important requirement for the scientific study of disease, particularly if their pattern-recognition skills are not well developed.

The size of this textbook was decided upon before pen was put to paper or the word-processor booted up. This has had its effect: each author has had to define the core of their subject. Subjects such as immunology are not covered to any great extent as we believe that these are best learned from specific textbooks, many of which are referenced in the further reading list provided. We have also attempted to use the illustrations to teach, and have tried not to duplicate facts in texts and figures. Other innovations are perhaps more obvious. There is a chapter on multisystem disease to encourage the student to think about how pathogenic mechanisms may result in differing effects in different tissues, and we have included case studies to make the clinical relevance of pathology that much clearer.

The challenge to the modern doctor or medical student is to keep up with those advances which influence his or her practice, in whatever discipline. The aim of this book is to give the student a thorough grounding in the basic mechanisms of disease and to illustrate the effects of these mechanisms system by system. No attempt has been made to cover all diseases, although we have tried to include examples of those that are important either because they are common, or because they show mechanisms well.

It is of course impossible to please everybody, but I hope that this textbook will at least meet some of the criticisms levelled at pathology and make it a more popular subject with students.

I. A. Cree
London, 1996

Acknowledgements

When I was asked to edit this book, I had little idea of what I was taking on. I must first and foremost thank my long-suffering wife and family who put up with frequent absences as it neared completion. That it has appeared at all is a great tribute to the efforts of the authors, all of whom are busy consultants who have constantly to juggle demands from many sources.

I have been aided by a number of people behind the scenes at Chapman & Hall, particularly Paul Remes, Nick Dunton and Sharon Duckworth. Much of the editing has been done by Kathleen Lyle and Jane Sugarman. Most of the line illustrations were drawn by Barking Dog Art Ltd from authors' rough diagrams, and the diagrams that accompany most of the histological sections were drawn by Louise Perks. Photographs were provided from a large variety of sources to me or to authors; many were specially taken for this book. I am immensely grateful to all those involved in collecting these together, but particularly to Bill Guthrie and Ron Fawkes, who taught me all I know about how to obtain decent macroscopic and microscopic images. Finally, I am most grateful to Professors F. Walker, W. Lee and J.S. Beck for their advice and encouragement.

Ian A. Cree

Chapter 1 The basis of disease

Learning objectives
❏ Appreciation of the role of pathology in defining the causes, progression and effects of disease
❏ Ability to define the aetiology of disease and classify the causes of disease
❏ Understanding of what is meant by pathogenesis and the factors involved in determining disease progression
❏ Understanding of the possible effects of disease on cells and tissues

Pathology is most simply defined as the study of disease, and as such it is the basis of scientific medical practice. Scientific treatment or prevention of disease depends upon an understanding of the causes of disease and how these relate to the patient.

The stages of disease formation can be summarized in terms of cause (**aetiology**), progression from cause to disease (**pathogenesis**) and effects. Descriptions of the effect of disease on tissues hardly alter over the years, but understanding of aetiology and pathogenesis is increasing at a phenomenal rate. This is having an increasing impact on medical practice and makes an appreciation of pathology more and more important.

The aetiology of disease

The causes of disease can be divided into several different groups as shown in Table 1.1, and this list also forms a convenient way of classifying disease. Faced with a particular appearance in a tissue or clinical syndrome, this classification can be helpful in organizing the approach to diagnosis and treatment. A mass in the lung seen on a chest radiograph may be infective (an abscess), inflammatory (a granuloma) or neoplastic (a tumour).

Stages of disease formation

Aetiology	Cause of the disease
Pathogenesis	Sequence of mechanisms leading to disease
Pathological features	Effects of pathogenic mechanisms on tissues
Macroscopic	Visible to the eye
Microscopic	Invisible to the eye
Prognosis	Probable outcome of disease

Table 1.1   A classification of disease causation (aetiology)

Cause	Disease example
Inherited (genetic)	
Congenital	Cystic fibrosis
Late appearing	Huntington's disease
Consequent upon growth or ageing	Senile dementia
Infective	Pneumonia
Inflammatory	Eczema
Vascular	Myocardial infarction
Metabolic/toxic	Diabetes
Physical or chemical trauma	A burn
Neoplastic	Lung cancer
Environmental	Starvation
Idiopathic (unknown)	Sarcoidosis

Causes of disease are usually multiple, although one may have greater significance than the rest. Some causes may also result in more than one disease: tobacco smoking is a known cause of both lung cancer and vascular disease. In all disease, there should be a clearly identifiable pathway from cause to clinical presentation and outcome. However, the causes of some diseases are still not known: in these, there may be associated risk factors which occur commonly in people with these disorders and may point to causes which need research to find out their relevance. Diseases of unknown cause are usually qualified by an adjective such as 'idiopathic', 'primary' or 'cryptogenic'.

Discovery of causative relationships

Only two centuries ago, the causes of disease were largely unknown. Ideas on disease we now regard as fanciful were commonplace – such as the idea that bad smells caused disease. Paradoxically, one of the greatest advances was made without knowledge of the cause of disease, when in 1855 John Snow traced the source of an outbreak of cholera to a contaminated water supply and brought it to an end. The invention of the microscope stimulated many early scientists to look at the problems of disease, the most famous being Louis Pasteur. Robert Koch discovered the cause of anthrax and developed a set of rules for deciding whether an organism was the true aetiological agent. The success of this approach has led others to use similar rules in deciding whether any postulated pathological mechanism is operating in disease. This is particularly important for sorting out the significance of test tube effects, which may not even occur in the patient.

Koch's postulates
- Organism should be found in all cases of the disease, localized with lesions
- Organism should be maintained in pure culture in vitro for several generations
- Isolated organism should be able to produce disease in other susceptible animals

Much of medical research is aimed at clarifying the aetiology and pathogenesis of disease, since once the cause is known it may be avoided, and once mechanisms are known they may be interrupted. Such research can be divided into three areas:

- **Descriptive research:** The classification of living organisms by Linnaeus, the histological typing of lymphoma and the first description of AIDS fall into this category. Such work is the basis of all medical research.
- **Hypothesis-driven research:** Classically, scientists formulate hypotheses (ideas) and then test them. Then they try again! Ideally this results in a progressive narrowing down of possibilities until the right one is found.
- **Technical research:** To test hypotheses one needs methods or techniques. Often scientific progression stalls until someone invents a new piece of equipment (such as the microscope) or method (such as monoclonal antibody production).

In the last few years, a combination of all three types of research, the basis of which was careful clinical observation, has resulted in the identification of many genes and the consequence of their malfunction in both inherited disease and cancer.

Inherited (genetic) disease

The recent identification of many genes which cause inherited disease is just the start of a revolution in our approach to disease. The well-characterized diseases such as cystic fibrosis are already being joined by a large number of other newly recognized disorders in which the outcome is not a specific disease, but an increased susceptibility to disease. These include syndromes in which affected individuals have increased susceptibility to cancer, diabetes or infections.

Discovering how these genetic defects result in disease (Fig. 1.1) should ensure the future of many medical researchers for years to come. It is often more practicable to alter the disease process before the disease becomes clinically apparent than to wait and act later. The newly discovered genetic markers will allow populations to be screened for potential problems and at-risk individuals to be treated accordingly. This raises ethical issues, but some screening for genetic disease has been practised in many countries for years as part of childhood screening.

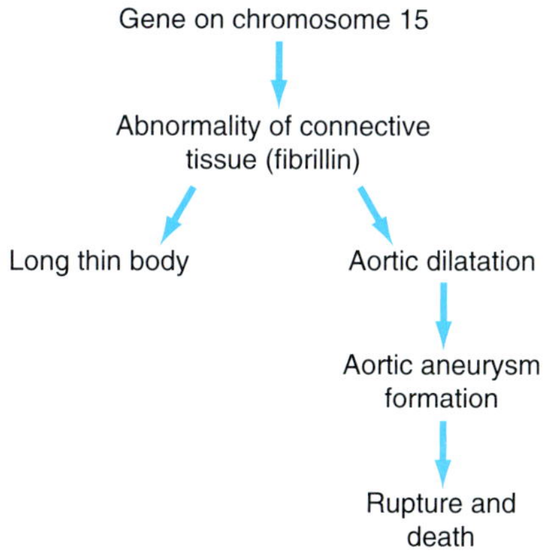

Growth and ageing

The changes which occur in the body from conception to old age are thought to be regulated by the switching on and off of genes, modified by the influence of many environmental factors including diet, radiation and infection. Yet the inevitability of many changes currently associated with ageing is far from certain. For instance, although failure of the immune system is thought to be responsible for the increased incidence of infections in elderly people, healthy aged people rarely show many differences from younger subjects. Many patients over 80 years old admitted to our hospital wards are written off as having multiple pathology because they are old – not because they have had time to accumulate more medical problems.

Does a pathological mechanism lead to disease?

- Is the disease always associated with the mechanism?
- Is it less prominent in those with mild disease and more prominent in those with severe disease?
- Does restoration of normality lead to disappearance or cessation of the mechanism?
- Can similar mechanisms cause abnormalities in animal or in vitro models?
- Is there a clear pathway from cause to disease via this mechanism?
- Does interruption of the mechanism prevent or resolve the disease?

Gene on chromosome 15

↓

Abnormality of connective tissue (fibrillin)

↙ ↘

Long thin body   Aortic dilatation

↓

Aortic aneurysm formation

↓

Rupture and death

Fig. 1.1 Genetic disease: Marfan's syndrome.

Infections

It has been said that human beings stay alive by being one jump ahead of the bacteria. This may be true, but it is hardly in the interests of the large number of species of bacteria which live on humans for *Homo sapiens* to die out! Nevertheless, parasitic and infectious diseases remain a major threat to human civilization and to individuals. There is little doubt that the two most troublesome methods of spread of micro-organisms are the **faecal–oral** and **respiratory** routes. The difference is that it is possible by means of sanitation and water services to prevent those infections which depend upon faecal–oral transmission almost entirely. Indeed, where there is no safe water supply and no sanitation, the impact on disease levels in the population is such that life expectancy at birth is halved and infant death rates may be 30% or more.

Even in wealthier societies, the problems of infection cannot be ignored: newly virulent organisms may appear from time to time and well-known pathogens may reappear if antibiotic resistance occurs or levels of immunization fall. At present, AIDS and tuberculosis are good examples of this process.

Transmission of pathogenic micro-organisms
Direct
- Droplet spread to lung/nose
- Touch
- Venereal

Indirect
- Fomites (infected objects)
- Water-borne
- Food-borne

Inflammation

Inflammation occurs as the body's response to injury from any cause and requires an intact immune system to operate correctly. If the immune system malfunctions, then disease can result from inappropriate inflammation. In addition, the body's attempts to cure an injury are sometimes worse than the injury itself. Inflammation can therefore be the direct cause of many of the clinical effects observed in disease.

Vascular causes

Just as inflammation is rarely alone responsible for disease, so vascular events may be responsible for many clinical effects without necessarily being the root cause of the problem. Changes in vessel walls known as atheroma underlie most myocardial infarctions, but the aetiology and pathogenesis of atheroma are still not entirely clear.

Metabolic or toxic causes

This varied group of disorders may be primary (usually due to genetic abnormalities), secondary to other disease, or caused by doctors (iatrogenic). Many can be dealt with either by replacement therapy or by treating the underlying cause. The frequency of iatrogenic disease underlines the need for careful medical practice. *Primum non nocere* – first do no harm – is a good principle to follow in medical treatment.

Neoplastic disease

Cancer is often thought of as a single disease, when in fact it is many different diseases, all of which are characterized by abnormal and unlimited cell growth. Advances in molecular biology and genetics mean that we now understand many of the mechanisms which control cell growth, but in general this has not yet been translated into improved treatment.

Metabolic diseases
Primary
- Phenylketonuria

Secondary
- Diabetes mellitus
- Hypercalcaemia

Iatrogenic
- Drug reactions
- Electolyte imbalance

In the next few years, it is likely that increased knowledge of the differences between normal and cancerous cells will lead to the production of new drugs with greater efficacy and fewer side effects. However, every tumour has a different genetic make-up and the heterogeneity of drug sensitivity which results often means that one treatment does not suit all patients, even if they have the same type of cancer.

Physical or chemical trauma

Physical trauma, whether accidental or intentional, is dealt with by the body in a highly organized fashion. The primary problem is systemic – usually blood loss, respiratory failure or loss of mobility. Immediate cardiovascular changes and damage limitation give way, if the patient survives, to healing processes within tissues which are dealt with in their appropriate chapters.

Environmental causes

There is increasing awareness of the importance of environment for disease. We are in constant interaction with our environment, whether it is obvious, such as extreme heat or cold, or insidious, such as holes in the ozone layer. In most countries, water, food and air pollution are major problems, and efforts to control such risks are of considerable health benefit.

Adaptation to environmental changes is a key requirement for health. Hypothermia is avoided by increasing physical activity, wearing insulation (clothes) and maintaining good nutrition. Less obvious examples include the adaptation to high altitude in which the cardiovascular system changes and numbers of circulating erythrocytes increase.

The pathogenesis of disease

The course of any disease is modified by a host of different factors, including those determined genetically and those resulting from previous exposure to the environment or pre-existing disease. Individual factors include sex, age, race and genetic polymorphism, whereas environmental factors such as previous immunological experience of antigens determine the outcome of many infections.

Age

The age of the patient is an important consideration for many diseases, as shown by the graph of death rates against age in Fig. 1.2. Some ageing changes are apparent even in the 30s, when many athletic careers end as mild changes in muscle or neural functions reduce competitiveness. Changes in skin may be more related to the degree of sun exposure, and may also occur in the 30s, but ageing itself does lead to progressive changes with thinning and wrinkling of the skin.

The role of hormones in this process is well understood: in women the menopause results from a sudden decrease in oestrogen secretion by the ovaries leading to changes in the uterus, breasts and bones. The causes of ageing may differ between different cell types. Accumulation of genetic defects in rapidly dividing cells as a result of both random and acquired mutations may result in abnormal function, including an increased incidence of cancer.

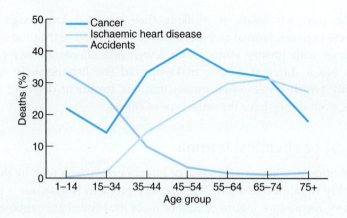

Fig. 1.2   Age and cause of death.

Highly specialized tissues in which the cells do not divide may have a different problem. Loss of these cells over time may lead to functional deficiencies.

Genetic polymorphism

Individuals differ in appearance because of their differing genetic makeup. Racial characteristics are one example of this, but even at the level of families, the genetic heterogeneity may be sufficient to influence the susceptibility of individuals to disease. Knowledge of racial background and family history is therefore an important part of a clinical history.

Environmental effects

Disease expression is altered substantially by the general fitness of the individual. Factors which determine this include nutrition, intercurrent disease, housing, exercise, mental attitude and preventive health care. Appreciation of the influence of environment on health has been highlighted by the changes in the incidence of fatal infectious disease among children in Western society in comparison with the last century. The problems which improved living standards have overcome include measles, tuberculosis, diarrhoeal disease and pollution-related emphysema.

It has become clear that there are requirements for optimum health which can have a substantial impact on disease: the cure for a dripping tap is a new washer, not a bucket beneath it!

Requirements for health

Homo sapiens has proved itself to be an adaptable species, able to respond to new infective threats to health by means of an effective integral (passive) immune system and active (cerebral) measures. It has been said that the difference between a civilized society and an uncivilized one is possession of a clean water supply and sanitation. Together with adequate balanced nutrition, these are undoubtedly the main needs for health.

The risk of disease can, however, be further reduced by attention to family planning (restricting population pressure on resources), immunizing against disease and preventing pollution. The ability to remove carcinogens from the environment is becoming ever more important as our understanding of them grows. However, the cost-effectiveness and economic impact of environmental intervention must be assessed carefully before intervening.

Requirements for health: interventions in order of cost-effectiveness
- Water and sanitation
- Nutrition
- Family planning
- Immunization
- Removal of environmental dangers

Chapter 2　　Molecular and genetic disease

> ### *Learning objectives*
> ❏ Appreciation of the relationship between DNA structure and function
> ❏ Understanding of the process of gene expression, including transcription, translation and modification
> ❏ Understanding of mitosis and meiosis and their implications for gene inheritance
> ❏ Knowledge of how gene defects arise and cause disease
> ❏ Appreciation of the methods used to detect such defects
> ❏ Understanding of the possible approaches to gene therapy
> ❏ Appreciation of the ethical dilemmas involved in screening for abnormal genes and treating patients with genetic disease

The genetic blueprint

DNA is the genetic material of almost all living organisms (Fig. 2.1). The only exceptions are the very smallest viruses, which have an RNA genome. When a cell divides, the DNA must replicate and be distributed in exact aliquots to the daughter cells (Fig. 2.2). There is an important exception, the formation of **germ cells** (sperm or ovum) where the daughter cell has only half the DNA content of its precursor. Normal cell division is accompanied by the process of mitosis, but underlying the phenomena visible with the light microscope is the chemical process of DNA replication. In essence, the two strands of the double helix separate and a new strand is added to each of the originals, using the original base sequence as a template. This is known as **semi-conservative replication** because each of the DNA molecules produced is half new, half old.

A complex series of biochemical reactions is involved in DNA replication. A **helicase** enzyme begins the uncoiling, a primase attaches a few complementary bases to each strand at the origin of replication and a series of **DNA polymerase** enzymes attach further bases to the primer, always extending the growing chain in the 5′ to 3′ direction and using the original strand as template so that the A–T and G–C pairings are preserved in the new double helix. As the original double helix unwinds, one of the new daughter strands can be synthesized continuously since the unwinding allows progressive elongation 5′ to 3′. The other strand, however, is in the opposite orientation and therefore it can only be elongated by a series of 'jumps' on the part of the primase, repeatedly adding starter bases to the template strand as it is exposed and then filling-in the new strand backwards (Fig. 2.3).

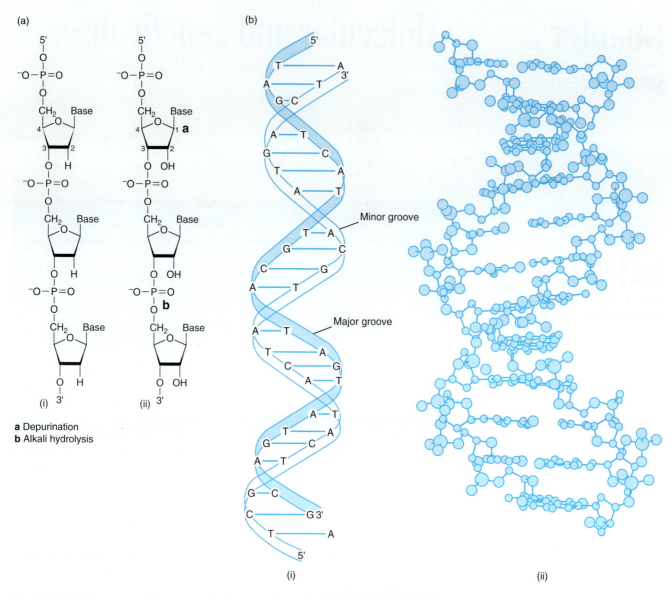

Fig. 2.1   DNA structure: (a) covalent structure of the 'backbone' of (i) DNA (bases: A, adenine; G, guanine; C, cytosine; T, thymine) and (ii) RNA (bases: A, adenine; G, guanine; C, cytosine; U, uracil). (b) The DNA double helix in the usual B-DNA configuration. (i) Diagram of the arrangement of the two strands; (ii) atomic structure. Note the major and minor grooves in the double helix, and the base pairs perpendicular to the axis of the molecule.

DNA replication enzymes	
Function	**Enzyme**
Uncoiling	Helicase
Attachment of a few bases along length of DNA	Primase
Extension of bases	Polymerases
Joining of strands	Ligase

The bases attached by the primase system are actually in the form of RNA rather than DNA. These must be removed and replaced by DNA bases before replication is complete. Furthermore, in the case of the strand copied in a series of short fragments, these must be linked up by a **DNA ligase**. Finally, some of the DNA polymerases have an **editing** function – that is, they check for and correct any errors in base-pairing as replication proceeds.

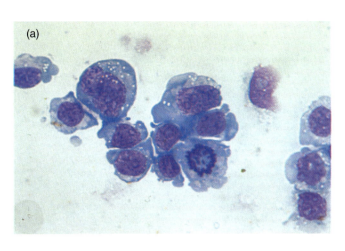

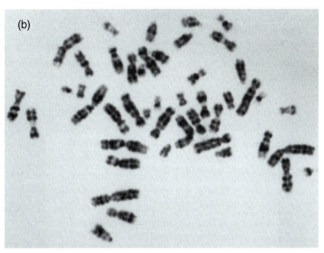

Fig. 2.2 (a) A mitotic cell (centre of clump): note that the nuclear membrane has gone and chromosomes have formed. (b) A human metaphase spread. The dividing cell has been fixed in suspension and dropped on to a slide. The chromosomes spread out as the fixative dries. They have been processed and stained to display the G-banding (Giemsa) pattern that allows individual members of the chromosome set to be identified.

Gene structure

Only about 5% of DNA in most higher organisms (including humans) is used to encode genetic information (genes). The rest is of unknown function. In most instances the encoded information is broken up into several blocks (**exons**) separated by non-coding stretches (**introns**). In addition, most genes have other important elements which are not expressed as gene products but serve to regulate the activity of the gene. These include **promoter** sequences lying upstream (i.e. in the 5' direction, because a gene is always read from 5' to 3') and **enhancers** which can be either upstream or downstream and may be a considerable distance away (Fig. 2.4). Some promoters have easily recognized sequences, such as CAAT or TATTAA. They, together with the enhancers, interact with regulatory peptides in the nucleus and such interactions control gene expression according to the state of cellular differentiation and/or activation.

Fig. 2.3 Events at the replication fork: (a) binding of the helicase–primase complex. (b) Local uncoiling of DNA double helix. A short complementary RNA 'primer' sequence is synthesized at the start point on each strand. (c) These primers are extended by DNA polymerase, synthesizing a DNA-complementary sequence on each strand. (d) Elongation proceeds steadily in the 5' to 3' direction on the 'leading' strand but, on the 'lagging' strand, a series of new RNA primers must be added at intervals as the duplex unwinds. As each Okazaki fragment is completed (between successive RNA primers), the DNA polymerase removes the RNA primer from the preceding fragment, replacing it with DNA. A ligase enzyme completes the join to the newly synthesized DNA. (e) Polymerase on the lagging strand jumps back to initiate the next Okazaki fragment.

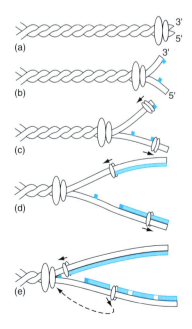

The structure of DNA

The structure of DNA (Fig. 2.1a) comprises a continuous 'backbone' of pentose sugar, deoxyribose, phosphorylated on the 5' carbon atom and linked by 3'–5' phosphodiester bonds. This linkage gives the backbone, and hence the whole molecule, directional polarity which is important in all aspects of DNA function. Covalently attached to the 1' carbon atom is an organic base, which can be a purine (adenine or guanine) or a pyrimidine (cytosine or thymine). Conventionally, these are referred to by the single-letter codes A, G, C, T. The bases project from the backbone at right angles and two strands of this type can 'hybridize' or 'anneal' to form a double helix with the sugar phosphates on the outside and the bases linking up like the rungs of a ladder. This configuration is only possible if the bases on one strand are exactly **complementary** to those on the other. Guanine must always lie opposite cytosine and adenine opposite thymine. This means that the base sequence on one strand specifies the precise sequence on the complementary strand. The absolute requirement for complementarity is the basis of DNA replication – and hence the basis of all genetics. Watson and Crick, who first solved the structure of DNA, called its base complementarity 'the secret of life'.

Note that in a DNA double helix, the two strands run in opposite directions: 3' to 5' and 5' to 3'.

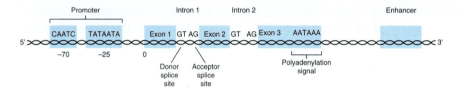

Fig. 2.4 Structure of a typical eukaryotic gene. Note that some genes (possibly those that are continuously active) do not have recognizable promoters with CAAT and TATA boxes. An enhancer, if present, may be within the structural gene itself, or several kilobases distant and either 5' or 3' to it.

TRANSPOSONS

Certain DNA sequences are believed to be capable of being excised from one site in the genome and re-inserted elsewhere, often undergoing duplication in the process. These mobile elements or **transposons** can influence the expression of genes by physically disrupting their coding or control sequences and in both plant and animal species (maize and drosophila fruit flies are the most widely studied) have the effect of generating genetic instability. The presence of long DNA repeats contributes to the ease of re-insertion in other parts of the genome because when DNA is replicating during cell division, single strands from different regions of the genome may 'accidentally' form a transient double helix where the sequences happen to be homologous. In human genetics the strongest candidate for a transposon is known as Kpn or LINE-1 (long interspersed repeat element). Many thousands of copies of LINE-1 are found in the human genome, distributed on all chromosomes.

Gene expression

TRANSCRIPTION

When a gene is expressed, the information it encodes must somehow be conveyed to the rest of the cell. This happens in two stages. First a replica of the DNA is made, in the form of RNA (**transcription**), and then that is converted into a corresponding protein (**translation**). The transcription process is very similar to DNA replication except that the new strand formed on the DNA template uses ribose phosphate (rather than deoxyribose phosphate) as the backbone and, among the bases, thymine is replaced by its analogue uracil. The resulting product is ribonucleic acid (RNA) rather than DNA (Fig. 2.1b).

Just as in the case of replication, for transcription the two DNA strands separate, but only over a short distance, and an RNA polymerase copies one of them from its 3' end. Note that RNA too has polarity, so that the RNA

Gene expression
- Transcription (formation of RNA from DNA template)
- Processing of RNA transcripts
- Translation of RNA to form protein
- Modification of gene products

transcript will be in the opposite orientation to the template and its base sequence will be complementary – i.e. where the template strand reads CCT, the RNA copy will read GGA. In both respects, the RNA transcript will be virtually identical to the opposite strand of the DNA helix. We therefore refer to that as the **coding strand**, to distinguish it from the template (Fig. 2.5).

Fig. 2.5 Transcription of DNA into mRNA: (a) binding of RNA polymerase to the template strand. (b) RNA polymerase reaches the promoter site. (c) The DNA strands separate at the point of transcription and, as the RNA polymerase moves relative to the template, the double helix reforms behind it. (d) The methylguanosine cap is added as the RNA chain elongates.

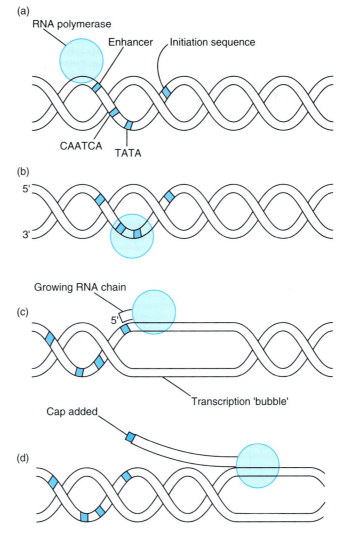

Transcription factors

Nuclear proteins that bind to specific promoter and/or enhancer DNA sequences and thereby regulate gene transcription are termed **transcription factors**. They generally have at least two functional domains, one that interacts directly with DNA and a second that interacts with other proteins, such as hormones, conveying signals from the cell's environment. The DNA-binding region typically has a high content of cysteine and basic amino acids. It may form repeating motifs that interdigitate with the DNA helix ('zinc finger' and 'helix–turn–helix' are descriptive terms for such motifs). Often quite complex chains of both positive and negative transcription signals are built up by interacting nuclear proteins.

Some hormones, such as the steroids (including sex hormones) and thyroid hormones, bind to receptor proteins in the cytoplasm which then enter the nucleus and function directly as transcription factors. Many other hormones (catecholamines, insulin, glucagon, ACTH, TSH, etc.) are recognized by receptors on the cell surface. Their binding triggers signalling via **second messengers**, usually by activation of protein kinases and phosphatases which transmits a wave of change through the cytoplasm and ultimately alters the quantity or distribution of specific transcription factors, thus indirectly influencing gene expression.

Transcript processing

Transcription is continuous, starting from a point downstream of the promoters and reading through all the exons and the introns of the gene. However, the RNA copy does not remain bound to the template DNA strand. They separate, and the original double helix of DNA re-forms. The single-stranded RNA then undergoes major engineering within the nucleus. This is accomplished by a series of small nuclear ribonucleoproteins (snRNPs) which cut out the non-coding (intron) sequences and splice the exon sequences (Fig. 2.6). At the 5′ end a cap of 7-methylguanosine is added to provide an important recognition signal for later translation into protein (Fig. 2.7) while at the 3′ end a long string of adenine residues is attached. This spliced, capped, polyadenylated RNA is known as **messenger RNA (mRNA)** because it now moves from the nucleus to the cytoplasm (the AAAA tail is important in this transport process) carrying the information originally present in the gene.

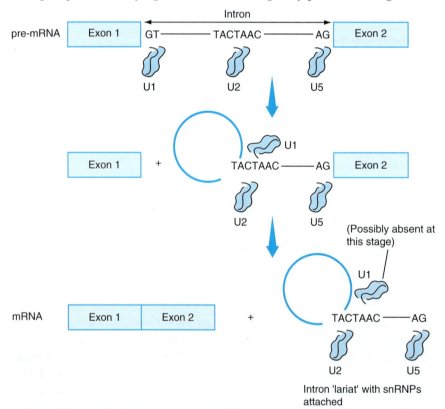

Fig. 2.6 Processing of the primary RNA transcript to form messenger (m)RNA. Small nuclear ribonucleoproteins (snRNPs) catalyse the excision of non-coding sequences (introns) and the splicing of coding sequences (exons) to form contiguous mRNA.

Reverse transcription

Certain small viruses which have an RNA rather than a DNA genome are able to reverse the normal process of transcription, making a DNA copy from an RNA template. This is necessary before they can become integrated into the host cell genome and either use the synthetic machinery of the cell to replicate themselves or subvert the normal regulation of cellular growth and differentiation in a process known as **transformation**. The **reverse transcriptase** enzyme from such a virus is used experimentally to make

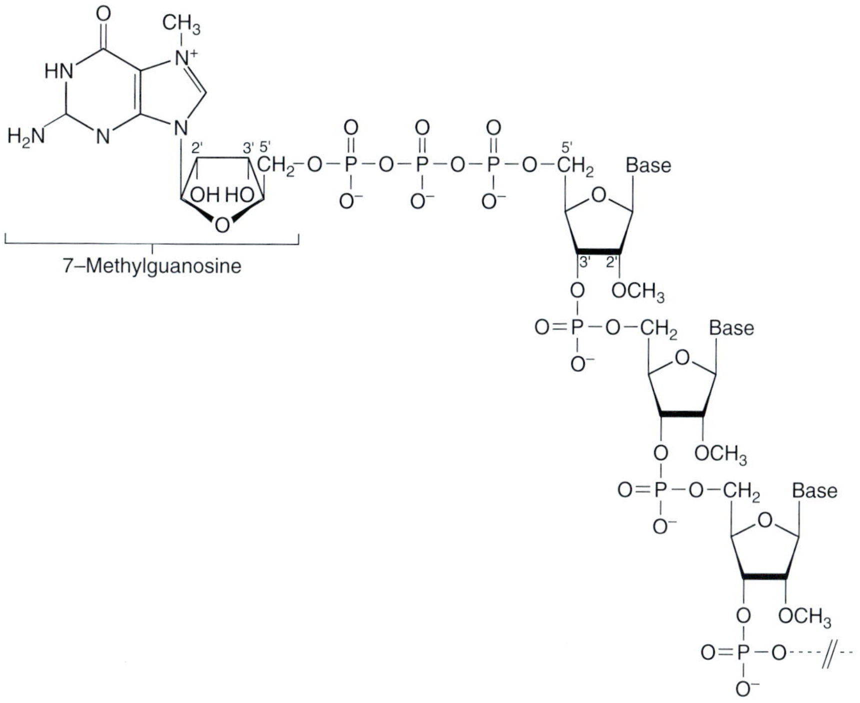

Fig. 2.7 The 7-methylguanosine cap at the 5′ end of mRNA.

7–Methylguanosine

complementary DNA (cDNA) copies of mRNA sequences. The cDNA copies are useful for studying the detailed structure of genes and for generating shortened versions of genes that can be manipulated in vitro, for example, by insertion into bacterial or eukaryotic cells.

Pseudogenes

Within the genome of all higher organisms, including humans, there are many near-copies of functional genes. These generally lack control elements necessary for transcription and are often incomplete or defective in other ways – hence the term **pseudogenes**. They invariably consist of a single recognizable exon with no introns and are thought to be derived from mRNA transcripts that, at some point in evolution, underwent reverse transcription and re-insertion into the DNA, often close to the site of the corresponding functional gene.

TRANSLATION

What genes actually specify is the sequence of amino acids in proteins and the conversion of information in the chemical form of nucleic acid to the chemical form of protein requires the reading of one language or code into another, hence the term 'translation'. Now the only significant variation in DNA structure lies in the sequence of bases, of which there are only four, while the major variation in proteins lies in the sequence of amino acids of which there are 20 (plus others formed by chemical modification of that set). The solution to this apparent discrepancy is to read the DNA (or RNA) bases in sets of three, which gives a total of $4 \times 4 \times 4$ (= 64) possible permutations. Each triplet of bases is termed a **codon** and the code is said to be redundant because in several cases two or more codons specify a single amino acid (Table 2.1). In these cases it is usually the third base (reading from 5′ to 3′) that is variable, for reasons that will become apparent. Three codons (UGA, UAA and UAG) are 'stop' signals for translation.

Table 2.1   The genetic code: identity of codons in mRNA (read in the 5′ to 3′ direction)

First base	Second base				Third base
	U	C	A	G	
U	Phe	Ser	Tyr	Cys	U
	Phe	Ser	Tyr	Cys	C
	Leu	Ser	Stop	Stop	A
	Leu	Ser	Stop	Trp	G
C	Leu	Pro	His	Arg	U
	Leu	Pro	His	Arg	C
	Leu	Pro	Gln	Arg	A
	Leu	Pro	Gln	Arg	G
A	Ile	Thr	Asn	Ser	U
	Ile	Thr	Asn	Ser	C
	Ile	Thr	Lys	Arg	A
	Met	Thr	Lys	Arg	G
G	Val	Ala	Asp	Gly	U
	Val	Ala	Asp	Gly	C
	Val	Ala	Glu	Gly	A
	Val	Ala	Glu	Gly	G

Fig. 2.9   Structure of a transfer RNA. Shaded nucleotides are common to tRNAs. Abbreviations for unusual (modified) nucleotides: Ψ, pseudouridine; D, dihydrouridine; T, ribothymidine; Y, a hypermodified purine; M, methylated base; m, methylated ribose. Other abbreviations are as in Fig. 2.1.

Fig. 2.8   Structure of a eukaryotic ribosome.

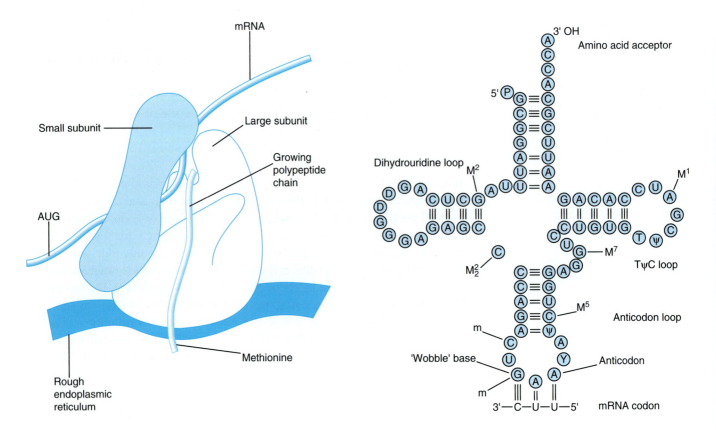

Translation itself takes place in the cytoplasm, specifically within small electron-dense particles called **ribosomes** (Fig. 2.8). These comprise two major subunits; a substantial proportion of both is RNA (but distinct from mRNA). The two subunits have to attach to the methylguanosine cap of mRNA. They then move along the mRNA in the 5' to 3' direction reading off one codon at a time and catalysing the attachment to each codon in the sequence of another form of RNA, termed **transfer RNA** (tRNA). These small RNA molecules, conventionally shown as having a cloverleaf structure (Fig. 2.9), carry a specific anticodon on one face that is complementary to one of the triplet base sequences of mRNA. Thus AUG on the mRNA will interact with UAC on the corresponding tRNA.

That particular tRNA will carry the amino acid methionine attached to its 3' tail. The last few bases of tRNA actually specify the amino acid that will be carried and it is clearly essential that the match between the triplet anticodon and the attached amino acid is faithfully observed for all tRNAs.

Fig. 2.10 Protein synthesis in eukaryotes: (a) the elongation phase of translation on an mRNA molecule containing three codons, the initiator codon, AUG, followed by UUU (Phe) and UGG (Trp). Elongation proceeds through three steps: (1) binding of the aminoacyl-tRNA, tRNAPhe, to the A site; (2) peptide bond formation, catalysed by peptidyl transferase, and the formation of peptidyl-tRNA in the A site; (3) translocation of the peptidyl-tRNA to the P site, catalysed by translocase, leaving the A site empty and displacing the initiator tRNA. The ribosome monomer moves along the mRNA in the 5' to 3' direction, ending one cycle of elongation. Binding of the next aminoacyl-tRNA, tRNATrp, would begin the next cycle of elongation. (b) Detail of the formation of the peptide bond in (a) between methionine and phenylalanine.

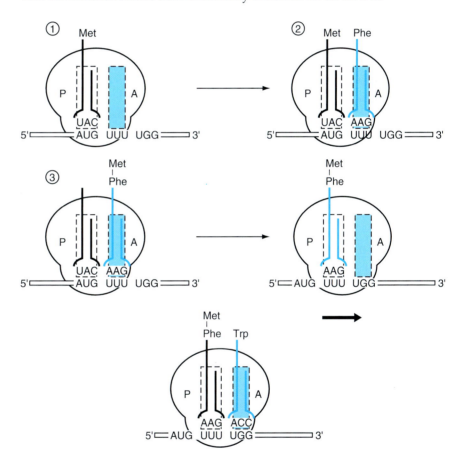

Within the ribosome–mRNA complex, a succession of tRNAs meet their anticodons and release their amino acids to join a growing peptide chain (Fig. 2.10). As the mRNA is read from 5' to 3', the peptide chain elongates from C terminus to N terminus. The anticodon of tRNA is represented as curved so that the fit with the mRNA codon is imperfect, particularly at the third 'wobble' base, hence the variability of the genetic code at the third base position.

MODIFICATION OF GENE PRODUCTS

Some genes have more than one possible initiation and/or termination site so that the primary transcripts may be of different lengths, depending on the arrangement of transcription factors. Similarly, **differential splicing** of the transcript may generate a variety of mRNAs. This applies, for example, to some peptide hormones which are encoded in adjacent exons of the same gene complex.

Post-translational modification of gene product (i.e. at the stage of protein assembly) is almost universal and takes many forms. For example, proteins are often directed to specific intracellular sites, or exported from the cell, by means of signal or targeting peptides which are cleaved away as the protein reaches its destination. Many proteins only become functionally active after partial digestion (this is true, for example, of proinsulin and other prohormones and proenzymes). The majority need to acquire a stable tertiary and quaternary structure that involves glycosylation, oligomerization or specific interaction with other proteins (Fig. 2.11). These modifications are often specific to the organism in which synthesis normally occurs, or at least they are properties of eukaryotic as distinct from prokaryotic cells. Thus protein synthesis by genetic engineering in cell-free systems or in bacteria cannot always be carried through to the point of a fully functional end product.

INHIBITORS OF MOLECULAR PROCESSES

Many chemical compounds, including a number of poisons found in nature, such as the toxins produced by some pathogenic organisms, interfere with DNA replication, transcription, translation or post-translational modification

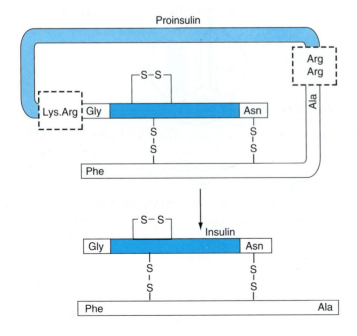

Fig. 2.11 The activation of proinsulin to insulin. Proteases act on proinsulin in the storage granules of pancreatic β cells. The A and B chains of insulin are shown in solid and open areas, respectively; the connecting C-peptide is indicated by the hatched area, with the basic amino acids excised by proteolytic activation within the dashed boxes.

of gene products. Apart from their relevance to pathogenicity, such substances have been of value in the development of experimental systems to examine these processes.

Inhibitors of DNA replication include aphidicolin and anti-topoisomerases (such as camptothecin and etoposide). Many anti-cancer drugs such as 6-mercaptopurine and the nitrogen mustards result in the incorporation of modified bases into the DNA and eventually generate sufficient errors to block successful replication. The antibiotic actinomycin D and the peptide amanitin (from the death cap mushroom, *Amanita phalloides*) are potent inhibitors of transcription. Protein synthesis is blocked by the interferons, cycloheximide, diphtheria toxin and many antibiotics including puromycin, neomycin, tetracyclines, kanamycin and erythromycin (Table 2.2).

Table 2.2 Some inhibitors of molecular processes

Inhibitor	Process affected	Comment
Mitomycin C Bleomycin	DNA replication	Anti-cancer antibiotics
Acridine dyes Ethidium bromide	DNA replication: intercalate in double helix	Can cause frame-shift mutations
Actinomycin D	DNA and RNA synthesis	Anti-fungal antibiotic and cytotoxic
Dideoxynucleoside triphosphates	DNA chain growth	Used in DNA sequencing techniques
Methotrexate	Dihydrofolate reductase (hence purine synthesis)	Anti-cancer agent
Amanitin	RNA polymerase (mainly mammalian)	From death cap mushroom
Puromycin Cycloheximide	Translation (eukaryotes and prokaryotes)	

Deficiencies of vitamins and of trace elements such as zinc can have serious consequences because post-translational modifications of many proteins (attachment of prosthetic groups, formation of tertiary structure) and hence their function, for example, as enzymes, structural proteins or transcription factors, is compromised.

Molecular organization of DNA

Repetitive DNA

Much of the non-coding (i.e. non-gene) DNA is in the form of multiple copies of repeated sequences. The components of these repeats may range from dinucleotides (e.g. CACACACA) up to 50 or more base pairs and sometimes there are groups of distinct elements assembled in complex patterns which are then repeated in long tandem arrays. These multiple repeated sequences probably serve a structural role. They form a very large proportion of the DNA close to the centromeres of most chromosomes which appears as densely staining C-band heterochromatin in metaphase preparations. Specialized repeat elements are also characteristic of the ends of chromosome arms (the telomeres) and repetitive sequences are relatively over-represented in the 'dark' regions of G-banded chromosomes (Figs 2.2b and 2.12).

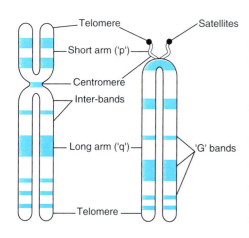

Fig. 2.12 Structure of human chromosomes at metaphase. The ideogram shows a metacentric (centromere near-central) and an acrocentric (centromere near-terminal) chromosome stained by the G-banding procedure.

Z-DNA

Surprising as it may seem, some physical variation is permitted in the arrangement of the double helix. Most of our DNA is in the form known as B-DNA (Fig. 2.1) where the helix has a right-hand thread with 10 nucleotide pairs to a complete turn. A more compressed form of this structure (A-DNA) is found in certain circumstances, for example, when RNA is pairing with DNA as in the process of transcription. Z-DNA, in which the helix adopts a left-hand thread, occurs rarely and then only where there are stretches of alternating purines and pyrimidines in the base sequence. Since protein–DNA interactions depend upon the geometry of the helix, these structural variations can be functionally important.

DNA packaging

In **eukaryotic** cells (i.e. those with a nucleus and cytoplasm) the nuclear DNA is intimately associated with a set of small highly basic proteins, the histones. An octamer of **histones** H2A, H2B, H3 and H4 (two molecules of each) forms a core round which the DNA double helix wraps itself twice. This DNA–histone complex is termed a **nucleosome** and electron micrographs of

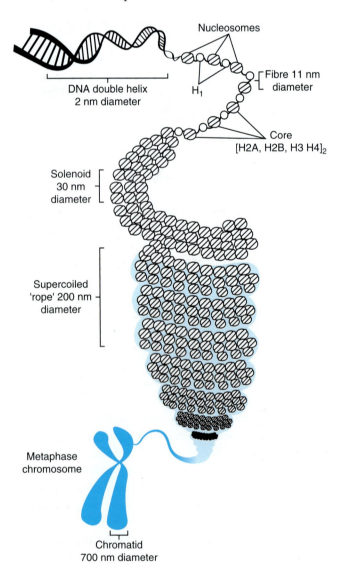

Nucleosomes

DNA double helix
2 nm diameter

H₁

Fibre 11 nm
diameter

Core
[H2A, H2B, H3 H4]₂

Solenoid
30 nm
diameter

Supercoiled
'rope' 200 nm
diameter

Metaphase
chromosome

Chromatid
700 nm diameter

Fig. 2.13 Organization of DNA into chromatin showing the multiple levels of ordered structure.

teased-out chromatin (the DNA/protein contents of the nucleus) show the appearance of beads on a string because of the regularly spaced nucleosomes. In the process of **apoptosis** ('programmed' cell death) activation of endogenous nucleases leads to a characteristic ladder pattern of DNA on an electrophoretic gel. The spacing between rungs of the ladder, 200 base pairs, corresponds to the spacing of nucleosomes. Histone H1 contributes to the stability of the overall structure, one molecule being associated with each nucleosome but outside the octamer core (Fig. 2.13).

The 'beaded' DNA/histone complex is further packaged into a 'solenoid' and the solenoid supercoiled into a 'rope'. This degree of ordering in chromatin is necessary because in its native state the DNA double helix of a single human cell would stretch for some 3 m. During transcription, the histone core opens to allow access of the RNA polymerase to the template strand of DNA but the basic nucleosome structure remains intact.

At mitosis, the chromatin condenses still further to form visible **chromosomes**, whose characteristic sizes and proportions (relative lengths of long and short arms) are determined by structural 'scaffold' proteins. The DNA is attached to the scaffold at intervals and hangs from it in a series of loops. Individual chromosomes can be identified by their banding patterns after fixation and a variety of staining procedures. As noted earlier, the bands are produced by the non-uniform distribution of condensed highly repetitive non-coding DNA sequences.

The centromere of each chromosome includes a trilaminar protein structure, the kinetocore, which provides attachment for the spindle fibres that pull the chromatids apart as the daughter cells form and separate at the end of mitosis.

Mitochondrial DNA

In addition to its nuclear DNA, every cell also contains a second component of the genome, in the mitochondria. These organelles are believed to have evolved from free-living prokaryote ancestors and their DNA is in the form of multiple copies of a closed double-stranded circle, like a bacterial chromosome. They also have their own ribosomes, their own version of the genetic code, their own transfer RNAs and their own enzyme systems for transcription and translation. Only a few proteins are encoded by mitochondrial DNA, most mitochondrial proteins being imported after synthesis in the cytoplasm. Nevertheless the mitochondrial genes determine some functions that are important in oxidative phosphorylation and a few human disorders are attributed to defects in these genes. Since the sperm contributes no mitochondria to the zygote, all mitochondrial genes are inherited from the female line.

Mitosis and meiosis

At mitosis (Fig. 2.14a), the DNA condenses into visible chromosomes, of which there are 23 pairs in humans (44 autosomes + XX or XY). One half set (**haploid**) is derived from each parent to form the total (**diploid**) set. Before the chromosomes become visible, the DNA has already replicated so that each chromosome, consisting of a pair of **chromatids** (Fig. 2.12), is actually two complete DNA molecules, each several centimetres in length. At anaphase, the chromosomes line up along the axis of division. The spindle fibres

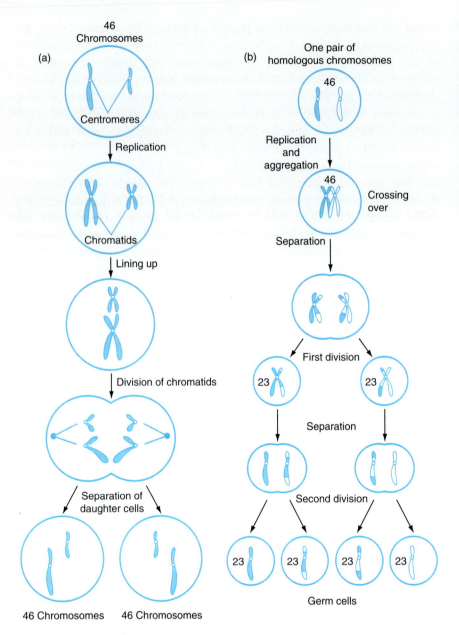

Fig. 2.14 Comparison of mitosis and meiosis. (a) Mitosis. Only two chromosomes (belonging to different pairs) are shown, though the same pattern applies to all 46 human chromosomes. (b) Meiosis. Only one chromosome pair is shown. In the male all four cells finally formed, each with a haploid complement of 23 chromosomes, develop into mature sperm, but in the female three of the four cells are discarded as polar bodies and only one of the four cells forms a mature ovum.

attached to the kinetocore (where the two chromatids join) pull the **chromatids** apart so that one molecule of each pair goes to each daughter cell.

Formation of a germ cell (sperm or egg) requires a reduction step since the daughter cells in this instance are haploid (i.e. they contain a half set of chromosomes). At the first meiotic (reduction) division (Fig. 2.14b), the chromosomes form homologous pairs (i.e. the number 1 chromosomes from each parent come together, the number 2 chromosomes likewise, and so on) and interchange material. When the paired elements separate, they no longer represent the maternally and paternally derived chromosomes: each is a mosaic of parts from the two parents. This greatly increases the amount of **genetic heterogeneity** in the population and also has important consequences for the study of genetic disease (see below).

After this interchange of material, the entire chromosomes segregate to separate daughter cells so that each of these cells has only 23 including, in the case of sperm, either an X or a Y. There follows a second meiotic division in which the chromatids segregate to four granddaughter cells.

Chromosomal map locations of genes and other DNA sequences

Within any species, a given gene is always located at precisely the same position on the same chromosome. In fact this is true for all specific DNA sequences, whether coding or non-coding. There are exceptions in the case of transposons already mentioned, and considerable variation is found between individuals in the size of highly repeated blocks of DNA, for example, of heterochromatin. In general, however, the structural anatomy of the genome is very precisely defined and much current effort is devoted to constructing detailed maps of the human chromosomes. Once completed, these will be valid for all healthy individuals. The stability of the genetic map is illustrated by the fact that large segments of the chromosomes of other species (e.g. mouse) correspond closely, in terms of the collection of genes they carry and the relative order of these genes, to parts of human chromosomes, implying that the underlying structures have been conserved throughout millions of years of evolution (Fig. 2.15).

Fig. 2.15 The human X chromosome with the map locations of some of the genes responsible for X-linked disorders.

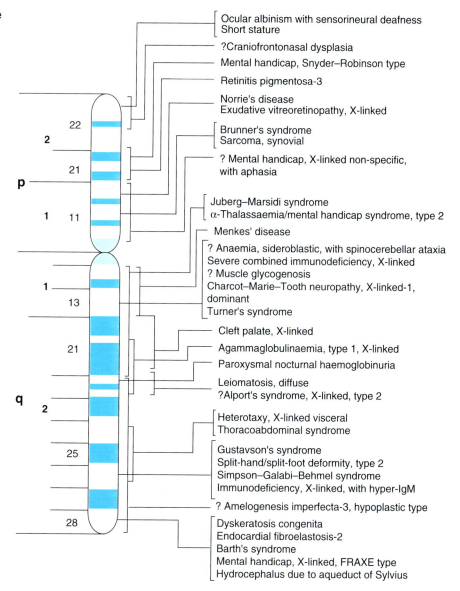

Why do genes change?

Mutation

Errors in the specification or the reading of the genetic code can arise in several ways.

DELETIONS

Large or small gaps in the DNA will obviously disrupt those genes that are partially or totally missing. Occasionally a deletion may be sufficiently large to be visible at the chromosome level. This is rarely compatible with life if it affects the whole organism but it may arise as an accident of somatic cell division, particularly in tumour cells.

INSERTIONS

Extra DNA sequences may be inserted as a result of unequal chromosome exchange at meiosis or mitosis or through the activity of mobile elements in the genome or of viruses. Again, if this happens within a coding sequence, translation is likely to be seriously disrupted.

BASE SUBSTITUTION

Despite the editing function of DNA polymerase, small errors can creep into the DNA sequence and a single base may be miscopied. Certain mutagens (DNA-damaging chemicals or radiation) can also lead to the exchange of one base for another. Because the genetic code is redundant, some base substitutions have no effect (e.g. changing UUA to UUG still specifies leucine). Others will cause a change in one amino acid in the protein product – a **mis-sense** mutation – the consequences of which will vary from the trivial to the catastrophic. If the base substitution results in the reading of a stop codon (UGA, UAA or UAG) – a **nonsense** mutation – then there will be premature termination of translation and a shortened protein product.

FRAME-SHIFT

The ribosome has no means of recognising successive codons except by reading bases in sets of three from the start sequence AUG. If a small deletion or insertion occurs, other than in a multiple of three bases, then the **reading frame** will be shifted and all the codons downstream of the lesion will be read incorrectly. The effect will be to produce a nonsense sequence of amino acids and (usually) premature termination when a spurious stop signal is reached (Fig. 2.16).

LARGE OR UNSTABLE OLIGONUCLEOTIDE REPEATS

The presence of an unusually large tandem array of repetitive DNA can interfere with the expression of adjacent structural genes by mechanisms that are not yet understood. This phenomenon is now known to cause at least four human genetic disorders: Huntington's disease, fragile-X syndrome, myotonic dystrophy and spinobulbar muscular atrophy. In each case, the repeat element is a trinucleotide (CAG, CGG, CTG and CAG respectively). These tandem oligonucleotide arrays can show meiotic instability – i.e. they can change in length during spermatogenesis and oogenesis. Hence the offspring may inherit a segment of different length from either parent. Such a change is a true mutation and in two of the diseases mentioned (fragile-X

Types of mutation
- Deletion
- Insertion
- Base substitution (point mutation)
- Frame-shift
- Expanding oligonucleotide repeat

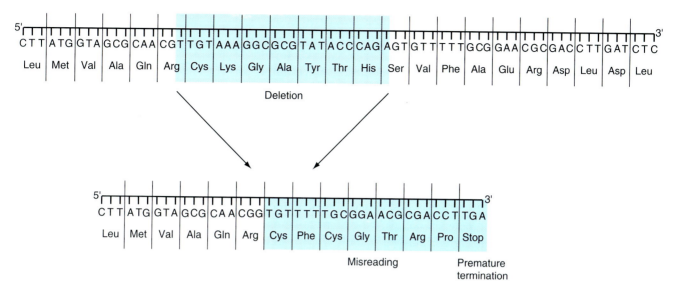

Fig. 2.16 Frame-shift mutation caused by deletion of 23 bases from coding DNA. When the 23 bases in the boxed segment are deleted from the upper sequence a new reading frame is generated, starting with a CGG codon which still specifies the correct amino acid (arginine). The next seven codons, however, specify incorrect amino acids (in terms of the original peptide sequence) and the eighth is a stop codon which will terminate protein synthesis.

syndrome and myotonic dystrophy), meiotic instability increases as the segment expands. Since disease is associated with large repeat segments, the condition tends to become more severe and the age of appearance of symptoms tends to become younger with successive generations. This is termed **genetic anticipation**.

Chromosome abnormalities

ANEUPLOIDY

Errors of chromosome segregation can result in germ cells with too few or too many chromosomes. When one of these contributes to the fertilized zygote, there may be 45, 47 or some other chromosome number. Such errors are actually quite common in humans (perhaps affecting 30% of zygotes) but it is estimated that the great majority are aborted spontaneously at a very early stage of pregnancy and only about 1% result in viable offspring. The best known examples are 47XX (or XY) + 21 (Down's syndrome) and the sex chromosome anomalies 45XO (Turner's syndrome), 47XXY (Klinefelter's syndrome) and 47XYY. The 45XO and 47XXY phenotypes are almost invariable infertile. Some numerical chromosome aberrations, particularly Down's syndrome, are associated with advanced maternal age.

STRUCTURAL ANOMALIES

Major chromosome deletions are rarely compatible with life, although the *cri-du-chat* syndrome (small deletion on the short arm of chromosome 5) is an exception.

TRANSLOCATIONS

A translocation in which there is (usually reciprocal) interchange of parts of two different chromosomes may have little apparent effect so long as all the chromosome material is still present in normal amounts (**balanced translocation**), although specific translocations occurring in somatic cells can disrupt important genes and therefore can be features of certain malignancies. A balanced translocation can cause problems at meiosis since the different parts of a chromosome that have been separated from each other by the translocation may not segregate correctly to the daughter cells. This can give rise to partial trisomy or partial monosomy in the germ cell and hence to an **unbalanced translocation** in the offspring.

Numerical and structural chromosome aberrations may arise in the very early stages of embryogenesis rather than in the germ cell. As a consequence the individual may be composed of a *mosaic* of cells with 45, 46 and 47 chromosomes. This is a relatively common phenomenon, for example, in Turner's syndrome. Major chromosome abnormalities account for about 0.3% of all live births in most populations.

DNA repair

DNA replication is error-prone, but the editing function of DNA polymerases corrects most mistakes before the copying is complete. The most important element of the editing process seems to be 3'–5' exonuclease activity which excises mismatched bases in the new strand, allowing them to be replaced with the correct ones. The reverse transcriptase of small RNA viruses has no exonuclease activity and the associated error frequency in DNA copies is about 1 in 600 bases. This compares with about 1 in 10^5 bases for mammalian DNA polymerases.

Mutations arise, however, as a result of DNA damage from ultraviolet light, mutagenic chemicals or ionizing radiation, even when DNA is not replicating. There is low background level of **unscheduled** DNA synthesis, mainly accounted for by repair processes. A series of enzymes is required to scrutinize the DNA, identify and excise damaged bases, insert new ones and ligate the patch to the strand at each end.

The type of damage arising in the DNA is often characteristic of the agent causing it. X-rays, for example, tend to produce single- or double-stranded breaks. Ultraviolet light causes crosslinking between adjacent thymidines to produce dimers. Nitrogen mustards generate covalent bonds between adjacent guanines. Nitrous acid deaminates adenine to hypoxanthine and cytosine to uracil. Defects in particular components of the repair system also have distinctive consequences. In **xeroderma pigmentosum** (an autosomal recessive deficiency of the enzyme that excises thymidine dimers) there is excessive sensitivity to sunlight (ultraviolet) and a high risk of skin cancers. Other genetic repair deficient syndromes such as **ataxia telangiectasia** and **Fanconi's anaemia** are associated with altered sensitivity to X-rays and often with increased susceptibility to malignant disease but the precise molecular lesions are not yet known. In one particularly rare condition of this type, **Bloom's syndrome**, there is believed to be a defect in DNA ligase, the enzyme which joins segments of DNA together during replication.

Amplification and reduplication of genes

Duplication of a segment of a chromosome can arise through a rare double breakage and misrepair event, the homologous chromosome being left without that segment. If such a reduplication becomes fixed in the daughter cells then further expansion of the segment can occur at subsequent divisions through unequal crossing-over, particularly during meiotic recombination, since misalignment of the homologous repeated segments may happen rather easily. Thus if the paired chromosomes each have two copies of the segment, after separation one may have three copies and the other only a single copy. Throughout evolution this process has generated blocks of repetitive DNA, which, as mentioned above, show wide variations in copy number. Sometimes the reduplicated segment may include one or more expressed genes and in higher organisms, including humans, many genes are now present in multiple copies. These have often diverged slightly from one another by point mutations so that the properties of the different globin, actin or collagen gene products, for example, are sufficiently distinct to subserve a wider range of specialized functions than any single protein. Thus gene duplication and divergence contribute to the evolution of the species. Initially the process of duplication tends to maintain the cluster of gene copies close together in tandem array on the same chromosomal segment. However, transposition or major breakage and recombination events can lead to dispersal of gene copies throughout the chromosome set. For example, separate clusters of immunoglobulin genes, clearly derived from a common ancestral sequence, are now found on human chromosomes 2, 14 and 22.

RAPID EXPANSION

Occasionally, a rapid increase in the copy number of a particular expressed gene confers a marked growth advantage on the cell in which it occurs, so much so that the gene may become amplified many hundred or even a thousand-fold in the course of relatively few cell generations. This applies particularly to a few **oncogenes** in certain tumour cells, for example, N-*myc* in neuroblastoma, c-*erb B2* in some breast cancers. The mechanisms involved in such rapid amplifications are not fully understood but in addition to unequal sister chromatid crossing-over during mitosis, there may be over-replication, i.e. repeated separation and copying of the DNA strands over a short region of the chromosome.

DNA changes and evolution

It is clear that mutations, generating genes with new properties, contribute to evolution. Indeed in the Darwinian view they are the very basis of evolution. As already mentioned, however, non-coding DNA also undergoes mutations, reduplication and amplification. In fact, within the population there is much greater variation in non-coding DNA than in expressed genes. The generally accepted explanation is that changes in the former are neutral with respect to survival of the organism whereas mutations in genes are much more likely to be disadvantageous. There is therefore a selective pressure for conservation of the DNA of genes, not only within a single species but even between species. Thus the genes of men, mice and even fruit flies, worms or yeast are often remarkably similar at the DNA level, whereas the intervening non-coding sequences have little in common (other than being composed of the same four bases). Variation within a population (**polymorphism**) is of considerable value for tracing the inheritance of particular DNA segments. One application is in forensic pathology where **DNA fingerprinting** is applied to identify unique individuals and to establish family relationships. Another is in **linkage analysis** where the co-segregation, within families, of polymorphic DNA markers and specific genetic traits is used to localize the relevant genes. Both topics are discussed below.

Effects of genetic variation

Polymorphisms at protein and DNA level

THE MHC REGION GENE PRODUCTS

The most variable expressed gene system known is the **major** histocompatibility complex (MHC) located on the short arm of human chromosome 6. Many of the genes belonging to this cluster encode histocompatibility (HLA) antigens which determine the difference between self and non-self. This has important implications for organ transplantation, but their biological functions are related to the physical presentation of foreign antigens (e.g. derived from invading organisms). Other genes within the MHC are also involved in immune reactions. They include complement components, cytokines (TNF-α and TNF-β) and enzymes that participate in antigen processing and the movement of protein molecules within the cytoplasm. The

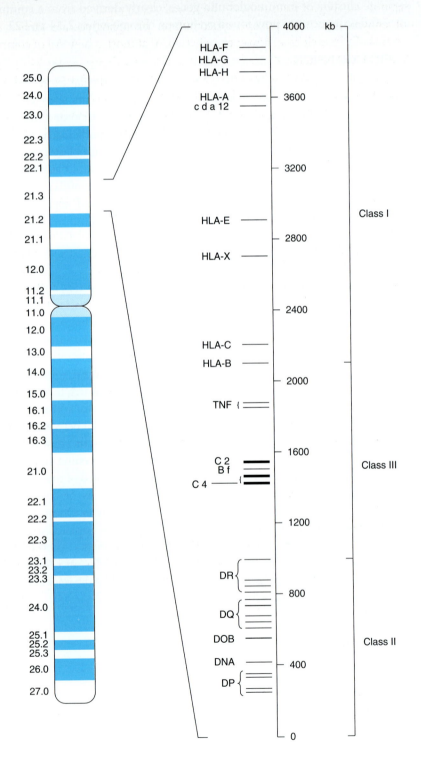

Fig. 2.17 The human major histocompatibility complex (MHC) region on chromosome 6. From the ideogram of chromosome 6, the MHC region of band p21.3 is shown expanded on the right. The principal subregions containing class I, class II and class III genes are indicated and the positions of individual genes are marked by bars. The scale is in kilobases of DNA (i.e. thousands of base pairs). Class I and class II genes comprise the HLA, A, B, C, DR, DP and DQ 'tissue type' cell surface determinants. Among the class III genes are those encoding several complement components (C2, C4, Bf) and tumour necrosis factor (TNF).

most polymorphic of these elements are the structural chains of the histocompatibility antigens HLA class I (A, B and C) α chains and class II (DR, DP, DQ) α and β chains. It is calculated that known variants of these molecules can generate several hundred million different permutations. This gives an idea of the odds against finding two humans (other than identical twins) who are completely identical at the major histocompatibility locus (Fig. 2.17).

OTHER PROTEINS

Other well-known protein polymorphisms include the ABO, rhesus and 'minor' blood group systems, the haptoglobins, α_1-antitrypsin and a number of enzymes such as phosphoglucomutase, phosphoglycerate kinase and esterase D. In each case, however, only two, or at most, a handful of common variants are recognized. In fact, variation of this degree is probably very frequent and is often overlooked because the different forms of the gene product occurring in the population are functionally equivalent under most conditions. The presence of such polymorphism may, however, declare itself under abnormal conditions, for example, when an enzyme is required to metabolize a drug, as discussed below.

VARIATION IN DNA SEQUENCES

All of the above polymorphisms can be identified by detailed chemical analysis of the proteins involved though, in many instances, immunological procedures (e.g. serotyping for blood groups and histocompatibility antigens) are preferred in practice. By definition there must be underlying differences at the DNA level. Indeed the DNA variability is often found to be greater than that recognized in the proteins. For example, several MHC antigen specificities each defined by a single antiserum can be 'split' into genetically distinct components on DNA sequencing. Furthermore, as discussed above, some single base changes in a gene sequence do not change the amino acid specified, particularly if the base occupies the third position in the codon. Thus DNA polymorphism exceeds protein polymorphism even in expressed sequences.

In non-coding sequences, there is no opportunity for protein polymorphism and the DNA, as explained earlier, is highly variable. It is, however, not necessary to sequence long stretches of DNA to demonstrate the variation. Two major categories of DNA polymorphism are demonstrable by relatively simple procedures. One depends upon the property of certain

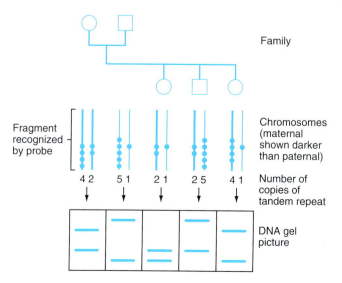

Family

Fragment recognized by probe

Chromosomes (maternal shown darker than paternal)

4 2   5 1   2 1   2 5   4 1   Number of copies of tandem repeat

DNA gel picture

Fig. 2.18 A VNTR polymorphism. For the members of the family illustrated, the regions of a pair of chromosomes bearing a VNTR locus are shown underneath the symbol for each individual. Each element of the tandem repeat is shown as a dense block. Both parents are heterozygous for different copy numbers of this repeat (Mother 4 2: Father 5 1). Each passes one of the chromosome pair to every child, generating the heterozygous patterns indicated. When DNA is cut with a restriction endonuclease and run out in an electrophoresis gel, then probed to reveal the fragment bearing the repeat element, these are found to be of different sizes, according to the number of copies of the tandemly repeated sequence.

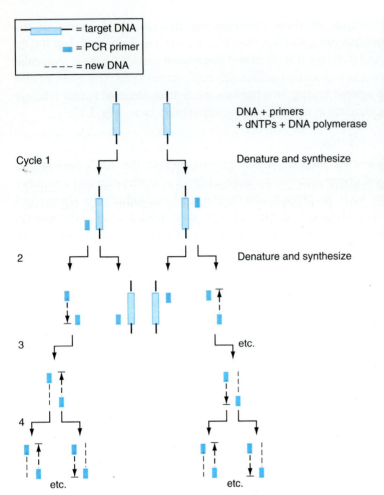

= target DNA

= PCR primer

- - - - = new DNA

DNA + primers
+ dNTPs + DNA polymerase

Cycle 1   Denature and synthesize

2   Denature and synthesize

3   etc.

4

etc.   etc.

Fig. 2.19   The polymerase chain reaction (PCR). The key to this technique for almost unlimited amplification of a specific DNA sequence is a form of DNA polymerase that is heat stable. The 'target' DNA (light colour) and polymerase are mixed with free nucleotides (dNTPs) and with two oligonucleotide primers (darker colour) – short stretches of synthetic DNA complementary to different ends of the target sequence and to opposite strands. On heating, the target strands separate and on cooling, the primers hybridize to them; the polymerase extends them, incorporating the free nucleotides into new double-stranded copies of the original target (dotted lines). Heating and cooling are repeated cyclically and with each round the copy number of target DNA is doubled. After 20 cycles, the theoretical amplification is about a million-fold and actual yields are not far short of this.

(restriction) endonucleases, commonly found in bacteria, to cleave double-stranded DNA only where specific sequences of four or more bases occur. Any mutation – even a single base change – that alters such a sequence will cause loss of the **restriction site** and hence a change in the length of DNA fragment generated from that region of the genome by digestion with the corresponding endonuclease. The second depends upon the presence of a tandem repeat array between adjacent restriction sites, variation in the number of copies of the repeating unit generating a range of possible fragment lengths (**v**ariable **n**umber of **t**andem **r**epeats – VNTR) when the appropriate restriction endonuclease is used (Fig. 2.18). The **microsatellite** polymorphism is a particular case of the latter principle, where the repeat unit may be a simple dinucleotide (e.g. –CACACA–) which may be short enough overall to be amplified by the **polymerase chain reaction (PCR)** (Fig. 2.19) and hence capable of detection using trace amounts of DNA – from a dried blood spot, for example – as the starting material. Fixed tissue from pathology blocks also yields DNA suitable for PCR analysis.

Both protein and DNA polymorphisms can be used for genetic characterization of individuals and are of considerable value in forensic practice (establishing paternity, tracing suspects from 'scene of the crime' specimens of blood or sperm, and identification of human remains) but nowadays DNA analysis is much more widely applied. It reaches its apotheosis in the technique of DNA fingerprinting, mentioned above, which, in essence, sets out a whole series of VNTRs from different regions of the genome within a single gel track (Fig. 2.20).

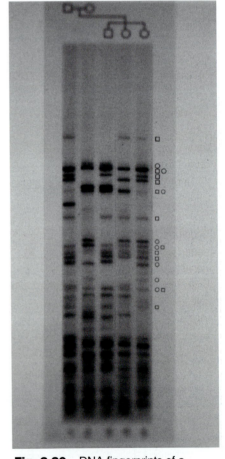

Fig. 2.20   DNA fingerprints of a family, after digestion with H inf I and hybridization with λ 33-15 probe. Fragments present in the mother's (lane 2) DNA fingerprints are indicated by a circle (○) and paternal fragments by a square (□). Approximately half of the polymorphic fragments in the offspring (lanes 3–5) are derived from the father (lane 1) and the rest from the mother.

The significance of meiosis: linkage and association

The interchange of material between homologous chromosomes during the reduction division of meiosis greatly increases the rate of dispersion of new genetic traits and adds to the diversity of the human species. It also has practical implications for gene mapping since DNA sequences will be inherited together through several generations only if they lie physically so close together on the same chromosome arm that meiotic crossing-over rarely occurs in the interval between them. Rates of crossing-over are not identical for oogenesis and spermatogenesis, nor are they uniform over the whole genome so that physical map distances along a given chromosome do not correspond exactly to **genetic distances** (i.e. measures of separation based on

---

CASE STUDY 2.1

The family tree illustrated in Fig. 2.21 shows an apparent 'cluster' of breast cancer (seven cases in three generations). The possibility of a familial predisposition to the disease was made even more likely by the fact that most of the women affected had been under age 55 at diagnosis – some as young as mid-30s. Furthermore, there was one instance of colorectal cancer and two of prostate cancer, all presenting before age 60. The association of these three tumours in a family is well recognized and many examples can now be attributed to inherited mutations in the *BRCA1* gene on the long arm of chromosome 17. Even before the gene was cloned, it was possible, in large families such as this one, to demonstrate **linkage** of the trait to the appropriate chromosomal region. The vertical bars below several of the symbols represent part of the long arm of chromosome 17 on which four polymorphic markers have been typed. Since each person carries two copies of chromosome 17, there are two alleles identifiable at each marker locus but it is evident that all the breast cancer patients have inherited a particular combination of alleles (4, 6, 8, 1) on one of the chromosomes. This set of adjacent alleles is called a **haplotype** and there is a very strong likelihood that the mutant *BRCA1* gene in this family is carried on the chromosome bearing that haplotype (i.e. that the cancer trait is 'linked' to the 4, 6, 8, 1 allele set).

Three members of the current generation of the family (arrowed), aware of the possible familial risk, sought genetic counselling and, after the situation had been explained to them, opted to undergo screening for the linked markers. As shown, two of them carried the high-risk haplotype while one did not. On the strength of this evidence, the male carrier was advised that, in due course, he might wish to undergo regular screening for prostate cancer and, if he had children, that there would be at 50% risk of carrying the mutant gene. The carrier woman decided to seek bilateral prophylactic mastectomy, even though linkage data leave some room for doubt as to the exact genetic status. The apparent non-carrier woman was offered cautious reassurance that she probably did not have the 'cancer gene'. Some years later, when *BRCA1* was isolated, the mutation in this family was identified and, on definitive genetic testing, the predictions with regard to carrier status in these three individuals were confirmed. Several additional members of the family then came forward requesting *BRCA1* screening.

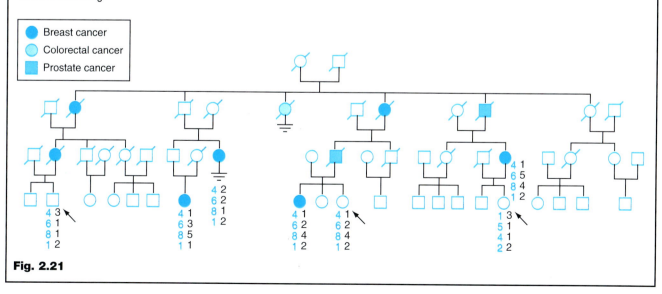

Fig. 2.21

cross-over frequency). The latter, however, are useful in linkage analysis in which the position of a given gene is estimated relative to known DNA sequences by estimating the frequency with which they separate at meiosis. For the purpose of tracing inheritance over several generations it is essential to be able to distinguish the alleles of the chosen markers and the more polymorphic they are, the better. VNTR sequences are therefore particularly useful in this context.

It is important to distinguish between the phenomena of **linkage** and **association**. Genetic linkage between gene and marker implies only a physical relationship and use of the principle, for example, to identify carriers of a genetic disorder, requires a knowledge of which marker allele is linked to the disease gene in one particular family. Other families with the same disorder will show linkage to the same marker locus but to different alleles at that locus. The rationale cannot therefore be applied to population screening for the defective gene (Fig. 2.22).

By contrast, some disorders with a genetic component may show association with the same allele at a polymorphic locus in almost all affected individuals. This is clearly illustrated in the case of HLA association (e.g. ankylosing spondylitis with HLA-B27 or coeliac disease and DQA*0501, DQB*0201). While the precise mechanisms for these associations are not yet clear, physical proximity of an 'ank spond' or a 'coeliac' gene with the MHC complex probably is not the explanation. Instead we must conclude that the particular MHC alleles involved play some functional role in the aetiology of the diseases.

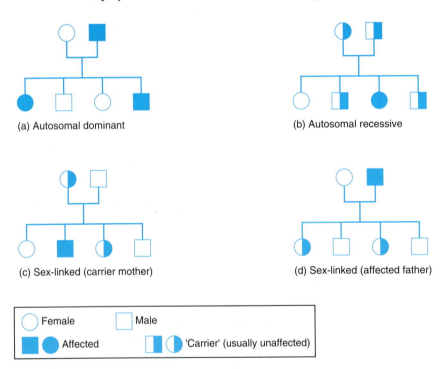

(a) Autosomal dominant

(b) Autosomal recessive

(c) Sex-linked (carrier mother)

(d) Sex-linked (affected father)

| ◯ Female | ☐ Male |
| ■ ● Affected | ◨ ◖ 'Carrier' (usually unaffected) |

Fig. 2.22 Mendelian patterns of inheritance. The four pedigrees illustrate families (two parents, four children) in which genetic disorders are segregating. The proportions of carrier and affected members are as predicted by Mendel's laws but, of course, segregation of genes at meiosis is random and the actual number of affected and carrier individuals in a real family might be greater or less than shown. For example, if a couple have a child with cystic fibrosis – an autosomal recessive condition – they must both be carriers and any child of theirs has a one in four chance of being affected. It does not mean, unfortunately, that their next three children are guaranteed to be unaffected. The one in four risk applies to each child, regardless of the distribution of the genes in their brothers and sisters.

MENDELIAN GENETICS

Our understanding of the rules of eukaryotic genetics derives from the work of the nineteenth-century Moravian monk Gregor Mendel. He postulated that we inherit two copies of the gene determining any given trait, one from each parent. Many genes exist in different forms (**alleles**). The **phenotype**, i.e. the property resulting from expression of a given allele (eye colour, ability to taste DEPC, hair texture, etc.) may be **dominant**, **co-dominant** or **recessive**, depending on the properties of the allele in relation to another allele of the same gene.

CASE STUDY 2.2

A married couple sought counselling because the husband's brother had recently been found to have carcinoma of the colon at the age of 38 and examination had revealed thousands of adenomas throughout the large bowel. There was no previous family history of polyposis coli. The parents of the affected patient were alive and well in their 60s. Molecular analysis of blood from the patient showed a mutation in one copy of the *apc* (polyposis coli) gene on chromosome 5, but this was not present in his parents or in any of his sibs. It was therefore a new mutation. The couple seeking advice were reassured that the husband and their children were not at risk; however, the affected brother had two sons aged 13 and 11 who also underwent blood screening. The younger was found to have inherited the mutation from his father. Although he had not yet developed any adenomas, arrangements were made for him to have annual colonoscopic examinations from the age of 15 so that prophylactic colectomy could be planned before the onset of malignant change. As the older boy had not inherited the *apc* mutation, he was spared the anxiety and discomfort of regular endoscopic examination.

Hardy–Weinberg distribution
If p and q are the frequencies of two alleles of the same gene, the distribution of p and q homozygotes and heterozygotes among fertilized zygotes (and therefore within the population) will be $p^2 + 2pq + q^2$

We can add, to Mendel's concepts, the idea that genes carried on the sex chromosomes show special patterns of inheritance because one sex (the male in *Homo sapiens*) does not have a pair of identical sex chromosomes. Furthermore, we now know that the genes occupy fixed positions on the chromosomes and that, unless they lie physically very close together on the same chromosome arm, the alleles of different genes segregate from each other at random in forming the germ cells.

Armed with the foregoing knowledge we can now interpret the underlying processes in the inheritance of diseases caused by **single gene defects**.

DOMINANTLY INHERITED DISORDERS

Diseases such as adenomatous polyposis coli, Huntington's disease or achondroplasia must be **autosomal** – i.e. carried on one of the 22 chromosomes other than X or Y, because both sexes are equally affected and transmit the trait with equal efficiency. The disease phenotype is **dominant** over the normal because affected parents have affected offspring and the proportion of children affected is about 50%. In other words, if you have one copy of the mutant gene, that is enough to cause the disease and there is a 50 : 50 chance that you will pass on the mutant to any child. Those children who do not inherit the mutation cannot pass the disease on to their own offspring.

Serious autosomal dominant conditions are likely to be rare (indeed, they are rare!) because they will probably reduce **reproductive fitness**. In most instances there is a special reason why the mutant gene has not disappeared:

- the disease may present after reproductive age (Huntington's disease)
- there may be a high rate of new mutations (achondroplasia, adenomatous polyposis coli)
- the gene sometimes escapes being expressed at all (**limited penetrance**) as in familial retinoblastoma
- its expression sometimes results in only a mild form of the disorder (**variable expressivity**) as in neurofibromatosis type 1 (von Recklinghausen's disease – Fig. 2.23).

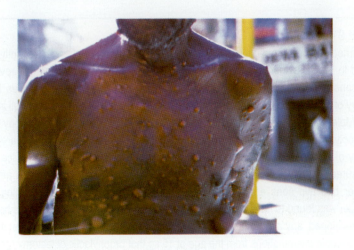

Fig. 2.23 Neurofibromatosis.

CASE STUDY 2.3

An officer captured during the Second World War hatched an ingenious plan to escape by making an army uniform out of blankets dyed with paints provided for scenery at the prison camp Christmas concert. He would then march out through the main gates, hoping to take advantage of the lowered vigilance associated with the festive season. Unfortunately he had inherited the common X-linked form of red–green colour blindness and was totally unaware of it, like many affected individuals. When making his dye, what he considered to be a close match for the grey uniform of the guards (which has a slight green tinge) was in fact a bright and bilious green which failed to deceive even the most mellow guardroom squad. Happily he was more successful on a subsequent occasion, using a plan which did not rely on perfect colour vision.

If two people both suffering from an autosomal dominant disorder, such as achondroplasia, have children, it is possible to predict the outcome on the basis that half the ova and half the sperm will carry the mutant (disease) allele, while the other half will carry the normal one. The possible combinations of zygote will be MM **(homozygous mutant)**, MN **(heterozygous mutant/normal)** and NN **(homozygous normal)**. The ratios will follow the Hardy–Weinberg distribution (which also applies to populations). Applying this to the achondroplasia example, within the family p and q are each equal to 1, so the ratios of MM, MN and NN will be $1:2:1$. The homozygous mutant (MM) phenotype is non-viable so if a child is born to such a couple there is a two-thirds chance that he or she will be achondroplasic (MN) like both parents and a one-third chance that he or she will be normal.

CASE STUDY 2.4

Albinism is commonly inherited in an autosomal recessive pattern. Visual impairment is one of its features. A young albino couple met at a college for partially sighted students, married and had a child who was normally pigmented and had perfect eyesight. Delight was tinged with some consternation, but the explanation was shortly provided by demonstrating that the father was homozygous for tyrosinase deficiency while the mother had normal tyrosinase levels and must be homozygous for a different enzyme involved in melanin synthesis. Thus their child (and any subsequent offspring) carries one normal copy of each enzyme and, being heterozygous, shows no phenotypic effect.

RECESSIVELY INHERITED CONDITIONS

Autosomal recessive disorders are commoner because, by definition, the normal allele is dominant over the mutant so that only the homozygous mutant individual is severely affected. In practice it is often possible to detect a mild abnormality in the heterozygous carrier. The thalassaemias, point mutation haemoglobinopathies (such as sickle cell and haemoglobin C disease) and cystic fibrosis are all examples of common autosomal recessive disorders. Typically, both parents appear healthy but on average one in four offspring (of either sex) will be affected. There is less selection against genes with recessive expression; nevertheless there must be some reason why they have become so common in many populations. In certain instances this can be explained because the populations are highly inbred – in other words they have a small gene pool. The Ashkenazi Jews and the Hutterite communities of the eastern central USA are classic examples. Most recessive disorders are commoner among the offspring of cousin marriages since the parents will have an eighth of their total genome in common, and hence have an appreciable risk of sharing the same potentially adverse mutation.

The haemoglobinopathies (including the thalassaemias) have probably been maintained because heterozygotes suffer from mild anaemia, sufficient to protect then from cerebral malaria (which depends upon a very high parasite load in the red cells). Hence the distribution of the corresponding mutations in those parts of the world where malaria is (or was) endemic. Conversely, the cystic fibrosis mutation which, in one form or another, is carried by 1 in 25 white people, is virtually unknown in Africans. One likely explanation is that heterozygotes have a higher than normal sweat chloride and sodium content and thus are ill-adapted to conserve water in a hot climate. We still do not know what positive selection may have been operating in colder parts of the world.

SEX-LINKED (OR X-LINKED) DISORDERS

Sex-linked disorders typically affect males only but are transmitted by carrier females. They are caused by mutant genes on the X chromosome which are recessive in the presence of a normal allele on the other X but are expressed as if dominant in the male because there is no counterpart on the Y chromosome. An affected male will have only unaffected sons but all his daughters will be carriers. An unaffected male cannot pass the disorder on to any of his children and a carrier mother will pass it to half her sons. Half her daughters will also be carriers.

Because this pattern of inheritance is so distinctive, a very large number of genes has been mapped to the X chromosome. These include the ones responsible for Duchenne and Becker muscular dystrophy, chronic granulomatous disease, at least two forms of retinitis pigmentosa, red–green colour blindness, haemophilia A and B, fragile-X mental handicap and Fabry's syndrome (Fig. 2.15).

X-linked dominant disorders would be expected to affect females twice as commonly as males and to show absence of male-to-male transmission. One form of pseudohypoparathyroidism and a very few other rare conditions do seem to be inherited in this fashion but there remains room for argument about the underlying genetics.

Mitochondrial genes have been mentioned earlier. They are inherited only from the mother (in the cytoplasm of the egg) but are distributed to all offspring, regardless of sex. Mutations in mitochondrial genes involved in the respiratory complexes are associated with Leber's hereditary optic neuroretinopathy and with a syndrome of ataxia, retinitis pigmentosa and peripheral neuropathy. Other mutations in mitochondrial tRNA genes appear to cause a variety of myopathies, with or without central nervous system involvement. They include 'ragged red fibre' myopathy with myoclonus epilepsy (MERRF), mitochondrial encephalomyopathy, lactic acid and strokes (MELAS) and a recently described syndrome of maternally inherited myopathy and cardiomyopathy.

It is obvious that some broad categories of disorder, such as mental handicap, myopathy, pathological short stature or deafness, may have many different causes, both genetic and non-genetic. The same applies, however, to some very specific clinical syndromes. Albinism, retinitis pigmentosa and adrenal hyperplasia are all examples of genetic conditions in which the same, or a very similar, phenotype can result from a number of quite distinct genetic lesions. This is understandable since the phenotype is generated by failure of one or more metabolic pathways which can be interrupted at several different points. These clinically similar but genetically distinct conditions are termed phenocopies and it is important to be aware of the phenomenon when investigating the genetics of what may appear to be a homogenous disorder affecting more than one family.

Polygenic inheritance

So far we have considered only single gene diseases. Individually, however, these tend to be rare and the total impact of hereditary illness owes more to the contributions of multiple genes in common disorders such as hypertension, coronary heart disease and diabetes. In these cases, the pattern of inheritance is seldom as clear cut as for single gene diseases. Nevertheless familial clustering is usually obvious. Measures of the relative contributions of genes and environment (eating habits, level of activity, etc.) to common disorders can be obtained by measuring the relative **concordance rates** for monozygotic versus dizygotic twins. If concordance (i.e. the frequency with both members of the pair are affected) is higher for **monozygotics** (who are genetically identical) than for **dizygotics** (who have only 50% of genes in common) then this suggests a genetic contribution. It is not always possible to collect large series of twins for such studies, and similar, though more complex, calculations can be carried out by comparing concordance with closeness of relationship within families (e.g. **first-degree relatives** are parents or sibs; **second-degree relatives** are grandparents, aunts, uncles, nephews, nieces, half-sibs; **third-degree relatives** are cousins, etc.).

Genes and environment

Few disorders can be attributed exclusively to the influence of inherited factors. In most cases (e.g. heart disease, haemoglobinopathies) diet, infection and other aspects of the environment modify the clinical picture.

In a few instances, a mutant gene may be totally silent until exposure to some environmental factor 'uncovers' it. Thus a variant form of acetylcholinesterase is harmless until the short-acting muscle relaxant suxamethonium (succinylcholine) is given. Homozygotes for the mutation cannot metabolize suxamethonium and remain paralysed for hours rather than minutes. The detoxification or inactivation of several drugs (particularly via acetylation) is a common genetic variable and this can have a profound effect on the therapeutic index, for example, of isoniazid. Acute intermittent porphyria triggered by sulphonamides or barbiturates is another instance of the importance of **pharmacogenetics**. We have already seen how environmental factors can influence the frequency of mutations such as haemoglobin S or thalassaemia, and it is not altogether fanciful to suggest that genes have changed the world environment. They have certainly made their mark on history. In the nineteenth century, for example, most of the royal houses of Europe were related to each other and within this gene pool haemophilia A was present. The disease contributed to the downfall of the ruling dynasties of Russia and of Spain and may therefore have hastened both the Russian revolution and the Second World War.

Tracing genes through family studies

When a disease is seen to cluster within a family, study of its distribution should tell us whether it is likely to be a single gene disorder following mendelian rules. Due allowance must be made for variable penetrance, variable expressivity, possible non-paternity and variable age of onset. Nevertheless in most instances the answer will be clear and if we seem to be dealing with an autosomal single gene defect, linkage analysis is the logical way to locate the gene.

Ideally we require large families (so that at least some first indication of linkage may be obtained without combining multiple families where quite different genes may be involved) and they should be accessible (i.e. alive and cooperative). Tracing distant members of scattered families can be demanding but is a crucial element in genetics. As already mentioned, the advent of PCR has allowed us to include deceased family members from whom paraffin-embedded pathology blocks are available.

THE USE OF DNA MARKERS IN LINKAGE ANALYSIS

It is preferable to use highly polymorphic markers that are already accurately mapped within the human chromosome set. In many instances this information is already available through catalogues such as the reports of successive International Gene Mapping Workshops. The actual mapping of these probes can involve several steps, notably demonstration of the complementary sequence in interspecific hybrid cells containing only a single human chromosome, linkage to other markers already mapped and **in situ hybridization**, i.e. annealing of labelled probe to its complementary sequence on a metaphase chromosome spread.

Through inspired guesswork, luck or simply hard and repetitive toil, eventually linkage between the disease gene and one polymorphic marker will be established. The next step is to extend the analysis to more families and to 'saturate' the relevant chromosomal region – i.e. to test for linkage to other polymorphic markers that map to that area. By a complex series of computations known as **multi-point linkage analysis**, a genetic map showing the relative positions of the disease gene and all adjacent markers can be drawn. It is particularly valuable to have at least one informative marker on either side of the disease gene because a single meiotic crossing-over event may separate one flanking marker from the disease gene but two such events would be required to separate the gene from both flanking markers and this is extremely unlikely. Thus, when we use markers to trace inheritance of the gene for family counselling purposes, the existence of two

Some conditions now amenable to antenatal diagnosis

Note that several conditions may be amenable to antenatal diagnosis by more than one technique.

- By biochemical assay of maternal serum and/or amniotic fluid
  - Open neural tube defects (high AFP)
  - Down's syndrome (low AFP, low unconjugated oestriol, high HCG)

- By high resolution ultrasound scans of fetus
  - Anencephaly; microcephaly; hydrocephalus
  - Skeletal abnormalities: achondroplasia, severe osteogenesis imperfecta
  - Major congenital heart defects
  - Polycystic kidneys; renal agenesis; bladder outflow obstruction
  - Cleft lip/palate; oesophageal atresia; exomphalos; imperforate anus
  - Down's syndrome and other major chromosome abnormality syndromes

- By biochemical analysis of amniotic fluid cells or chorionic villus biopsies
  - Adrenogenital syndromes
  - Albinism
  - Familial hypercholesterolaemia
  - Galactosaemia
  - Gangliosidoses (e.g. Tay–Sachs disease)
  - Gaucher's disease
  - Glycogen storage diseases types I–IV
  - G6PD deficiency
  - Homocystinuria
  - Hypothyroidism
  - Marfan's syndrome
  - Mucolipidoses
  - Mucopolysaccharidoses
  - Niemann–Pick disease
  - Phenylketonuria
  - Porphyrias

- By fetal blood analysis
  - Agammaglobulinaemia
  - α_1-Antitrypsin deficiency
  - Chronic granulomatous disease
  - Fragile-X syndrome
  - Haemoglobinopathies
  - Haemophilias A and B
  - Rhesus incompatibility
  - Von Willebrand's disease

- By DNA analysis of amniotic fluid cells or chorionic villous cells
  - Adrenogenital syndromes
  - Agammaglobulinaemia
  - Chronic granulomatous disease
  - Cystic fibrosis
  - Duchenne and Becker muscular dystrophy
  - Familial hypercholesterolaemia
  - Familial polyposis coli
  - Fragile-X syndrome
  - Friedreich's ataxia
  - G6PD deficiency
  - Haemoglobinopathies
  - Haemophilias A and B
  - Hereditary angio-oedema
  - Huntington's disease
  - Lesch–Nyhan syndrome (HPRT deficiency)
  - Marfan's syndrome
  - Mucopolysaccharidoses types II, IIID and VII
  - Myotonic dystrophy
  - Neurofibromatosis type 1
  - Osteogenesis imperfecta
  - Phenylketonuria
  - Retinoblastoma
  - Tay–Sachs disease
  - Tuberous sclerosis
  - Von Willebrand's disease

informative flanking markers will alert us to the occurrence of any meiotic recombination event close to the gene.

'HOMING IN' ON THE GENE

In many cases, close flanking markers are acceptable surrogates for the gene itself in identifying affected family members. This is so, for example, in haemophilia A even though the factor VIII gene has been cloned. The advantage of good markers is that the same technology can be applied to almost all affected families whereas the site of the actual mutations (in the same gene) can vary enormously from one family to another. If the gene is very large (as in haemophilia A, cystic fibrosis, neurofibromatosis or adenomatous polyposis coli) a disproportionate effort may be required to pinpoint each individual mutation.

Of course, when any genetic disorder is first attributed to a lesion in a defined chromosomal region, through linkage to mapped markers, that becomes the signal for an intense effort to find and characterize the gene itself for only then can the pathogenesis of the disease be understood. It really requires filling in the detail of the map outlined by the adjacent flanking markers.

Normally genomic libraries (particularly YAC libraries, constituting very large stretches of DNA) are screened for fragments that are recognized by the probes mapping closest to the disease gene. These fragments (or sections of them) may then be used themselves as probes to find additional fragments extending further away from the original probes, a process termed **chromosome walking**. Ultimately the question is asked: 'Do we have a gene, or genes, among this collection of genomic DNA?' Now genes are structurally like all the rest of the DNA but they do have certain relatively distinctive properties. They are expressed as mRNA, so one approach is to probe the RNA from a tissue where you would expect the disease gene to be expressed (e.g. myoblast in the case of a muscular dystrophy gene). Each genomic fragment is tested in turn to see which of them carries a sequence recognized by the mRNA.

Genes also tend to be highly conserved in evolution so that mouse, frog, fruit fly and even yeast DNA may retain similar expressible **gene** sequences while non-coding DNA has diverged to the point where the species do not 'recognize' each other. Hence, hybridizing each genomic DNA fragment to total DNA from a succession of lower animals (a so-called 'Zoo' or 'Noah's ark' blot) may identify conserved sequences.

Finally, many structural genes have clusters of very characteristic hypomethylated bases, rarely found elsewhere, just upstream of the promoter regions. These so-called **CpG islands** may be identified because they generate easily recognized patterns on digestion with restriction enzymes such as Not I.

DEFINING THE CAUSAL MUTATION

Very often more than one gene will be found in the vicinity of a disease locus. Which one is the disease gene? That may be answered by finding mutations in affected individuals confined to only one of the genes, but ultimately the gene must be sequenced, the structure of its protein product deduced and its function demonstrated, for example, by inserting the gene into a suitable indicator cell.

By all of these means, we are approaching an understanding of the nature of more and more genetic diseases. This undoubtedly has a clinical impact in diagnosis and in prevention. The real challenge of the future lies in treatment, perhaps by pharmacological alleviation of the consequences of a gene defect and more distantly, but not unrealistically, by direct intervention at the gene level to reverse the abnormality.

Management of genetic diseases

Whenever a genetic disorder is recognized several questions must be addressed:

- How great is the risk to any given member of the family and to his or her offspring?
- Can the genetic status be defined by laboratory tests?
- Can such tests be applied to fetal tissue for prenatal diagnosis?
- Is any treatment available to alleviate the condition?

Although the principles of genetics do not change, it should be obvious from the preceding sections that clinical practice is evolving rapidly and today's answers to the above questions will often differ from yesterday's or tomorrow's.

The **counselling** of affected families requires, first, confirmation of the diagnosis and of the mode of transmission, by a combination of careful family history, examination of affected individuals and appropriate laboratory (increasingly nowadays molecular) tests.

Prenatal diagnosis

A growing list of genetic disorders can now be diagnosed in the fetus by sampling cells shed from the fetal skin, respiratory or urinary tract. These cells can be recovered by tapping the amniotic fluid, usually after an ultrasound scan to establish the position of the placenta (Fig. 2.24). Even with this precaution, **amniocentesis** carried a small risk (<1%) of precipitating abortion. It cannot normally be carries out before week 16 of gestation and is commonly undertaken at about week 18. An alternative method of obtaining fetal tissue is **chorionic villus biopsy** which is possible from about week 11 of gestation but has been associated in a number of instances with damage to the fetus (particularly partial agenesis of limbs).

Fig. 2.24   (a) Amniocentesis (at weeks 16 – 18). (b) Chorionic villus sampling (at week 11).

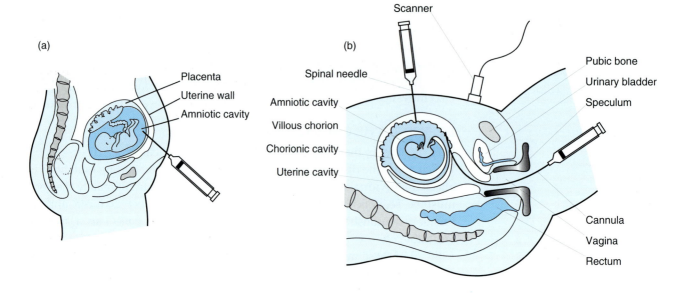

These procedures are appropriate when the family history or known carrier status of the parents suggests the fetus is at substantial risk of a genetic disease. The risk may come to light because a previous child has been born affected, for example, with an unbalanced chromosome translocation.

In the special case of Down's syndrome (trisomy 21) many centres advise screening of all pregnant mothers over the age of 35 but amniocentesis may be reserved for those mothers with low plasma α-fetoprotein (AFP) and unconjugated oestriol levels and/or suspicious features on detailed ultrasound scan of the fetus.

Prevention of genetic disease

The application of prenatal diagnostic techniques implies that selective termination of pregnancy may be carried out if the fetus is affected. Where this is considered acceptable, it is an effective method of preventing genetic disease in individual cases but it is important to recognize that it has negligible impact on the frequency of deleterious genes in the population since that is determined largely by the existence of heterozygous carriers of recessive disorders and by new mutations in the case of serious dominant conditions. The same applies to the decision taken voluntarily by some couples, on genetic grounds, not to have children. It is equally true that improvements in medical care that permit people with genetic disorders to survive and have children, in general, will probably not have a measurable effect on the global incidence of these diseases in future years.

The phenotypic expression of some genetic disorders may be modified dramatically by preventive measures. In the autosomal recessive condition phenylketonuria, where symptoms can be extremely variable, affected mothers are advised to adhere to a very low phenylalanine diet throughout pregnancy to avoid the damaging effects of hyperphenylalaninaemia on the developing brain of the fetus. A similar restriction is applied throughout childhood for infants diagnosed as phenylketonuric shortly after birth. The Guthrie card (blood spot) scheme in the UK is designed to identify such infants since many of them would suffer neurological damage if raised on a normal diet.

Homozygotes for the more severe forms of α_1-antitrypsin deficiency are susceptible to emphysema, but deterioration of lung function can be slowed very dramatically if they avoid smoking and if respiratory infections are treated promptly. Total proctocolectomy, at the stage of multiple adenomatosis, will prevent the development of colorectal cancer in familial adenomatous polyposis and there is current interest in the possibility that non-steroidal anti-inflammatory drugs may inhibit the growth of adenomas in this condition. A rather special example of preventive therapy is the administration of anti-rhesus D antibody to rhesus-negative mothers who have just delivered rhesus-positive infants, so that fetal red cells can be eliminated rapidly from the maternal circulation thus avoiding sensitization against subsequent fetuses genetically incompatible at the *Rh* locus.

Replacement therapy

Many of the genetic syndromes characterized by failure of development or function of endocrine organs (e.g. thyroid or adrenal cortex) can be treated very successfully by appropriate hormone replacement, which must of course be lifelong. Most forms of diabetes mellitus have a genetic component, so, in a sense, insulin can also be regarded as genetic replacement therapy. The same is true of blood clotting factors (notably VIII and IX) for the haemophilias, pooled immunoglobulins for X-linked agammaglobulinaemia, adenosine deaminase (ADA) for the less common ADA-deficient severe combined immunodeficiency syndrome and many other specific treatments for defined deficiencies.

Anaemia associated with severe haemoglobinopathies or with less common genetic defects in erythropoiesis can be managed by regular blood transfusions but this creates problems of iron overload which are difficult to overcome even with the use of potent (and costly) chelating agents.

Gene therapy

The concept of direct 'repair' or replacement of defective genes has caught the public imagination, partly as a result of advances in genetic manipulation of mice and other species. There is, however, a fundamental difference between **transgenic animal** technology and correction of a genetic lesion in a human patient. The former involves genetic manipulation of an embryonic stem cell in vitro, insertion of the modified cell into a very early embryo (usually about the eight-cell stage), implantation of that embryo into a surrogate mother, production of a live animal which is a mosaic (i.e. its tissues are derived from both the normal and the genetically manipulated cells), then breeding from that mosaic mouse to generate offspring in which every cell of the body carries the 'engineered' genetic change. Further rounds of breeding between such heterozygous mice will be required to produce animals that are homozygous for the altered gene (Fig. 2.25).

Fig. 2.25   The steps involved in producing a transgenic mouse.

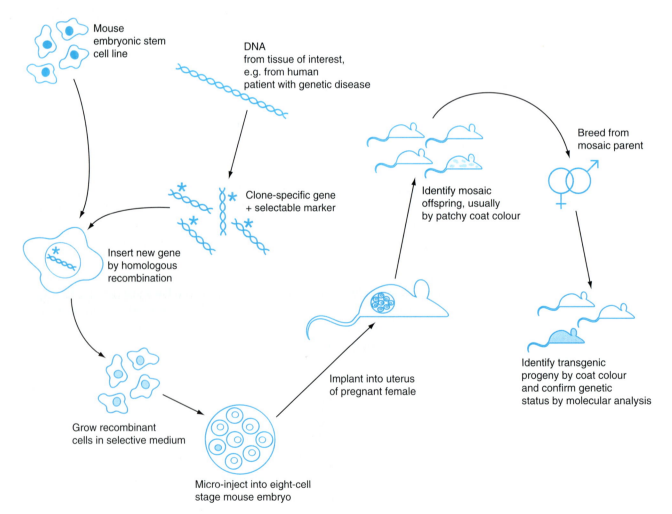

Mouse embryonic stem cell line

DNA from tissue of interest, e.g. from human patient with genetic disease

Clone-specific gene + selectable marker

Insert new gene by homologous recombination

Grow recombinant cells in selective medium

Micro-inject into eight-cell stage mouse embryo

Implant into uterus of pregnant female

Identify mosaic offspring, usually by patchy coat colour

Breed from mosaic parent

Identify transgenic progeny by coat colour and confirm genetic status by molecular analysis

PRACTICAL LIMITATIONS OF HUMAN GENE THERAPY

In theory a related approach might be possible to enable a couple affected with a serious genetic disorder to have a child in whom the defect has been corrected at the germ-line level, but it raises immense difficulties, both ethical and practical. For most purposes, discussion of human gene therapy centres upon methods of delivering a 'replacement' gene to a sufficient number of somatic cells to ameliorate the disorder. The simplest way to achieve this may be to transplant living cells from a genetically normal histocompatible donor. Genetically determined organ failure (e.g. polycystic kidney disease) is an indication for organ transplantation, but 'incomplete' tissue replacement may be appropriate if the donor cells are capable of growing and repopulating the host or of producing sufficient functioning product (e.g. an enzyme) for the rest of the body. This approach has achieved some success, for example, in cases of total thymic agenesis (fetal thymus grafts) and has also been attempted in some aplastic anaemias (using marrow or stem cell grafts) and in the mucopolysaccharidoses (using cultured fibroblasts). The possibility of infiltrating the dystrophin-deficient muscle of muscular dystrophy patients with normal fetal myoblasts is currently being debated. In this, as in many other situations, the establishment of animal models of human genetic diseases for direct testing of therapeutic options is a most important application of transgenic animal technology.

Most strategies for human gene therapy, including the few which are already being attempted and the somewhat greater number for which protocols are currently being devised (Table 2.3), rely upon the isolation of cells from the

Table 2.3   Some current gene therapy protocols

Disorder	Approach to gene therapy
Adenosine deaminase deficiency	Insertion of *ADA* gene into patient's marrow or peripheral blood stem cells
Cancers	Insertion of TNF, IL-2, GM-CSF, or other cytokine genes into patient's tumour-infiltrating lymphocytes (TIL)
	Insertion of thymidine kinase gene into tumour cells to activate pro-drug ganciclovir
Melanoma	Insertion of HLA-B7 gene into tumour cells
Familial hypercholesterolaemia	Insertion of LDL receptor gene into patient's liver cells
Cystic fibrosis	Aerosol delivery of *CFTR* gene to airways epithelium
Gaucher's disease	Insertion of glucocerebrosidase gene into patient's marrow cells

body, culture in vitro, genetic manipulation and re-implantation into the original host. A variety of cell types can be employed: fibroblasts, lymphocytes, hepatocytes, bone marrow and muscle cells. The genetic manipulation usually involves insertion of an intact 'normal' copy of the defective gene, including the relevant regulatory elements, together with a selectable 'marker', such as the gene for neomycin resistance, which allows those cells carrying the new insert to outgrow the remainder of the culture (Fig. 2.26).

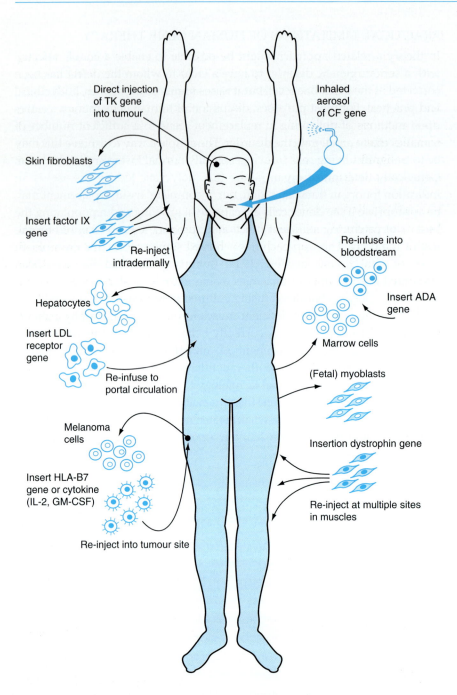

Direct injection
of TK gene
into tumour

Inhaled
aerosol
of CF gene

Skin fibroblasts

Insert factor IX
gene

Re-inject
intradermally

Re-infuse into
bloodstream

Insert ADA
gene

Hepatocytes

Insert LDL
receptor
gene

Re-infuse to
portal circulation

Marrow cells

(Fetal) myoblasts

Insertion dystrophin gene

Melanoma
cells

Insert HLA-B7
gene or cytokine
(IL-2, GM-CSF)

Re-inject at multiple sites
in muscles

Re-inject into tumour site

Fig. 2.26   Some approaches to human gene therapy.

The three major practical difficulties in this technology are:

- the low efficiency of DNA 'transfection' (i.e. only a few cells will take up the genetic 'package')
- instability of the insert (which may be lost or inactivated during the lifetime of the altered cell or of its immediate progeny)
- imperfect regulation of expression of the new gene.

The last of these poses the greatest challenge for the future of gene therapy since many disorders that might be candidates for this approach (the haemoglobinopathies, insulin-dependent diabetes and other peptide hormone deficiencies, etc.) require very accurately controlled expression of the replacement gene. Too much of the correct product could be as damaging as deficiency.

IN VIVO GENE THERAPY

In a few situations it may be possible to transfect an intact and functioning gene directly into the appropriate cells in the body – i.e. without prior isolation and culture. This is an attractive proposition, for example, in cystic fibrosis where strategies for delivering the *CF* gene, in aerosol form, to the cells of the respiratory tract, are currently being assessed. There is good evidence that only a proportion of cells need be targeted successfully to achieve significant improvement in chloride flux across the whole of the epithelium of the airways.

MUTATION REVERSAL

As an alternative to replacement of a defective gene by insertion of normal copy, a direct attempt may be made to reverse the mutation that has caused the defect. This would have the advantage that the corrected gene would be in its normal genetic context, amenable to normal regulatory processes and presumably as stable as any other DNA sequence in the cell.

By a process termed **homologous recombination**, a short segment of exogenous DNA can be exchanged for a similar sequence already in the genome. If the introduced segment differs slightly from the one it replaces, **site-directed mutagenesis** is achieved. In the context of gene therapy, of course, the new mutation would restore the **wild-type** gene sequence. Unfortunately, despite the enormous theoretical attractions, mutation reversal is unlikely to become a realistic option for human gene therapy in the foreseeable future since the efficiency of precise site-directed mutagenesis is still extremely low.

GENE THERAPY FOR CANCER

Cancer is a disorder of accumulated mutations, affecting **oncogenes** and **tumour suppressor genes** in somatic cells. In addition, for a significant proportion of common tumours such as breast, colon and ovarian cancers, there is a heritable component that can be attributed to mutation in a single gene. Overall, therefore, cancer represents the most widespread category of disorder for which gene therapy might be appropriate. In order to be fully effective, however, direct modification of the genome would have to be achieved in 100% of the tumour cells and no current in vivo delivery system can ensure this.

Nevertheless a number of approaches are being tested. Some are indirect, for example, the 'arming' of tumour-infiltrating lymphocytes (TIL), after culture in vitro, with potentially tumoricidal cytokines such as tumour necrosis factor (TNF), interleukin-2 (IL-2), or interferon to boost natural immunity to the tumour. Alternatively, the gene encoding an active enzyme such as thymidine kinase may be introduced into tumour cells by means of a virus modified in such a way that its infectivity cannot spread beyond the site of inoculation. An inert prodrug activated to a cytotoxic agent by the 'foreign' enzyme (e.g. ganciclovir in the case of thymidine kinase) can then be given systemically and will destroy those cells in which the transfected gene is expressed and perhaps their immediate neighbours, but not distant cells.

More direct gene therapy can be applied via **anti-sense oligonucleotides**, short synthetic stretches of single-stranded DNA, often with chemically modified bases to enhance stability, which are complementary to sequences found in the target cells. In the case of tumour cells the anti-sense oligomer may be directed against an oncogene that is over-expressed (such as N-*myc*, c-*erb* B2 or B*cl2*) or mutant (e.g. *p53*, *ras* or c-*myc*). It is usually designed to form a short double helix with the corresponding mRNA and hence both block translation and accelerate nuclease digestion of the message. Accessibility of the cancer cells in vivo to systemically delivered anti-sense oligonucleotides remains a limiting factor but the technique has been shown to cause selective inhibition of tumour growth in vitro and will probably have an early place in the 'purging' of autologous bone marrow taken from cancer patients and stored for re-infusion after very high-dose chemotherapy.

These are just a few examples of the directions that human gene therapy, now in its infancy, is likely to take in the course of the twenty-first century. While genetics, as a medical speciality, is obviously in a phase of rapid and exciting technical development, it is also at a stage of serious ethical uncertainty.

Ethical issues in genetics

The whole area of human genetics has always given rise to fierce arguments which have gained new urgency through advances in scientific knowledge. By its nature, genetic disease affects not only an individual patient but his or her entire family (including future generations), so there can be difficulties in applying the normal rules of medical confidentiality. In many instances at present, the genetic status of a patient can only be established by testing a number of relatives. Even if these are willing to cooperate, they may not wish to know the results of their own tests, yet these results may be inferred rather easily from the information eventually given to the original patient.

Decisions about whether to have children, to terminate an at-risk pregnancy or to undertake major prophylactic surgery (for example, in women with a bad family history of breast cancer) are best taken after prolonged and detailed counselling of the patient or couple which ensures that they have an understanding of the genetic principles involved.

There is an increasing trend for third parties – life assurance or health insurance companies and employers – to ask for access to the results of genetic tests. While this is understandable, given the financial implications of serious genetic disorders, there is a real risk that it will inhibit apparently healthy family members from participating in investigations that may help, for example, to establish the diagnosis in an affected relative. While so much of molecular genetics is at the research stage, it is particularly undesirable that families participating in studies for altruistic reasons should be penalized financially, or in any other way.

Because of the potentially serious implications of genetic testing, it should not be undertaken without careful discussion of the pros and cons with the individual to be tested. Indeed, that is a requirement for consent to be valid and without valid consent, even the taking of a blood sample for testing could be an indictable offence.

Codes of practice for the obtaining and recording of genetic information are still evolving. This is also true for the applications of gene therapy. These will rightly be controlled closely by statute but there will be individual situations where ethical dilemmas are not easily resolved by consulting a rule book. One firm principle to be upheld in all circumstances is that no one should suffer discrimination – in terms of provision of medical or social care – on the grounds of their genetic constitution.

Chapter 3

Cell and tissue communication

Learning objectives
- ❏ Appreciation of the role of cell and tissue communication in health and disease
- ❏ Ability to identify the problems of communication which contribute to disease

Even the simplest of multicellular organisms requires its cells to act in concert to sustain its existence, and the human body is no exception. Cells have internal programmes to which they work, but the basic structure of the body requires them to communicate with each other. However, this local communication network is not sufficient: cells form tissues which in turn need to communicate with other tissues to attune their functions. Disease as a result of communication difficulties between cells and tissues is common.

In this chapter, the mechanisms of communication are described under the main headings of cell–cell communication, tissue mediators, organ-specific hormones and the nervous system.

Cell–cell communication

Evolution of multicellular organisms probably arose from the association of unicellular organisms in colonies: in organisms these cells become specialized and cooperate. In the simplest organisms, cells do not totally separate at mitosis, but remain joined by cytoplasmic connections. They also secrete molecules which stick cells together and form an extracellular matrix. Sponges passed through a sieve will first aggregate and then form sheets of cells which are effectively epithelia. Although highly evolved in comparison, human cells still exploit direct cell–cell interaction through adhesion, secretion of extracellular molecules, and some are joined by channels known as gap junctions which permit the transfer of small cytoplasmic molecules.

Intercellular junctions

Cells within epithelia or other tissues are joined together by molecules on their surfaces (Fig. 3.1). **Desmosomes** and **hemidesmosomes** are examples of structural joins – rather like the welds holding a car together.

Gap junctions (Fig. 3.2) have no structural role, but are tiny opposing holes about 1.5 nm in diameter within the cell membrane of adjacent cells which permit small cytoplasmic molecules to pass by diffusion from cell to cell. Gap junctions can open and close in the same way as ionic channels: increases in calcium ions or decreases in pH close gap junctions reversibly within seconds.

surfaces of leukocytes, endothelial cells and intercellular matrix. These events are modulated by **mediators** – cytokines and others – produced locally within the tissue.

Three members of the **selectin** family (Table 3.1) have been recognized which share a **lectin**-like domain (a carbohydrate-binding region at the N-terminus) which is critical for adhesion to endothelial cells. Recent evidence indicates that different selectins may be involved in the adherence of leukocytes to different type of endothelial cells such as resting, activated endothelial cells and endothelial cells of high endothelial venules of Peyer's patches and lymph nodes.

Table 3.1   Adhesion molecules: selectin family

Selectin	Cell distribution	Target	Previous nomeclature
P-selectin (CD62)	Activated erythrocytes	PMN	GMP-140
	Platelets	Monocytes	
		Some lymphocytes	
L-selectin	PMNs	High erythrocyte	MEL 14
	Monocytes	venules of lymph nodes	LAM-1
	Some lymphocytes	Activated erythrocytes	LECAM-1
			Leu 8
E-selectin	Cytokine-activated	PMN	
	erythrocytes	Monocytes	
		Some lymphocytes	

PMN, polymorphonuclear leukocyte.

INTEGRINS

Integrins (Table 3.2) are heterodimers which share a common β subunit of 95 kDa (identified by monoclonal antibodies to CD18) and have select α subunits (CD11a, CD11b, CD11c) ranging from 150 to 180 kDa. They bind to **ICAM-1** and **ICAM-2** (immunoglobulin-like intercellular adhesion molecules), receptors present on endothelial cells. In addition, CD11b–CD18 (previously called Mac-1 and MO-1) also bind to matrix proteins such as laminin and activated complement iC3b. The very late activation (VLA) molecules are also heterodimers with a common β_1 chain (CD29) and selective chains (CD49), identifiable by monoclonal antibodies. These molecules help in binding of leukocytes to **collagen** and **laminin**.

Immunoglobulin-like molecules such as ICAM-1 and VCAM-1 are ligands for integrins which are expressed on the surface of endothelial cells. They can be up-regulated by cytokines to increase the likelihood of firm adhesion between leukocytes and endothelium leading to migration of leukocytes into tissues.

Tissue mediators

Mediators within tissues are divided into several groups, some of which are lipid derived *(arachidonic acid metabolites)*, while others are proteins or peptides secreted by cells or produced by the action of enzyme cascades on plasma proteins (Fig. 3.4).

Table 3.2 Adhesion models: examples of integrin family members

Integrins	CD	Genes	Cell distribution	Target	Previous nomenclature
β_2-Integrins	CD11a–CD18	$\alpha_L\,\beta_2$	Leukocytes PMN Monocytes Some lymphocytes	ICAM-1 ICAM-2	LFA-1
	CD11b–CD18	$\alpha_M\,\beta_2$	PMN Macrophages	ICAM-1 C3bi ?matrix proteins	Mac-1 Mo-1 CR3
	CD11c–CD18	$\alpha_X\,\beta_2$	PMN Macrophages	ICAM-1 iC3b	gp150, 95 CR4
VLA-1	CD49a–CD29	$\alpha_1\,\beta$	Leukocytes	Laminin Collagen	
VLA-2	CD49b–CD29	$\alpha_2\,\beta$	Leukocytes	Laminin Collagen	
VLA-3	CD39c–CD29	$\alpha_3\,\beta$	Leukocytes	Fibronectin Laminin Collagen	
VLA-4	CD49d–CD29	$\alpha_4\,\beta$	Leukocytes VCAM-1	Fibronectin	LPAM-2
VLA-5	CD49e–CD29	$\alpha_5\,\beta$	Leukocytes	Fibronectin	
VLA-6	CD49f–CD29	$\alpha_6\,\beta$	Leukocytes	Laminin	

PMN, polymorphonuclear leukocytes; VLA, very late activation.

Cytokines

Cytokines are glycoproteins which are produced by diverse cell types. They are considered to be **pleiotrophic**, as they are produced not only by different cells but also act on many target cells. Though they were initially identified as products of immune cells acting on leukocytes **(interleukins)**, it is now clear that they are also important products of non-immune cells. Cytokines influence the synthesis and functions of other cytokines and many functions may be mediated by one cytokine. They may antagonize or synergize with each other.

Cytokines function in three ways. They may act:

- on the same cell that produces them – **autocrine** function
- on a cell in the immediate neighbourhood – **paracrine** function
- on a distant target cell in a hormone-like fashion – **endocrine** function.

A single cytokine may have all three functions. Cytokine secretion is usually brief and self-limited; however, the response of the target cells may take many hours as it often involves synthesis of new mRNA and protein.

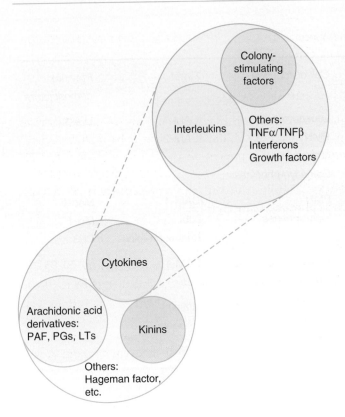

Fig. 3.4 An ever-increasing number of mediators is known to be involved in inflammation. Many also have other functions. They can be classified as shown on the basis of their structure and speed of function: arachidonic acid metabolites usually act faster but are destroyed more quickly than cytokines. LT, leukotriene; PAF, platelet-activating factor; PG, prostaglandin; TNF, tissue necrosis factor.

Table 3.3 Cytokines involved in inflammation

Cytokine	Source cells	Endothelial cell response	Function in vivo
IL-1	Macrophages	PGI$_2$ production of PCA and PAI	Vasodilatation
TNF-α	Endothelial cells		
	Natural killer (NK) cells	TM	Thrombosis cell adhesion
		PAF	
		ICAM-1	Leukocyte cell adhesion
		ICAM-2	Extravasation
		ELAM-1	
		Stimulation of IL-8, MCP-1, IL-1, IL-6	
IL-6			Stimulation of acute phase proteins
IL-8			PMN adhesion
			Activation
			Migration
TNF	Macrophages		Giant cell formation
IFN-γ	Macrophages	MHC class II expresssion	Antigen presentation
	Activated T cells		
	NK cells		
IFN-γ + TNF	Macrophages	MHC class I	Antigen presentation
	Activated T cells		
	NK cells		
TGF-β	Macrophages	Endothelial cell proliferation and migration	Angiogenesis
	Activated T cells		Collagen synthesis
PDGF	Activated macrophages	Fibroblast proliferation	Granulation tissue

Table 3.3 gives the cell source, the targets involved and the functions mediated by some inflammatory cytokines.

Arachidonic acid metabolites

Oxygenated arachidonic acid metabolites have an important role in pathological processes such as inflammation. **Arachidonic acid** is a polyunsaturated fatty acid which in its esterified form is present on the cell membrane (5,8,11,14-eicosatetraenoic acid). It is not found in the free form and has to be released from the plasma membrane. This is achieved through activation of cellular phospholipases such as **phospholipase A_2** (PLA_2).

PHOSPHOLIPASE A_2

PLA_2 has proinflammatory effects as it helps in synthesis and release of chemical mediators. PLA_2 is activated by complement, proteases, toxic oxygen intermediates, bacterial products and cytokines. Several human tissues and cells contain mRNA transcripts of the PLA_2 gene. Therefore, the release and activation of PLA_2 from the cell membranes affects many pathological situations, by leading to hyperaemia, oedema and accumulation of PMN, as in rheumatoid arthritis, adult respiratory distress syndrome, endotoxic shock and malaria, for example.

Tumour necrosis factor (TNF) and interleukin-1 (IL-1) induce the activation of membrane-bound PLA_2 and promote the synthesis and release of soluble PLA_2. IL-1 has maximal effects whereas TNF only acts at a higher concentration.

FORMATION OF ARACHIDONIC ACID METABOLITES

The arachidonic acid metabolites are formed by one of two pathways (Fig 3.5).

■ The products of the **cyclo-oxygenase** pathway are:
  - **thromboxane A_2** released by thromboxane synthetase, which has a half-life of seconds, is a strong vasoconstrictor and also aggregates platelets
  - **prostacyclin (PGI_2)**, released by prostacyclin synthetase, which has the opposite effect, inhibiting platelet aggregation and leading to vasodilatation, and is present mainly in blood vessel walls
  - **prostaglandins PGE_2, PGF_2 and PGD_2**, which have longer half-life and also cause vasodilatation and increase vascular permeability and extravasation of serum into tissue.

The anti-inflammatory effect of drugs like **aspirin** and **indomethacin** is due to their inhibitory effects on cyclo-oxygenase. Cytokines also influence arachidonic acid metabolism. IL-1, IL-2, TNF-α and TNF-β increase prostacyclin production by increasing prostacyclin synthtease in endothelial cells and thereby cause vasodilatation, an important process in inflammation. Prostaglandin E, a strong mediator of vasodilatation, is also produced in large amounts from endothelial cells stimulated by cytokines IL-1 and TNF.

■ In the **lipoxygenase** pathway arachidonic acid is converted into hydroperoxyeicosatetraenoic acid (HPETE) and then to **hydroxy-eicosatetraenoic acid (HETE)**, which is a potent chemoattractant for PMN and also gives rise to a series of **leukotrienes**. Leukotriene A_4 is unstable

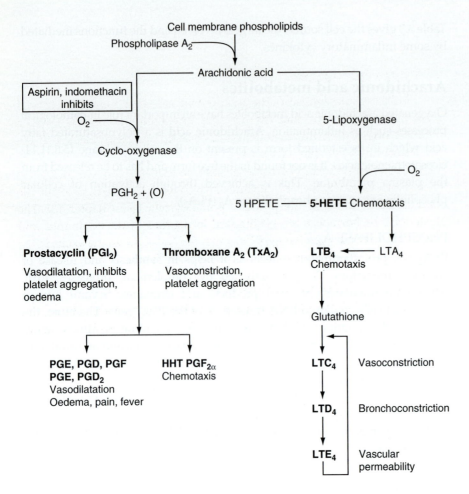

Fig. 3.5   Arachidonic acid metabolites.

and is converted to leukotriene B_3 which is a potent chemoattractant and platelet aggregator. On addition of glutathione it is converted first to leukotriene C_4, then leukotriene D_4 and finally leukotriene E_4. These leukotrienes cause vasoconstriction, bronchospasm and vascular permeability, which are responsible for symptoms seen in immediate hypersensitivity reactions such as asthma. Mast cells are a rich source of leukotrienes C_4, D_4 and E_4 whereas leukotriene B_4 is produced by blood-derived leukocytes.

Other mediators

Gases have only recently been discovered to act as messengers. It is now clear, however, that nitric oxide is an important messenger which dilates blood vessels, acts as a neurotransmitter, relaxes smooth muscle in the gut, and inhibits platelet activation. It is produced by the reaction of the amino acid L-arginine with oxygen to form L-citrulline and nitric oxide. Phagocyte production of nitric oxide may be important in killing micro-organisms, but tissue damage caused by overproduction may be an important facet of the pathogenesis of shock.

In inflammation, important mediators are produced from the kinin, clotting, fibrinolysis and complement pathways which are linked via **Hageman factor**: these are dealt with in Chapter 6.

Organ-specific hormones

Pituitary hormones

The pituitary gland consists of the anterior lobe **(adenohypophysis)**, derived from the primitive gut, and the posterior lobe **(neurohypophysis)** which takes its origin from the central nervous system and is connected to the **hypothalamus** by the pituitary stalk.

The secretion of hormones from the anterior lobe is controlled mainly by chemicals released by the hypothalamus, which reach the anterior lobe by the vascular connections of the pituitary portal system (see Chapter 18). The posterior lobe hormones are synthesized in neurons of the supraoptic and paraventricular nuclei in the hypothalamus and travel down the axons in the pituitary stalk to be released into the systemic circulation.

ANTERIOR PITUITARY HORMONES

The anterior pituitary gland produces six classic hormones, which have effects either on specific target glands or directly on general metabolism. These are:

- **growth hormone (GH)**
- **adrenocorticotrophin (ACTH)**
- **prolactin (PRL)**
- **thyroid-stimulating hormone (TSH)**

and the gonadotrophins:

- **follicle-stimulating hormone (FSH)**
- **luteinizing hormone (LH).**

The gland also produces a wide range of other peptides which may have a paracrine role in regulating the secretion of the classical hormones.

The release of GH is controlled by the integrated action of two hypothalamic factors: (1) growth hormone-releasing factor (GRF) which stimulates and (2) somatostatin (SMS) which inhibits release.

Growth hormone directly alters the level of protein synthesis in liver and muscle, and induces lipolysis in fat stores. It has an indirect action on skeletal growth via the stimulation of production of **insulin-like growth factor-1** (IGF-1) by the liver. IGF-1 also exerts negative feedback on GH secretion by the pituitary. ACTH is derived from a large precursor, pro-opiomelanocortin (POMC). ACTH mainly controls the secretion of glucocorticoids from the adrenal cortex. The synthesis and secretion of ACTH are stimulated by the hypothalamic peptides corticotrophin-releasing factor (CRF) and, to a lesser extent, vasopressin (VP). Glucocorticoids exert negative feedback.

POMC also gives rise to other peptides which have been shown to stimulate steroidogenesis and adrenal growth in animals, and to **melanocyte-stimulating hormones (MSH)**. The role of these peptides in humans is unclear.

FSH, LH and TSH are glycoproteins and each comprises two subunits. The α subunit is common to all three, the β subunit specific to each individual hormone. FSH and LH are synthesized by the same cells within the pituitary. In males, FSH stimulates spermatogenesis, while LH regulates Leydig cell function. In the female, FSH controls follicle growth while LH is involved in ovulation and the maturation of the corpus luteum. The release of both is stimulated by gonadotrophin-releasing hormone (GnRH) from the hypothalamus, and sex steroids exert negative feedback. The complex interactions which control the differential secretion of the two hormones throughout the menstrual cycle are unclear. TSH regulates thyroid hormone secretion, stimulated by hypothalamic thyrotrophin-releasing factor (TRH), with negative feedback by thyroid hormones.

PRL, a polypeptide hormone, is involved in the regulation of the breast in lactation. Although basal circulating levels are similar in males and females, its role in the male is unclear. In contrast to the major stimulatory role of the hypothalamus on the other pituitary hormones, the dominant hypothalamic influence on PRL secretion is inhibitory, mainly via dopamine.

POSTERIOR PITUITARY HORMONES

- **Oxytocin** causes contraction of the smooth muscle of the uterus and ejection of milk in response to suckling.
- **Vasopressin (antidiuretic hormone)** stimulates reabsorption of water by the distal tubules and collecting ducts of the kidney, and thus plays a role in water balance.

Thyroid hormones

The thyroid gland consists mainly of the thyroid **follicles** which produce the hormones derived from the iodination of tyrosine:

- **tetra-iodothyronine or thyroxine** (T_4)
- **tri-iodothyronine** (T_3) (Fig. 3.6).

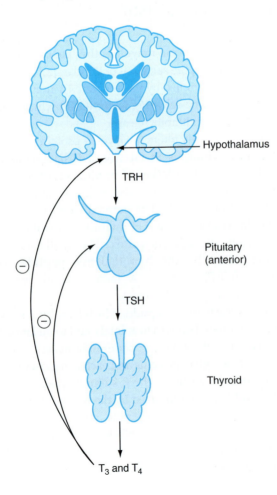

Fig. 3.6 The hypothalamic–pituitary–thyroid axis. Thyrotrophin-releasing hormone (TRH) stimulates the anterior pituitary secretion of thyroid-stimulating hormone (TSH) into the peripheral blood. This then stimulates the synthesis and secretion of thyroxine and tri-iodothyronine by the thyroid gland. These have multiple peripheral actions and also exert negative feedback at both pituitary and hypothalamic levels.

Hypothalamus

TRH

Pituitary
(anterior)

TSH

Thyroid

T_3 and T_4

These are synthesized on tyrosine residues on a large protein, thyroglobulin, stored as **colloid** in the thyroid follicles. Inorganic **iodine** is actively trapped and oxidized by the follicular cells by thyroid peroxidase enzyme, situated at the apical membrane of the follicular cells. It is then bound to thyroglobulin tyrosine residues as mono- and diiodotyrosine. Coupling of these iodotyrosines produces T_3 and T_4. TSH stimulation results in endocytosis of thyroglobulin into follicular cells, fusion with lysosomes and release of T_3 and T_4 into the systemic blood. Uncoupled iodotyrosines are deiodinated by a dehalogenase enzyme and the iodine recycled.

Circulating T_4 and T_3 are mainly bound to **thyroxine-binding globulin (TBG)** and thyroxine-binding prealbumin (TBPA). Only a small proportion circulate in the free active form. Peripheral tissues metabolize T_4 to T_3 or reverse T_3, T_3 being the metabolically active hormone. This has wide-ranging effects on general metabolism via modulation of fat, protein and carbohydrate metabolism, and regulation of key enzymes in metabolic pathways.

The thyroid also contains **C cells**, dispersed focally among the follicles, mainly in the upper third of the gland, These secrete **calcitonin**, a calcium-lowering hormone, which acts by inhibiting bone resorption, and calcium absorption by the gastrointestinal tract and by increasing renal excretion of calcium and phosphate. These actions are of only minor physiological importance in human metabolism.

Adrenal cortex

The adrenal cortex synthesizes a range of steroid hormones from cholesterol (Fig. 3.7). It consists of three zones (see Chapter 18). The zona glomerulosa produces **mineralocorticoids**, mainly **aldosterone**, and is regulated by the **renin–angiotensin system**. The zona reticularis and zona fasciculata act as a unit, producing mainly **glucocorticoids** with **cortisol** the most important in humans. The zona reticularis acts as the physiologically functional zone with the zona fasciculata as reserve. Sex steroids are also produced in small quantities, most probably only by the zona reticularis. These zones are stimulated by ACTH.

Aldosterone has a major role in the regulation of potassium balance and plasma volume homeostasis. It increases renal tubular secretion of potassium and reabsorption of sodium and chloride. **Glucocorticoids** have a significant

Fig. 3.7 Biosynthetic pathway for steroid hormones synthesized in the adrenal cortex, showing the enzyme pathways involved. DHEA, dehydroepiandrosterone.

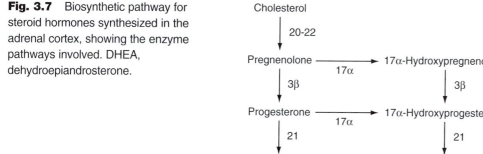
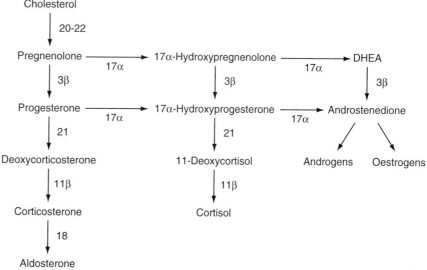

role in regulating general metabolism and, in excess, cause well-recognized pathological effects. They are antagonistic to insulin, promote gluconeogenesis, inhibit protein synthesis and stimulate protein catabolism. Their actions on vascular smooth muscle increase blood pressure. In the immune system they are cytotoxic to lymphocytes, particularly T cells, and inhibit the phagocytic and bactericidal actions of polymorphs and macrophages. They delay healing by inhibiting the normal formation of granulation tissue and collagen maturation. Osteoporosis may be induced via effects on bone formation and calcium absorption.

Adrenal medulla

The phaeochromocytes of the adrenal medulla secrete catecholamines, mainly **adrenaline** and **noradrenaline**. These also help regulate a variety of physiological functions interacting with local sympathetic innervation in control of vascular tones, cardiac rate, gastrointestinal mobility, fluid and electrolyte transport across cell membranes, and effecting a role in aspects of cell proliferation and immune responses. The adrenal medulla also produces various peptide hormones, including **enkephalins**, but their roles are largely unknown.

Parathyroid glands

The parathyroid glands secrete **parathyroid hormone** (**parathormone**), the primary function of which is to control calcium concentration in extracellular fluid. This action is effected by stimulating reabsorption of calcium in the kidney, increasing calcium reabsorption from bone and increasing **vitamin D**-mediated calcium absorption from the gastrointestinal tract.

Pancreas

The islets of Langerhans secrete a number of peptide hormones, including **glucagon**, **insulin**, **pancreatic polypeptide** and **somatostatin**. Glucagon is secreted by the α cells, insulin by the β cells. Insulin is the main regulator of glucose metabolism. It stimulates glucose uptake by liver, fat and muscle and inhibits glycogen breakdown and gluconeogenesis in liver. Glucagon opposes the action of insulin by stimulating glycogenolysis and gluconeogenesis in the liver. In addition, insulin suppresses glucagon secretion, while glucagon stimulates insulin secretion. Somatostatin suppresses both insulin and glucagon. The role of pancreatic polypeptide is not fully elucidated.

Neural communication

In order to function as an efficient and self-contained unit within the body, the structural complexities of the nervous system require a highly developed cell–cell communication system. This is of paramount importance in the central nervous system (CNS), where the smooth integration of functional activity places a high requirement for sensitive and rapid intercellular communications. Furthermore, the integration of functionally diverse pathways within the CNS requires not only rapid communication but specific feedback mechanisms in order to ensure a sensitive functional organization.

Implications for structural organization

The requirement for rapid and sensitive cell–cell communication in the CNS is reflected in its architectural organization, particularly in the arrangement of the neurons, which are responsible for the electrical activity of the brain and spinal cord. The cerebral cortex is arranged in six horizontal layers which vary relatively across the hemispheres. In the **primary motor cortex**, the large pyramidal cells of Betz are located in layer V, representing the major source of the corticospinal motor tract. In the **visual cortex** of the occipital lobe, cortical layer V is not so prominent, but layer IV is particularly well developed and includes a prominent band of myelinated nerve fibres (the band of Gennari). The nerve cells in the cerebral cortex are also arranged in a series of columns, in which the constituent cells are able to communicate between themselves and with adjacent groups in the same hemisphere by longitudinal fibres, and with other groups in the opposite hemisphere by special bands of nerve fibres known as the commissures, for example the corpus callosum.

The organization of nerve cells in the deep grey matter structures (basal ganglia, thalamus and hypothalamus) varies markedly from region to region, with functionally related nerve cells occurring in groups known as **nuclei**. This arrangement allows related cells to be located in close proximity, and provides a well-defined 'target' for afferent fibres. The myelinated fibres within the white matter are also arranged in related groups, particularly within the spinal cord. This form of functionally related structural organization is well demonstrated in the motor pathway of the CNS (Fig. 3.8).

Cellular communication

Neurons are distinct structural and functional cellular units within the CNS. They have no direct connections, but they have specialized features which allow the reception of nerve impulses from other neurons (which may be either inhibitory or excitatory), and the conduction of nerve impulses. These specialized functions are reflected in the cellular anatomy of neurons (Fig. 3.9), where the multiple short branching processes known as **dendrites** form the main receptive area of the cell, and the single **axon** conducts impulses away from the perikaryon, usually to other neurons in the CNS. Within this basic cell structure there is enormous variation in the relative size and complexity of the dendritic tree and axon between neurons in different regions of the CNS, many of which relate to the functional diversity of neurons at these various sites. In the CNS, neuronal intercellular communication occurs at sites known as **synapses**, which were first visualized by light microscopy as small projections on the branches of the terminal axon which lie in close contact with the dendrites or perikarya of other neurons. Synaptic development begins *in utero* and continues into postnatal life; synaptic remodelling in the adult CNS is thought to be partly responsible for functional plasticity in both normal and disease states, allowing partial clinical recovery following a stroke, for example.

A nerve impulse can be propagated in many directions on a neuronal cell surface, but in vivo the direction of nerve impulses is determined by a constant polarity at synapses, where transmission occurs from the axon of one neuron to the cell surface of another. Most synaptic junctions in the CNS are chemical synapses in which a substance, the **neurotransmitter**, is released from the terminal axon and diffuses across the narrow space

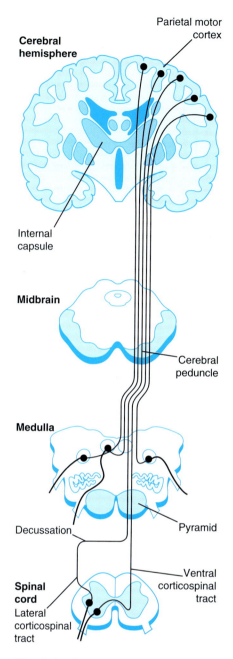

Fig. 3.8 Corticospinal motor pathway. Main motor fibres are black, grey matter is blue.

between the two cells to become bound to specific receptors in the postsynaptic membrane of the adjacent cell. Electron microscopic studies have revealed much more information on the structure of synapses, the main features of which are illustrated in Fig. 3.10. A synapse is composed of three main constituents:

- The **presynaptic element**, comprising the axon terminals which contains the synaptic vesicles filled with neurotransmitter, while the surrounding cytoplasm contains other organelles, including mitochondria, smooth endoplasmic reticulum, microtubules and neurofilaments.
- The **synaptic cleft**, usually 20–30 nm wide, which is often surrounded by glial cell processes.
- The **postsynaptic neuronal membrane**, which contains an accumulation of dense material on its surface and specialized receptors for specific neurotransmitters.

A large number of substances have been identified as **neurotransmitters** in the CNS (Table 3.4), including **acetylcholine** and the monoamine neurotransmitters **noradrenaline**, **adrenaline** and **dopamine**. A number of amino acids act as neurotransmitters, including **glutamate**, a potent excitatory neurotransmitter, and the inhibitory neurotransmitters γ-**aminobutyric acid** and **glycine**. A large variety of **neuropeptides** may also act as neurotransmitters, including pituitary peptides, intestinal hormones and opioid peptides. Recent researches on neurodegenerative disorders have demonstrated an abnormal distribution of neurotransmitters and neuro-peptides in a variety of disease states, e.g. cortical acetylcholine deficiency in **Alzheimer's disease**, and dopamine deficiency in the basal ganglia in **Parkinson's disease**. Therapeutic replacement of dopamine by **levodopa** in Parkinson's disease is a standard form of treatment which helps alleviate the clinical signs and symptoms of this disorder.

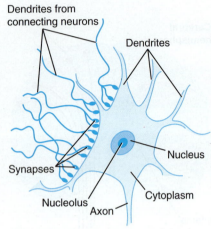

Fig. 3.9 Cytoarchitecture of a neuron demonstrating the specialized cell processes and synapses.

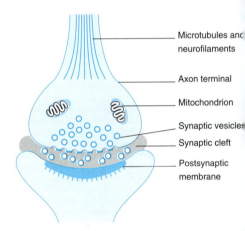

Fig. 3.10 A chemical synapse.

Table 3.4   Distribution of neurotransmitters in the cerebral cortex

Chemical group	Afferent fibres	Cortical neurons
Monoamines	Dopamine	Dopamine
	Noradrenaline	
	Serotonin	
	(5-hydroxytryptamine)	
Cholines	Acetylcholine	
	γ-Aminobutyric acid	γ-Aminobutyric acid
	Glutamate	Glutamate
	Aspartate	Aspartate
Neuropeptides		Somatostatin
		Chiolecystokinin
		Vasoactive intestinal peptide

Neuron transport and conduction mechanisms

Neurons in the CNS act as secretory cells, the products of which form the chemical signals for intercellular communication at synapses. Neurotransmitters and neuropeptides are synthesized in the perikaryon, and then transported along the axon to be stored in vesicles in the presynaptic axonal terminals. The axonal terminals can be far removed from the site of transmitter synthesis, so **axonal transport** mechanisms are vital for the maintenance of cellular communication in the CNS. Fast axonal transport (50–500 nm/day) carries organelles, e.g. mitochondria, vesicles and membrane-bound neurotransmitters which are essential for synaptic activity. Slow axonal transport mechanisms (0.2–8 nm/day) transport larger compounds which are involved in the growth and maintenance of the axons. Retrograde transport mechanisms also exist, for the recovery and recycling of vesicle proteins following neurotransmitter release, for instance. Axonal transport is an active mechanism which can be blocked by a variety of agents, including drugs which inhibit microtubule function: an example is the cytotoxic drug vinblastine.

Whereas axonal transport mechanisms are involved in the supply of neurotransmitters to axonal terminals, transport of electrical impulses depends on an intact functional cell membrane. The neuronal cell membrane is semipermeable, and in the resting state potassium ions diffuse from the cytoplasm to the outer surface of the membrane, which acquires a **resting potential** of around 80 mV with respect to the inside. During excitation the membrane potential is reduced by 10–15 mV to threshold value, accompanied by a functional alteration allowing a selective increase in permeability to sodium ions. This creates a local **action potential** which is self-propagated along the cell membrane as the nerve impulse.

Rapid **conduction** of the nerve impulse in the CNS is facilitated by the process of saltatory conduction, which in turn depends on the presence of myelin around axons. **Myelin** in the CNS is produced by **oligodendrocytes**, which form a tightly spiralled sheath derived from cytoplasmic processes. Myelin has a characteristic constant structure within the CNS, and the thickness of the myelin sheath is related to axonal diameter. One oligodendrocyte may provide myelin for many axons; myelin is arranged in segments along the axon between **nodes of Ranvier**. Membrane depolarization at these nodes allows rapid conduction along the axon. Damaged myelin in the CNS cannot be effectively resynthesized by oligodendrocytes and consequently many demyelinating disorders in the CNS, such as multiple sclerosis, are characterized by a reduction in nerve impulse velocity. This can be of diagnostic value in the measurement of **visual evoked responses**, which are characteristically delayed in multiple sclerosis.

The role of glial cells

It is evident that the satisfactory function of intercellular connections in the CNS depends on the structural and functional integrity of neurons. However, the **glial cells** of the CNS also play a major role in facilitating neuronal function. **Astrocytes** establish close contacts with nerve cells, including perikarya and dendrites, with numerous astrocytic processes around areas of synaptic activity. This helps protect receptive neuronal surface from non-specific stimulation. Astrocytes are also thought to play a role in synaptic remodelling in the adult CNS and may influence neuronal functional plasticity. They are also involved in ion transport and neurotransmitter metabolism, particularly in the uptake of glutamate released by neurons at synapses.

Oligodendrocytes synthesize and maintain myelin, which is required for rapid axonal conduction of nerve impulses. Oligodendrocytes may influence neuronal metabolism, particularly the satellite oligodendrocytes which are situated immediately adjacent to neuronal perikarya. **Microglial cells** also maintain a close functional relationship with neurons and axons, and are thought to play a role in the regulation and transport of ions and fluid in the extracellular space.

Chapter 4   Disorders of growth

Learning objectives
- ❏ Appreciation of how cells grow and divide
- ❏ Understanding of the cell cycle and the basic factors controlling it
- ❏ Appreciation of the importance of stem cells in tissue homeostasis, and the mechanisms involved in hypoplasia and hyperplasia
- ❏ Understanding of differentiation and metaplasia
- ❏ Appreciation of the factors involved in cellular ageing
- ❏ Ability to distinguish apoptosis from necrosis and understanding of the causes involved

The cell cycle

There has been a great increase in the knowledge of the **cell cycle** and its control over the past 20 years. This is probably in part due to the interest in its role in disorders of cell proliferation and cancer. Much of the detail of the eukaryotic cell cycle has been obtained from study of various yeast species and it has been shown that there are fundamental similarities at the molecular level in all eukaryotic cells.

The term 'cell cycle' refers to a sequence of events which occur consistently between successive mitoses (Fig. 4.1). It may be divided into five major phases: G_1, S, G_2, M and cytokinesis.

The length of the cell cycle differs depending on the type of cell and varies from a few hours to days. **Interphase**, consisting of successive G_1, S and G_2 phases, normally takes up the majority (about 90%) of the cell cycle time. In human cells S, G_2 and M together are of fairly constant length (usually about 12 hours). Most of the variability in the cell cycle therefore resides in the duration of G_1.

Cells in an apparently non-proliferative or a quiescent G_1 condition are often said to be in G_0. The capacity for cell division varies between different cell types in the human body.

Neurons and skeletal muscle are incapable of division and therefore form a **static cell population**; some cell populations such as keratinocytes in the skin or surface epithelial cells in the gut are continually renewing their numbers because of constant cell loss and their precursor cells have a relatively rapid cell division rate; other cell types normally have a slow turnover rate but when the need arises, for instance to replace cells lost by injury, cell division may be stimulated. These are known as **conditional renewal populations**, an example being hepatocytes. It is therefore apparent that cells in G_0 can be triggered into passing through the cell cycle

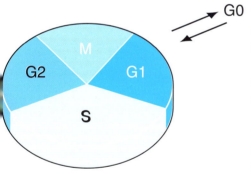

Fig. 4.1 The cell cycle.

Phases of the cell cycle
- **G_1 phase** (Gap 1) is the interval between M phase and S phase
- **S phase** is the period of DNA synthesis
- **G_2** (Gap 2) is the interval between the end of the S phase and the next M phase
- **M phase** is mitosis
- **Cytokinesis** is the formation of two daughter cells

in response to certain environmental factors, not only cell loss but also to hormones and growth factors.

If the conditions are not favourable for growth – for example, nutrition is inadequate – then the cell may come to rest in G_1. There is a point in G_1 known as **start** beyond which the cell is committed to divide. A gene, *cdc2* (cell division cycle), was isolated from fission yeast and its product, p34cdc2, appeared to be required at two points in the cell cycle: **start** and **mitosis**. Similar substances are involved in the regulation of the human cell cycle and they have protein kinase activity. A protein whose concentration fluctuated during the cell cycle was discovered originally in sea urchin eggs and given the name **cyclin**. Cyclins bind to p34cdc2 and together they form the **mitosis (or maturation) promoting factor (MPF)**. The cyclins act as regulatory subunits for protein kinases including p34cdc2, a serine/threonine kinase. p34cdc2 is only active as a protein kinase when associated with its cyclin subunit.

Phosphorylation is also important in the regulation of protein kinase activity in the cell cycle. p34cdc2 becomes increasingly phosphorylated during S and G_2 (when it also becomes complexed with cyclin) and activation of its kinase activity occurs as a result of subsequent dephosphorylation. The progression of the cell cycle therefore depends on fluctuations in the activity of these cyclin-dependent kinases (CDKs) (Fig. 4.2).

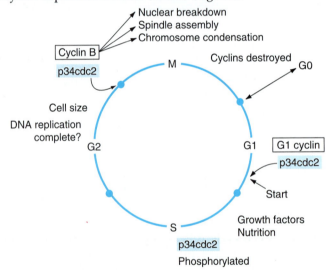

Fig. 4.2 Regulation of the cell cycle. See text for details.

There are two main checkpoints in the progression of the cell cycle and these are at the G_1/S and G_2/M transitions. The G_1/S checkpoint is sensitive to extracellular signals such as growth factors, whereas passing beyond the G_2/M checkpoint depends more on the cell's internal environment – whether DNA replication is complete and the cell is an appropriate size.

Activity of p34cdc2 is required for the promotion of the G_1/S and at the G_2/M transitions, and particular cyclins are complexed with it at each stage. The *cdc25* gene is a positive regulator of p34cdc2 and it is thought to be through this that the cell determines whether or not DNA replication is complete. On the other hand, the gene called *wee1* negatively regulates p34cdc2 and this is associated with the recognition of cell size and nutrition.

The exact function of the protein kinase activity of p34cdc2 is unclear, but it is almost certainly involved in the breakdown of the nuclear envelope and may also contribute to chromosome condensation and spindle formation possibly through histone H_1 kinase activity.

It is possible that the cell cycle checkpoints are the points at which oncogene products act. Certain oncogene products such as c-abl protein have been shown to be phosphorylated by p34cdc2 kinase, but the exact significance of this is uncertain. Cyclin D_1 is one of the cyclins active in G_1 phase. It is carried on chromosome 11q13 and is the gene also known as *BC11* and *PRAD1*. The 11q13 region is amplfied in several types of cancer. Increased cyclin D_1 may be significant in these tumours. Tumour suppressor genes are probably also intimately involved in the control of the normal cell cycle. The product of the retinoblastoma (*RB*) gene for instance is a nuclear phosphoprotein and it would appear to be responsible for inhibiting proliferation in response to growth inhibitory signals. This activity is also likely to be controlled by the phosphorylation state of the protein. The RB protein appears to be inactivated by hyperphosphorylation and only becomes active when the phosphate groups are removed during G_1.

Growth factors

Even in a multicellular organism the individual cells are not isolated from their environment and are subjected to a variety of signals, some of which result in the stimulation of cell division. A complex set of reactions processes and conveys these signals from the cell surface to the nucleus; this is known as signal transduction. One of the main mechanisms utilized in **signal transduction** also involves protein phosphorylation using the diverse family of protein kinases.

Growth factors are polypeptides which bind to cell surface receptors resulting in a variety of responses including alterations in proliferation rate. They tend to have short half-lives and act locally in an autocrine or paracrine manner. They are active at extremely low concentrations. There are a number of growth factor families (Table 4.1) and their target cells are characterized by specific transmembrane receptors, many of which have

Table 4.1   Growth factor families

Family	Examples
Epidermal growth factor family	EGF
	TGF
	Amphiregulin
Heparin-binding growth factor family	Fibroblast GFs a and b
	Keratinocyte GF
Platelet-derived growth factor family	PDGF
Insulin-like growth factor family	IGF-1
	IGF-2
Nerve growth factor family	NGF
Transforming growth factor beta family	TGF-β
Hepatocyte growth factor	HGF

cytoplasmic tyrosine kinase domains, such as epidermal growth factor receptor (EGF-R). Ligand binding activates the tyrosine kinase, which sets off a sequence of events within the cell resulting in biochemical changes. These include:

- protein phosphorylation
- production of cyclic nucleotides, inositol phosphate and diacylglycerol (DAG) which in turn affect the intracellular release of calcium ions and activation of protein kinase
- alkalization of the cytoplasm.

Then follow morphological and metabolic alterations within the cell and cell cycle progression. The immediate substrates for this tyrosine kinase activity are somewhat unclear, but one candidate is the **ras GTPase-activating protein** (ras-GAP) which stimulates the GTPase activity of the products of the *ras* proto-oncogene. GAP is known to be physically associated with the platelet-derived growth factor (PDGF) receptor. These ras proteins are a common relay point for many of the growth factor receptors and are probably important messengers in the signal transduction process leading to stimulation of cell proliferation. This may explain the mechanism by which mutations in the *ras* gene lead to uncontrolled cell proliferation in many types of cancer. There are relatively few groups of cell surface receptors. Their basic structure is similar with an extracellular portion responsible for ligand binding, a short component within the membrane and an intracellular portion which passes on the signal.

In addition to the membrane-spanning tyrosine kinases there are transmembrane receptors coupled to G proteins. The G proteins are GTP-binding proteins and one subunit has GTPase activity which detaches from the receptor complex to initiate the next step within the cytoplasm.

A series of protein kinases conveys the signal within the cell. **Mitogen activated protein (MAP) kinases** are a family of serine/threonine kinases and they are known to be rapidly activated following application of growth factors to cells. It is thought that such a protein kinase cascade ultimately leads to phosphorylation of key nuclear proteins involved in cell cycle control. These proteins include products of proto-oncogenes such as c-*jun* and c-*fos* which are able to affect transcription by interaction with certain DNA sequences. Phosphorylation of these proteins may produce either stimulation or inhibition of their activity and therefore induction or suppression of gene expression with effects on cell proliferation and/or differentiation. Other transcription factors include **cyclic AMP response element binding protein (CREB)** and the products of c-*myc* and c-*myb*. CREB is interesting in that it is involved in the stimulation of gene expression resulting from an increase in cyclic AMP in the cell. Various substances, in particular hormones, can produce such an increase in cyclic AMP and thus CREB forms a direct link between hormone stimulation and cell proliferation.

It is therefore apparent that there is quite a lot of information relating to the events at the cell surface and within the cytoplasm in signal transduction. Relatively little is known, however, about the nuclear events which couple the cytoplasmic events to the eventual long-term response of the cell. Attention has been focused recently on a set of genes known as **immediate early** or **primary response genes**. These genes are rapidly and transiently induced upon stimulation of cell proliferation and their transduction is not dependent upon de novo protein synthesis. Many of these genes and the targets of their products are known. Of particular interest with regard to control of cell proliferation are those genes which encode transcription factors, such as c-*fos* and c-*jun*, as these are able to control the expression of other target genes that lead to the cellular responses necessary for cell division and differentiation.

Growth factors may also have an inhibitory effect on cell proliferation. **Transforming growth factor (TGF)** is an example. A number of genes (*gas, prohibitin, IND1* and *IND2*) associated with growth arrest have recently been described but their exact function is unclear.

Stem cells

In order to maintain a relatively constant tissue volume during adult life, cells must be replaced at a rate equivalent to that of cell loss. This is a constant process in continually renewing tissues such as the haemopoietic system, the skin and the intestine. At these sites cell division is confined to a population of **stem cells**. These give rise to daughter cells, some of which become a new generation of stem cells and some undergo terminal differentiation and are destined to die. The stem cell therefore has a high capacity for self-renewal and has a less differentiated phenotype than its daughters. Some stem cells can give rise to a variety of differentiated progeny, and these are said to be **pluripotential stem cells**. A good example of a pluripotential stem cell is that found in the bone marrow, which can give rise to both myeloid and lymphoid cells through a series of intermediate precursor populations (**transit amplifying population**) (Fig. 4.3). The division rate in the stem

Fig. 4.3 Stem cells are a self-renewing population giving rise to transient amplifying cells from which the terminally differentiated cells arise.

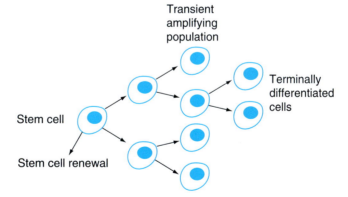

cell 'compartment' is actually less than that in the transit compartment, and relatively minor changes in the rate of cell division in the transit compartment can have a great effect on the tissue as a whole. The regulation of stem cell activity and lineage must be very precise in order to maintain a balanced cell population. The exact mechanisms remain unknown, but it is clear that the microenvironment (stromal factors, cell adhesion and cell–cell signalling) of the cell may well be important in determining differentiation.

An abnormality in the control of cell proliferation is central to many disease processes. Neoplasia is an obvious example (see Chapter 5) but there are many instances when a tissue responds to sublethal trauma by increasing cell production. One example of this is increased thickness of the epidermis in response to chronic irritation.

Psoriasis is another chronic inflammatory skin disorder and is characterized by hyperproliferation of the epidermis. Keratinocyte turnover is extremely rapid and whereas in normal epidermis the cell cycle time is about 200 hours, in psoriatic skin this is reduced to 50 hours.

As well as showing hyperproliferation the keratinocytes display abnormal differentiation. There is prominent parakeratosis (persistence of nuclei into the keratin layer) and a loss of the normal granular cell layer. TGF-α, which acts on the EGF-R present on keratinocytes, may have an important role to play in the pathogenesis of this condition. This growth factor acts in an autocrine manner and is present in greater amounts in psoriatic epidermis than in normal epidermis.

CASE STUDY 4.1

A man first developed psoriasis at the age of 21 years. This manifested itself as chronic plaques affecting the elbows, knees, scalp and sacral area (Fig. 4.4a and b). This was controlled initially with topical treatments such as tar-based preparations, dithranol creams and mild steroids. Intermittent flare-ups required hospital admission.

At age 40 he was found to have an increasingly large alcohol intake, and with this in addition to depression his psoriasis became more unstable. The decision was taken to progress to systemic therapy. He was unable to take methotrexate because of his alcohol dependence and was therefore started on Tigason (etretinate) 30 mg daily. His psoriasis became much improved and his alcohol intake subsequently decreased.

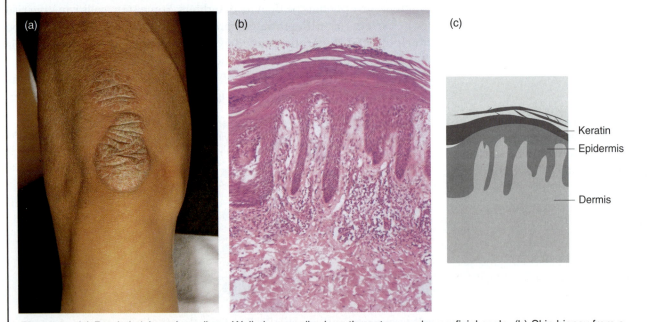

Fig. 4.4   (a) Psoriatic 'plaque' on elbow. Well-circumscribed, erythematous and superficial scale. (b) Skin biopsy from a psoriatic lesion. Note the regular thickening (acanthosis) of the epidermis with overlying increase in keratin (hyperkeratosis).

Hyperplasia

Hyperplasia refers to growth by an increase in cell number. Usually there is an obvious stimulus to the hyperplastic process and the endocrine system provides some good examples. Excess production of a trophic hormone will produce hyperplasia of the target organ, therefore overproduction of ACTH by a pituitary adenoma leads to bilateral adrenal cortical hyperplasia. Primary dysfunction of the thyroid gland can stimulate thyroid-stimulating hormone (TSH) production by a negative feedback mechanism, and goitrous enlargement of the thyroid might ensue. Hyperplasia of the breast is a physiological response to the hormonal milieu of pregnancy. In certain tissues hyperplasia of uncertain pathogenesis such as prostate gland enlargement (Fig. 4.5) can have unwelcome effects, in this case disturbances in urination and urine retention.

Fig. 4.5 Prostatic hyperplasia. Glands are lined by tall columnar epithelium with papillary infolding.

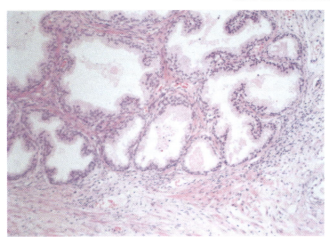

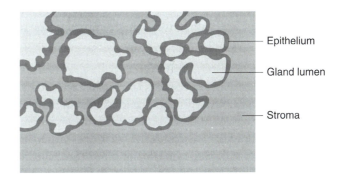

Hyperplasia may occur when cell loss has occurred within an organ owing to severe injury. The liver provides a good example, as it has very good regenerative properties. The stimulation of cell division is due to the production of a growth factor. As mentioned above, repetitive trauma to the skin such as constant abrasion can stimulate keratinocyte production and epidermal hyperplasia.

Hypertrophy

Growth in certain circumstances results from the capacity of cells to respond to a demand for increased work by increase in size (**hypertrophy**) rather than number. One of the most familiar examples is the hypertrophy of skeletal muscle induced by regular exercise, as in weight-lifting, for example. Cardiac muscle also undergoes hypertrophy as a result of increased pressure load as in systemic hypertension or aortic valvular stenosis or as a result of increased volume load as with mitral valve regurgitation (Fig. 4.6). Ventricular hypertrophy occurs following dilatation

Fig. 4.6 Left ventricular hypertrophy. Compare the thickened left ventricle (arrow) with the normal.

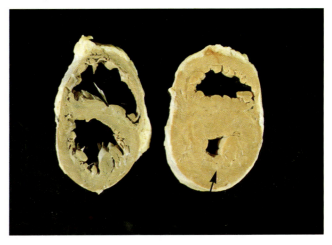

of the chamber which appears to stimulate protein synthesis within the muscle cells. Recent studies have shown that changes in cardiac gene expression take place in the hypertrophic process. One of the earliest changes noticed is the expression of certain immediate early genes such as c-*fos*, c-*jun* and *EGR1*. The details of the signal transduction mechanisms remain unclear, but it is thought that activation of protein kinase C may be one of the earliest responses in the cells to a variety of autocrine and paracrine factors. The contractile protein gene *MLC2* is induced resulting in accumulation of the protein within the myocardial cell.

Hyperplasia and hypertrophy may occur together, as for example in the enlargement of one kidney following removal of the other.

Atrophy

Decrease in size or number of cells leading to a reduction in tissue mass is often referred to as atrophy. This can occur physiologically, as in the involution of organs following cessation of prolonged hormonal stimulation – decrease in breast size following pregnancy, for example. Other hormonally responsive tissues such as the endometrium may also undergo atrophy following the menopause. Osteoporosis can be considered an important form of atrophy of bone which can have serious consequences leading to crush fractures of the vertebral bodies and fractures of the femoral neck and wrist. This is particularly seen in postmenopausal women, but the exact pathogenesis is unknown.

Atrophy may occur as a result of decreased workload, such as skeletal muscle atrophy in the bedridden patient. Muscle may also atrophy following denervation and almost any organ will atrophy upon sublethal chronic reduction in blood supply.

Metaplasia

A change from one cell type to another is known as **metaplasia**. It is most often observed in epithelia but can occur in other cell types.

There is always an abnormal stimulus associated with the process. For instance, in the bronchus the columnar epithelium is replaced by squamous epithelium due to chronic irritation, by cigarette smoke for example. This is termed **squamous metaplasia** and is also commonly seen in the uterine cervix (Fig. 4.7) where, due to the natural eversion of the cervical os during puberty, the endocervical mucin-secreting columnar epithelium becomes exposed to the lower pH environment of the vagina and undergoes

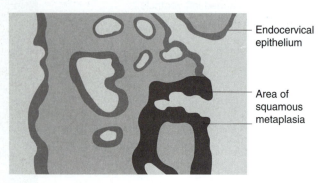

Fig. 4.7 Squamous metaplasia in the uterine cervix.

Endocervical epithelium

Area of squamous metaplasia

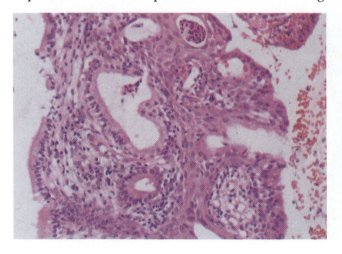

squamous metaplasia. In both of these sites the metaplastic epithelium may form the site of neoplastic change and squamous cell carcinoma formation. Metaplasia, however, is not always a precursor of malignancy.

The change does not take place between terminally differentiated cells but arises because of a change in the differentiation of precursor cells. Indeed, the process of metaplasia shares many similarities with that of the normal differentiation process.

Cellular ageing

There is an increasing amount of interest in the factors affecting the ageing process within the cell and the possible role in the ageing process of the individual.

- It is well known that cells in culture have a limited lifespan. The actual time in culture does not appear to be the important factor, but rather the number of cell divisions completed. In the case of human fibroblasts, if they have been taken from an embryo they will complete about 50 divisions and the number will decrease according to the increasing age of the donor. As the cells age they undergo several changes in cell contents and metabolism.

There are two basic theories which try to explain cellular ageing:

- The first is that errors in cellular material such as nucleic acids and proteins caused by a variety of environmental agents accumulate, and that this is compounded by a decreasing capacity of the inherent cellular repair mechanisms. It has been suggested that oxygen free radicals may be important injurious substances in this respect. Free radicals carry an unpaired electron and can therefore readily oxidize DNA, lipids and proteins. It is of interest that the antioxidant superoxide dismutase is produced in greater amounts in the cells of longer-lived species, including humans. Glycosylation of certain proteins such as collagen may lead to mechanical alterations which may play a role in ageing.

- The second theory proposes that ageing is in fact a 'programmed' process due to alteration of gene expression. Activation of a gene or set of genes following a number of cell divisions could for instance prevent entry into S phase of the cell cycle. It has been suggested that *p53* or *RB* genes could fulfil such a purpose, but there is no evidence for this. Another possibility is that cellular ageing might be related to telomere shortening. Telomeres are the portions of DNA that cover both ends of the chromosome, and it has been shown that these progressively shorten on successive divisions of somatic cells. It would appear that the cell eliminates a part of the telomere with every cell division and that in this part of the genetic material may lie the factor which produces the loss of proliferative capacity in cells. On the other hand there do appear to be genes which can confer longevity to certain species. In the nematode *Caenorhabditis elegans*, mutation of a gene *age-1* produced a significant increase in lifespan. These worms produced higher levels of superoxide dismutase than normal.

> **Changes in cellular ageing**
> - Increasing numbers of abnormal proteins and nuclei
> - Increasing numbers of chromosome abnormalities
> - Increasing deposition of substances such as lipofuscin
> - Decreasing transcription and proteolysis
> - Decreasing expression of the c-*fos* immediate early gene
> - Decreasing expression of the *cdc2* gene

Cell death

Cell death is important in pathology as the end result of a variety of noxious stimuli ranging from physical injury to infections.

Cell death may be defined as the permanent loss of cellular activity and function together with the irreparable disorganization of its structure. Until relatively recently cell death was synonymous with the term **necrosis**, but it became clear that death of cells was an important process in normal development and physiology. Eventually the concept of **apoptosis** was developed.

Apoptosis

Apoptosis is a term derived from the Greek meaning 'dropping off', like leaves from the trees in autumn. Unlike necrosis, this form of cell death occurs in isolated cells leaving the surrounding healthy cells undisturbed. This process has sometimes been referred to as **programmed cell death** as it does not appear to be a passive process but often requires active protein synthesis and as such is a direct consequence of gene expression. In development apoptosis plays a crucial role in the remodelling of tissues and organs and is thought to be the method by which the lumina of some hollow organs are formed. In normal tissue maintenance of a relatively constant cell population size is achieved not only by control of proliferation but also through apoptosis and apoptotic cells can be seen, for instance, in normal intestinal epithelium.

In the immune system it has been suggested that apoptotic cell loss may be the mechanism by which autoreactive T lymphocytes are deleted during thymic maturation and is thus a safeguard against autoimmunity. In the B-cell population, selection of clones which produce high-affinity antibodies may also utilize this process. Cell-mediated cell death via natural killer (NK) cells and cytotoxic T lymphocytes is also an example of apoptosis. The population of neutrophils which accumulates in an inflammatory reaction undergoes apoptosis and phagocytosis by macrophages. The nature of the apoptotic process allows the safe disposal of these enzyme-rich cells which could potentially cause massive tissue destruction if their contents were allowed to spill indiscriminately into the extracellular space. Certain tissues undergoing involution following hormonal stimulation do so with apoptosis: the endometrium, for example. Apoptosis is not confined to the physiological role, however; it also comes into play following a variety of injurious stimuli such as the administration of cytotoxic drugs and ionizing radiation. Apoptosis is not uncommonly seen in tumour cells.

Apoptotic cells may be identified by light microscopy as having dense nuclear chromatin with a little eosinophilic cytoplasm. They are typically surrounded by a clear halo which separates these individual cells from the surrounding normal cells (Fig. 4.8). They may fragment into several

Fig. 4.8 Endometrium showing apoptotic cells within glandular epithelium.

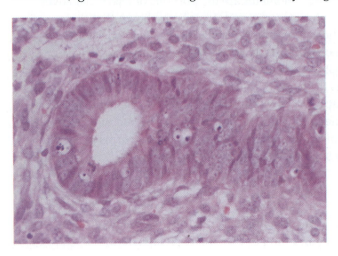

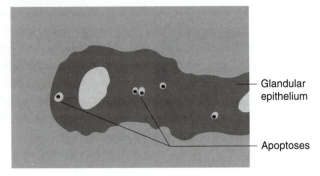

Glandular epithelium

Apoptoses

apoptotic bodies and these are readily recognized and phagocytosed by macrophages or adjacent parenchymal cells.

The process viewed by the electron microscope shows a consistent sequence of events. The specialized features of the cell membranes such as microvilli or intercellular junctions are lost. The cytoplasm undergoes condensation with a reduction in water content resulting in crowding of organelles. Unlike necrosis, the morphology and function of organelles remains relatively intact until late in the process. The nuclear chromatin becomes arranged into dense crescents at the periphery of the nucleus. Degradation of the material within phagosomes proceeds as usual (Fig. 4.9). The nuclear changes result from a specific cleavage of DNA resulting in oligonucleosome fragments which on electrophoresis produces a

Fig. 4.9 Apoptosis: (a) condensation of cytoplasm, rearrangement of chromatin, organelles intact; (b) fragmentation and phagocytosis by adjacent parenchymal cells and macrophages.

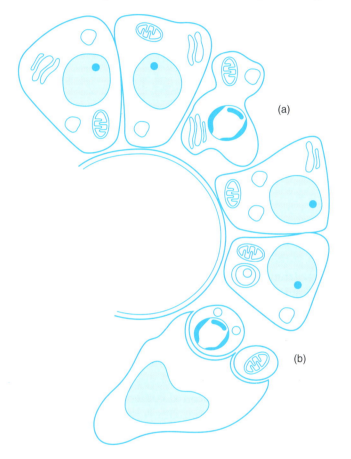

characteristic ladder pattern as opposed to the smear produced by necrotic cellular DNA. The nucleosome is a protein unit of eight histones around which the DNA helix is wrapped. This DNA fragmentation requires a sustained increase in intracellular calcium ion concentration which appears to activate the endonuclease that digests the linker DNA between the nucleosomes. The process of apoptosis is regulated by many genes including *p53*, *bcl2*, *RB1*, c-*myc* and *ras*.

Necrosis

Necrosis is the process which usually occurs following severe cellular injury. The trauma may be directed towards the cell membrane or energy-producing systems within the cell. The usual effect is the loss of control of ion movement across the plasma membrane. Sodium and calcium tends to enter the cell and potassium is lost. This leads to one of the first changes recognized in cells undergoing necrosis – cellular swelling due to the influx of water. Intracellular organelles such as the smooth endoplasmic reticulum swell and membranes eventually rupture. The reduction in oxidative metabolism leads to lactic acidosis and this reduction in intracellular pH activates the hydrolytic enzymes released from lysosomes and this further disrupts the fabric of the cell. In the nucleus the chromatin pattern becomes coarse, the nucleus may shrivel (pyknosis), break up into fragments (karyorrhexis), or completely lose its staining property (karyolysis) (Fig. 4.10).

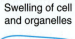

Swelling of cell
and organelles

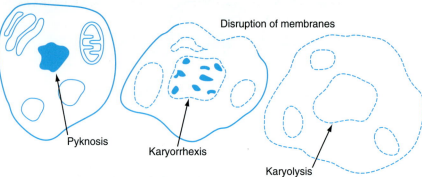

Disruption of membranes

Pyknosis

Karyorrhexis

Karyolysis

Fig. 4.10   Necrosis.

Unlike apoptotic cells, necrotic cells are usually found in sheets and provoke, in life, an inflammatory response.

Disruption of the cell by its own constituents is called autolysis and this results largely from the spillage of hydrolytic enzymes. After death of the individual all of the tissues of the body begin to undergo autolysis and this process is most rapid in those cells (pancreas, gastric mucosal cells) with the highest concentration of such enzymes.

Heterolysis is the term used to describe disruption of one cell by another. This is exemplified by phagocytosis of cells (often dead or dying) by macrophages or neutrophils. Heterolysis does not necessarily require phagocytosis, however, as lysosomal contents released from polymorphs can have the same effect on surrounding cells.

The patterns of necrosis within tissue may provide a clue to the agent or type of damage responsible:

- **Coagulation necrosis** is usually caused by reduction in blood supply, usually sudden and complete. Cells in areas of coagulative necrosis lose staining with haematoxylin (the usual histological stain is haematoxylin and eosin). This is as a result of loss of RNA and DNA from the cell. The tissue therefore shows staining predominantly with eosin. Protein is retained within the dead cell and therefore the basic tissue architecture remains and the eosinophilic outlines of the cells can be seen (Fig. 4.11) .
- **Infarction** is the term used to describe the process of tissue death due to a sudden and permanent cessation in blood supply. The area of dead tissue is referred to as an infarct. Because the blood vessels within an infarct suffer the same fate as the rest of the tissue, they become leaky and red cells tend to extravasate. The extent to which this happens

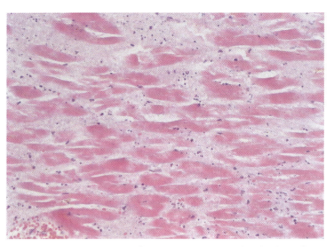

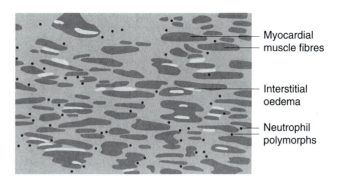

Myocardial
muscle fibres

Interstitial
oedema

Neutrophil
polymorphs

Fig. 4.11   Myocardial infarction. Note loss of definition of myocardial fibres and interstitial oedema with neutrophil polymorph infiltration.

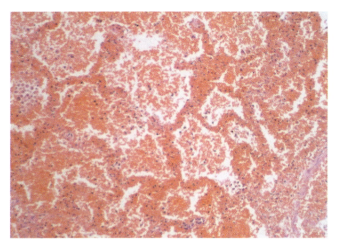

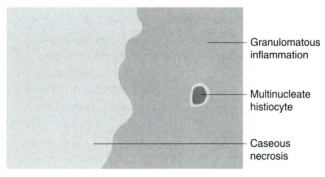

Blood-filled
alveolus

Interstitium

Fig. 4.12   Pulmonary infarct. Blood fills the alveolar spaces.

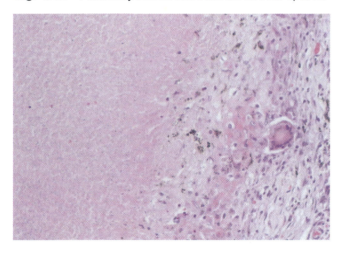

Granulomatous
inflammation

Multinucleate
histiocyte

Caseous
necrosis

Fig. 4.13   Caseous necrosis. Note peripheral granulomatous inflammation with multinucleate histiocyte.

depends on the type of tissue affected. For instance in pulmonary infarcts this is prominent (Fig. 4.12) whereas it is unusual in more solid organs such as the kidney.

- **Caseous necrosis** is severe disintegration of tissue and is typical of the necrosis which occurs as a consequence of infection by the tubercle bacillus (*Mycobacterium tuberculosis*). In caseous necrosis the architecture of the tissue is completely lost and it appears on microscopy as an amorphous protein-rich eosinophilic material (Fig. 4.13).

Chapter 5   Neoplasia

Learning objectives
❑ Knowledge of the features of neoplasia and understanding of the difference between benign and malignant neoplasia
❑ Familiarity with the terms used to describe neoplasia, including adenoma, carcinoma, sarcoma
❑ Appreciation of the importance of cellular transformation and oncogenes in the pathogenesis of neoplasia
❑ Awareness of the main routes and mechanisms involved in tumour invasion and metastasis
❑ Understanding of the importance of interactions between neoplastic cells and other cell types, particularly those belonging to the immune system

The term **neoplasia** (plural of neoplasm) refers literally to 'new growth' by cell proliferation. It is generally accepted that the constituent cells of a **neoplasm** display abnormal growth and do not respond normally to regulatory factors which control cell proliferation. Recent research suggests that these features are the result of mutations affecting the genes which control cell growth and proliferation, and that these mutations are the cause of the abnormal growth exhibited by neoplastic cells.

A **tumour** is a swelling or mass, and the term can be applied to inflammatory lesions as well as neoplastic ones; however, in practice tumour and neoplasm are used synonymously.

The essential distinction between a **benign** and a **malignant** neoplasm is that a malignant tumour has the ability to spread to a distant part of the body. This process is known as **metastasis**. These differences are further described later in the chapter. This does not mean that benign tumours cannot be harmful: their growth may disturb local structures, or their cells may secrete substances such as hormones which can produce metabolic abnormalities.

Tumours generally arise from continuously renewing cell populations (such as haemopoetic cells or gastrointestinal epithelial cells) or from conditional renewal tissues such as hepatocytes, and rarely from stable cell populations such as neurons.

Features of neoplasia
● Abnormal and excessive cell growth
● Lack of control
● Persistence of abnormal growth
● Mutations in genes which control cell growth and proliferation

Classification

The classification of neoplasms, and consequently the names given to them, is based largely on the cell or tissue from which the tumour is thought to have arisen. In practice the name given to a neoplasm reflects the differentiation of its constituent cell type. By convention the name given to the tumour also reflects its likely behaviour. For instance, the suffix '-oma' is usually applied to benign tumours. A benign tumour of adipose tissue is therefore referred to as a **lipoma**; an **adenoma** is a benign neoplasm of glandular tissue. There are of course exceptions to this basic rule, such as **hepatoma** (more correctly termed hepatocellular carcinoma), a malignant tumour of hepatocytic origin.

A **carcinoma** is a malignant tumour of epithelial cells. The name may be further qualified by the addition of a prefix such as **'adeno-'**, an **adenocarcinoma** thus being a malignant tumour of glandular tissue. Alternatively the term may be preceded by the specific type of epithelium (for example **squamous cell carcinoma**, **transitional cell carcinoma**).

The macroscopic morphology, particularly of epithelial tumours, may also be described using terms such as **polyp** to describe the localized projection of a tumour beyond a mucosal surface or **papilloma** referring to a warty outgrowth with finger-like projections. A **sarcoma** is a malignant tumour of mesenchyme or connective tissue and its specific differentiation may also be conveyed in the nomenclature: for example a **leiomyosarcoma** is a malignant tumour showing smooth muscle differentiation. A **teratoma** is a neoplasm which contains a variety of tissues normally derived from all three germ cell layers. It may therefore contain skin or nervous tissue (ectoderm), gastrointestinal or respiratory epithelium (endoderm), and cartilage or even teeth (mesoderm). These tumours most commonly occur in the gonads, and both benign and malignant types exist. A particular group of neoplasms which occur almost exclusively in childhood are the **blastomas**, highly malignant tumours formed of cells which resemble the primitive cells present in development. One of the most common examples is the **nephroblastoma** or Wilms' tumour of the kidney.

Neoplasms of lymphoid cells, the **lymphomas**, are basically separated into Hodgkin's disease (although here the precise cell of origin is unknown) and non-Hodgkin's lymphomas (B- and T-cell types).

All of the above are sometimes referred to as **solid tumours** to distinguish them from the neoplasms of haemopoietic cells known as **leukaemias**. Although leukaemic cells do tend to replace the normal bone marrow they do not usually form tumour masses but are characterized by large numbers of neoplastic cells within the circulation (Table 5.1).

Tumour typing

The correct identification of the type of tumour is of great practical importance in assessing its likely behaviour and in influencing the choice of treatment, as well as the likely response. However, sometimes it can be difficult to be certain of the exact nature of a malignant tumour in which the cells do not display any particular pattern of histological differentiation. In this case the tumour is said to be **undifferentiated**. Tumours of very different origins (carcinoma, malignant melanoma, lymphoma) may appear very similar on light microscopy. A clue to the

Table 5.1   Classification of tumours

Tissue of origin or differentiation	Benign	Malignant
Epithelium		
Glandular	Adenoma	Adenocarcinoma
Squamous	Squamous papilloma	Squamous carcinoma
Transitional	?Transitional cell papilloma	Transitional cell carcinoma
Melanocytes	Melanocytic naevus	Malignant melanoma
Mesenchyme		
Fibroblast	Fibroma	Fibrosarcoma
Adipose tissue	Lipoma	Liposarcoma
Smooth muscle	Leiomyoma	Leiomyosarcoma
Skeletal muscle	Rhabdomyoma	Rhabdomyosarcoma
Nerve sheath	Neurilemmoma Neurofibroma	Malignant nerve sheath tumour
Blood vessels	Angioma	Angiosarcoma
Cartilage	Chondroma	Chondrosarcoma
Bone	Osteoma	Osteosarcoma
Central nervous system		
Glia		Astrocytoma Oligodendrocytoma Ependymoma
Meninges	Meningioma	
Neuroendocrine cells		Oat cell carcinoma
		Carcinoid tumour
	Islet cell tumours (pancreas)	
Chromaffin tissue	Phaeochromocytoma Paraganglioma	
Haemopoietic		
Lymphoid		Lymphoma Leukaemia Myeloma
Embryonal		
Germ cell		Teratoma Seminoma Dysgerminoma
Kidney		Nephroblastoma
Liver		Hepatoblastoma
Retina		Retinoblastoma
Adrenal medulla		Neuroblastoma
Trophoblast		Choriocarcinoma

This is not intended to provide a comprehensive list, merely to illustrate some of the principles.

differentiation may be found by ultrastructural examination by electron microscopy. In the example given, melanosomes were seen within the tumour cells indicating that the neoplasm was in fact a malignant melanoma (Fig. 5.1).

Fig. 5.1 Melanosomes within a malignant melanoma are seen as black cytoplasmic granules by transmission electron microscopy. The nucleus (N) contains a nucleolus (nuc). Some of the granules have been indicated by arrows.

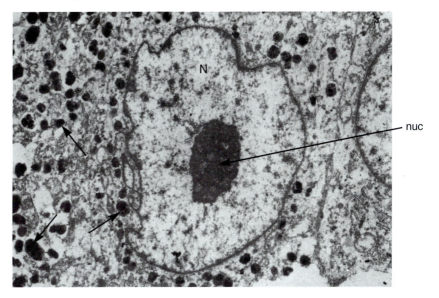

Another way to determine the nature of an undifferentiated neoplasm is by **immunocytochemistry**. An unstained section of the tumour is exposed to an antibody directed against an antigen usually found in a particular type of neoplasm. This antigen may be very specific, such as prostate-specific antigen, or less so as is the case with the leukocyte common antigen found on the membrane of most lymphoid cells. Binding of the antibody can be made visible by a variety of methods. By application of a panel of different antibodies the type of tumour can be identified (Fig. 5.2).

It is generally accepted that most tumours arise from a single abnormal stem cell. In other words, the proliferation is **clonal**. However, this does not mean that all of the cells are the same, as further mutations within the rapidly proliferating population of tumour cells may lead to considerable functional and genetic heterogeneity.

It is important to be aware that tumours are not composed of pure populations of cells, but contain a variety of cell types. Not only are the neoplastic cells themselves heterogeneous in structure and behaviour, but there are also supporting tissues such as collagen and the fibroblasts which produce it, blood vessels essential for the nutrition of the tumour, and macrophages and lymphocytes, which may possibly form part of an immune reaction against the neoplastic cells.

Morphology of tumours in relation to behaviour

The basic property which demonstrates that a tumour is malignant is its ability to **invade** tissue and, in most cases, to **metastasize**. Apart from this there are no absolute rules which allow the distinction between a benign and malignant tumour to be made on morphological grounds. Nevertheless there are features which are more in keeping with a benign tumour rather than a malignant one and allow discrimination.

Benign tumours tend to have relatively slow growth and are well circumscribed, often surrounded by a collagenous capsule (Fig. 5.3). They

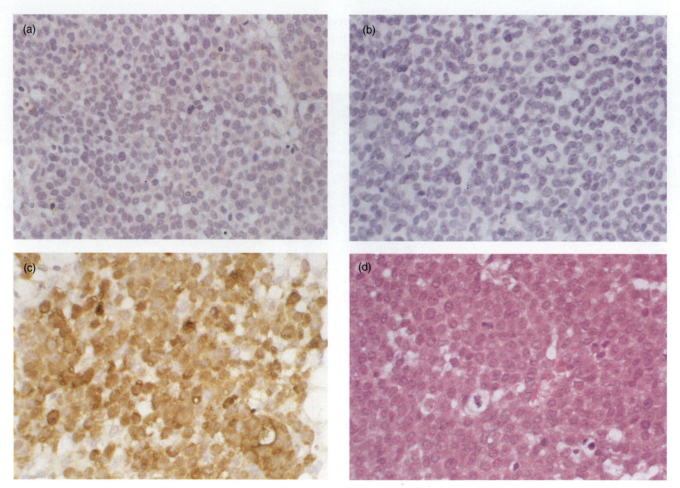

Fig. 5.2   A lymphoma stained with a panel of antibodies: (a) S100 protein (positive for neuroectodermal and some other cells). (b) Cam 5.2 (cytokeratin S, present in most epithelia). (c) Leukocyte common antigen. (d) H&E. The brown stain deposit seen in (c) indicates the positivity of lymphoma cells for leukocyte antigen, whereas (a) and (b) are negative.

usually do not infiltrate the surrounding tissues but grow in an expansile, pushing manner. At the microscopic level a benign tumour often closely resembles the normal tissue, the cells being little different from the normal organ cells (Fig. 5.4).

In contrast, **malignant** tumours display rapid growth, are poorly circumscribed and unencapsulated (Fig. 5.5). The tumour is invasive

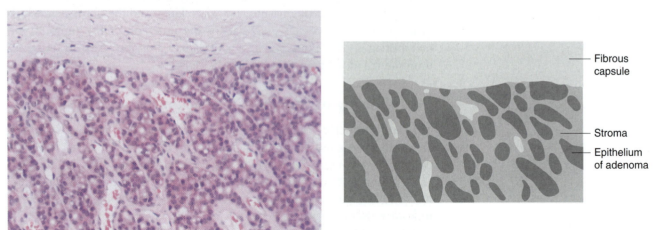

Fig. 5.3   Fibrous capsule (arrow) surrounding a benign adenoma.

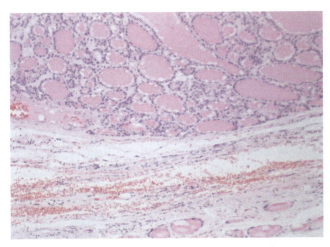

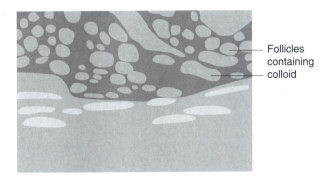

Follicles
containing
colloid

Fig. 5.4   Thyroid adenoma (arrow) showing follicular structures.

Fig. 5.5   Longitudinal slice through a kidney containing a large carcinoma.

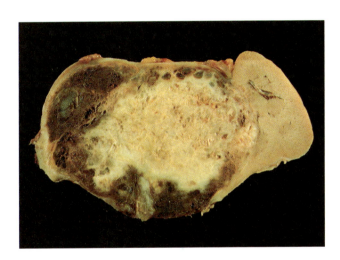

with an infiltrative growth pattern and there may be tumour cells within vascular or perineural spaces. Necrosis is more commonly seen in malignant tumours as the blood supply is often inadequate to maintain the rapidly increasing mass. Malignant cells are often clearly abnormal and very different from those in the tissue of origin (Fig. 5.6).

CULTURE OF NEOPLASTIC CELLS IN VITRO

Cells in culture may be stimulated to acquire some or all of the characteristics of cancer cells. This is known as cellular **transformation**. Certain viruses, chemicals and irradiation can transform certain cultured cell lines. Transformation may also be achieved by experimentally introducing foreign DNA into the cell so that the DNA integrates into its genome. This process is known as **transfection** and can provide valuable information about the ability of specific genetic material to induce transformation.

Morphologically the transformed cells show similar features to those described above in malignant cells. Transformed cells often have an abnormal chromosome complement and chromosome rearrangements, as do malignant tumour cells. For a cell to be fully transformed it must be capable of producing a tumour when inoculated into an appropriate animal host (**tumorigenicity**).

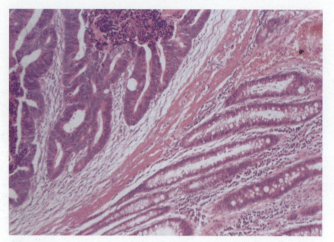 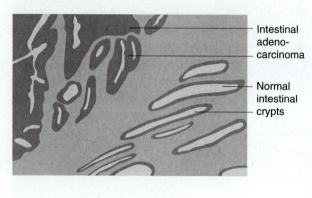

Fig. 5.6 Intestinal adenocarcinoma. Compare the neoplastic glands with the adjacent normal intestinal crypts.

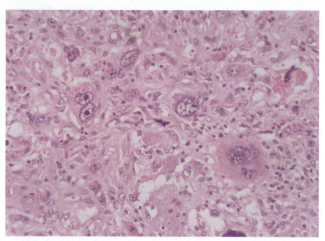 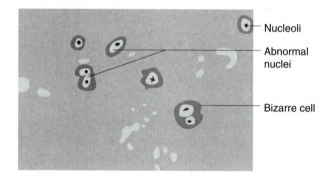

Fig. 5.7 Poorly differentiated carcinoma containing bizarre cells.

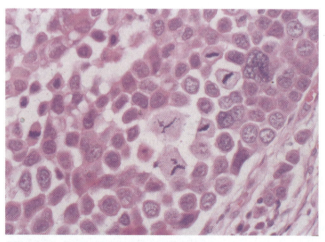 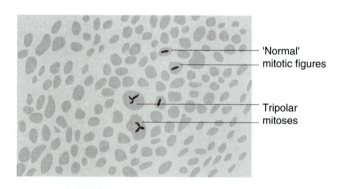

Fig. 5.8 Atypical mitoses: tripolar forms.

Cytological features indicating that a cell is likely to be malignant
- Increase in the size of the nucleus relative to the amount of cytoplasm (increased nuclear/cytoplasmic ratio)
- Variation in shape and size of the cells and/or nuclei (pleomorphism); sometimes very bizarre forms (Fig. 5.7)
- An abnormal pattern of nuclear chromatin and often increased intensity of nuclear staining (hyperchromasia).
- The presence of cells in division (mitotic figures), especially abnormal forms (Fig. 5.8)

Transformed cells also show certain behavioural characteristics. Whereas normal cells in culture require anchorage to a solid substrate before they are able to form a colony, transformed cells tend to be able to grow and divide in suspension in a semi-solid medium (**anchorage-independent growth**). Anchorage independence correlates well with tumorigenicity. Unlike normal cells in culture, which are capable of only a finite number of cell divisions before death, transformed cells can be maintained in culture for a considerable period of time.

Prognostic factors

The main factor influencing survival in patients with malignant neoplasia is the extent of tumour spread at the time of diagnosis. Clinical staging is performed to determine this and it is the staging results which then determine the appropriate treatment.

However, other factors are also important determinants of prognosis. The degree of differentiation shown by a malignant tumour can be graded histologically. Low-grade tumours which are well differentiated tend to be slowly growing and have a better prognosis, whereas high-grade tumours are usually rapidly proliferating, aggressive neoplasms with a poor prognosis. For example, breast carcinomas may be assigned to one of three grades depending on the extent of tubule formation, the degree of cytological pleomorphism and the number of mitoses seen. In breast cancer and several other tumour types, the grade of the tumour has been shown to correlate with survival (Fig. 5.9).

The grade of the tumour may also influence the choice of treatment. This is of particular importance in the chemotherapy of malignant lymphomas. To allow consistency from one centre to another there is a general agreement internationally on systems of tumour grading.

Carcinoma in situ

Epithelial cells normally rest on a basement membrane. Epithelial cells showing the morphological characteristics of malignancy, i.e. carcinoma

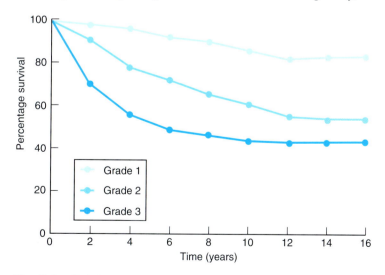

Fig. 5.9   Relationship between breast cancer grade and survival. (From Elston, C.W. and Ellis, I.O. *Histopathology* **19** (1991), 403–10, with permission.)

cells, may be seen to occupy the epithelium but remain resting on and confined by the basement membrane. This is **carcinoma in situ**. It is generally believed that a carcinoma usually begins as a focal–clonal overgrowth of stem cells near the basement membrane and expands within the epithelium before invading through the basement membrane. This process may take several years. In addition to the cytological features of malignancy the epithelium shows disordered or absent maturation.

Carcinoma in situ does not have the ability to metastasize; it is only when the basement membrane is breached that distant spread can occur. Diagnosis of carcinoma in situ is therefore of great importance, since it is often amenable to curative treatment. Sites where carcinoma in situ is frequently diagnosed include the uterine cervix, the breast and the skin (Fig. 5.10).

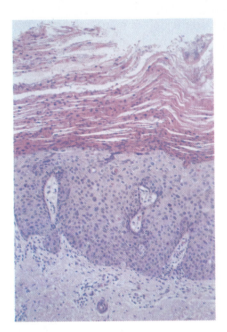
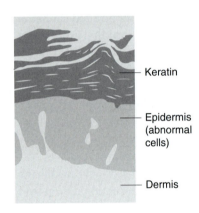

Fig. 5.10 Sections of skin showing squamous carcinoma in situ. Note the lack of normal stratification and presence of atypical keratinocytes.

In the uterine cervix, identification of abnormal epithelial cells scraped from the epithelial surface forms the basis of population screening for detecting precancerous (dysplastic) changes known as **cervical intraepithelial neoplasia** (CIN). It is recognized that, in the cervical epithelium and other epithelia in the body, dysplastic changes occur within the epithelial cells prior to the development of carcinoma in situ.

The effects of tumours on patients

Both benign and malignant neoplasms may cause local effects due to the expansion of the tumour mass. Although tissue destruction by an invasive malignant tumour is often greater, benign tumours can cause serious local effects particularly when the growth occurs within a confined space such as the pituitary fossa. Not only may a benign pituitary adenoma damage local structures such as the optic chiasma by pressure effects, but loss of the normal pituitary tissue could result in hypopituitarism (Fig. 5.11).

Fig. 5.11 Pressure effects of a pituitary adenoma.

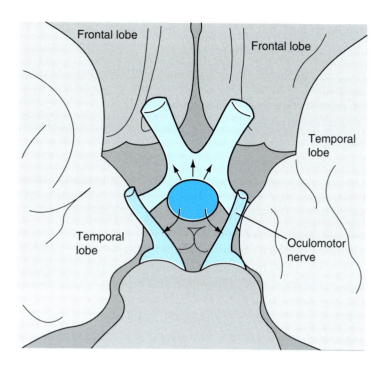

Paraneoplastic effects of tumours
- Cachexia
- Hormone secretion
- Cushing's syndrome (ACTH)
  - inappropriate ADH secretion (SIADH)
  - gynaecomastia (HCG, LH)
  - appropriate (pituitary adenomas . . . prolactin)
- Hypercalcaemia
- Hypertrophic osteoarthropathy and clubbing
- Hypoglycaemia
- Neurological complications
  - cerebellar dysfunction
  - peripheral neuropathy
  - Eaton–Lambert syndrome (myasthenia-like)
- Haematological effects
  - anaemia
  - polycythaemia (renal carcinoma)
  - Increased clotting
- Skin manifestations
  - canthosis nigricans
  - dermatomyositis

The vascular system may be affected by tumour growth either by compression of blood vessels leading to **ischaemia** or **thrombosis** (pelvic masses leading to deep vein thrombosis in the leg veins, for example) or by invasion of vessels leading to **haemorrhage**. The haemorrhage may be massive and catastrophic, such as from a large pulmonary vessel invaded by a carcinoma of the bronchus or gradual, as may be seen with carcinoma of the caecum in which iron deficiency anaemia is not an uncommon presenting feature. A tumour may produce **obstruction** of the lumen of the bowel or bile duct either by compression from outside the wall or by origin within the wall. Bile duct obstruction is very common in carcinoma of the head of the pancreas and rectal adenocarcinomas often produce bowel obstruction. Tumours may **ulcerate** as a result of cell death often due to ischaemia, and this may become the focus of infection particularly in tumours on the surface of the body.

PARANEOPLASTIC SYNDROMES

A tumour may exert distant or systemic effects not directly related to metastatic events; these are often referred to as **paraneoplastic** syndromes. One of the most obvious is hormone production by the tumour cells. In some situations such as a pituitary adenoma, one or more pituitary hormones may be produced in excess, the most common being prolactin leading to amenorrhoea and infertility in the female. Hormones may be produced inappropriately by a variety of tumours derived from tissues not normally associated with endocrine function. This is probably the result of derepression of genes responsible for hormone synthesis. One such example is anaplastic small cell carcinoma of the bronchus which may produce adrenocorticotrophic hormone (ACTH).

Hypercalcaemia is a relatively common paraneoplastic phenomenon. It may present with features of constipation, mental confusion or depression, muscular weakness, cardiac abnormalities or renal failure, but it is often subclinical and detected by routine blood analysis. There are two mechanisms by which malignancy may induce hypercalcaemia.

- Release of factors by the tumour which act on osteoclasts to promote bone resorption, increase intestinal absorption of calcium or increase calcium reabsorption by the renal tubules.
- Bone resorption stimulated by the presence of adjacent metastatic deposits.

The humoral mechanism is usually the most important and has features similar to hyperparathyroidism. Isolation of substances with parathyroid hormone-like activity from tumours has resulted in the discovery of a new hormone, **parathyroid hormone-related protein**. Increased osteoclast activity as a result of cytokine production and effects mediated indirectly via osteoblasts may also play a role. Tumours associated with this humoral mechanism include squamous cell carcinomas of the head and neck region and bronchus, breast cancer and renal cell carcinoma.

The mechanism by which metastases stimulate bone resorption is poorly understood. However, the neoplastic cells or macrophages associated with the tumour may produce hydrolytic enzymes, or the neoplasm may release paracrine factors such as prostaglandin E_2 (PGE$_2$). Some tumours have a predilection for metastasis to bone, for instance breast, prostate and lung cancers.

Some rare paraneoplastic syndromes affect the central nervous system and these may appear before the tumour is detected. Peripheral neuropathies, cerebellar dysfunction, visual disturbances and the myasthenia gravis-like Eaton–Lambert syndrome are all examples. The pathogenesis of these syndromes is unknown but it has been suggested that the immune response against the tumour may be involved, since immunoglobulins raised against tumour antigens can cross react with neuronal antigens.

CACHEXIA

Cachexia is common particularly in advanced malignancy but may occur relatively early in some cancers, such as lung cancer. It is characterized by weight loss, anorexia, muscle weakness and anaemia (hypochromic, microcytic). Although the anorexia suffered by many cancer patients may contribute to weight loss, this is insufficient to account for the accelerated weight loss typical of cachexia. The pathogenesis of cachexia is unknown, but is probably multifactorial. There are a variety of metabolic abnormalities involving carbohydrate and protein metabolism, but these are not consistent. There may also be an element of intestinal malabsorption. It has also been postulated that tumour products such as tumour necrosis factor (TNF) may be involved.

TUMOUR SPREAD

Tumours may spread by direct invasion from the primary site into surrounding tissues, or metastasize to distant sites via body cavities, the lymphatic system or the circulation (Fig. 5.12).

Invasion and metastasis

The ability to invade tissues and to metastasize is an integral part of malignancy. This process is complex and involves a number of steps:

Fig. 5.12   Modes of tumour spread.

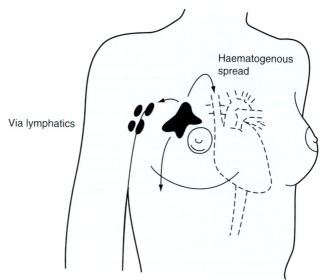

Haematogenous spread

Via lymphatics

Direct spread to adjacent structures and body cavities

CASE STUDY 5.1

A 62-year-old woman developed a fixed painless lump in the soft tissues adjacent to the right knee. This was excised and histological examination revealed it to be a malignant fibrous histiocytoma (a type of sarcoma) of low grade; excision was incomplete. Three years later this recurred and again it was incompletely removed. She suffered a further recurrence four years later and again tumour was seen at the resection margin. She received radical radiotherapy to the site but one year later tumour appeared in the middle of the treatment site. After removal of this she remains well one year on.

1. Progressive growth of tumour cells.
2. Tumours smaller than about 2 mm can receive nutrition via diffusion. Above this size new blood vessel growth must occur to supply the tumour. This **angiogenesis** occurs as a result of the production and secretion of certain angiogenesis factors by the tumour.
3. Invasion of the adjacent stroma and thin-walled vascular channels (venules and lymphatics) allows access to the circulation for malignant cells.
4. Many of the circulating tumour cells do not survive. Experiments have shown that less than 1% of cells remain viable after 24 hours in the circulation, and less than 0.1% eventually produce metastatic deposits.
5. The viable tumour cells lodge in the circulation at a distant site and migrate into the tissue.
6. Cell proliferation occurs to form a metastatic deposit.

Cell adhesion molecules probably play a major role in the process of invasion and metastasis. However, the process is complex and it seems that the tumour cells require decreased cell adhesion at one stage and an increased ability to adhere to cells and stroma at another.

In vivo and in vitro experiments suggest that **integrins** play a role in invasion and metastasis, but this role is not a simple one. Integrin-like receptors are found on the cell surface of many tumour cells. The

The three basic mechanisms of metastasis

- **Direct spread across body cavities:** The surfaces of the pleural and peritoneal spaces are frequently seeded by cancer cells from adjacent organs such as the lung and ovaries. This process is often accompanied by fluid exudation and its accumulation as pleural effusion or ascites.

- **Lymphatic spread:** Carcinomas often spread via lymphatic channels to the draining lymph nodes. Therefore carcinoma of the breast, particularly if located laterally, would be expected to metastasize to the axillary lymph nodes. It is important to note that clinical enlargement of lymph nodes may not only be due to tumour deposition but also to reactive hyperplasia induced by infection of the tumour or an immune response to the tumour itself. Lymphatic channels may sometimes become occluded by the tumour and lymphoedema can result. Lymph nodes may serve as a temporary barrier to tumour dissemination but this is controversial. Cells within the lymphatic channels may ultimately gain access to the bloodstream via the various connections between the two systems.

- **Haematogenous spread:** Haematogenous spread usually occurs via the venous system and some tumours such as renal cell carcinoma have a particular propensity for venous invasion. Sarcomas appear to spread more commonly via the bloodstream than the lymphatics. Common sites for haematogenous metastases include the liver and lungs.

integrins are a family of membrane glycoproteins consisting of two subunits. This large group contains cell–cell and cell–matrix receptors. Many of these receptors recognize ligands with the amino acid sequence Arg–Gly–Asp, also known as the **RGD motif**. Molecules containing the RGD sequence include fibronectin, vitronectin, thrombospondin, von Willebrand's factor and collagen, especially type I. The $\alpha_5\beta_1$ integrin binds fairly specifically to fibronectin and it is interesting that studies have shown that tumorigenic cells lacking this receptor lose the ability to migrate on surfaces and this is restored on transfer of the appropriate gene. In experimental animals injection of a synthetic peptide bearing the RGD sequence which blocks $\alpha_5\beta_1$ binding to fibronectin inhibited the formation of metastases by melanoma cells injected at the same time. On the other hand, some integrins seem to be associated with an increased capacity for invasion.

The calcium-dependent cell adhesion molecules **cadherins** are also implicated in the ability of tumour cells to invade. It appears that E-cadherin if introduced into a carcinoma cell line can inhibit their ability to invade. Invasion seems to correlate in some tumour cell lines with loss of E-cadherin expression, and loss of E-cadherin has also been related to more aggressive behaviour in some squamous cell carcinomas of the head and neck.

Studies of metastatic colon carcinoma cells discovered that a gene termed *DCC* (**d**eleted in **c**olonic **c**ancer) was absent in about 70%. This gene in fact codes for a member of the **immunoglobulin superfamily** of cell adhesion molecules. This finding therefore suggests that the expression of this molecule prevents invasion and metastasis. It appears therefore that tumour progression requires the neoplastic cells to display either increased or decreased adhesion depending on the stage of the process.

The mechanism of invasion

How does invasion actually occur? The tumour can expand into the adjacent tissue merely by the pressure effect of the cellular proliferation. Nevertheless it is apparent that successful invasion requires additional factors. Barriers such as the basement membrane have to be breached. Attention has been focused on several hydrolytic enzymes including the **metalloproteases** (for example type IV collagenase), **cathepsins**, **elastases** and **plasminogen activator**. There is good correlation between the capability of a tumour to metastasize and the secretion of such enzymes. Metalloproteases may also be produced by the adjacent stroma. Many malignant neoplasms produce high levels of lytic enzymes compared to normal or benign tumour cells. Cell motility may also play its part but it has been shown that inhibition of cell motility inhibits invasion in only some tumours.

Tumour cells can invade lymphatic vessels and capillaries very easily, but only rarely penetrate arteries or arterioles. It is thought that this is related to the presence of elastic tissue in arteries and also the possibility that antiproteolytic factors are present within them which inhibit the action of the proteases.

Survival of metastatic cells

Once they have gained access to the circulation, factors which increase the survival of the tumour cells include the formation of multicellular **emboli** and the ability of the cells to undergo deformation within the small vessels of the microcirculation. The death of tumour cells within the circulation is attributable to either non-specific immune surveillance by macrophages, NK cells or neutrophils and specific immunity mediated by antigen-dependent cytotoxic T cells and antibodies. The presence of large numbers of cells within the circulation does not necessarily increase the risk of metastasis. The insertion of peritoneovenous shunts into patients for the alleviation of malignant ascites led to the entry of large numbers of viable tumour cells into the circulation via the jugular vein without a concomitant increase in the incidence of metastatic disease.

The pattern of metastases is non-random. Two major theories have been put forward to explain this, but they are not mutually exclusive (Fig 5.13).

- The **anatomical** theory suggests that the pattern of metastases depends on the distribution of the circulating cells and therefore the first organ encountered will be a frequent site of metastases.
- The **'seed and soil'** hypothesis suggests that conditions at the metastatic site must be favourable for the particular circulating cell. In other words the process of metastasis is not merely passive but selective.

It is certainly true that some tumours have a predilection for metastasis to certain sites independent of the distribution of tumour cells to each organ. The cells within a malignant tumour are heterogeneous in many respects and this includes their ability to metastasize. The fact that certain clones of malignant cells are much more able to produce metastatic deposits must depend on their ability to interact with factors at the metastatic site. Tumour cells may selectively adhere to endothelial cells at the metastatic site. Cytokines produced within certain organs have also been shown to influence the proliferative capacity of the entrapped tumour cells. Local immune defences may also be able to prevent the growth of certain clones of cells.

Fig. 5.13 The metastatic process.

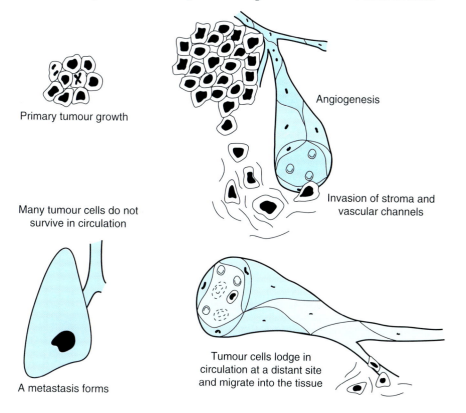

Primary tumour growth

Angiogenesis

Invasion of stroma and vascular channels

Many tumour cells do not survive in circulation

A metastasis forms

Tumour cells lodge in circulation at a distant site and migrate into the tissue

Whatever the mechanisms of spread, the identification of metastatic deposits is of enormous importance in determining the prognosis and appropriate treatment regimen in a particular patient.

TUMOUR STAGING

The extent of spread of a tumour is assessed by tumour staging. As with tumour grades, there are internationally recognized systems of tumour staging. One of the most commonly employed is the **TNM system** developed by the Union Internationale Contre Cancer (UICC).

The general principles of this system are that T1–T4 denote increasing size of or local infiltration by the primary tumour, N0–N3 increasing nodal involvement and M0–M1 the absence or presence of metastases.

This classification obviously relies upon accurate clinical examination without necessarily relying on histological confirmation of, for instance, nodal involvement.

A commonly used staging system which uses histological data is that devised by Dukes for carcinoma of the large bowel (see Chapter 11). This pathological staging provides very good prognostic information.

TNM staging system for breast cancer

- **T**: Primary **T**umour
- **N**: Regional lymph **N**ode involvement
- **M**: Distant **M**etastases
- **T1**: Tumour of 2 cm or less in its greatest dimension
- **T2**: Tumour more than 2 cm but not more than 5 cm
- **T3**: Tumour more than 5 cm

These categories may be further qualified depending on the presence or absence of fascial and/or muscle fixation.

- **T4**: Tumour of any size with direct extension to chest wall or skin
- **N0**: No palpable homolateral axillary lymph nodes
- **N1**: Movable homolateral axillary lymph nodes
- **N2**: Homolateral axillary lymph nodes fixed to one another or to other structures
- **N3**: Homolateral supra-clavicular or infraclavicular lymph nodes considered to contain growth or oedema of the arm

---

CASE STUDY 5.2

A 38-year-old woman presented with a firm, non-mobile breast lump with overlying skin dimpling. A Tru-Cut needle biopsy confirmed invasive carcinoma and she underwent a mastectomy. One node out of 12 found in the axillary contents contained metastatic carcinoma. Five years later she suffered a local recurrence of tumour in the scar and was beginning to experience back pain. Tamoxifen therapy was commenced. She remained reasonably well for the next 4 years when a bone scan revealed abnormal uptake in the sacrum. This, however, appeared to settle both radiologically and clinically but 2 years later a lytic lesion was visible on radiography of the sacrum and she was given a course of chemotherapy. Over the next couple of years she developed many bone metastases and eventually died from her disease (Fig. 5.14).

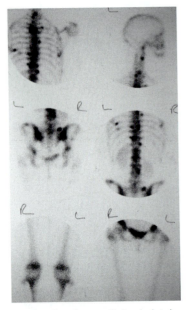

Fig. 5.14   A bone scan showing multiple skeletal metastatic deposits.

Basic cancer epidemiology

Epidemiology basically refers to the study of disease in relation to populations. This approach has proved extremely useful in providing clues to the causes of cancer. Information is often gained from the comparison of the incidence of a particular cancer in defined populations. Cancer incidence refers to the number of cases arising each year: **prevalence** indicates the number of individuals with a history of cancer who are alive at a specified time. In the UK there is no statutory requirement to register cases of cancer and therefore the statistics available are only an estimate of the actual figures. The most common cancers in the UK are shown in Fig. 5.15. Some of these, for instance the majority of skin cancers, do not commonly lead to the death of the patient, therefore the most common causes of cancer death are slightly different (Fig. 5.16).

Fig. 5.15 Commonest cancers in men and women in the UK. (Data taken from CRC Factsheet 1.1, 1990.)

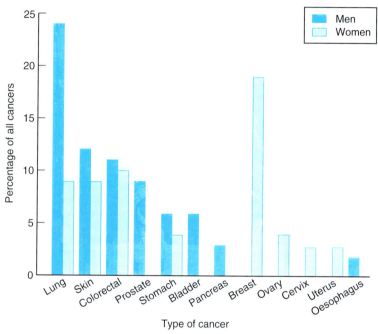

Fig. 5.16 Cancer deaths in men and women in the UK. (Data taken from CRC Factsheet 3.1, 1989.)

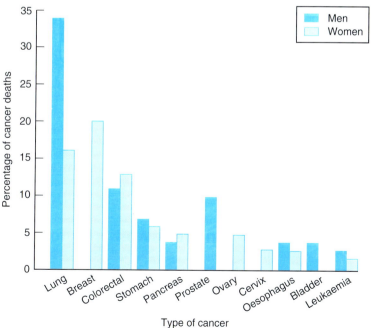

There may be geographical variation, for instance in the high incidence of stomach cancer found in Japan compared with that in the USA. There may of course be many possible reasons for this difference, including racial and environmental influences. One way of attempting to investigate the importance of environmental factors is to look at the incidence of the disease in migrants. One such group is Japanese migrants to Hawaii, in whom there is a clear change in the incidence of several common tumours, with higher incidence of carcinoma of the colon and breast but lower incidence of stomach cancer. These results suggest that environmental factors such as dietary constituents may be important in the aetiology of these tumours (Fig. 5.17).

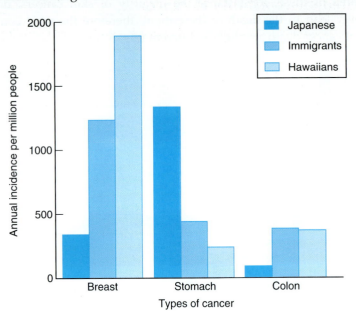

Fig. 5.17 Comparison of cancer incidence rates in Japan, in Japanese immigrants to Hawaii and in indigenous Hawaiians. (Data taken from Doll, R. and Peto, R., *The Causes of Cancer*, Oxford University Press, 1981.)

Trends in the incidence of cancers over periods of time may also provide useful information. There is often some difficulty in assessing this accurately because of variations over time in the methods of data collection, but in some circumstances, such as the steady increase in lung cancer incidence attributed to cigarette smoking during this century, the conclusions appear valid.

Cancer screening

Screening of the population at risk from certain common cancers is an attractive proposition as the early diagnosis of some tumours or their precursor lesions provides a very real opportunity of successful treatment. In order to be acceptable, the screening test must be reliable in terms of sensitivity and specificity, and must be safe, simple to perform and without unacceptable unpleasantness for the individual. There are national programmes for breast cancer (mammography) and cervical precancer (smear test) in operation in the UK at present. There is a considerable body of evidence from trial programmes in other parts of the world which show that, in time, with reasonably complete coverage of the population to be screened, a reduction in mortality from these important causes of cancer death can be expected. Screening for large bowel cancer is possible by testing for trace amounts of blood (occult blood) in the stools. However, this has so far met with some resistance from trial populations.

Molecular biology of cancer

Epidemiological studies have come to the conclusion that up to 80% of cancers are caused by environmental factors. At the cellular level genetic damage is fundamental to the process of tumorigenesis, and there is a great deal of evidence that there is increasing genetic instability within cells as they proceed towards the malignant phenotype.

Cancer cells have abnormal karyotypes, many are aneuploid and there are also abnormalities of individual chromosomes. Cancer can therefore be considered a genetic disease of somatic cells.

Inherited susceptibility to cancer

There are two main ways in which a predisposition to cancer development may be inherited:

- The abnormal genes that are directly involved in tumour development may be inherited through the germ line.
- A condition may be inherited which renders the individual more susceptible to a variety of cancers as a secondary phenomenon.

RETINOBLASTOMA

Retinoblastoma (Fig 5.18) is probably the most familiar and most important example of the first group. Retinoblastoma is a malignant tumour of the

Fig. 5.18 The retinoblastoma gene: familial retinoblastoma; sporadic retinoblastoma. There is congenital loss of one allele in the familial type, whereas the sporadic type results from two events leading to loss of both alleles.

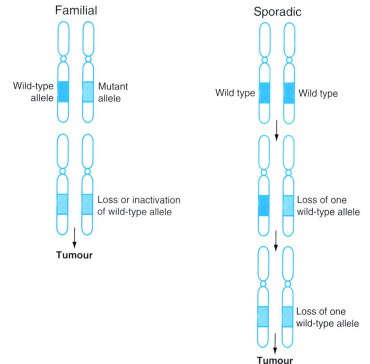

eye occurring in childhood. About 40% of cases are familial and the pattern of inheritance is autosomal dominant. Whereas the inherited tumours tend to be bilateral, and the individuals are at risk of developing a second cancer, usually osteogenic sarcoma, those with the sporadic form tend to be unilateral. In an attempt to explain this difference it was postulated that both alleles of the gene involved (the *RB* gene) must be abnormal for the tumour to occur, in other words the gene was in fact acting in a recessive manner. In the inherited form one abnormal allele is transmitted through the germ line and therefore only one more mutation in the normal allele is required for tumour development. In the sporadic type, however, two mutations are required and the chances of this happening are much less likely. The reason that the inheritance appears of dominant type is that in the presence of one inherited mutation the likelihood of the second allele being mutated is such that tumour formation is almost a certainty. Further studies have supported this by the recognition that the *RB* gene is one of a series of genes known as tumour suppressor genes. The *RB* gene is located on the portion of chromosome 13 deleted in retinoblastoma cells.

FAMILIAL ADENOMATOUS POLYPOSIS

A similar situation is found in familial adenomatous polyposis (FAP), a rare inherited condition in which those affected develop numerous adenomatous polyps of the large bowel and subsequently colonic carcinoma. The gene involved here is located on the long arm of chromosome 5.

FAMILIAL BREAST AND OVARIAN CANCER

A history of breast cancer in a first-degree relative confers an increased risk of development of the disease. Breast cancer often with ovarian cancer aggregates in certain families. Studies have shown that the inherited gene responsible for this susceptibility is located on the long arm of chromosome 17. The gene is called *BRCA1* and is thought to be a tumour suppressor gene. A woman who inherits a mutated *BRCA1* gene has a 60% risk of developing breast or ovarian cancer by the age of 50 compared with a risk of 2% in the general population.

DNA REPAIR AND TUMOUR SUSCEPTIBILITY

If DNA is the major target of the carcinogenic agent then it is not surprising that inherited syndromes resulting in defects in DNA repair are associated with an increased risk of tumour development. These syndromes include the autosomal recessive conditions **xeroderma pigmentosum**, in which affected individuals develop skin cancers such as squamous cell carcinomas and malignant melanomas because of the mutagenic effects of ultraviolet light, and **Bloom's syndrome**, in which there is a defect in a DNA ligase which is involved in joining DNA fragments. Sufferers are at risk from acute leukaemia and other cancers.

IS CANCER A GENETIC DISORDER?

Cancer can be regarded as a genetic disorder affecting somatic cells which requires more than one genetic error for its development. A series of mutations occur by which a normal stem cell becomes a clone of cells abnormal in their control of proliferation. It appears that the genetic damage directly involved in the development of the cancer cell phenotype is found in two particular classes of gene: **oncogenes** and so-called **tumour suppressor genes** (also known as antioncogenes).

ONCOGENES

It has been known for some time that certain viruses are capable of malignant transformation of cells. **Acutely transforming retroviruses** can rapidly transform cells in culture and induce tumours in experimental animals in short periods of time. It was found that viral genes termed oncogenes were necessary for tumorigenesis. An oncogene is a gene which by abnormal expression or alteration of the gene product directly leads to the production of the malignant phenotype. The viral oncogene is derived from mutated forms of normal vertebrate cellular sequences termed **proto-oncogenes**. The oncogene may therefore be regarded as the activated form of the proto-oncogene, and has acquired activities that induce malignancy.

By the study of oncogenic retroviruses various oncogenes were discovered, their DNA isolated, and subsequently homologous sequences were identified in human tumours. Using molecular biological techniques which had by then become available, it was shown that the malignant phenotype could be transferred to cultured cells using DNA transfection and thus the first transforming gene was identified. This oncogene was H-*ras* and was activated by a mutation.

Oncogenes function in a dominant fashion. Altered cellular oncogenes have been found in a large proportion of human cancers. The three-letter nomenclature used for oncogenes may refer to the retrovirus (*sis*: **si**mian **s**arcoma virus), the tumour in which it was first isolated (*neu*: **neu**roblastoma), or the type of oncogene product (*trk*: **tr**opomyosin receptor **k**inase).

This has prompted a search for the physiological functions of the proto-oncogenes. It appears that most proto-oncogene products are components of the signal pathways involved in the control of cell division. These products act either by phosphorylation of proteins, transmission of signals by GTPases and control of DNA transcription. Oncogenes can be classified according to the cellular location and function of their products (**oncoproteins**):

- **Growth factors:** Some oncoproteins show structural similarity to growth factors. The *sis* oncoprotein is similar to the chain of PDGF, for example. It is interesting to speculate that autocrine stimulation of tumour cells might result from overexpression of this type of oncogene, although no primary abnormalities have been demonstrated in the genes coding for these growth factors in human tumours.
- **Growth factor receptors:** *Erb* B encodes the kinase domain of the epidermal growth factor receptor. Overexpression of this oncogene is frequently found in breast and other cancers and correlates with a poor prognosis. The fms oncoprotein is homologous to the colony stimulating factor-1 receptor (CSF-1R).
- **Signal transduction proteins:** Some oncoproteins are located in the internal portion of the cell membrane and are likely to be involved in signal transduction. Oncogenes encoding these proteins include *ras*, mutation of which is one of the commonest oncogene abnormalities in human cancer, being found in pancreas, colon and thyroid carcinomas. The normal p21 ras proteins are able to bind and hydrolyse GTP and therefore function in a similar fashion to G proteins coupling extracellular stimluli to intracellular second messenger systems.

Other oncoproteins in this location possess tyrosine kinase activity but unlike growth factor receptors do not have a ligand-binding domain. The most important gene coding for this type of protein so far identified is *ABL*. This oncogene is located on the long arm of chromosome 9 and in chronic myeloid leukaemia is translocated to a region in chromsome 22 occupied by a gene *BCR*. The hybrid gene so formed codes for an altered protein product with increased protein kinase activity and growth signal.

- **Nuclear factors:** Oncoproteins located in the nucleus include those encoded by *myc*, *myb*, *fos* and *jun* proto-oncogenes. Most are probably transcription factors involved in the regulation of DNA replication and cell division. Oncogenic versions of c-*fos* and c-*jun* have been identified.

It can therefore be seen that defects of proto-oncogenes at any point in the signal transduction pathways can disturb the normal growth regulatory mechanisms within the cell and contribute to tumorigenesis. Activated oncogenes are found in 15–30% of human cancers. Some such as those encoding growth-factor-like substances are found in a restricted group of tumours whereas those such as *fos* and *myc* encoding nuclear factors are less tumour specific.

Oncogene activation

How can proto-oncogene activation occur by non-viral mechanisms? There are three main mechanisms:

- **Chromosome translocations** may result in an oncogene, for example, c-*abl* in chronic myeloid leukaemia, coming to lie in proximity to another gene which results in its overexpression.
- **Amplification:** Some tumours carry abnormally amplified domains of DNA that can include proto-oncogenes and therefore increase their expression. In neuroblastoma, for instance, N-*myc* may be overexpressed in this way and this correlates with poor prognosis, as also appears to be the case with amplification of c-*erb* B2 in breast cancer.
- **Point mutations** usually result in the substitution of a single amino acid leading to a change in the function of the protein. Proto-oncogenes may be activated by specific point mutations, for example *ras* in many tumours and *fms* in myelomonocytic leukaemia.

Deletions play little part in the activation of proto-oncogenes, being much more important in loss of tumour suppressor genes.

A single oncogene does not seem to be sufficient for the transformation of normal cells. Certain oncogenes may complement the activity of each other, a process known as **oncogene cooperation**. The H-*ras* gene product can stimulate the phosphorylation of c-*jun*, thereby increasing its ability to activate transcription. In combination these two oncogenes can transform rat embryo fibroblasts, whereas neither alone is able to do this. The actions of H-*ras* can also be increased by expression of another oncogene such as c-*myc*. It has recently been shown that apoptotic cell death induced by c-*myc* can be inhibited by *bcl2*. A single oncogene activation may be only capable of a temporary increase in cell proliferation, further genetic lesions, possibly sequential activation of oncogenes, being required for the development of the full malignant phenotype.

TUMOUR SUPPRESSOR GENES

Mutations may result in the loss or gain of function within the cell which can lead to loss of normal control of cell proliferation and therefore tumour development. Following the study of inherited tumours such as retinoblastoma, genes have been discovered which upon inactivation result in tumorigenesis. Naturally occurring inherited forms of oncogene mutations are not known.

The terms used to describe these genes include **tumour suppressor genes** or **antioncogenes**. The use of these terms has met with some resistance, because it is unlikely that tumour suppression is their sole physiological function.

The RB gene

Studies on hereditary cases of retinoblastoma discovered in some a small deletion in chromosome 13. It was subsequently revealed that tumour development depended on the loss of both alleles of a gene near 13q14. This *RB* gene seems to play a part in cell cycle control and it is interesting that DNA-virus-transforming proteins such as SV40, adenovirus E1a and HPV E7 all bind and probably inactivate *RB*. This may well underlie the ability of these viruses to transform cells. Inactivation of the *RB* gene has been found in a variety of human tumours including bladder, breast and bronchial small cell carcinomas.

The p53 gene

Loss of chromosome material at specific loci in the cells of certain tumours suggested the existence of other tumour suppressor genes. One of these and perhaps the most important is the *p53* gene. Sporadic mutations in this gene which encodes a nuclear phosphoprotein are one of the most common genetic lesions seen in human cancer and are particularly common in small cell carcinoma and colonic carcinoma. Mutations of this gene are much more common than complete deletions and these missense mutations produce abnormal proteins which have greater stability and therefore a longer half-life than their normal counterparts. The concentration of these proteins is thus much higher in the tumour cell than the concentration of normal p53 protein in the normal cell. This can be demonstrated immunocytochemically and can be used as evidence for the presence of abnormal *p53* expression within the tumour.

Inheritance of *p53* gene mutation is important in the rare **Li–Fraumeni syndrome**. This syndrome involves the occurrence within a family of a proband who develops a sarcoma, usually in childhood, and two first-degree relatives with cancer occurring before the age of 45 years.

Chromosome 11 holds a probable tumour suppressor gene for **Wilms' tumour**. The *NF1* gene on chromosome 17 is a site of frequent mutation in patients with **neurofibromatosis** type 1 (Table 5.2).

Table 5.2   Chromosomal deletions and tumour suppressor genes (TSG) associated with cancers

Chromosomal deletion	TSG	Neoplasm(s)
13q	RB1	Retinoblastoma Osteosarcoma
17q	p53	Small cell carcinoma of the lung Breast cancer Colorectal cancer
11p	WT1	Wilms' tumour Transitional cell cancer of the bladder Breast cancer Rhabdomyosarcoma
18q	DCC	Colorectal cancer
17q	NF1	Neurofibroma
5q	FAP	Colorectal cancer
11q	MEN-1	MEN-1[a]

[a]Multiple endocrine neoplasia syndrome type 1.

The physiological role of tumour suppressor genes

What are the normal functions of tumour suppressor genes? The *RB* gene appears to play an important part in cell cycle control. Phosphorylation of the *RB* gene protein precedes entry into S phase. This protein is a 110–114 kDa nuclear protein associated with DNA-binding activity. The p53 protein is also a phosphoprotein located within the nucleus. It appears to be a transcription factor which blocks the progress of cells that have undergone DNA damage through the cell cycle at the end of G_1. However, cell lines without *p53* are capable of survival and mice deficient in *p53* develop normally but suffer spontaneous tumour formation at an early age. In contrast, mice deficient in the *RB* gene die in utero, the cause of death appearing to be related to deficiencies in differentiation of certain tissues such as the central nervous system and erythrocytes. These studies suggest that, although important, tumour suppressor genes are not indispensible in all cell types for proliferation control.

Are multiple genetic events required?

Several tumours have been studied with regard to the requirement of multiple or sequential genetic defects for development of the malignant phenotype. Colon cancer provided a useful model, as it has been recognized for some time that this tumour tends to arise following a sequence of identifiable morphological stages involving adenoma formation preceding the development of invasive carcinoma. Four chromosome loci have been shown to be deleted or mutated at high frequency in colon carcinoma (Fig. 5.19).

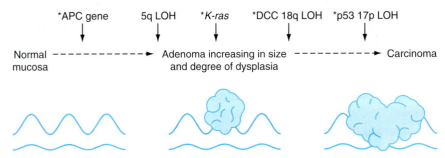

Fig. 5.19 Possible sequence of genetic events in the development of colorectal cancer. *, mutation; LOH, loss of heterozygosity.

Chromosomes and cancer

Chromosomal abnormalities appear to be of fundamental importance in tumorigenesis. Karyotypic analysis of malignant tumours (and some benign ones) show increase in ploidy and structural abnormalities when compared to normal cells. Indeed, in comparison to cells from the primary tumour metastatic cells often show a more severe degree of karyotypic aberration. Increasingly abnormal genotype therefore seems to be associated with biologically and clinically more advanced tumours. This supports the concept of clonal evolution.

Banding techniques have allowed the recognition of specific changes within individual chromosomes. In many tumours characteristic non-random chromosomal abnormalities can be identified. **Translocations** are of importance in haemopoietic malignancies. In solid tumours, **amplification** units (multiple copies of particular gene sequences) and **deletions** are more common.

Amplification units are visible on chromosomes in metaphase preparations of the tumour cells as homogeneous staining regions (HSRs) or abnormal banding regions (ABRs). Double minutes (DM) are multiple small paired bodies which contain chromosome material. DMs and HSRs

Some chromosomal abnormalities identified in tumour cells
- Translocation
- Inversion
- Interstitial deletion
- Amplification units

are thought to represent alternative forms of amplification of the same gene within the cell population and are only found in tumour cells, never in normal cells. Deletions are of particular significance if the lost genetic material contains a tumour suppressor gene.

It has been discovered that certain locations within chromosomes are particularly liable to break. These have become known as **fragile sites**, and they can be induced by a variety of insults; they also appear to be linked to translocation breakpoints where many oncogenes and tumour suppressor genes are also found.

Chromosomal abnormalities within a tumour cell may fall into one of three categories:

- In **primary abnormalities** the aberration is thought to be essential in the establishment of the tumorigenic process and tends to have a strong correlation with tumour type.
- **Secondary abnormalities** are a manifestation of tumour progression and clonal evolution and are not as tumour specific as the primary abnormalities.
- **Cytogenetic noise** is a manifestation of the genetic instability of the tumour cell. These abnormalities are randomly distributed throughout the genome.

CHARACTERISTIC CHROMOSOME ABNORMALITIES FOUND IN SOME COMMON MALIGNANCIES

In addition to providing valuable information regarding the genetic basis of certain tumours, chromosome abnormalities may have useful clinical application. Molecular probes for the hybrid *BCR/ABL* gene have been shown to be of some value in monitoring patients for relapse following bone marrow transplantation for chronic myeloid leukaemia (CML). The identification of certain translocations may be of use in the differential diagnosis of some tumours (Table 5.3).

Table 5.3   Common chromosome abnormalities in tumours

Leukaemias	
Acute myeloid leukaemia	t(6;9)(p23;q34)
	t(9;11)(p22;q23)
	t(15;17)(q22;q12)
Chronic myeloid leukaemia	t(9;22)(q34;q11)
Acute lymphocytic leukaemia	t(9;22)(q34;q11)
Chronic lymphocytic leukaemia	Trisomy 12
	t(11;14)(q13;q32)
Lymphomas	
Burkitt's lymphoma	t(8;14)(q24;q32)
Other non-Hodgkin's lymphomas	t(11;14)(q13;q32) t(14;18)(q32;q21)
Solid tumours	
Lung carcinoma (small cell)	del 3p
Breast carcinoma	Translocations 1q
Colorectal carcinoma	Trisomy 7
	Trisomy 12
	Structural changes in 1 and 17
Renal carcinoma	Structural changes in 3p
Bladder carcinoma	Structural changes in 1 and 11
Liposarcoma	t(12;16)(q13;p11)
Ewing's sarcoma	t(11;12)(q24;q12)

Myeloid neoplasms

In nearly every typical case of chronic myeloid leukaemia there is a small 22q− chromosome which is known as the **Philadelphia chromosome**, first described in 1960. This represents the result of a t(9;22) translocation. The c-*abl* proto-oncogene is located on the long arm of chromosome 9 and is translocated to a region of chromosome 22, the breakpoint cluster region (*BCR*), occupied by a gene of unknown function. This region is so called because it was noticed that in patients with Philadelphia chromosome-positive CML the breakpoints on chromosome 22 were confined to a small DNA segment. A hybrid gene is formed between the proto-oncogene and *BCR* and, in some way, this is crucial to the development of CML. The appearance in CML of a clone of blast cells with further karyotypic abnormalities is referred to as blast crisis. One of the additional abnormalities contributing to this progression involves the loss of the short arm of chromosome 17, the site of *p53* gene; mutation in the homologous gene results in the loss of *p53* function from the cell.

B-cell lymphomas

In about 75% of Burkitt's lymphoma cells there is a t(8;14)(q24;q32) translocation. The remainder of the cases also have translocations involving the same region of chromosome 8 but involving either chromosomes 2 or 22. The c-*myc* gene is located on the long arm of chromosome 8 and this is brought into proximity with immunoglobulin heavy chain gene sequences on the long arm of chromosome 14 (in the other translocations this involves the κ light chain gene on chromosome 2 and the λ light chain gene on chromosome 22). This arrangement leads to overexpression of the *myc* gene and affects the normal growth regulation of the B-cell clone. In other B-cell neoplasms such as follicular lymphomas there is a translocation involving chromosomes 14 and 18. A gene *bcl2* is moved from chromosome 18 to chromosome 14. It is of considerable interest that the gene product of *bcl2* is found on the mitochondrial membrane and exerts its effect not by increasing cell proliferation, but by preventing programmed cell death in the tumour.

Colorectal cancer

A series of chromosomal deletions involving chromosomes 5, 17 and 18 have been identified. Because of the inherited nature of some colonic cancers, particularly those arising in familial adenomatous polyposis (FAP), it was suggested that the short arm of chromosome 5 could be the site of a tumour suppressor gene as deletion of this region was seen commonly in the early stages of tumour development. The crucial region is 5q21, and the *APC* gene has been identified here. The *APC* gene is mutated in the germ line of some patients with FAP and Gardener's syndrome. The deletion of chromosome 17 involves the p53 gene, once again emphasizing the importance of this in human neoplasia and that on chromosome 18 is associated with the *DCC* gene which codes for a protein in the integrin family.

Lung cancer

Many small cell carcinomas of the lung have deletion of the short arm of chromosome 3.

Breast cancer

The chromosome most commonly affected in breast carcinomas is chromosome 1, many involving translocations of 1q.

Renal adenocarcinoma

The characteristic chromosomal lesions in renal adenocarcinoma involve rearrangements of the short arm of chromosome 3.

Wilms' tumour (nephroblastoma) occurs as a result of deletion or inactivation of a tumour suppressor gene located in 11p13. Other abnormalities found in this tumour affect chromosome 1.

Growth factors and neoplasia

Growth factor genes have been implicated in cellular transformation and tumour progression. There is no doubt that secretion of growth factors by tumour cells is common and may act in an autocrine fashion to stimulate tumour growth. The effect of growth factors on increasing cell proliferation rate will itself also lead to an increased risk of spontaneous mutation as the time for DNA repair is reduced during S phase and mitosis in rapidly growing cells.

Growth factors are also important in tumour angiogenesis and a variety of substances capable of stimulating **neovascularization** are released by tumour cells. These include TGF-α, TGF-β, EGF, PDGF and the family of heparin binding growth factors (HBGFs). The factor BFGF activates endothelial proliferation and production of enzymes such as collagenases and plasminogen activator which participate in capillary penetration into the tumour substance. Growth factors produced by tumour cells may also affect local immune responses and may be responsible for attracting some of the infiltrating lymphoid cells found in tumours.

Carcinogenesis

Carcinogenesis is a general term used to denote the development of malignancy. Having established the importance of genetic damage in neoplasia, it is necessary to consider the various environmental agents which possess the potential to cause such lesions. Despite the many types of human cancer known, relatively few established carcinogenic agents have been identified (Table 5.4).

Chemical carcinogens

Since the discovery, in the late eighteenth century, that there was an association between chronic exposure to soot and the development of scrotal carcinoma in chimney sweeps, many chemical agents have come under scrutiny as potential carcinogens.

Most chemicals which are known to be carcinogenic have also been shown to cause mutations – they are **mutagens**. The **Ames test** is a rapid mutagenicity assay in which bacteria (*Salmonella typhimurium*) are treated with suspected carcinogens. The culture medium utilized incorporates rat liver extract containing microsomal enzymes. This is necessary because some chemicals require metabolic activation before they become effective carcinogens. Most procarcinogens are activated by cytochrome P450 mono-oxygenases. The bacteria are normally unable to synthesize histidine. If some organisms acquire mutations resulting in their ability to do so, as a result of their exposure to the test substance, then the test is positive.

Table 5.4   Carcinogenic agents

Agent	Site of cancer
Aflatoxin	Liver
Alcohol	Mouth
	Oesophagus
	Liver
Aromatic amines	Bladder
Arsenic	Skin
Asbestos	Pleura
	Lung
Hardwood dust	Nasal sinus
Oestrogens	Endometrium
Anabolic steroids	Liver
Tobacco	Mouth
	Pharynx
	Lung
	Larynx
	Oesophagus
	Bladder
Ultraviolet light	Skin
Ionizing radiation	Bone marrow
	Thyroid
Hepatitis B virus	Liver
Schistosomiasis	Bladder

It has become customary to think of chemical carcinogenesis as a multistage process mirrored by a progression of genetic abnormalities as discussed in previous sections. Much information has been gained from studies of the experimental induction of tumours by chemicals in animals.

1. **Initiation** is the first step in the carcinogenic process and involves the short-term exposure of the cell to a carcinogen. These chemicals damage DNA – they are genotoxic at extremely low levels, and therefore there is virtually no threshold. Initiation is irreversible.

2. **Promotion** requires the long-term administration of a substance which is usually non-genotoxic (although some compounds can act as both initiators and promoters, so-called **complete carcinogens**). Tumour promoters show some tissue specificity and cause a clonal expansion of the initiated cells, their effects are reversible and there is a threshold level below which they are ineffective. Among the promoting agents which have been identified are the phorbol esters which activate members of the protein kinase C family of serine/threonine kinases, and okadaic acid, a potent inhibitor of protein phosphatase. The effect of both is to increase the phosphorylation of protein kinase C targets leading to DNA synthesis and cell division.

3. **Progression** is the term used to describe the increasing severity of abnormality seen in the evolution of a tumour.

These concepts may also be applied to other forms of carcinogenesis, for example tumours induced by radiation.

Chemical carcinogens interact with DNA in a variety of ways: by binding to DNA and forming carcinogen–DNA adducts, by alkylation of bases, by causing DNA strand breaks and by cross-linking between strands. It is likely that normally much of this damage is repaired by cellular enzymes such as DNA ligases. In individuals where the repair mechanisms are deficient (such as those suffering from xeroderma pigmentosum or Bloom's syndrome), there is an increased risk of the development of certain cancers.

THE SOURCE OF CHEMICAL CARCINOGENS

Some chemicals have been firmly established as having a role in the development of human cancer (Table 5.5).

Table 5.5   Chemical carcinogens

Compound	Cancer
Organic compounds	
Polycyclic aromatic hydrocarbons (require activation)	
Aromatic amines e.g. naphthylamine, benzidine	Bladder cancer
Nitrosamines	?Stomach cancer
Alkylating agents e.g. busulphan, cisplatin (no activation) cyclophosphamide (activated in liver)	Lymphomas and leukaemias
Vinyl chloride monomer	Hepatic angiosarcoma
Aflatoxin B1	Hepatocellular carcinoma
Cigarette smoke	Lung, mouth, larynx, oesophagus
Inorganic compounds	
Arsenic	Skin, lung
Chromium and nickel	Lung
Asbestos	Lung, pleura, peritoneum

Diet

The diet is a potential source of carcinogens and, although many putative dietary carcinogens have been identified, few specific substances have been proven to actually cause human cancer. However, known carcinogens can be present in natural foodstuffs: **cycasin** in the cycad nut, **pyrrolizidine alkaloids** in *Senecio* sp. and bracken fern. Most of these have not been shown to be related to human cancer, but bracken fern is consumed in Japan and appears to be related to an increased risk of oesophageal cancer. **Aflatoxin** is produced by the fungus *Aspergillus flavus* which contaminates stored nuts and other foodstuffs, and this is an important cause of hepatocellular carcinoma in some countries, particularly in Africa. The risk is further increased in individuals with chronic hepatitis B virus infection, suggesting a synergistic effect.

N-Nitroso compounds are extremely powerful mutagens and can be formed in the body from nitrites and nitrosable compounds. Nitrites themselves are formed by bacteria from ingested nitrates present in vegetables and nitrosable compounds are present in meat and fish. Gastric cancer in particular has been linked to the formation of N-nitroso compounds.

Apart from identifiable carcinogens, common components of the diet to have received most attention with regard to their impact on the incidence of cancer are salt and fat. Salted fish, which forms a substantial part of the diet in southern China, is linked to nasopharyngeal carcinoma in that region. **Salt-preserved foods** appear to promote the development of gastric cancer.

Fat consumption has been implicated in various cancers including breast, colorectal, endometrium, ovary, prostate and gallbladder. It has been suggested that it is by increasing the amount of faecal bile acids, which act as tumour promoters, that fats contribute to the development of colorectal cancer. There is also speculation that mutagens produced by the pyrolysis of meat, as in barbecuing, might also contribute to colorectal carcinogenesis.

Although there is little experimental evidence to show a role for **alcohol** in carcinogenesis, and the mechanisms of its action remain unclear, there have been many epidemiological studies which implicate the consumption of alcoholic beverages in oral, pharyngeal, oesophageal and hepatocellular cancers. There is also a suggestion that a moderate intake of alcohol increases the risk of breast cancer.

Dietary factors may also play a protective role against cancer. The role of **dietary fibre** in reducing the risk of colorectal carcinoma is complex in view of its many constituents and the lack of hard evidence. It would appear that the consumption of fruit and green vegetables reduces the risk of stomach and lung cancer in epidemiological studies. This has led to interest in the possible protective role of **carotenoids**, in particular carotene.

Tobacco smoking

Tobacco, particularly in the form of cigarette smoke, is probably one of the greatest single avoidable causes of cancer. Cancers of the lung, mouth, pharynx, larynx, oesophagus, bladder and possibly pancreas and kidney can be attributed to the habit. Which of the many components of cigarette smoke is responsible is unknown, but it contains undoubted carcinogens such as polycyclic aromatic hydrocarbons. The possibility that there is a genetic susceptibility to lung cancer has been considered and it may be that there are inherited differences in the activity of the enzymes which activate the chemical carcinogens involved.

The impact of cigarette smoke inhaled by non-smokers (**passive smoking**) has received considerable attention recently and there is a great deal of evidence to suggest that this sort of exposure increases the individual's risk of developing cancer. **Chewing tobacco** is related to oral cancer.

Hormones and cancer

Hormones play a significant role in certain human cancers. **Steroids**, particularly the sex hormones, have been implicated in carcinomas of the endometrium, breast and prostate. The evidence for this comes largely from epidemiological studies and clinical observation. The unopposed (by progestogens) action of **oestrogens** on the endometrium initially produces hyperplasia which increases the risk of cancer development. This effect can be seen with exogenous oestrogen administration as well as endogenous oestrogen production by, for instance, a hormone-producing ovarian tumour. Although the exact part played by hormones in breast cancer remains unclear, the evidence points to excess oestrogen exposure. Similarly, in prostatic cancer, although there does seem to be an influence of androgens on the development and progression of the disease the precise mechanism remains to be found. It is a well-established concept that the steroid hormone interacts with a cytoplasmic protein receptor which results in a product that binds to DNA leading to protein transcription and stimulation of growth. Hormones thus tend to act as promoting agents by increasing cell division in their target organs and are not mutagenic. One exception may be an initiating role in the development of vaginal adenocarcinomas in the female offspring of women prescribed diethyl **stilboestrol** during pregnancy. Hormone manipulation can be useful in the treatment of certain cancers.

Radiation carcinogenesis

All forms of radiation – electromagnetic and particulate – are carcinogenic. There is epidemiological evidence strongly implicating ultraviolet light in the causation of the common forms of skin cancer. Occupational exposure to particle radiation from inhaled **radon** gas has been observed to produce an increased incidence of lung cancer in uranium miners, and osteosarcomas of the jaw were induced in workers involved in painting the dials of luminous watches with substances containing isotopes of radium (who were in the habit of licking their brushes to produce a fine point). Early and misguided applications of radiation in medical practice, in which children received therapy for enlarged thymus glands and fungal infection of the scalp, have been shown to be associated with an excess of thyroid cancers.

Survivors of the atomic bomb explosions in Japan have unfortunately provided vivid evidence of the power of **radiation** as a carcinogen, with increased rates of lung, breast and thyroid cancers and leukaemias. The effects of high LET (linear energy transfer) particulate radiation on cells are much greater than weakly ionizing low LET radiations, such as X-rays and γ-rays.

Radiation exposure leads to breaks within DNA. Cells are most vulnerable during mitosis and very early in G_1 phase when chromosomal damage such as deletions occur. Cells that naturally have a rapid proliferative rate like haemopoietic and intestinal epithelial cells are therefore most radiosensitive.

The biological damage caused by particulate radiation seems to be mediated by free radicals liberated by their interaction with intracellular molecules.

Ultraviolet radiation is a low-energy emission and therefore penetrates little, exerting its effects mainly in the skin with the formation of basal cell and squamous carcinomas and also malignant melanomas. This form of radiation induces pyrimidine dimer formation in DNA, and the importance of adequate cellular DNA repair mechanisms is exemplified by the occurrence of skin cancer in individuals with xeroderma pigmentosum.

Viral carcinogenesis

In 1908 Bang discovered that a 'filtrable agent' could induce erythroid leukaemia (erythroblastosis) in chickens. Three years later Peyton Rous showed that such agents could produce sarcomas in chickens. Bittner in 1936 demonstrated that the breast tumours found in some strains of mice were due to the transmission of a virus to the offspring. It was not until relatively recently that such discoveries were directly related to human carcinogenesis. It is now generally accepted that over one-fifth of human cancers can be attributed at least in part to viral infection (Table 5.6).

Table 5.6   Viral causes of cancer

Virus	Disease
EBV	Burkitt's lymphoma and nasopharyngeal carcinoma
HBV	Hepatocellular carcinoma
HPV	Cervical, penile and anal carcinoma
HTLV-I	Acute T-lymphoblastic leukaemia
HIV	Non-Hodgkin's lymphoma

The ability of certain viruses to transform cells in culture provided researchers with an invaluable tool for investigating not only the mechanisms of viral carcinogenesis but also the basic molecular genetics of cancer in general.

RNA VIRUSES

Only one group of RNA viruses, the **retroviruses**, are able to cause tumours. On infection of the host cell the RNA genome of the virus is copied into double-stranded DNA by an enzyme, DNA polymerase. The DNA is then integrated into the host cell DNA. One of the important discoveries to have evolved from studies of the retroviruses is that of oncogenes. There are three replicative genes:

- *gag*, which encodes the internal core structures
- *pol*, encoding the DNA polymerase, reverse transcriptase
- *env*, which encodes the envelope proteins.

Some members of the retrovirus family have the ability to induce tumours very rapidly in experimental animals. These viruses differ from the majority of retroviruses which induce tumours after a long latency period, in that they do not possess some of the genes required for their replication. In place of this material are sequences responsible for the rapid transformation. These sequences are the **viral oncogenes (v-oncs)**. It was subsequently found that highly conserved homologous sequences, **proto-oncogenes**, are present in normal vertebrate cells. The viral oncogenes are derived from and mutated forms of their cellular counterparts. As discussed earlier, proto-oncogenes may become cancer-forming genes either by transduction into retroviruses giving rise to v-oncs or by their activation in situ.

Studies of the **Rous sarcoma virus (RSV)** revealed that the part of its genome involved in cellular transformation was the oncogene *src*. Unlike the rapidly transforming retroviruses, RSV is unique in that the oncogene is present together with the replicative genes (Fig. 5.20).

Fig. 5.20 Retroviral genomes: (a) basic retoviral genome; (b) Rous sarcoma virus genome; (c) rapidly transforming retroviral genome; (d) integrated virus.

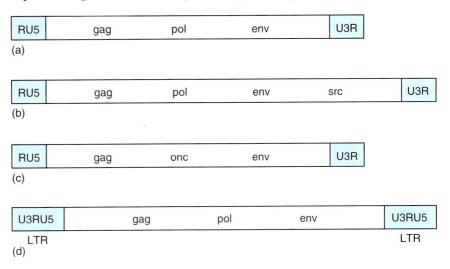

The structure of the integrated viral DNA shows duplication of regulatory sequences at the 3′ and 5′ ends. These sequences are called **long terminal repeats** and are important for the integration of the DNA copy (provirus) into chromosomal DNA. It is important to understand that these regulatory sequences can also serve as promoters or enhancers for adjacent cellular genes.

The various types of retroviruses induce malignancy by different mechanisms.

- The **acutely transforming retroviruses** possess oncogenes and are therefore able to transform cells by integration into the host genome.
- The **slowly transforming retroviruses** do not contain oncogenes and cannot transform cells in culture. **Avian leukosis viruses (ALV)** belong to this group and these produce neoplasia by a process known as insertional mutagenesis. The site of proviral integration allows increased transcription of an adjacent proto-oncogene because of the retroviral promoters or may induce structural alteration in the cellular gene
- The third mechanism is exemplified by that employed by **human T-cell leukaemia virus (HTLV-I)** which is important because it was the first human retrovirus isolated and is the only retrovirus aetiologically linked with a human cancer. It is associated with a T-cell lymphoma/leukaemia which is endemic in the West Indies and southern islands of Japan. This virus does not have an oncogene nor is its site of integration in the neoplastic cells consistent, which would be in keeping with an insertional mutagenesis type of activation. Like other retroviruses it has three structural genes flanked by long terminal repeats, but in addition it has another gene (*tax*). This gene is able to activate IL-2 and IL-2 receptor genes (there is also a possible effect on IL-3 and the *fos* oncogene). This activation causes autocrine stimulation of polyclonal T-cell proliferation but is alone insufficient for malignant transformation. Further genetic events may be more likely to occur under these circumstances and further emphasizes the importance of multiple events in neoplasia.

The **human immunodeficiency virus (HIV)** is another major human retrovirus and is also associated with the development of malignancy (non-

Hodgkin's lymphoma, Kaposi's sarcoma and squamous carcinoma of the mouth and anus). Unlike HTLV-I, however, HIV probably exerts its effect because of the immunodeficiency which it induces.

DNA VIRUSES

The first oncogenic DNA virus to be discovered was the **wart papilloma virus**, a papovavirus in rabbits. Other papovaviruses such as **simian virus 40 (SV40)**, **polyoma virus** and the **BK** and **JC** viruses can all cause tumours in experimental animals, although so far they have not been linked to human cancer.

Papillomaviruses, on the other hand, have long been known to be tumorigenic. There are many different types of papillomavirus, some of which cause the familiar viral wart and others have been implicated in carcinoma of the uterine cervix. Chronic infection with **hepatitis B virus (HBV)** is strongly associated with the development of hepatocellular carcinoma. This is extremely important on a worldwide basis as several hundred million individuals are affected.

The **adenoviruses** can also cause tumours in rodents but have not been associated with human neoplasia. **Epstein–Barr virus**, a herpesvirus, was the first virus linked to human cancer – **Burkitt's lymphoma**. Other tumorigenic herpes viruses include **Marek's disease virus** which causes a lymphoma-like condition in chickens.

There are a number of possible oncogenic mechanisms by which these viruses act. It would appear that in most oncogenic DNA viruses there are certain 'early genes', those transcribed prior to viral DNA replication, which are essential for cell transformation. The proteins encoded by these transforming genes have been extensively studied in polyoma virus and SV40 and are called **T proteins**. The interaction of these proteins with the products of tumour suppressor genes may be of relevance to transformation. In SV40 one of these, 'large' T, is present in the nucleus and binds p53 protein. The transforming protein of adenovirus E1B also has this property. SV40 T protein, adenovirus E1A protein and papillomavirus E7 protein bind the RB protein.

Epstein–Barr virus

This virus was first discovered in the cells of Burkitt's lymphoma, but its clinical effects are more familiar as those of infectious mononucleosis. Epstein–Barr virus is able to immortalize B cells in culture and they become phenotypically like lymphoblasts. It is likely that in this state they are more susceptible to translocations including the characteristic t(8;14) translocation discussed earlier. Burkitt's lymphoma is endemic in regions of Africa where malaria is also endemic. This has led to the suggestion that malaria may play a part in the development of this neoplasm, possibly through its immunosuppression effect.

This virus is also found in the cells of nasopharyngeal carcinomas, a tumour common in China and southeast Asia. The exact role of the virus in this tumour is uncertain.

Hepatitis B virus

There is a very high incidence of hepatocellular carcinoma (HCC) in Africa and southeast Asia, where young men are particularly affected. This high incidence mirrors that of HBV infection. Like Epstein–Barr virus it is possible that HBV integration produces an activated state which renders the cells more susceptible to subsequent genetic errors. Although there does not appear to be a specific site of insertion for viral DNA there is some evidence that HBV inserts adjacent to a region similar to the *erb*A oncogene. It is likely that HBV is only required for events early in transformation and further factors such as exposure to aflatoxin may be necessary for the development of HCC.

Human papilloma virus

Certain types of HPV are associated with clinical entities such as the common viral wart or genital warts, while some, such as HPV-16, have been implicated in cervical carcinoma. These viruses are double-stranded DNA viruses. All of the major open reading frames are on one of the strands and this is the only strand expressed as mRNA. Two genes which are capable of transformation in vitro are known as E_6 and E_7. The products of these genes have been shown to bind to the *RB* gene product, and the E_6 gene product of HPV-16 binds to p53 protein. This property of essentially inactivating these tumour suppressor genes may underlie the oncogenicity of these viruses.

It is apparent therefore that a variety of different mechanisms of viral carcinogenesis exist. It is important to be aware that only a small proportion of infected individuals (often after a considerable incubation period) eventually develop the tumours and that other genetic and environmental factors may be required for tumorigenesis. For instance, oesophageal tumours associated with bovine papilloma virus infection in cattle appear to require ingestion of bracken fern for their development.

The immune system and cancer

The possibility that tumour cells express antigens which may elicit immune responses and that these responses might be protective or potentially useful in a therapeutic role has been of considerable interest for some time. Experiments using tumour models in animals have demonstrated that T cells are able to recognize tumour-specific antigens and under certain circumstances can produce tumour rejection. These antigens are known as **tumour-specific transplantation antigens** (**TSTA**), and although their presence in human tumours is strongly suspected there is as yet no hard evidence to support this. Cancer cells, potentially, can become immunogenic through the expression of a variety of protein classes. These include proteins encoded by mutated oncogenes such as *erb*B2, proteins encoded by transforming viruses such as Epstein–Barr virus or HPV, and normal proteins which happen to be overexpressed such as the melanoma-associated gene in melanoma. A lymphocytic infiltrate is not uncommonly present within a tumour suggesting a possible immune response and certain cancers, for instance melanomas and renal cell carcinomas do occasionally undergo spontaneous regression, possibly immune-mediated.

The cellular infiltrate within tumours contain many T cells. These may be cytotoxic T cells which recognize foreign or abnormal antigens in association with MHC antigens on the surface of the cells or NK cells which are not MHC restricted. In vitro it has been shown that cells with features of NK cells are capable of lysing tumour cells, these cells have been defined functionally as **lymphokine-activated killer cells** (**LAK**) but it is doubtful whether these play a significant role in vivo. Other cells include macrophages which may affect the function of the tumour-reactive lymphocytes or may have a direct action, their activity being enhanced by interferon and TNF produced by activated NK cells. Macrophages themselves are important sources of some cytokines and these may affect the actions of other inflammatory cell types in the tumour-associated infiltrate. At the present time, however, our knowledge of the role of inflammatory cells and immune responses in established human tumours is rather limited (Fig. 5.21).

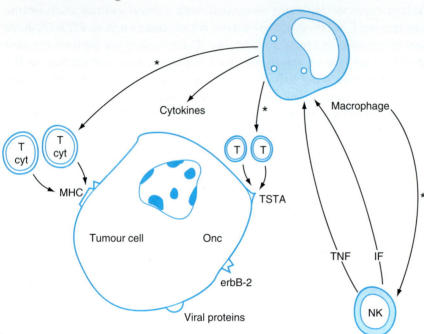

Fig. 5.21   The immune system and cancer. The asterisks indicate a direct effect on function by cytotoxic T lymphocytes and by cyotkines produced by inflammatory cells.

Treatment

Removal of tumour tissue surgically has long been the mainstay of cancer treatment, but it is now well established that, for many tumours, when they have attained a size sufficient to be apparent clinically then they have probably already spread to other parts of the body. Successful treatment therefore often requires systemic therapy. Unfortunately, so far, any systemic therapy has the potential to destroy normal as well as neoplastic cells with the consequence of unacceptable side effects.

Surgery and tumour diagnosis

Surgical therapy is more likely to be effective if the tumour is diagnosed at an early stage in its development, particularly if it is at the in situ cancer stage. The resected tumour must always be subjected to **histopathological examination**. Usually the diagnosis has been made prior to definitive surgery, either by removal of a small piece of tissue (**incision biopsy**), or increasingly by the use of cytological preparations made by aspirating cells from the tumour with needle and syringe (**fine needle aspiration**, **FNA**) or by scraping cells from the surface of the tumour (**exfoliative cytology**). Cytological techniques have the advantage that they are often less traumatic for the patient and the specimen is more quickly available for examination allowing a more rapid answer than conventional histology (almost immediately rather than about 48 hours). This preoperative diagnosis is necessary in order to avoid mistakes in diagnosis, as certain benign conditions can mimic malignancy clinically. It also allows proper planning of definitive treatment. Occasionally tissue obtained during a surgical procedure will be sent to the laboratory where a rapid histological section will be cut from frozen tissue, stained and examined while the patient remains anaesthetized. This technique enables additional surgery, if necessary, to be performed without having to resort to a further operation.

Histological examination of the surgically removed tissue enables the diagnosis to be confirmed and additional information with regard to staging, such as the involvement of lymph nodes and the presence or absence of vascular invasion, can be obtained. Completeness of excision can also be assessed by examining the margins of the specimen. Other important prognostic information such as tumour grade may also be more accurately recorded from the excision specimen.

Aside from a potential cure, surgery may also be necessary to alleviate some of the symptoms associated with the presence of the tumour. Thus dysphagia resulting from oesophageal carcinoma, obstructive jaundice from pancreatic cancer or bowel obstruction from rectal carcinoma may be relieved, and these palliative procedures are important in improving the patient's quality of life even if a cure is unattainable.

Radiotherapy

Radiation therapy was originally used for those tumours thought to be inoperable, but nowadays combined regimens of treatment are commonplace with radiotherapy being used in conjunction with surgery and chemotherapy. Newer techniques have allowed better targeting of therapy to the tumour with reduced risk of damage to adjacent healthy tissues.

Systemic therapy

Because of the disseminated nature of malignant disease the concept of systemically administered antineoplastic drugs is an attractive one, but the nature of most chemotherapeutic agents is such that normal cells are damaged in the process leading to dangerous side effects such as bone marrow suppression.

CHEMOTHERAPY

A variety of cytotoxic drugs are used clinically (Table 5.7) and many act at various points in the cell cycle. Despite the empirical nature of the treatment and the potential drawbacks some tumours have been successfully treated, in fact cured, with cytotoxic drugs. These include acute leukaemias, testicular tumours and some childhood tumours such as neuroblastoma and Wilms' tumour. These drugs are often used in combinations which have been found to be more effective than the use of individual drugs alone. Some agents have been shown to increase survival in certain tumours, for example breast cancer, when used as an adjuvant, although in general the response of the common solid cancers to chemotherapy is poor. One of the reasons for failure of treatment is the development of drug resistance. There are various mechanisms of drug resistance. The genetic instability of the tumour cell population can lead to

Table 5.7   Chemotherapy of malignancy

Alkylating agents	Cyclophosphamide	Lead to alkylation of sites within DNA and interfere with replication
	Chlorambucil	
	Busulphan	
	Melphalan	
Nitrosoureas	CCNU (lomustine)	Inhibit synthesis of DNA, RNA and protein
	BCNU (carmustine)	
Antimetabolites		
Folic acid antagonists	Methotrexate	Inhibits dihydrofolate reductase and blocks purime and thymidylate synthesis
Base analogues	5-Fluorouracil	Inhibit nucleic acid biosynthesis
	Cytarabine	Act in S phase
	6-Mercaptopurine	
Mitotic inhibitors	Vincristine	Bind to tubulin and lead to metaphase arrest
	Vinblastine	Act at mitosis
	Etoposide	
Antibiotics	Bleomycin	Intercalate between base pairs in DNA and inhibit replication
	Doxorubicin	
	Actinomycin D	
Others	Cisplatin	Binds to DNA and protein
	Procarbazine	Inhibits synthesis of DNA, RNA and protein
	Asparaginase	Asparagine is an essential amino acid for some cancer cells that require asparagine for growth

alterations in gene products which in turn can affect drug uptake by alterations at the cell surface, increased drug efflux, altered drug metabolism or intracellular binding and more efficient repair of the drug-induced damage. **Multidrug resistance (MDR)** refers to the situation in which a cancer becomes resistant to a number of drugs with apparently unrelated modes of action. The drugs often involved include doxorubicin, vinca alkaloids and mitomycin C. MDR is associated with the overexpression of a membrane-associated glycoprotein, **P-glycoprotein**, which belongs to a family of transport proteins. The normal substrate and function of P-glycoprotein is unknown but in drug-resistant cells it appears to bind to the drug and actively remove it from the cancer cell. Several strategies have been proposed in order to overcome this form of drug resistance including the use of cytotoxic agents to which MDR cells show increased sensitivity, agents which inhibit P-glycoprotein function such as calcium channel blockers and immune mechanisms using monoclonal antibodies to P-glycoprotein.

There is a growing number of novel potential targets for chemotherapeutic agents and some of these such as **paclitaxel**, which has an action against microtubules, have already been shown to be of value in clinical trials.

HORMONE THERAPY

Hormone manipulation may be used therapeutically in endocrine-dependent tumours. **Progestogens** may be of value in the oestrogen-dependent endometrial carcinomas, **stilboestrol** is used to slow the progress of prostatic carcinoma and the antioestrogen **tamoxifen** has both oestrogenic and antioestrogenic properties and causes breast cancer cells to accumulate in G_0 and G_1 of the cell cycle; it is used widely in the treatment of breast cancer and is being evaluated as a potential preventative agent.

IMMUNE THERAPY

The advent of monoclonal antibodies aroused a great deal of interest in cancer treatment research because of the potential for targeting specific antigens within cancer cells and being able to more specifically direct cytotoxic agents without harming normal cells. Theoretically the antibodies themselves could have antitumour effects by triggering complement or activating antibody-dependent cytotoxicity, or they could be used to enhance the effects of other substances such as interferon or interleukin. Some monoclonal antibodies, such as those directed against antigens, e.g. CAMPATH-1, have been used for the treatment of human lymphomas with some positive response, but studies with monoclonal antibodies directed against antigens on solid tumours have shown less encouraging results. An immune response can be mounted against determinants (idiotypes) in the antigen-binding sites of antibodies. Antibodies which are themselves directed against these determinants are known as **anti-idiotype antibodies**. When the original antigen is on the surface of the malignant cell the anti-idiotype antibody can mimic this antigen and so potentially immunization against this antibody will also produce immunization against the tumour. This approach is under investigation as a method of tumour vaccine production.

A greater cytotoxic effect might be expected if the monoclonal antibody directed to the tumour is conjugated to antineoplastic drug molecules, and this also has the advantage of greater selectivity. Clinical trials are already under way with conventional cytotoxic drugs such as anthracyclines. Cancer treatment by conjugation of monoclonal antibodies with other natural toxins such as ricin is also under investigation.

Radionucleotide-conjugated monoclonal antibodies would have the advantage of exerting their effect on cells adjacent to those to which attachment occurred, and therefore tumour cells which did not express the antigen would also be subjected to the cytotoxic effect. One of the problems still to be overcome in these techniques is that of the development of immune responses to repeated doses of foreign immunoglobulins. The toxicity of monoclonal antibody administration has so far been slight, with a small risk of anaphylaxis (Fig.5.22).

Cytokines have also been used therapeutically. Interleukin-2, when used alone or in combination with LAK cells, has been shown to decrease tumour growth in animal models and has some effect in clinical trials in human melanoma. The lymphocytes are harvested from the patient by leukopheresis and activated using recombinant IL-2. They are then reinfused into the patient together with more IL-2. Responses to interferon have also been reported in hairy cell leukaemia, myeloma and renal cell carcinoma.

GENE THERAPY

Developments in gene therapy have provoked much interest recently, and clinical studies are already under way in the USA. Techniques being

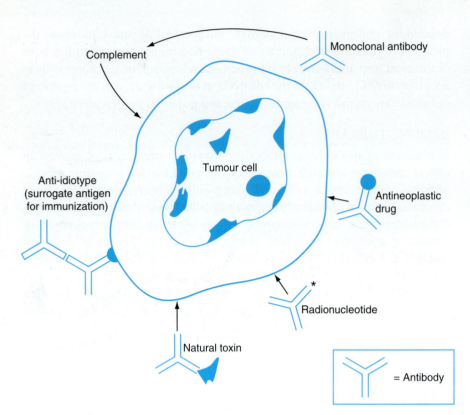

Fig. 5.22 Monoclonal antibody therapy, showing the way in which various anticancer agents can be linked to antibodies to target them towards specific tumour cell antigens.

evaluated include the transfer of tumour-infiltrating lymphocytes, infected with retroviruses containing human cytokine genes into patients with cancer. These lymphocytes will then effectively deliver large doses of interferon, TNF and IL-2 directly to the tumour. Alternatively, the coupling of a promoter region of a gene expressed in tumour cells with an enzyme that can activate an innocuous substance to a cytotoxic agent will produce targeted activity within the appropriate tumour cells. Genes encoding cytokines or MHC products may be inserted into the tumour cells in order to enhance their immunogenicity. Eventually even the oncogenes or tumour suppressor genes themselves might be manipulated and therapy can be directed at the genetic basis of cancer.

Chapter 6   Inflammation and healing

Definition of inflammation

'The sequence of changes which occur when a tissue is damaged but not destroyed, from the time of injury to the stage of healing.'

Names of inflammatory diseases

Inflammatory disease names often end in **'-itis'**, as in
- Appendic**itis** or
- Bronch**itis**

BUT there are exceptions, such as
- Pneumonia

Acute or chronic inflammation?

■ **Acute inflammation**
- Occurs quickly
- Cells involved:
  - Polymorphonuclear leukocytes (PMN)
  - Platelets
  - Endothelium

■ **Chronic inflammation**
- Takes a long time
- Cells involved:
  - Plasma cells
  - Lymphocytes
  - Macrophages

Signs of inflammation
- **Heat** (calor)
- **Erythema** (rubor)
- **Pain** (dolor)
- **Swelling** (tumor)
- **Loss of function**

Learning objectives

To appreciate and understand:
❏ The process of inflammation, its relationship to immunity and role in promoting healing
❏ The events involved in acute inflammation
❏ The events responsible for chronic inflammation and granuloma formation
❏ The relationship between immunity and hypersensitivity as the cause of disease
❏ The requirements for healing in soft tissues and bones

Inflammation is the body's response to injury from any cause. It occurs during the time between injury and healing and is of two major types – either acute or chronic inflammation. Acute inflammation differs from chronic inflammation in its timing (as the names suggest) and in the types of cells present in the affected tissue.

Acute inflammation

The cardinal signs of acute inflammation have been known for centuries: the affected tissue becomes hot, painful, red and swollen, with loss of function.

The extent and the constituents of the acute inflammatory response vary with its cause. This depends upon the type and amount of inflammatory mediators released from injured tissues. For instance, inflammation as the result of necrosis may result in production of a different set of mediators compared with infection, and even if the mediators themselves are similar, the levels produced may be different. Such differences in the **mediator profile** modulate the scale and character of the inflammatory response early in its development, and continue to do so as it develops into chronic inflammation.

The mediator profile

The mediator profile is determined by the production and degradation of mediators from a large variety of cellular and non-cellular sources.

Mediators of inflammation can be classified as **tissue-derived**, **plasma-derived** or **cell-derived**. The immediate response to injury usually involves the production of tissue-derived mediators from damaged or dying cells.

Mechanical forces may trigger mast cells to release histamine and leukotrienes, and the contribution made by neuropeptides released from nerve endings in the injured area should not be underestimated. Once the vascular part of the response begins to occur, plasma-derived mediators will act in concert with tissue and cell-derived mediators. Proinflammatory cytokines such as **interleukin-1 (IL1)** are produced by many cell types, including epithelial cells. If endothelial damage has occurred within the tissue, the contribution to the mediator profile by platelets may be particularly important. The time frame in which this occurs can be minutes: it is quite common to see mild acute inflammation in the peritoneum covering an otherwise normal appendix removed by a surgeon in under 15 minutes (Fig. 6.1).

Causes of inflammation
● Infection
● Physical or chemical trauma
● Adjacent necrosis
● Ischaemia
● Immunopathology

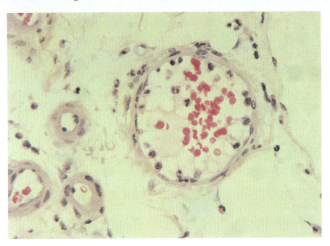

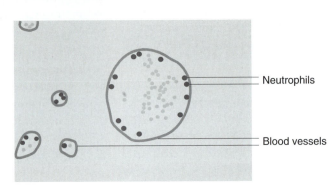

Neutrophils

Blood vessels

Fig. 6.1 Handling of appendix for a few minutes at operation can cause margination of neutrophils in peritoneal blood vessels, as shown here.

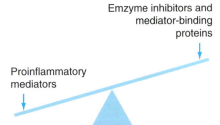

Emzyme inhibitors and mediator-binding proteins

Proinflammatory mediators

Fig. 6.2 The balance of mediators and down-regulators in inflammation.

The sequence of events so far described has concentrated on **up-regulators** of inflammation. However, even at an early stage in the inflammatory response, there will be a contribution from **down-regulators**: enzymes which inactivate mediators and proteins which bind to and reduce the amount of biologically active mediator present in the site of inflammation. Obviously, these mechanisms will be more successful at a distance from the site of injury than they are closer to the site of maximal proinflammatory mediator production. Even at an early stage, such down-regulation will tend to balance up-regulation and limit the extent of the response (Fig. 6.2).

The effects of mediator release

The clinical signs and systemic effects of acute inflammation depend on the responses induced in the tissue by mediators. Initially there is a vascular response with congestion and hyperaemia of the tissue, which is followed by exudation of plasma proteins, and then by cell emigration.

Vascular congestion at the site of injury is responsible for the affected tissue becoming reddened and hot to the touch, while the plasma exudate causes tissue swelling and loss of function. Pain is due partly to mechanical stimulation and partly to mediator-induced nerve stimulation.

Sources of inflammatory mediators
■ Dead tissue
● Kinins
Histones (from DNA breakdown)
■ Cellular
● Histamine
● Neuropeptides
● Leukotrienes
● Cytokines (IL1, IL6, IL8, TNF-α)
■ Plasma-derived
● Complement products (C3a and C5a, for example)
● Fibrin degradation products

HYPERAEMIA AND ERYTHEMA

The primary vascular event caused by neural reflexes and exposure of arterioles to mediators is **vasodilatation** (Fig. 6.3). This results in passive capillary congestion, opening of arteriovenous shunts, and slowing of blood flow. The mediators involved include histamine and arachidonic acid metabolites (prostaglandins, leukotrienes and platelet-activating factor, PAF). It has also recently become clear that another factor, which may be produced by nerve endings and was formerly known as endothelium relaxing factor, is actually **nitric oxide**. This highly reactive chemical is extremely transient, but plays an important part in the maintenance of vascular tone and is almost certainly involved in acute inflammatory responses. The relative importance of these various mediators is still not clear, but the mediator blocking drugs available at present have relatively little effect on models of inflammation and the story is far from complete.

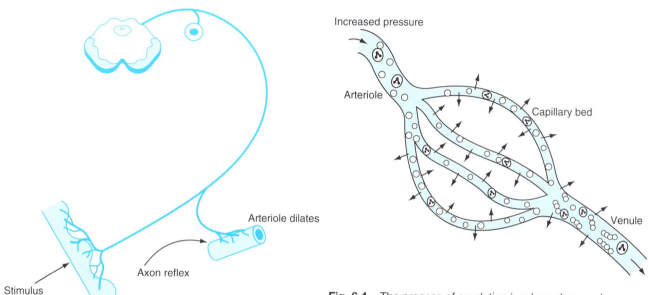

Fig. 6.3 Reflex vasodilatation is mediated by neural mechanisms.

Fig. 6.4 The process of exudation involves changes in hydrostatic pressure within the capillary bed.

The effect of these changes is to increase the amount of blood within the tissue, reduce the oxygen tension (after an initial rise as blood flow increases) and allow the local pH within the tissue to fall.

EXUDATION

The changes in blood flow (Fig. 6.4) combine with endothelial cell contraction to permit larger molecules than usual to leave the circulation and exude into the tissues. This is assisted by changes in osmotic and hydrostatic pressure.

Exudation has several effects on the injured tissue. The oedema causes clinically apparent swelling and will compress lymphatics and venules within the tissue. This further slows blood flow. Macromolecules escape from the circulation as a result of endothelial cell contraction and loss of the normal ultrafiltration mechanism (Fig. 6.5). These include large molecules such as IgM and fibrinogen, which are not normally present in tissues.

Components of the clotting cascade and fibrinogen are released into the tissue, allowing a fibrin mesh to form at the site of injury. This is particularly important as it forms the basic framework within which healing will occur.

Fibrin degradation products are potent mediators and are thought to stimulate angiogenesis. The exudate also contains antibody and complement in large amounts. These will attack foreign objects such as invading bacteria from the skin surface and help to protect the vulnerable injured area from infection.

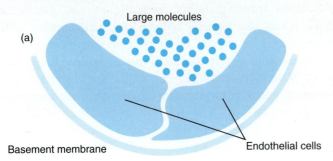

Fig. 6.5 Endothelial cell separation leads to enucleation of macromolecules which are normally restricted to the circulation.

Inflammatory exudate components
- Water
- Fibrinogen and coagulation proteins
- Immunoglobulins
- Complement components
- Macroglobulins and microglobulins

CELL EMIGRATION

The main cell type involved in acute inflammation is the **polymorphonuclear leukocyte (PMNL)**, while in chronic inflammation the **lymphocyte** is the predominant cell type.

The word polymorphic means 'having many shapes', and the term polymorphonuclear leukocyte includes three cell types, all of which have multilobed nuclei and granules in their cytoplasm. Most are **neutrophils**,

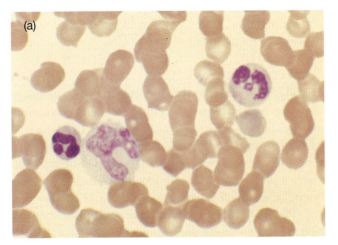

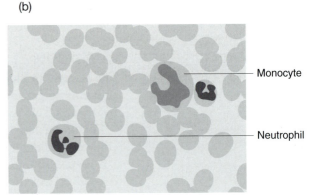

Fig. 6.6 (a, b) Neutrophils – blood stained to show their multiobed nuclei. (c, d) Electron micrograph of a neutrophil showing the lobed nucleus and prominent cytoplasmic granules. (e, f) Margination of PMNL within a blood vessel. (g, h) Massive neutrophil infiltration and congestion in acute inflammation.

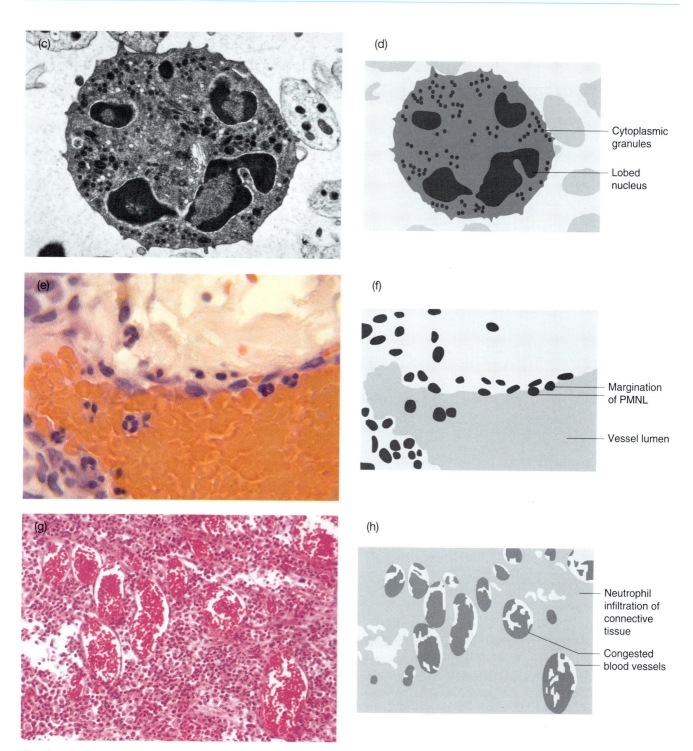

(c)

(d)
Cytoplasmic granules
Lobed nucleus

(e)

(f)
Margination of PMNL
Vessel lumen

(g)

(h)
Neutrophil infiltration of connective tissue
Congested blood vessels

Fig. 6.6 contd.

and it is this cell which is the first to arrive in acutely inflamed tissues – often within minutes of the injury occurring. If neutrophils are present within a tissue, then it is acutely inflamed and these distinctive cells are easily found in histological sections if they are present in any number (Fig. 6.6). The main role of the neutrophil is in fighting bacterial infection. Other types of polymorph are the **eosinophil** and the **basophil**. The eosinophil is particularly important in helminth infection and in atopic diseases such as asthma, while the function of basophils is still controversial.

CASE STUDY 6.1

A 22-year-old man is a keen and extremely fit amateur football player. In the course of a match he falls awkwardly after a hard tackle and presents to the accident and emergency department of the local district general hospital. He is clearly in pain and unable to bear putting weight onto his right foot. The nurse has some difficulty removing his football boot, and on examination his ankle is severely swollen and bruised with reddening (erythema) of the overlying skin. A radiograph reveals no fractures and he is allowed home with a firm adhesive strapping on his ankle from the ball of the foot to mid-calf which he is told to leave in place for two weeks. He is given a week's supply of a non-steroidal anti-inflammatory drug.

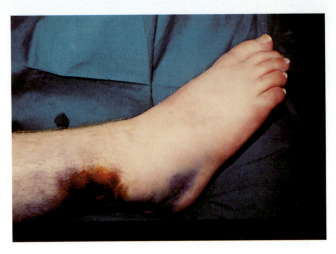

Fig. 6.7 A severely inflamed ankle with swelling and an area of bruising.

Cellular emigration requires:

- firm adherence of cells to the endothelium
- diapedesis of cells through the wall of the blood vessel
- chemotaxis-driven movement of cells to the site of inflammation.

Adherence of inflammatory cells to endothelium

Inflammatory cells are primed to adhere to endothelial cells by inflammatory mediators, and endothelium is stimulated by mediators to become more receptive to inflammatory cell adherence. The mechanism is simple: the mediators induce increased expression of adhesion molecules on the surface membrane of both circulating and endothelial cells. However, different mediators affect different cells and different adhesion molecules (see Chapter 3), so a complex series of interactions takes place within the blood vessel and the process can be finely controlled. This is an area of rapid scientific progress and it may soon prove possible to modulate inflammatory responses by influencing cell adhesion.

Owing to changes in blood flow as the first response to injury, neutrophils come in contact with the endothelial cells.

- The first movement that is seen is that of neutrophils **rolling** over the endothelial cells. This rolling is mediated by loose binding of neutrophils to P-selectin and possibly E- and L-selectin molecules which are on the surface of endothelial cells (see Chapter 3). E-selectin is also involved in adhesion as the time course of expression of this molecule parallels that of neutrophil adhesion.

Neutrophil functions in acute inflammation
- Production of mediators
- Phagocytosis and killing of invading micro-organisms
- Digestion of dead tissue
- Modulation of the immune response by interaction with other cells

- To **stabilize** endothelial cell–neutrophil interaction, further improvement in adhesion is necessary. Additional contact is established between the β_2-integrins (CD11–CD18) on the neutrophils and ICAM-1 on endothelial cells.
- This interaction facilitates the next event where neutrophils **tether** to endothelial cells and are seen to line the vessel wall like pebbles on a river bed.
- After anchoring to endothelial cells, neutrophils undergo **changes in shape** and become **activated**.

Though many factors such as surface charge and calcium ion concentration help in cell adhesion, it is becoming increasingly clear that the specific complementary adhesion molecules present on neutrophils and endothelial cells are of great importance in inflamed tissue. Moreover, these molecules can be rapidly altered qualitatively and numerically when stimulated by cytokines.

Endothelial cells also express PAF, the first molecule described on endothelial cells, which helps in adhesion to neutrophils. It is not constitutively expressed (that is, not seen on resting endothelial cells) but is rapidly synthesized within minutes after stimulation by histamine, thrombin and leukotriene C_4. After expression it acts as a signal for adhesion to integrins on leukocytes. This not only helps in tethering of neutrophils, but also improves their responsiveness to cytokines and chemoattractants which may be in the neighbourhood. Such activation mediated by membrane-anchored molecules on a neighbouring cell is called **juxtacrine activation**.

Endothelial cells activated by bacterial lipopolysaccharide, or cytokines such as TNF-α and IL1, produce another cytokine, IL8, which also upregulates integrins on neutrophils, thereby enhancing their adhesion. Both PAF and IL8 interact with specific receptors on leukocytes and mobilize integrins from the intracellular pool to the cell surface. IL8 also leads to change in shape, shedding of L-selectin and activation of PMNL. Endothelial cell selectins are also increased after activation by LPS and IL8.

Eosinophils and basophils also bind to vessel walls through β_2-integrins. Eosinophils bind to VCAM-1 on endothelial cells. VCAM-1 is a member of the immunoglobulin superfamily and is present on resting endothelial cells. Activation by cytokines enhances VCAM-1 expression. Thus both signalling and tethering are molecular events requiring bridging of complementary molecules on endothelial cells and leukocytes. Tightness of this adhesion is further improved in the presence of cytokines such as IL1, TNF-α and IL8.

Margination and diapedesis

Cell adhesion is enhanced by the reduction in the speed of blood flow through the tissue as a result of vascular congestion. This results in **margination** of cells at the edge of the blood vessel (see Fig. 6.6c), allowing them to adhere and emigrate by moving through the blood vessel wall between endothelial cells into the tissue. The potential barrier of the basement membrane is digested by enzymes secreted by the emigrating cell, leaving a small hole as it passes through which will eventually be repaired by the endothelial cells.

How do endothelial cells allow the extravasation of leukocytes and serum products during inflammation? Again, there is a series of controlling mediators. The cytokines IL1 and TNF-α increase the expression of enzymes in endothelial cells that synthesize prostacyclin (PGI_2), one of the metabolites of arachidonic acid in the cyclo-oxygenase pathway (see Chapter 3). This is a potent vasodilator and leads to exudation of fluids from the blood vessel. Other metabolites such as PGE_2, PGD_2 and PGE_1 have similar effects. However, thromboxane A_2, another product of the same pathway, has opposing effects and leads to vasoconstriction. The interplay of arachidonic acid metabolites regulates endothelial cell movement and controls the egress of cells and macromolecules during inflammation. Other cytokines and substances such as nitric oxide also have important effects.

Chemotaxis

Once in the tissue the cell will migrate towards the site of injury by responding to a chemical gradient – it moves towards the greatest concentration of mediators for which it has receptors on its membrane. This process is known as **chemotaxis**. One of the earliest changes which occurs is **polarization**: a change in the shape of the cell from a rounded mass to an oriented cone or triangular shape with the base pointing towards the origin of the chemoattractant (Fig. 6.8).

Chemotactic stimulus   Polarized cell   Resting cell

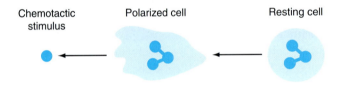

Fig. 6.8 Polymorphs respond to chemotactic peptides such as breakdown products of bacteria by polarization. This is the basis of a sensitive test for both cellular function and chemoattractants.

As well as responding to concentration gradients, cells such as polymorphs move in response to molecules such as IL8 bound to endothelial cells. This process is known as **haptotaxis** (movement over membrane-bound attractant) rather than chemotaxis (movement towards a soluble chemical). Though IL8 is usually in low concentrations in the blood, raised levels are seen in infections and inflammation. IL8 may then reach the lung tissues and cause sequestration of PMNLs in alveoli – a hallmark of the serious condition known as the **adult respiratory distress syndrome** (see Chapter 9). IL8 is a member of a family of cytokines known as **chemokines**, and is an important chemoattractant for eosinophils and basophils as well as neutrophils. Another cytokine called **monocyte chemotactic protein-1 (MCP-1)** acts mainly on monocytes.

The neutrophils migrating into the tissue have a variety of different functions, of which their ability to home in on and kill invading micro-organisms is probably the most significant. However, the mediators they produce have a major influence on the way in which the acute inflammatory response progresses.

In addition, changes in shape, phagocytosis and movement of leukocytes require alteration of cytoskeletal components such as actin, actinin and tropomyosin. Thus signals mediated by adhesion molecules on the surface also lead to intracellular signalling for cytoskeletal proteins.

Systemic effects of acute inflammation
- Acute phase response
- Increased protein turnover
- Fever – pyrogens
- Tachycardia
- Increased platelet adhesion
- Leukocytosis
- Neutrophil hypergranulation

INTERACTION BETWEEN LEUKOCYTES AND EXTRACELLULAR MATRIX

Leukocytes which have extravasated into the tissues come in contact with laminin and collagen through the β_2-integrins and VLA proteins (CD49–CD29). Cytokines promote the movement of leukocytes over intercellular matrix by increasing expression of the above adhesion molecules on leukocytes.

SYSTEMIC EFFECTS: THE ACUTE PHASE RESPONSE

Acute phase reactants consist of a large set of proteins synthesized in the liver and released into the serum during inflammation. They include the C3 component of complement, C-reactive protein, serum amyloid A, fibrinogen and some protease inhibitors. IL6, produced by lymphocytes, is the most important cytokine that stimulates hepatocytes to release acute phase proteins. Earlier studies had implicated IL1, but this cytokine does not induce all of the acute phase proteins.

During infection and inflammation IL1 and TNF may be detectable in the blood. Their presence coincides with high fever and hypotension characteristic of the endotoxic shock seen with Gram-negative bacterial infections. These cytokines act on the hypothalamus to produce PGI_2, which stimulates the vasomotor centre in the brain and thereby causes fever.

Macroscopic appearance of inflammation
- Fibrinous
- Serous
- Haemorrhagic

Progression of acute inflammation

Acute inflammation may either resolve or evolve into chronic inflammation over the course of time (Fig. 6.9). The period involved is very variable. It is influenced by the site, cause and extent of injury – and also by medical treatment.

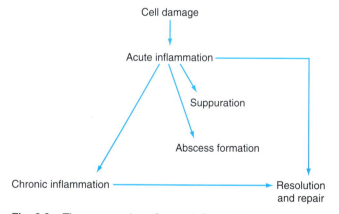

Fig. 6.9   The progression of acute inflammation.

SUPPURATION: PROLONGED ACUTE INFLAMMATION

Suppuration occurs when neutrophil emigration is prolonged and intense, leading to the formation of **pus** (Fig. 6.10). This is often a response to infection and can be prolonged. A localized collection of pus is known as an **abscess** (Fig. 6.11). Abscesses occur in virtually any organ and often form in areas of tissue destruction or in potential spaces such as the pleura (**empyema**). Attempted healing in the wall of the abscess isolates it from surrounding structures, but it may discharge pus into spaces such as the peritoneum or on to the skin surface.

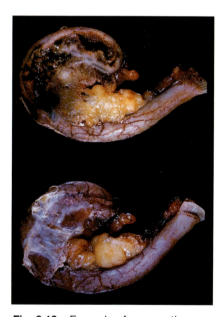

Fig. 6.10   Example of suppuration: a pus-filled appendix with exudate on its surface.

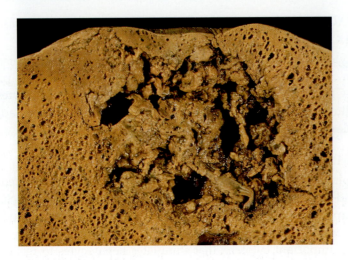

Fig. 6.11   A liver abscess showing the ragged edges and necrotic central cavity.

- Acute inflammation of mucosal surfaces is often **catarrhal** – simple inflammation with oedema, neutrophils, congestion and increased mucosal secretion.
- If it is more severe it may be **membranous**, in which case a membrane composed of fibrin with desquamated epithelial cells and neutrophils forms on the surface of the mucosa. This may slough off. If sloughing occurs in the larynx, as can happen in diphtheria, acute laryngeal obstruction can cause death.
- **Pseudomembranous** inflammation looks similar macroscopically, but histology shows that the epithelium is necrotic. The dead epithelial cells combine with fibrin and neutrophils to form a pseudomembrane.

Chronic inflammation

Chronic inflammation (Fig. 6.12) often evolves from acute inflammation, but it may also result from immune reactions in which neutrophils are not involved. As might be expected, the cells involved in the immune response are prominent in chronic inflammation, and chief among these is the lymphocyte.

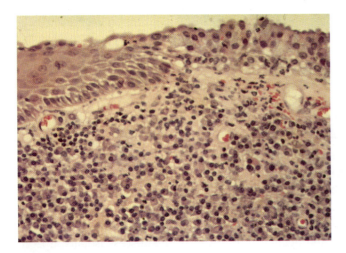
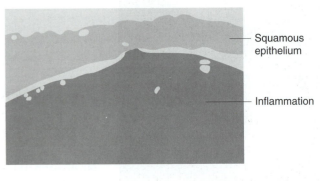

Squamous epithelium

Inflammation

Fig. 6.12   Chronic inflammation of the nasal mucosa showing a dense inflammatory infiltrate in the submucosa consisting largely of plasma cells and lymphocytes.

Lymphocytes

Lymphocytes are responsible for the control of immune reactions and are produced in the bone marrow like other blood cells. However, some (known as **T lymphocytes**) migrate to the thymus and undergo a complex cycle of differentiation during which they acquire distinctive properties which allow them to control immune reactions. Most of the remaining lymphocytes which do not go to the thymus are assigned to the antibody production arm of the immune response. These are known as **B lymphocytes** because in birds they undergo a differentiation step in the bursa of Fabricius. In humans there is no such organ, and it is thought that B-lymphocyte differentiation occurs in the bone marrow. Lymphocytes in the blood are small cells, slightly larger than a red blood cell, with dark-staining nuclei and little cytoplasm. In tissues they often enlarge a little, but many will still have the same shape and staining characteristics.

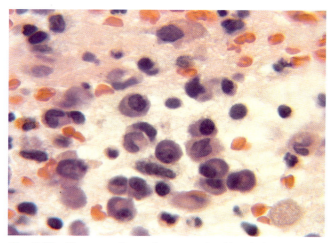
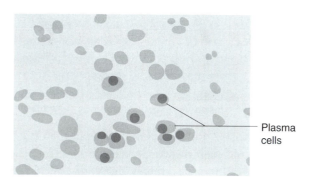

Plasma cells

Fig. 6.13 Plasma cells can be recognized by their peripherally placed nucleus, purple/blue cytoplasm in H&E-stained sections, distinctive 'cartwheel' nuclear chromatin pattern and a clear halo beside the nucleus, which represents the Golgi apparatus of the cell. Their function is antibody production.

Under appropriate stimulation by T lymphocytes, B lymphocytes can differentiate within tissues to form antibody-producing **plasma cells** (Fig. 6.13). These distinctive cells are often easy to recognize histologically and are diagnostic of chronic inflammation, although they may not be prominent in all types of chronic inflammation.

Macrophages

Macrophages are present in all tissues as part of the mononuclear phagocyte system. Some of these cells have become very specialized, but they are all thought to be derived at one time from monocytes. In inflammation, these cells may act as early warning systems which trigger immune responses by presenting foreign antigen to lymphocytes, but most macrophages present in inflamed tissue are derived from blood monocytes which migrate into the affected area. Monocytes also differentiate in tissues under the influence of T-lymphocyte-derived and other mediators to form activated macrophages.

PHAGOCYTE FUNCTIONS

Both polymorphonuclear leukocytes and macrophages are examples of phagocytes. As their name suggests, these cells are primarily concerned

---

Cells of the mononuclear phagocyte system: some examples

■ **Typical tissue macrophages**
- Kupffer's cells (liver)
- Alveolar macrophages (lung)
- Sinus histiocytes (lymph nodes)
- Splenic macrophages
- Histiocytes (connective tissue)

■ **Specialized macrophages**
- Microglia (brain)
- Langerhans' cells (epidermis)
- Dendritic reticulum cells (lymph nodes)

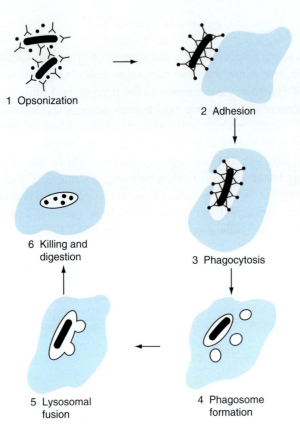

1 Opsonization

2 Adhesion

3 Phagocytosis

4 Phagosome formation

5 Lysosomal fusion

6 Killing and digestion

with phagocytosis – the ingestion of foreign material, micro-organisms or tissue debris, and their destruction (Fig. 6.14). The process of phagocytosis is often followed by a respiratory burst, in which the phagocyte takes in oxygen from its surroundings and produces a surge of reactive oxygen species (ROS). This is an energy-dependent mechanism dependent upon a chain of cytochrome enzymes in the membrane of the phagosome. ROS may also be expelled into the surrounding environment where they may produce bystander damage to endothelial and other cells.

Other tissue cells

Other cells present in tissues are also important in inflammation. Perhaps the most interesting are **mast cells**, which contain large amounts of histamine and other mediators of inflammation. However, **endothelial cells** and **fibroblasts** also play an important role. It is now established that changes in the membrane of both endothelial cells and blood-borne cells such as polymorphs or lymphocytes are required for cell migration to occur.

Types of chronic inflammation

Chronic inflammation is classified by its histological appearance into a number of types. In general these indicate specific causes, but often the pattern is 'non-specific' and will be reported by the pathologist as 'non-specific chronic inflammation' in a biopsy.

ACTIVE CHRONIC INFLAMMATION

Active chronic inflammation (sometimes known as acute-on-chronic inflammation) occurs when an acute inflammatory response is super-imposed on a background of established chronic inflammation. This is commonly seen in the gut and is characterized by the presence of both neutrophils and plasma cells in the same site. Recently, it has been discovered that many cases of gastritis result from an infection on the surface of the stomach with the bacterium *Helicobacter pylori*. This causes active chronic inflammation and often the organisms can be seen on the surface of the epithelial cells lining the stomach (Fig. 6.15).

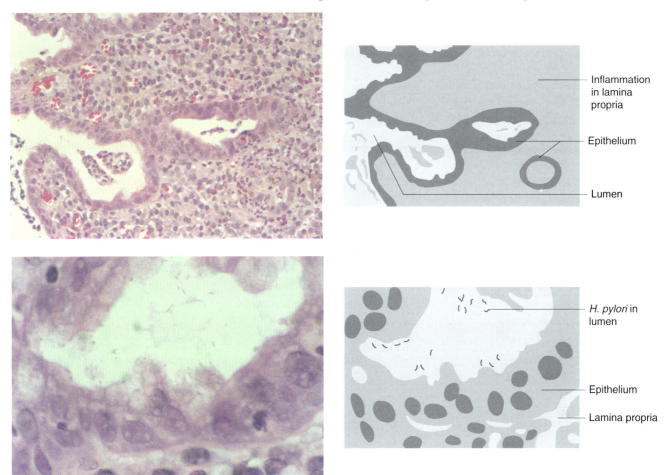

Fig 6.15   Acute-on-chronic inflammation – gastritis resulting from infection by *Helicobacter pylori*.

GRANULOMATOUS INFLAMMATION

A granuloma (Fig. 6.16) is perhaps best defined as an organized collection of macrophages showing evidence of activation in response to an agent localized within a tissue. The key points here are that:

- the agent must be non-removable by phagocytes, but not inert – it must be capable of exciting a cellular response
- there is evidence of macrophage activation with organization into a histological pattern, usually around the inciting agent.

Various types of granuloma are recognized, depending on their histological appearance, but all contain activated macrophages, usually in the form of epithelioid and/or giant cells.

Epithelioid cells are the cells typical of granulomata (Fig. 6.16). They are macrophages which have differentiated to become large cells with elliptical nuclei and copious cytoplasm. On light microscopy the cytoplasm of one epithelioid cell blends with adjacent cells and does not seem to have an

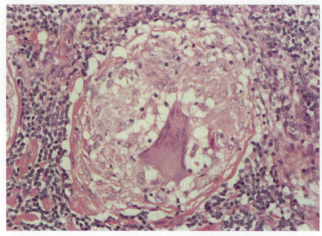
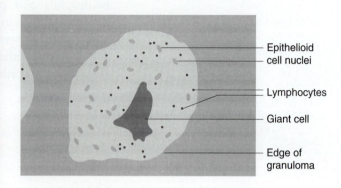

Fig. 6.16   Sarcoid granuloma with epithelioid and giant cells.

edge. Electron microscopy shows that the membranes of epithelioid cells interdigitate and that their intracellular structure suggests that they may have a secretory function. Nevertheless, they remain something of a mystery and just what they do is not completely understood.

Giant cells (Fig. 6.17) are described according to the distribution of nuclei within the cell, as shown above. It was thought that these were simply effete macrophages at the end of their lives which had joined together and had no special function. Recent evidence that they alter levels of their membrane receptors and contain mRNA for cytokines suggests that this may be simplistic.

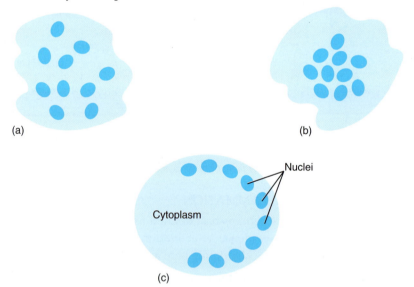

Fig. 6.17   Giant cell types. Giant cells have many nuclei within their cytoplasm and are classified by the location of these nuclei. (a) Foreign body giant cells (dispersed nuclei); (b) Touton giant cell (central nuclei); (c) Langhans' giant cell (horseshoe arrangement of nuclei).

Granuloma formation, maintenance and regression

Granuloma formation requires the presence of an inciting agent which is not removable, but otherwise appears similar to acute inflammation, with neutrophil involvement in the early stages. Aggregation of macrophages and their stimulation by T lymphocytes leads to the local production of lymphokines which cause the macrophages to differentiate into epithelioid and giant cells. TNF-α appears to be the principal cytokine that is responsible for the persistence of epithelioid cells. When macrophages are unable to phagocytose larger particles or handle mycobacteria, they fuse to form large multinucleated giant cells. This plasma membrane fusion is also

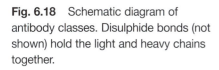

Types of granuloma
- ■ Non-caseating
  - ● Leprosy
  - ● Sarcoidosis
  - ● Beryllium
  - ● Zirconium
- ■ Caseating
  - ● Tuberculosis
- ■ Gummatous
  - ● Syphilis

mediated by TNF and IL1. Thus cytokines play an important role in the pathophysiology of granulomata. Since activated T cells are potent secretors of cytokines, it is easy to understand the link between the development of T-cell immunity and granuloma formation. Resolution of granulomata is less well understood, but it seems likely that removal of the epithelioid and giant cells occurs by apoptosis in simple granulomata, while caseation may occur in complex granulomata. The end-stage is usually fibrosis, although, in some granulomatous diseases, new granuloma formation, regression and fibrosis may occur simultaneously (as in fibrocaseous tuberculosis).

The consequences of granulomatous inflammation can be devastating, with tissue destruction and subsequent fibrosis contributing equally to progressive disease.

The immune response and inflammation

Inflammation is difficult to separate from immunity, in that many immune mechanisms are involved in both acute and chronic inflammation. These are covered in greater detail in textbooks of immunology – see the further reading list at the end of the book. In acute inflammation, the response to the initial injury does not often involve a specific immune response, but this is not the case with chronic inflammation. Even if it is histologically 'non-specific' in appearance, chronic inflammation usually involves highly specific immunological events.

Classically, the immune response is divided into two arms:

- ● the humoral or antibody-mediated response
- ● the cell-mediated immune response.

Humoral immunity

Antibody (Fig. 6.18) is produced in small amounts by all B lymphocytes and expressed in their cell surface membrane, but it is plasma cells derived

Fig. 6.18 Schematic diagram of antibody classes. Disulphide bonds (not shown) hold the light and heavy chains together.

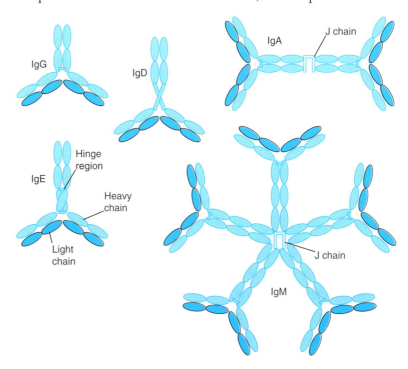

from B lymphocytes which produce the bulk of secreted antibody found in the circulation. Apart from blood and bone marrow, B lymphocytes are found in the lymphoid follicles of spleen, lymph nodes and mucosa-associated lymphoid tissue. These follicles are the powerhouses of humoral immune responses in which B cells come into contact with antigen and are stimulated by cytokines from other follicle cells to divide and form clones of lymphocytes, each of which can produce antibody on re-encountering that antigen.

Cytokines produced by T lymphocytes are responsible for B-lymphocyte differentiation (Fig. 6.19) and different cytokines can switch on the production of antibody classes.

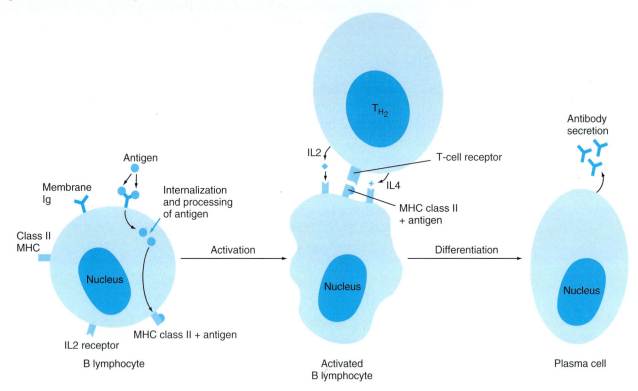

Defects of B lymphocytes lead to deficient antibody production. **Hypogammaglobulinaemia** (low or no IgG) is a serious hereditary condition in which the patients suffer from multiple infections in early life and often die prematurely, but IgA deficiency is quite common and compatible with normal life. The difference reflects the relative importance of these immunoglobulins within the immune system – IgM and IgG can fulfil many of the functions of IgA, but IgG cannot be quite so easily replaced.

Fig. 6.19 B-lymphocyte activation by antigen requires help from T-'helper' lymphocytes. These produce IL2 and IL4 which drive the B lymphocytes to become antibody-producing plasma cells.

Overproduction of antibody can also lead to disease, although it is the overwhelming growth of plasma cells which causes most of the problems in diseases such as **multiple myeloma**, in which neoplastic plasma cells take over the bone marrow and prevent other blood cells being formed.

The complement system

Complement proteins form an important part of the non-specific immune system and are also involved in inflammation via their breakdown products, several of which act as mediators. Activation of complement

(Fig. 6.20) may occur via two separate pathways, one of which (the classic pathway) requires the cooperation of antibody, while the other (the alternative pathway) is activated by micro-organisms.

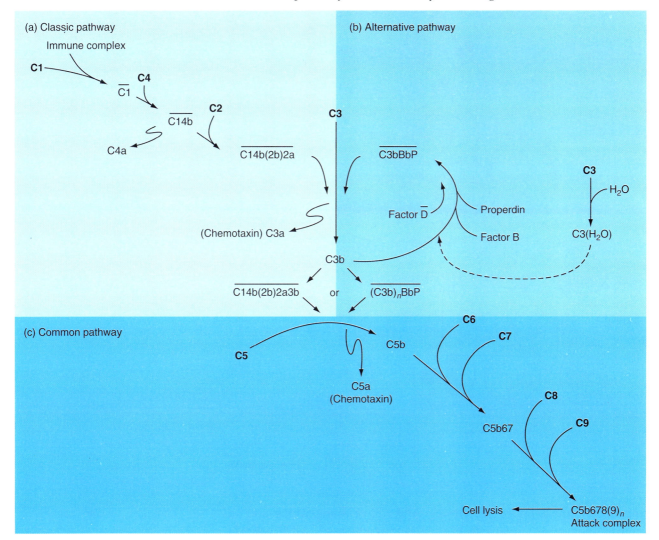

Fig. 6.20 Pathway of complement activation: (a) classic pathway; (b) alternative pathway. The key event is C3 activation to form C3b which triggers formation of the attack complex. C3b may be produced (i) from the classic pathway; (ii) by spontaneous hydrolysis; and (iii) by the action of other proteases.

Cell-mediated immunity

T lymphocytes are the cells which control the immune system – making sure that the immune mechanisms start and stop at the correct time, in the correct sequence. They are a complex group of cells with several subsets defined by their membrane proteins and by their function in producing mediators known as lymphokines. They interact with antigens via cell surface receptors. This T-cell receptor may be of two types: the type I or γ–δ receptor, and the type II or α–β receptor. Most T cells express the type II receptor.

These subsets interact with each other and with other cells to orchestrate immune reactions (Fig. 6.21). T lymphocytes do not produce antibody, but mediate their effects either by direct killing of cells or by inducing effector mechanisms in other cells, particularly macrophages and B lymphocytes.

Inherited T-lymphocyte deficiencies are rare and usually fatal. Until the emergence of the human immunodeficiency virus (HIV), T-lymphocyte deficiencies were very rare. HIV infection and the disease it causes (the

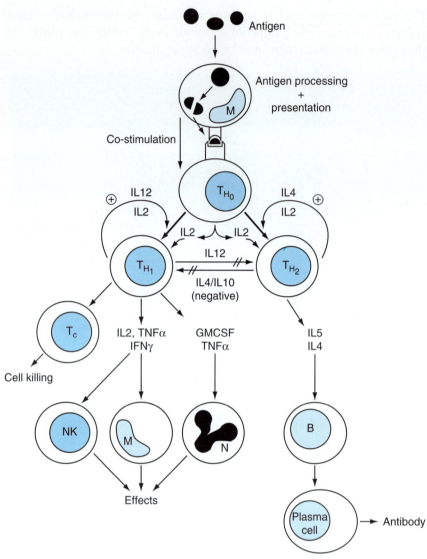

Fig. 6.21 Cell-mediated immunity showing the central role of helper T lymphocytes (T_H) in producing phagocyte activation and antibody production. T_H lymphocytes can be divided into two functional classes depending on their cytokine production. T_{H1} cells support cell-mediated immunity and macrophage activation while T_{H2} cells support B-lymphocyte differentiation to plasma cells.

acquired immune deficiency syndrome, AIDS) have changed this, and an understanding of T-lymphocyte biology is now essential. AIDS patients suffer from increasingly severe fungal and viral infections as their disease progresses and the number of circulating CD4-positive cells decreases (see Chapter 7).

Hypersensitivity

Many diseases in which immunity and inflammation are important fall into the category of hypersensitivity, in which immune responses get out of control and cause tissue damage.

TYPE I HYPERSENSITIVITY

Asthma and **hay fever** are examples of atopy in which IgE combines with antigen on the surface of mast cells to produce an acute inflammatory response (Fig. 6.22). Although neutrophils are present, eosinophils are particularly prominent in the cellular infiltrate that results (Fig. 6.23). The similarities and differences between this atopic response and 'normal' acute inflammation are best explained on the basis of differences in mediator profiles in the two situations.

Classification of hypersensitivity
- **Type I**   Immediate hypersensitivity (anaphylaxis)
  Type II   Cytotoxicity
  Type III   Immune complex formation
  Type IV   Delayed hypersensitivity

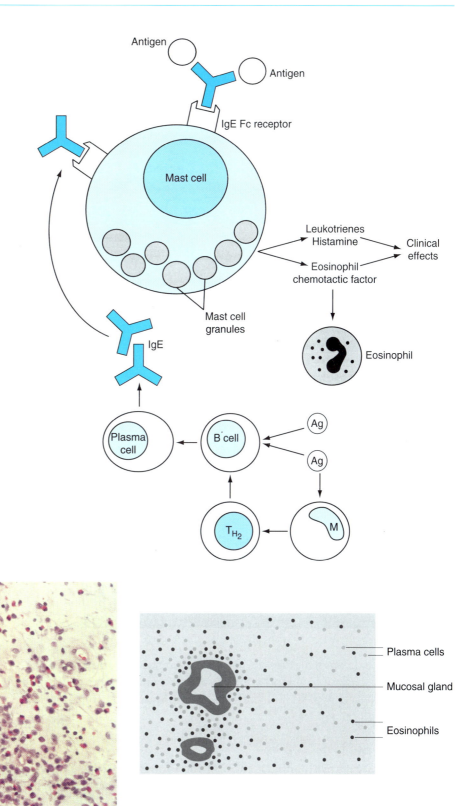

Fig. 6.22 Type I hypersensitivity, showing how the production of IgE leads to mast cell degradation and eosinophil attraction. T-lymphocyte responses are important as they drive this process.

Fig. 6.23 An allergic nasal polyp showing many eosinophils and plasma cells in an oedematous stroma around two mucosal glands.

TYPE II HYPERSENSITIVITY

The combination of antibody with antigen leading to complement activation can result in tissue damage (Fig. 6.24). When the antigen involved is part of the host or present in specific sites such as basement

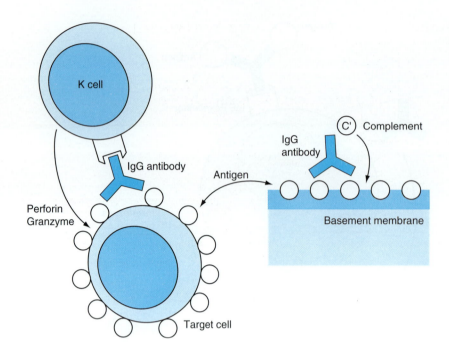

Fig. 6.24 Type II hypersensitivity, showing how antibody combines with antigen to cause inappropriate complement activation on membranes of cells or acts with K cells to kill target cells by lytic enzymes (perforin and granzyme).

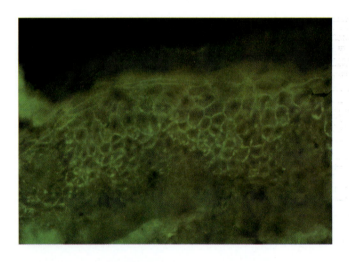

Fig. 6.25 In bullous pemphigus there is deposition of immunoglobulins and complement within the epidermis as shown here.

membrane, the damage that results can be considerable. **Pemphigoid** can be induced by drugs which bind to the basement membrane, as well as by antibodies directed against autoantigens. **Pemphigus** (Fig. 6.25) shows antibody within the epidermis.

TYPE III HYPERSENSITIVITY

Antibody combines with antigen to form **immune complexes**. Local or systemic immune complex formation happens frequently in perfectly healthy people and does not lead to disease. However, if it is prolonged or if large amounts of immune complexes are produced, the result may be inappropriate inflammation and tissue damage. The classic examples of this type of hypersensitivity (Fig. 6.26) are both experimental. If an animal is exposed to antigen and develops a high titre of circulating antibody, local injection of antigen will result in a local inflammation – an **Arthus reaction**. Systemic injection of antigen causes **serum sickness**, a much more serious condition in which shock and death may result.

Fig. 6.26 Type III hypersensitivity: immune complex deposition leads to complement activation and acute inflammation in which neutrophils release enzymes and reactive oxygen intermediates (ROIs) which damage bystander cells.

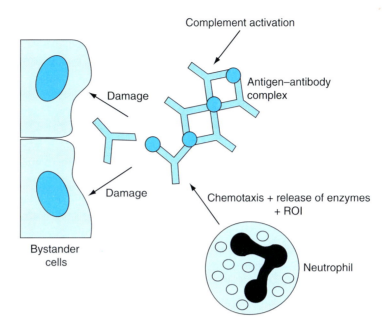

Fig. 6.27 Type IV hypersensitivity: the cell-mediated immune response is exaggerated leading to rapid and sustained macrophage activation which damages cells within the affected tissue.

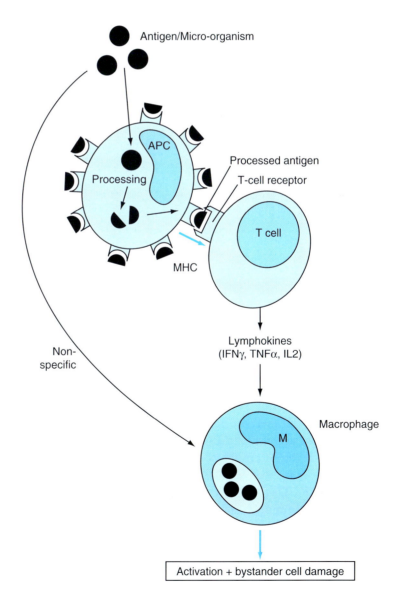

TYPE IV HYPERSENSITIVITY

This form of hypersensitivity (Fig. 6.27) is perhaps best understood as an exaggerated cell-mediated immune response, usually as a result of the sudden availability of a large amount of suitably presented antigen within a tissue. It occurs naturally during therapy for mycobacterial disease when treatment results in a sudden increase in the availability of mycobacterial antigen for presentation to circulating reactive T lymphocytes. The result is a large influx of lymphocytes into the tissue containing the bacteria with an increase in size of the granuloma. This may be sufficient to induce a sudden rise in intracranial pressure and death in patients with cerebral tuberculomas, and increased nerve damage in leprosy patients. Delayed-type hypersensitivity reactions have recently been associated with one subclass of T lymphocyte with a less common membrane antigen receptor type (γ–δ). Type IV reactions have proved useful for determining whether patients have been exposed to tuberculosis or not: they are the basis of the **Mantoux reaction** in which a small amount of soluble mycobacterial antigen is injected intradermally into the forearm (Fig. 6.28).

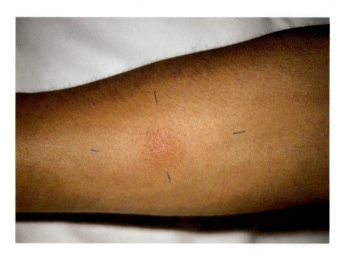

Fig. 6.28   Mantoux reaction at 72 hours. Note the central erythema and the extent of induration indicated by the pen marks on the arm.

Autoimmunity

Both humoral and cell-mediated immune mechanisms are carefully designed not to harm the host by a variety of central and peripheral tolerance mechanisms (Fig. 6.29). However, the potential for breakdown of these complex mechanisms always exists and when it occurs, autoimmune disease results. Examples of autoimmune disease include systemic lupus erythematosus, rheumatoid disease, insulin-dependent diabetes and thyrotoxicosis.

The breakdown of tolerance is closely linked to the genetics of immune response genes and the mechanisms of antigen presentation. Space does not permit a detailed account of this, and the student is referred to the list of further reading at the end of the book.

Autoimmunity may involve humoral or cell-mediated immune responses, or both. The effector mechanisms are similar to those involved in other immune responses (particularly hypersensitivity reactions) and the effects on tissues are equally predictable. By definition, such immune responses are highly specific, and so only one tissue or many may be affected depending upon the distribution of the antigen concerned.

Fig. 6.29 Mechanisms of tolerance: during T-cell development in the thymus cells are selected by positive and negative screening which do not permit self-reactive T cells to survive. Those that do are controlled in the peripheral tissues by similar mechanisms.

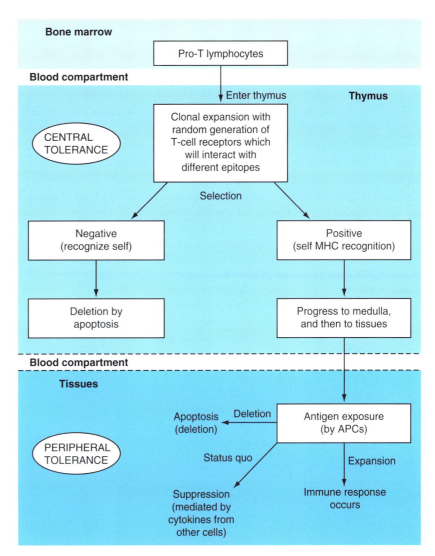

Treatment of hypersensitivity or autoimmunity tends to rely upon immunosuppression. Unfortunately, few drugs are specific to one part of the immune system and general immunosuppression may result in a risk of infection.

Amyloidosis

Amyloidosis is the term used to describe a distinctive type of protein deposition in tissues due to partial proteolysis of certain proteins. Deposits may be localized or systemic. While localized forms of amyloidosis are usually of little consquence, **systemic amyloidosis** can cause death as the deposits interfere with normal organ function. The key features of amyloid are shown in the box.

Systemic amyloid deposits are associated with chronic inflammatory disease or myeloma. The causative proteins are normally present in the plasma, but are often present in excess in patients with amyloid. This is most clearly demonstrated in myeloma, in which the neoplastic plasma cells secrete immunoglobulin light chains which are then deposited in many organs. The condition known as **primary amyloidosis** also results from abnormal light chain secretion. **Secondary** or **reactive amyloid** is deposited in patients with chronic inflammatory disease,

Features of amyloid
- Gives organs pale, waxy appearance
- Amyloid fibrils are composed of molecules with β-pleated sheet configuration
- Extracellular birefringent eosinophilic deposits stain metachromatically with Congo red
- Usually contains amyloid P protein (derived from plasma SAP protein made by the liver)

particularly rheumatoid disease, other autoimmune disorders and tuberculosis. Finally, some inherited conditions such as familial Mediterranean fever and familial amyloidotic polyneuropathy can cause amyloidosis.

The effects of amyloidosis are dealt with in the systematic sections. Virtually any organ may be involved, but heart and kidney involvement are the most serious, leading to cardiac failure and renal failure. Gastrointestinal involvement occurs from the tongue to the rectum – rectal biopsy may be useful for diagnosis. Hepatosplenomegaly may occur and give rise to clinical suspicion.

Localized amyloidosis occurs most notably in the thyroid (calcitonin-derived in medullary C-cell carcinoma), in the cerebral plaques of Alzheimer's disease and in many other tissues (Fig. 6.30).

Substances involved in amyloidosis	
Clinical cause	**Protein involved**
Reactive (secondary)	Serum amyloid protein (AA), secreted as part of the acute phase response
Senile	Prealbumin or atrial naturetic peptide (ASc)
Myeloma and primary	Immunoglobulin light chain (AL) amyloidosis
Haemodialysis-associated	β_2-Microglobulin (AH)

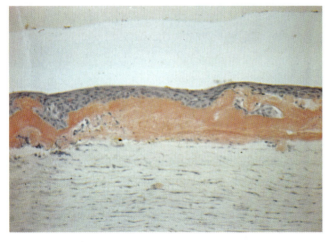 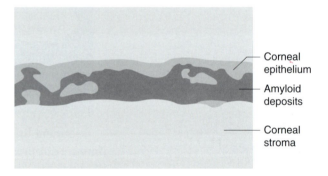

Corneal epithelium

Amyloid deposits

Corneal stroma

Fig. 6.30   Corneal amyloidosis. These localized amyloid deposits stain pink in this Congo red preparation.

Healing and fibrosis

Healing is usually required as a result of injury and therefore follows on naturally from inflammation. In the uncomplicated skin wound or bone fracture, once haemostasis has been established, an acute inflammatory reaction produces an ideal milieu for fibroblasts and endothelial cells to organize thrombus within the wound and lay down granulation tissue. This is then converted to scar tissue and covered by epithelium or converted to new bone as required. The process takes at least six weeks, and it is usually about three months before the tissue assumes its normal strength (Fig. 6.31). Some tissues heal better than others – in general non-specialized tissues in which cell division is common do best (such as skin), while those like muscle and brain do badly.

Fig. 6.31 Phases of wound healing. 1, haemostasis; 2, inflammation; 3, débridement; 4, maturation.

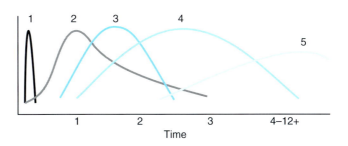

Haemostasis

Damage to blood vessels in wounds usually results in local bleeding into surrounding tissues, but if the wound is a break in the femur several litres of blood may be lost before haemostasis occurs. Haemostasis involves activation of the clotting system of plasma proteins and platelet aggregation. Endothelial damage in traumatized vessels leads to the release of mediators, particularly kinins, which activate aggregation of platelets which then plug small arterioles and are also involved in activation of the coagulation cascade (Fig. 6.32). Vasoconstriction assists this process.

Fig. 6.32 The coagulation cascade showing the extrinsic and intrinsic pathways.

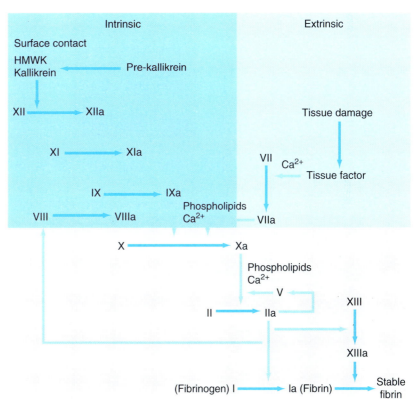

Macrophage enzymes used in débridement of tissues
- Enzymes which break down connective tissue:
  - Hyaluronidase
  - Collagenase
  - Elastase
- Enzymes which destroy dead cells and membranes:
  - Lipases
  - Proteases

Constituents of proliferation phase
- New blood vessels (angiogenesis)
- Fibrosis
- Re-epithelialization or formation of new tissue (e.g. bone)

Débridement

Removal of dead tissue and if necessary foreign material is accomplished by phagocytes which form part of the inflammatory infiltrate. Macrophages are the most significant cells in this process through their ability to secrete many different degradative enzymes, but neutrophils also play their part in liquefying necrotic tissue.

Débridement is effectively site clearance to make way for new building. The old is removed and the site prepared by the inflammatory process to receive new tissue. Often the débridement process is still going on at the top of a wound while the next step – proliferation – begins at the base.

Proliferation of new tissue: granulation

Granulation tissue is in reality part of the process of healing and is seen most often in open skin wounds. The fibrin mesh which forms from the inflammatory exudate is organized by migrating fibroblasts and endothelial cells in a distinctive histological and clinical pattern.

Similar processes occur in broken bones, in which a mixture of vascular granulation tissue with osteoid formation known as **callus** forms around the broken bone ends (Figs 6.33 and 6.34).

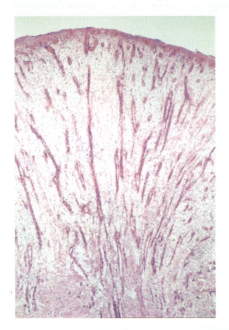

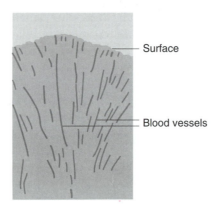

Fig. 6.33 Histopathological appearance of a granulating wound. Note the direction of the blood vessels which are oriented from the bottom to the top of the wound and the pale, oedematous texture of the intervening tissue.

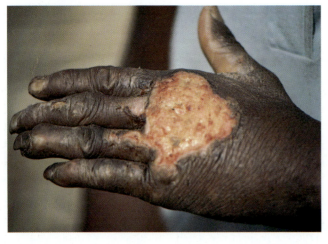

Fig. 6.34 A granulating wound following a burn one week previously. There is epithelialization at the edge of the wound.

Healing and inflammation are required to go hand in hand for early repair of damaged tissue. The hallmarks of healing are fibroblast growth, formation of new blood vessels and replacement of injured tissue by collagen. In recent years, several fibrogenic cytokines (Table 6.1) have been described which lead to fibroblast growth and collagen synthesis. Transforming growth factor-β (TGF-β) and platelet-derived growth factor (PDGF) are produced by the monocyte/macrophage family and are the most potent fibroblast growth factors. IL1 and TNF-α stimulate fibroblasts indirectly by inducing other secondary cytokines. This IL1 induces fibroblasts to secrete PDGF which then stimulates the cell to enter the cell cycle.

Table 6.1   Cytokines involved in healing and repair

Cytokine	Fibroblast proliferation	Connective tissue proliferation
IL1	Increase	Increase
TNF	Increase	Increase and decrease
TGF-β	Proliferation and inhibition	Increase
PDGF	Proliferation and inhibition	Increase
IFN	Decrease	Increase

IFN, interferon: IL1, interleukin-1; PDGF, platelet-derived growth factor; TGF-β, transforming growth factor-β; TNF, tumour necrosis factor.

Fig. 6.35 The influence of oxygen tension on the process of organization.

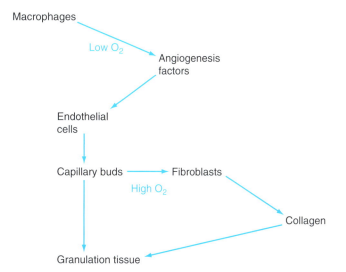

New blood vessel formation and collagen synthesis is also promoted by TGF-β (Fig. 6.35). Its presence has been associated with clinical states where fibrosis is a predominant feature, such as pulmonary fibrosis, peritoneal fibrosis, pneumoconiosis, sarcoidosis and fibrosis following peritoneal dialysis and immunotherapy. When TGF-β is injected into mice, endothelial cell proliferation and movement as well as basement membrane dissolution have been observed. The endothelial cells then move along the disintegrated membrane to form capillary buds. Recent research has implicated another important factor for the proliferation of endothelium. Vascular endothelial growth factor (VEGF), also known as

Fig. 6.36 Re-epithelialization occurs as epithelial cells migrate across the granulation tissue filling the wound.

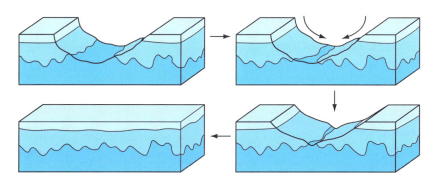

vascular permeability factor (VPF), is produced by macrophages and is the most potent stimulator of vascular proliferation yet found. The formation of new blood vessels and fibroblasts lead to the classic granulation tissue seen after local injury (Fig. 6.36). To prevent excessive collagen formation and to regulate the healing process interferons-α and -β turn off collagen gene expression.

Maturation and remodelling

Tissues under mechanical stress such as skin and bone undergo a realignment of collagen, fibroblasts and bone over a period of several months. Gradually the strength of the wound and its likeness to surrounding tissue increase. This process of maturation and remodelling requires energy and turnover of tissue components. It is not unusual to see mitoses and apoptoses in such sites, and this can give rise to diagnostic difficulty for the histopathologist if the history is not clear.

Disorders of healing

Many factors affect healing. The site, extent and type of wound, the health of the tissue and the effect of treatment are each important determinants of outcome (Fig. 6.37).

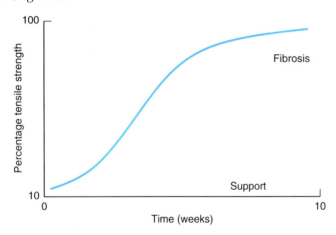

Fig. 6.37 Wound strength increases over the first 3 months.

Deficient healing may be due to infection of the wound (particularly important), or to a poor healing environment as a result of coexisting disease or poor nutrition, for instance. In skin wounds overlying joints and in bone fractures, mobility of the wound is a major problem. Successful healing often requires immobilization of the wound site by sutures or even plaster.

Occasionally, excessive healing responses occur, leading to disfiguring keloid formation in skin or contractures in other tissues.

CHRONIC ULCERATION

Chronic ulceration is the result of prolonged deficient skin healing and has as many causes as deficient healing itself. However, certain types of chronic ulcer are recognized and some are very common. An old woman hobbling along with bandages around her calves is a common site in Britain, and more often than not there is a varicose ulcer under the bandages. Varicose ulcers are an example of vascular ulceration due to poor blood supply or chronic venous congestion at the affected site.

Fig. 6.38 Varicose ulcer.

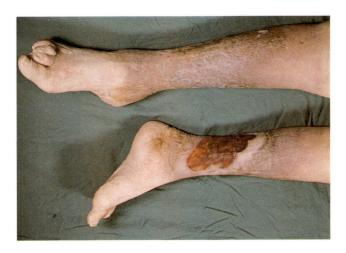

Neurogenic ulcers are also common, the classic example being the leprosy patient who has lost sensation in hands and feet, and who allows an injury which is not painful to turn into a chronic ulcer. this process is not helped by damage to the autonomic nervous system in the affected tissue, which comprises healing by interfering with the vasculature (Fig. 6.38).

The vasculature can also be compromised by pressure. Pressure sores are a difficult problem to prevent in patients who are immobilized for long periods of time or who become very weak and unable to move properly. They are more difficult to treat.

Metabolic abnormalities such as diabetes may lead to ulceration though a combination of vascular and neuropathic damage, together with systemic effects on immunity and local cell metabolism.

Finally, the increased cell turnover in skin at the margin of chronic ulcers appears to make the epidermal cells more susceptible than usual to carcinogens. Malignant transformation of ulcers which have been present for many years is a definite risk, albeit a rare event (Fig. 6.39).

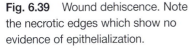

Factors affecting wound healing
- Local
  - Oxygen and blood supply
  - Infection
  - Impaired venous drainage
- General
  - Nutritional status
  - Age
  - Diabetes mellitus

Fig. 6.39 Wound dehiscence. Note the necrotic edges which show no evidence of epithelialization.

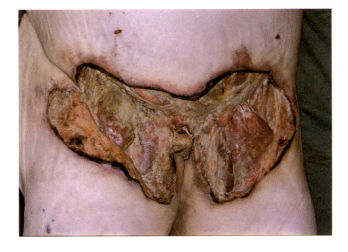

Bone healing

Healing of fractures is best regarded as a variant of the process described above (Fig. 6.40). In reality there are few differences – tissue damage leads to inflammation and there is usually haematoma formation around the

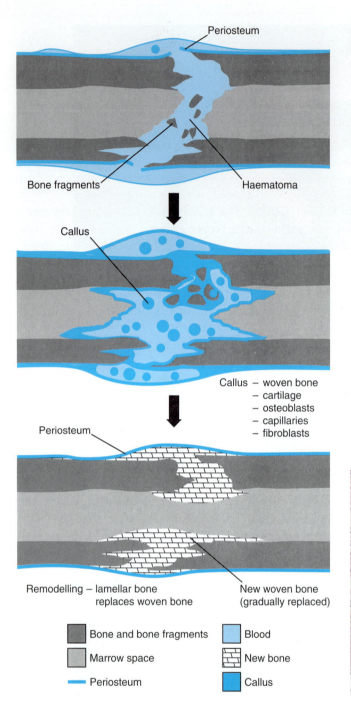

Periosteum

Bone fragments

Haematoma

Callus

Callus – woven bone
– cartilage
– osteoblasts
– capillaries
– fibroblasts

Periosteum

Remodelling – lamellar bone
replaces woven bone

New woven bone
(gradually replaced)

Bone and bone fragments   Blood

Marrow space   New bone

Periosteum   Callus

Fig. 6.40 Bone healing is a variant of tissue healing: for ganulation tissue read callus.

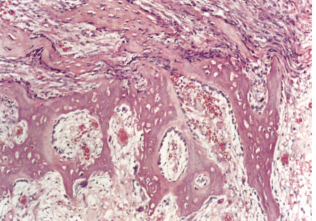

Fig. 6.41 Callus at the edge of a healing fracture.

broken ends of the bone due to rupture of blood vessels within and around the bone. The process of exudation produces intense oedema around the wound which is usually very painful. This helps to immobilize the wound and prevents further tissue damage by the bone ends moving about. The haematoma is invaded first by neutrophils (acute inflammation) and then by macrophages which begin an extensive demolition (débridement) phase. Small bone fragments are resorbed by osteoclasts, stimulated into activity by locally produced cytokines.

As the inflammatory process wanes, organization of the haematoma takes place with fibroblast and endothelial cell proliferation. Osteoid

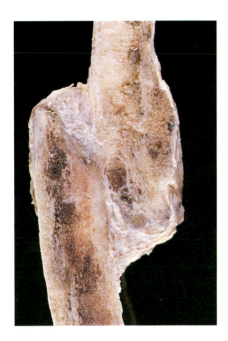

Fig. 6.42 Mass of callus.

appears as it is laid down by osteoblasts in the organizing haematoma, which is now known as **callus (Fig. 6.41)**. This may be thought of as the bony form of granulation tissue – it provides a suitable environment in which new bone can form to unite the fracture in a similar way to which granulation tissue allows epithelialization of skin wounds.

The final stage is remodelling, with haversian canals being laid down along stress lines as weight-bearing commences. Even dislocated bone ends can be stabilized by a mass of callus (Fig. 6.42) and will be remodelled to form a continuous shaft of bone.

Chapter 7　　Multisystem disease

Learning objectives

To appreciate and understand the aetiology, pathogenesis, effects and complications of six important systemic diseases:

❑ Human immunodeficiency virus (HIV) infection and aquired immune deficiency syndome (AIDS)

❑ Tuberculosis

❑ Sarcoidosis

❑ Rheumatoid disease

❑ Systemic lupus erythematosus (SLE)

❑ Septic shock

The aim of this chapter is to present six disease states which affect multiple tissues and do not fit the pattern of the subsequent chapters which deal in detail with individual organs or tissues. We have chosen diseases which highlight the interaction of inflammation-related pathogenic mechanisms with tissues to produce different effects. Many other diseases could of course be added to this list, but these are covered under the systematic sections into which they perhaps fit better.

The acquired immune deficiency syndrome

The acquired immune deficiency syndrome (AIDS) is a new disease, first seen in the late 1970s. It is the final phase of a chronic disease (**HIV disease**) that starts with infection by one of the human immunodeficiency viruses (HIV-1 and HIV-2). It is characterized by a progressive decline in cell-mediated immunity, the consequent development of opportunistic infections and tumours, and death (Fig. 7.1).

Aetiology and epidemiology

HIV-1 infection is now a global epidemic, with more than 12 million people infected. Although AIDS was first noted in homosexual men in industrialized countries, it is in developing countries (in Africa and Asia notably) that the major spread of infection is taking place. HIV-2 is mainly restricted to West Africa. Transmission of HIV occurs by four routes, the most important being heterosexual intercourse.

Pathogenesis

HIVs are RNA retroviruses: they incorporate their genes into a host cell's genome after making a matching DNA copy by means of their enzyme

Fig. 7.1 Course of HIV disease.

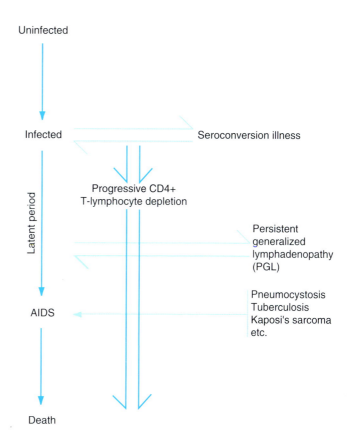

Routes of transmission of HIV
- Heterosexual intercourse
- Anal sexual intercourse
- Mother to child (pre- or perinatal)
- Transfusion or injection of infected blood or blood products

reverse transcriptase. This occurs after entry of HIV into a cell by binding of viral surface glycoprotein (gp120) to a CD4 receptor on the host cell. The cells that carry CD4 receptors are T-helper lymphocytes and macrophages – the two cornerstones of host cellular immunity – and it is impossible to remove the HIV from an infected cell (that is, to sterilize the infection).

Once HIV is incorporated into T-helper lymphocytes, the cells are progressively destroyed. The major sites of this action are the lymph nodes with the macrophage-like follicular dendritic cells being the reservoir of HIV infection. The precise mechanisms of cell destruction are still debated. The count of CD4+ T lymphocytes in the blood is an index of this depletion. Normal adult values are $500–2000 \times 10^6/l$. It is a mark of the substantial normal immune reserve that most of the important HIV-associated opportunistic diseases do not appear until the blood CD4+ T lymphocyte count is $200 \times 10^6/l$ (Fig. 7.2).

Before the phase of AIDS is reached, there are several defined clinicopathological states (Fig. 7.1).

- The initial infection is often marked by a short infectious mononucleosis-like illness (**seroconversion illness**). Plasma HIV viraemia peaks and the CD4+ T-lymphocyte count temporarily falls (Fig. 7.2).
- Then follows the **latent asymptomatic period**, which may last up to a decade, when the T-cell count drops but plasma viraemia is minimal.
- Interrupting this phase, many patients manifest a temporary hyperplastic immune reaction with enlargement of most lymph node groups. This **persistent generalized lymphadenopathy (PGL)** is histologically characteristic (Fig. 7.3).
- Finally, as the cellular immune system collapses, plasma viraemia returns and the **AIDS-characterizing diseases** develop.

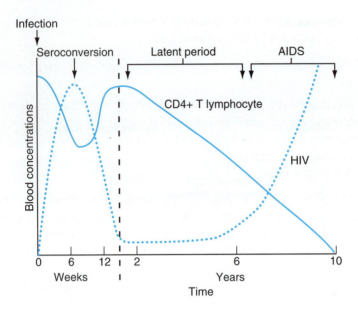

Fig. 7.2 Chronology of concentrations of CD4+ T lymphocytes and HIV in peripheral blood during HIV disease.

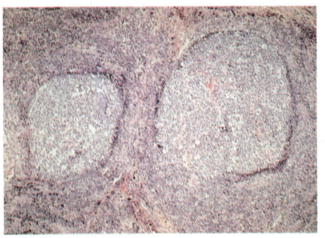

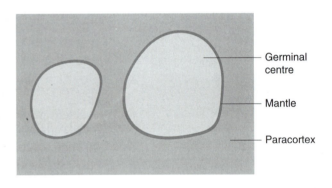

Fig. 7.3 Persistent generalized lymphadenopathy (PGL) lymph node: expanded hyperplastic germinal centres and little surrounding mantle, representing an immune response (ineffective) to HIV infection.

The diagnosis of HIV infection is readily made by serology; antibodies to HIV appear within 3–6 weeks of infection.

Pathology

Patients with AIDS usually have multiple diseases affecting multiple organs. Three important principles determine the patterns of disease.

- First, the more virulent infections (such as tuberculosis) appear before the less virulent (such as cytomegalovirus and *Mycobacterium avium*).
- Second, whilst some of the infections in AIDS are recently acquired (for example *Pneumocystis carinii*, *Cryptosporidium parvum* and the pyogenic bacteria), many are reactivations of infections that have lain latent and asymptomatic in the body. These include *Mycobacterium tuberculosis*, cytomegalovirus and *Toxoplasma gondii*.
- Third, HIV disease differs geographically according to the dominant latent and acquired infections: in the tropics, tuberculosis is the main associated infection, whilst in industrialized countries it is *Pneumocystis carinii*. Some HIV-associated infections are very focal: the fungus

Diseases that characterize AIDS in HIV-infected people

■ Opportunistic infections
- Viruses
  - Cytomegalovirus
  - JC virus
  - Herpes simplex
- Bacteria
  - *Mycobacterium tuberculosis*
  - *Mycobacterium avium*
  - Gram-negative rods (such as non-typhoid salmonellae)
  - Recurrent pyogenic pneumonias
- Fungi
  - *Pneumocystis carinii*
  - *Cryptococcus neoformans*
  - *Candida albicans*
  - *Penicillium marneffei*
- Protozoa
  - *Cryptosporidium parvum*
  - *Toxoplasma gondii*

■ Opportunistic tumours
- Kaposi's sarcoma
- High-grade non-Hodgkin's lymphoma

■ Direct effects of HIV
- HIV giant cell encephalitis
- HIV enteropathy

Penicillium marneffei is only acquired in south-east Asia, but is found in a high proportion of AIDS patients there.

Common to most patients is severe wasting; this is a complex process involving:

- gut infection by diarrhoea- and malabsorption-inducing agents such as *Cryptosporidium parvum* (Fig. 7.4) and HIV itself
- the hypermetabolic state induced by infections and the fever that all AIDS patients experience
- reduced caloric intake.

The **lungs** are major targets of opportunistic infection. The fungus *Pneumocystis carinii* proliferates to fill the alveoli and, in conjunction with an interstitial pneumonitis, produces hypoxaemia that is fatal without treatment (Fig. 7.5). Bacterial pneumonias (often due to streptococci) are frequent in AIDS and are often the final cause of death. Bacteraemias originating from the bowel, such as non-typhoid salmonelloses, are increasingly recognized as major diseases in AIDS.

The **central nervous system** is affected in more than half of AIDS patients. Cerebral toxoplasmosis causes multiple inflammatory lesions that raise the intracranial pressure (Fig. 7.6). This can also be mimicked clinically by cerebral lymphoma. *Cryptococcus neoformans* meningoencephalitis is another common disease, the fungus proliferating along and around the blood vessels without exciting a marked inflammatory response. The aetiology of the **HIV-associated dementia complex** is unclear. Many patients have widespread atrophy of grey and white matter associated with demyelination; and there is the lesion unique to HIV disease, a multinucleate giant cell encephalitis (Fig. 7.7), the giant cells developing from microglia (= macrophages in the brain) and containing HIV. Finally, a reactivation of JC virus, acquired universally during childhood, causes progressive multifocal leukoencephalopathy by destroying oligodendrocytes and myelin within the brain.

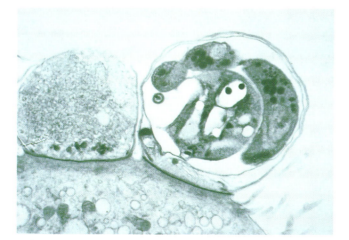

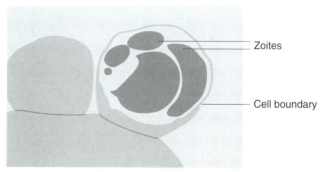

Fig. 7.4 Cryptosporidiosis: electron micrograph of a duodenal enterocyte with several zoites just within the cytoplasmic boundary.

Several infections are widespread throughout the lymphoreticular system (those organs containing abundant macrophages and lymphocytes, i.e. lymph nodes, gut mucosa, liver, spleen and bone marrow) because they are intracellular pathogens. These include *Mycobacterium avium,*

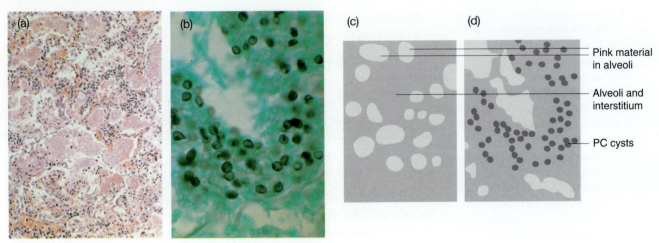

Fig. 7.5 *Pneumocystis carinii* pneumonia (PCP): (a, c) alveoli filled with pink-staining material; (b, d) *Pneumocystis carinii* cysts (high power).

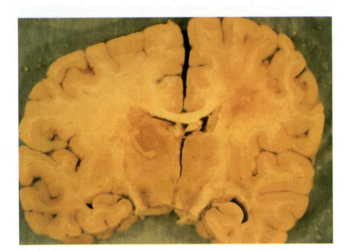

Fig. 7.6 Cerebral toxoplasmosis: space-occupying effect of the infection with secondary compression of ventricles.

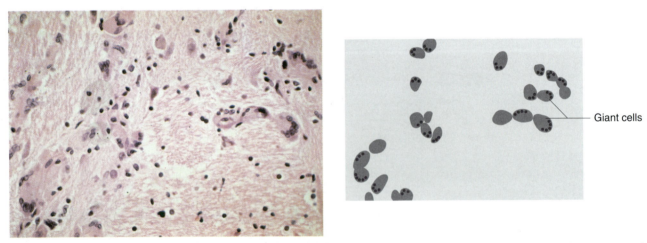

Fig. 7.7 HIV multinucleate giant cell encephalitis: nodule of giant cells within the white matter, which can be shown to contain virus.

Mycobacterium tuberculosis and *Penicillium marneffei*. *Mycobacterium avium* is relatively avirulent and simply proliferates to fill up macrophages (Fig. 7.8) and form space-occupying lesions. On the other hand, tuberculosis in AIDS patients is aggressive, miliary, necrotizing and very multibacillary – it is a much more virulent infection.

Fig. 7.8 *Mycobacterium avium* infection in a lymph node. There are vast numbers of acid-fast bacilli within macrophages and no necrosis.

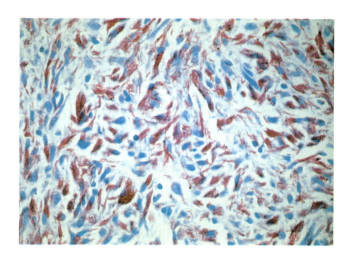

One of the most common HIV-associated infections is **cytomegalovirus (CMV)**, which is a universal latent infection. When immunosuppression is severe, many organs such as the lung, gut and eye show epithelial and endothelial cells with large intranuclear inclusions of CMV. This viral proliferation is not always pathogenic, but when it is associated with tissue necrosis, the CMV is cytopathic.

The two tumours associated with HIV disease are opportunist in that they are also encountered in patients with other causes of immunodepression, such as drug-induced states. **Kaposi's sarcoma** is a peculiar tumour-like proliferation of endothelial cells. It forms plaques and nodules in the skin, and also in the viscera such as lymph nodes, lungs, mouth and gut. As the lesions are very oedematous, pulmonary Kaposi's sarcoma is another important cause of death in AIDS.

The other important tumour in HIV disease is high-grade **B-cell (non-Hodgkin's) lymphoma**. Contrary to the usual nodal distribution in uninfected people, HIV-associated lymphoma is strikingly extranodal in location, with a high prevalence of primary intracerebral lymphoma.

Children and HIV infection

Children are infected pre- or perinatally from their mothers (see box on p. 145), and their development is affected. Failure to thrive, increased susceptibility to the common childhood illnesses, HIV encephalopathy, pneumocystis and bacterial pneumonias are typical events. Many die in the first two years of life.

Effects of treatment

Currently, there is no proven effective therapy directed against HIV itself, although the reverse transcriptase inhibitor **azidothymidine** (AZT) is commonly used. Specific therapy therefore consists of preventing opportunistic infections (prophylaxis), and treating infections and tumours when they develop.

As with all powerful chemotherapy, side effects are considerable. For example, AZT causes marrow suppression and anaemia. Anti-pneumocystis agents can delay or prevent lung infection but encourage the proliferation of the agent elsewhere, resulting in pneumocystosis of lymph nodes, bowel and even brain. Many of the anti-infection drugs are hepatotoxic, and liver biopsy is often needed to distinguish a drug reaction from an infection or tumour in the liver. Several infections are resistant to chemotherapy (*Mycobacterium avium* and cryptosporidiosis), although toxoplasmosis is highly sensitive. The responses of Kaposi's sarcoma and lymphoma to therapy are poor.

Ultimately, when the host's cell-mediated immunity is destroyed, no treatment can prevent the consequences of having ineffective defences against the multitude of infections by which we are surrounded.

Tuberculosis

Tuberculosis remains one of the world's most serious diseases. Although it virtually ceased to be a problem in many industrialized countries several decades ago, it has always been rife in developing countries with an annual estimated prevalence of around 4 million clinical cases, of whom some 25% will die of the disease. In the last few years, the trend of decreasing tuberculosis numbers in industrialized countries has reversed, and infection with highly antibiotic-resistant strains has become a significant clinical problem, particularly in North America.

Aetiology

Tuberculosis is a chronic infectious disease caused by *Mycobacterium tuberculosis* and characterized by necrotic granulomatous lesions with

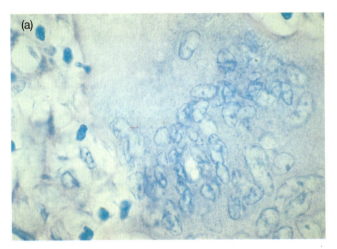
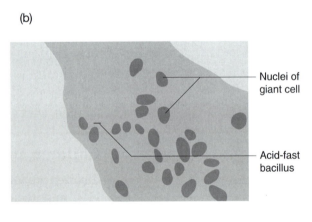

Nuclei of giant cell

Acid-fast bacillus

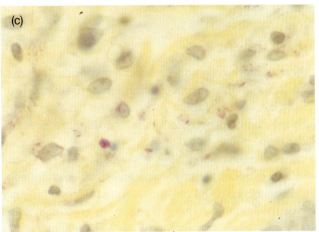

Fig. 7.9 (a, b) An acid-fast bacillus within a Langhans' giant cell (Ziehl–Neelsen stain). (c) Acid-fast bacilli in sputum (Ziehl–Neelsen stain).

Table 7.1 The annual incidence of active pulmonary tuberculosis cases per 100 000 of population

Area	Incidence
Africa	165
Asia	110
Latin America	80
Europe	24
North America	7

In some inner cities of the USA, the incidence is much greater than the overall figure for North America.

Factors predisposing to tuberculosis infection and disease
- Childhood and old age
- Race: African, Indian, North American Indian
- Impaired cell-mediated immunity: HIV infection, malignancy, diabetes, liver cirrhosis

---

tissue destruction. Of the dozens of mycobacterial species, most are environmental saprophytes. Two species are particularly adapted to humans – *Mycobacterium tuberculosis* and *Mycobacterium leprae*, the agent of leprosy (see below). Mycobacteria are aerobic Gram-positive bacilli with a waxy cell wall. They are referred to as **acid-fast bacilli** since they resist decolourization by acid after staining by fuchsin as in the Ziehl–Neelsen method (Fig. 7.9).

Tuberculosis is transmitted via inhalation of bacilli coughed up from a person with active pulmonary tuberculosis (by far the most important route). Oral ingestion and inoculation are much less common. The global prevalence of tuberculosis infection is more than one billion, most of those infected living in the developing world (Table 7.1). In the majority, the infection is latent and asymptomatic. Eight million incident (i.e. new) cases of tuberculosis present annually, with some three million deaths. In the tropics, tuberculosis is a major cause of premature mortality. In England and Wales in 1991, the incidence of tuberculosis was less than 10 000 cases with a fatality rate of less than 600.

Mycobacterium tuberculosis is a highly virulent organism capable of causing disease in anyone. However, certain groups of people are more susceptible to infection and consequent disease (see box). Although genetic factors are important, there is no single gene that conveys resistance to tuberculosis.

Pathogenesis

The course of tuberculosis is shown in Fig. 7.10. The initial infection causes lung and hilar node lesions. In 90% of those infected these heal spontaneously, but tubercle bacilli usually remain latent within the body, probably for a lifetime. The clinical sequelae within five years of the initial infection are termed **primary tuberculosis**.

The most frequent later event is **adult** (or **post-primary**) **pulmonary tuberculosis**. It is considered to be a reactivation of the latent infection due

---

Fig. 7.10 The course of tuberculous infection.

Features of primary tuberculosis: organs affected
- **Primary complex:** local lesion + larger lesion in draining node, e.g. lung + hilar node, mouth + neck node
- **Localized (end-organ) lesions:** adrenal, kidney, testis, fallopian tube, bone, brain
- **Miliary tuberculosis:** lung, liver, spleen, nodes, meninges

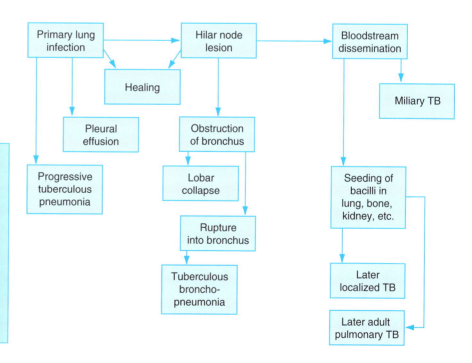

to a drop in the host defences against the tubercle bacillus. Under normal circumstances, this occurs as a 5–10% lifetime risk among those who have had earlier primary tuberculosis. Infection with HIV dramatically increases this risk of developing overt tuberculosis to 10% per year – hence tuberculosis is the most important opportunistic infection associated with HIV infection in developing countries.

PRIMARY INFECTION

Lung infection

Inhaled bacilli lodge in the alveoli under the pleura in any lobe, multiply and initiate the primary lesion. Bacilli are carried by lymphatics to the local lymph hilar nodes and cause a further lesion. Thus the **primary complex** consists of local plus nodal tuberculous lesions. Usually, the nodal lesion is the larger (Fig. 7.11). The appearance of these lesions is a white or yellow solid mass – cheese-like, hence the descriptive term **'caseous'**. In time, they usually heal, becoming smaller and leaving a fibrous scar. Often this calcifies, and residual subpleural calcification on radiography or seen at postmortem examination is a mark of earlier primary tuberculosis.

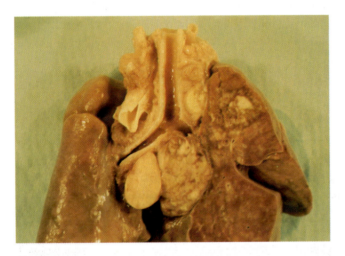

Fig. 7.11   Primary tuberculosis in a child.

Gut infection

A person ingesting tubercle bacilli can acquire a similar primary complex. Before the introduction of milk pasteurization, when tuberculous mastitis of cattle was common, drinking milk transmitted *Mycobacterium bovis* infection. The local lesion was in the mucosa and wall of the terminal ileum, with mesenteric nodes affected. This is now rare, and the more frequent disease is a small lesion in the oral mucosa associated with an enlarged tuberculous cervical lymph node.

Skin infection

Inoculation of *Mycobacterium tuberculosis* through the skin can cause infection. Surgeons and pathologists who dissect tuberculous tissues can acquire a skin ulcer by this route.

SPREAD OF PRIMARY INFECTION

In most people, the primary complex heals, but a minority develop further primary disease. The lung lesion can progress to a generalized pneumonia. The tuberculous inflammation in the hilar node can erode through bronchi, arteries and veins to disseminate the infection. Spread into the bronchus and inhalation of bacilli produce tuberculous bronchopneumonia with much caseation. Pleural effusions are often present early in the course of primary tuberculosis. Lymphatic spread to the local nodes may cause bronchial compression and causes collapse of the lobe.

Dissemination of bacilli in small numbers via a pulmonary artery or vein is a normal event in primary tuberculosis. It provides the source of later reactivation of infection (see Fig. 7.10). This may be in the lung itself in adulthood (see 'Pulmonary tuberculosis'), or in other organs (see box on p. 151).

Localized tuberculosis

The typical appearance of tuberculosis is of a white or yellow caseous mass lesion replacing the normal architecture. In the kidney, this can progress until the entire organ is a non-functioning mass of caseation, the infection retained within the renal capsule. Such a lesion is called a **tuberculoma**. In the spinal column, tuberculosis progressively destroys the vertebral bone which collapses and becomes angulated, often with compression of the spinal cord (**Pott's disease of the spine**).

Miliary tuberculosis

Heavy bloodstream infection results in disseminated, **miliary tuberculosis** (from the Latin *milium*, a seed). The lungs, liver, spleen and lymph nodes are studded with 1–2 mm white nodules (Fig. 7.12). The meninges are often infected this way, producing **tuberculous meningitis**. Without treatment, miliary tuberculosis is fatal.

Fig. 7.12 Miliary tuberculosis. Note the many small white dots of caseating granulomata throughout the lung, as well as the larger collections.

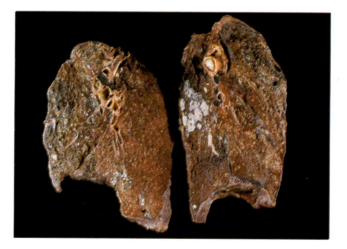

Clinically, the 90% of infected people with primary tuberculosis who heal without further progression or miliary disease are usually unaware of their infection.

Pathology

The lesions of tuberculosis have a characteristic histology. The most important feature is the presence of **caseating granulomata**, consisting of caseating necrosis surrounded by epithelioid cells, Langhans' giant cells and lymphocytes. Acid-fast bacilli are usually few in number (Fig. 7.13).

Tuberculosis in the immunosuppressed host is different from the usual course of the disease. Non-reactive tuberculosis is characterized by

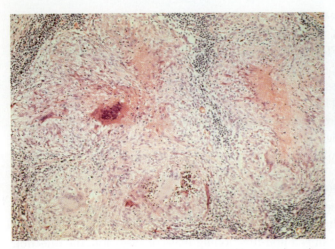

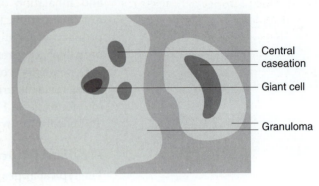

Central caseation

Giant cell

Granuloma

Fig. 7.13   Usual histology of tuberculosis with caseating giant cell granuloma.

multiple foci of necrosis throughout the lymphoreticular system (Figs 7.14 and 7.15). The histology is not that of activated macrophages, but of a rim of vacuolated macrophages, without giant cell formation, with necrosis containing much nuclear debris of dead cells. The **Ziehl–Neelsen stain** shows enormous numbers of acid-fast bacilli: unlike the heavy bacillation seen in *Mycobacterium avium* disease (see AIDS), these are extracellular bacilli.

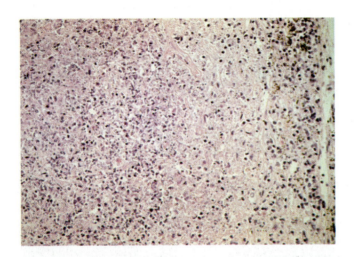

Fig. 7.14   Non-reactive tuberculosis showing granular necrosis with no granuloma formation.

The pathogenesis of the lesions has been described in Chapter 6. Langhans' and epithelioid cells form from migrating monocyte-derived macrophages under the control of lymphokines secreted by T-helper lymphocytes and autocrine cytokine production by epithelioid cells already present in the lesions. The mechanism of caseation is not known, but is thought to be linked closely with the strength of the delayed hypersensitivity response to the tubercle bacillus. Fibrosis follows successful antibiotic treatment or spontaneous healing of the primary focus.

Pulmonary tuberculosis

This is the major clinical problem of tuberculosis. It affects adults and is in most cases a reactivation of the latent infection. Reinfection from another

Fig. 7.15 Non-reactive tuberculosis (Ziehl–Neelsen stain): large numbers of extracellular acid-fast bacilli are present in the necrotic areas.

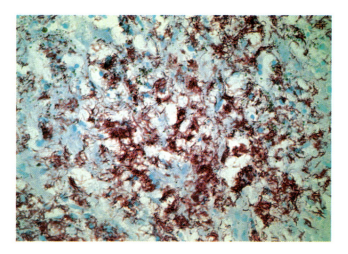

tuberculous patient also occurs. The lung lesion differs from that of primary tuberculosis. Robert Koch (who discovered the tubercle bacillus in 1882) observed a parallel pattern of experimental tuberculosis in the guinea pig.

The lung lesion is usually in the apex. There is rapid expansion of a caseous mass, which liquefies and is coughed up after communicating with a bronchus. At the same time, there is a vigorous peripheral fibroblastic response. The result is a ragged cavity: **cavitating fibrocaseous tuberculosis**. This time, the hilar nodes are not so affected by tuberculosis as they were in primary disease. As in the Koch phenomenon, this reflects the greater degree of immunity and hypersensitivity in the postprimary disease through previous infection.

The clinical effects of pulmonary tuberculosis are cough, fever and wasting. These patients are the source of tuberculosis infection to others.

Treatment

Modern antimicrobial agents are bactericidal and effective. The host macrophages resolve the lesions by phagocytosis of necrotic debris, leaving some residual scarring. However, not every tubercle bacillus in the body is killed: some may lie dormant in caseous material and reactivate after therapy stops. Recently, primary multidrug resistance of tuberculosis has become important in some countries (particularly the USA) rendering the management of tuberculosis more complicated.

On treatment, it is well recognized that in some patients the tuberculous lesions – pulmonary, or end-organ such as a cerebral tuberculoma – actually enlarge and worsen before resolving. This oedema and cellular infiltration are probably a delayed hypersensitivity reaction analogous to the phenomenon occurring in certain forms of leprosy on treatment.

Sarcoidosis

Sarcoidosis is a multisystem granulomatous disease of unknown origin in which granulomata are formed within many tissues. The clinical presentation and outcome are dependent upon the tissues affected and the severity of the disease. Sarcoidosis results in the death of about 15% of those affected and, as a chronic disease, causes much more morbidity than its low incidence would suggest. The lung and mediastinal lymph nodes are the most commonly affected sites, but skin, central nervous system and eye are also relatively common sites for sarcoid granulomata.

Aetiology: current hypotheses

The cause of sarcoidosis remains a matter of debate with protagonists for viral, bacterial and immunological alternatives. Since granulomata usually occur in response to an agent which cannot be removed from a tissue by macrophages, the concept of a chronic bacterial infection has always been strongly supported. However, recent use of very sensitive polymerase chain reaction methods to look for specific organisms such as mycobacteria have led to some rethinking. No organism has yet been demonstrated to date.

There is a predominantly lymphocytic interstitial infiltrate in the lungs of patients with pulmonary sarcoidosis. Examination of the T-lymphocyte receptor subsets has shown that these are oligoclonal, perhaps suggesting that there is an inciting agent. However, similar findings in a variety of autoimmune diseases suggest that this disease may turn out to be an autoimmune phenomenon.

Pathogenesis

Whatever its cause, sarcoidosis is characterized by the development of granulomata in many tissues (Fig. 7.16). Immunological studies in sarcoidosis patients suggest that the disease results from a cell-mediated immune response to an unknown antigen causing activation of T lymphocytes and phagocytes leading to granuloma formation, with subsequent fibrosis as these granulomata resolve.

In the lung and mediastinal lymph nodes, sarcoidosis is often found as a result of routine chest radiography. In skin, it may form indurated erythematous lesions which on biopsy show non-caseating granulomata in the dermis. Granulomata may be seen in the eye with an ophthalmoscope or turn up in a biopsy of an enlarged peripheral lymph node. Sarcoidosis in the central nervous system causes a variety of neurological complications, which may mimic other diseases. Whatever the site of the initial presentation, lung involvement is usually present to some extent. Diagnosis depends upon three main factors:

- chest radiograph appearances
- non-caseating granulomata on biopsy
- Kveim test.

The **Kveim test** was previously widely used to diagnose sarcoidosis. However, because of its origin from affected patients, worries about its safety have lead to a reluctance to use it in recent years. It has about an 80% positivity rate in sarcoidosis patients. Since non-caseating granulomata just like those seen in sarcoidosis may be found in many other diseases, the diagnosis of sarcoidosis is one of exclusion and is not easily made. The risk of missing a tuberculosis or leprosy patient is considerable.

Treatment and its effects

The primary aim of treatment is to suppress the cell-mediated immune

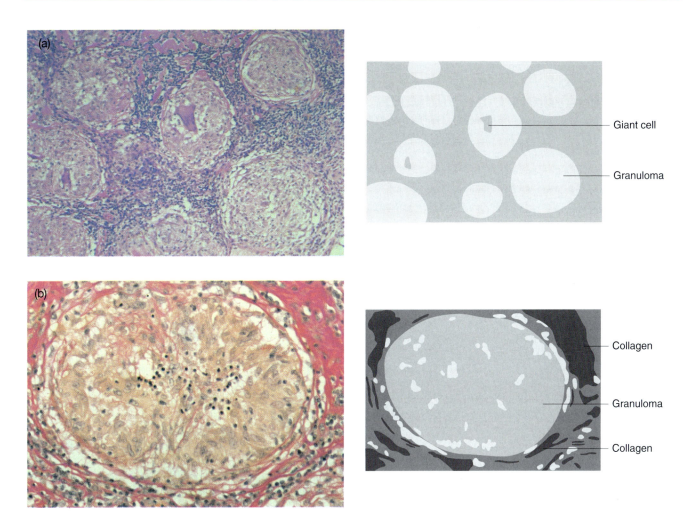

Fig. 7.16   (a) Sarcoid lymph node (low power) with (b) a single granuloma (high power, van Gieson's stain). Note the giant cells present towards the centre of some granulomata and the fine fibrous (red) around the single granuloma in (b)

response thought to be an early event in the pathogenesis of the disease, and to prevent fibrosis. This is currently achieved to some extent by the use of corticosteroids in immunosuppressive doses. The regimens used vary, but all carry the risk of toxicity.

Steroid treatment has consequences for the endocrine system (adrenal suppression), the musculoskeletal system (osteoporosis) and the immune system (susceptibility to viral and fungal infection). Most are problems of long-term, high-dose therapy and are not experienced by those who require short-term or low-dose treatment.

Rheumatoid disease

Rheumatoid disease is often preferred to the term rheumatoid arthritis because this disease is not just a problem with the joints. Other tissues which may be affected include the blood vessels, heart, lung and kidneys. It is regarded as a generalized autoimmune disease, rather than an organ-specific one, such as thyroiditis, and is the classic example of a 'connective tissue' disease. It is a common disease, affecting about 1% of the population in the UK, most of whom (about 75%) are female and in their 30s or 40s.

CASE STUDY 7.1

A 27-year-old woman presented with an erythematous rash on the anterior aspect of the lower legs which had been present for three weeks. The dermatologist suspected erythema nodosum and a chest radiograph (Fig. 7.17) showed a mottled lung appearance typical of sarcoidosis with mediastinal expansion due to lymph node enlargement. A Kveim test was positive. Various markers of inflammation were increased, including the erythrocyte sedimentation rate (ESR), serum angiotensin-converting enzyme (SACE) and soluble IL2 receptor level. Over the next 10 years, the patient was treated with 20–60 mg oral prednisolone daily according to laboratory and respiratory indicators of severity.

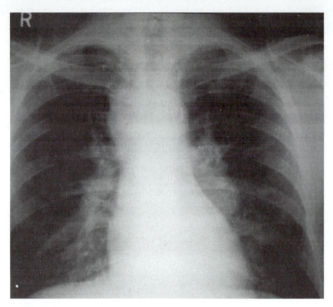

Fig. 7.17 Chest radiograph from a patient with sarcoidosis showing mediastinal expansion and hilar shadowing.

Aetiology

Like sarcoidosis, the aetiology of rheumatoid disease is unknown and a variety of different agents has been implicated at different times over the last 50 years. Patients with chronic inflammatory disease often have high titres of antibodies to a variety of agents to which they have earlier been exposed. Thus rheumatoid disease patients often have high levels of circulating antibodies to various viruses, many of which have at one time or another been blamed as the aetiological agent.

The idea that rheumatoid disease could be due to a viral or bacterial infection is far from dead. In the 1980s, a form of arthritis similar in many ways to rheumatoid disease occurred in the USA. Known as **Lyme disease**, after the town of Lyme in Connecticut, it was eventually tracked down to a form of borreliosis (*Borrelia burgdorferi*) transmitted by deer ticks.

Other research has implicated the idea that so-called 'superantigens' which occur in mycobacteria and other micro-organisms might be involved. These antigens have the capacity to bind non-specifically to the T-lymphocyte receptor and produce immune responses.

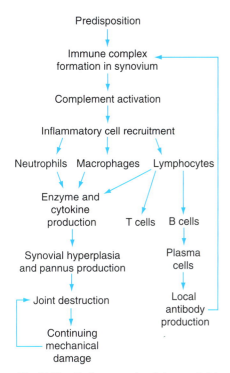

Fig. 7.18 Pathogenesis of rheumatoid arthritis. Immune complex formation leads to inflammation (chronic active type) and pannus formation. Damage to the joint is exacerbated by mechanical stress on the weakened bone and loss of cartilage.

Pathogenesis

The recognition of rheumatoid factors, usually IgM autoantibodies against parts of the Fc portion of IgG, led to the realization that the pathogenesis involved autoimmunity. More recent studies have shown up genetic associations with HLA-DR4 (MHC class II) molecules on the cell surface which control antigen presentation. The events which take place in the joints and lead to damage probably follow a course similar to that shown in Fig. 7.18.

In this model, it is suggested that the formation of immune complexes in the joints leads to a class III reaction with the activation of complement, causing tissue damage which is exacerbated by the attraction of phagocytes to the area. Chronic inflammation results.

Phagocytes are thought to be particularly important in this disease as they accumulate in the synovium in large numbers. They produce many cytokines, but one of the most important appears to be tumour necrosis factor-α (TNF-α). The involvement of TNF-α in the pathogenesis of rheumatoid joint damage has been shown by the efficacy of injected anti-TNF-α antibodies in ameliorating the pain and joint stiffness associated with active disease. This approach holds some hope for the future.

Effects on the tissues

Rheumatoid disease affects the joints in most patients, but the skin, vascular, and other tissue effects are significant in more severe cases (Fig. 7.19).

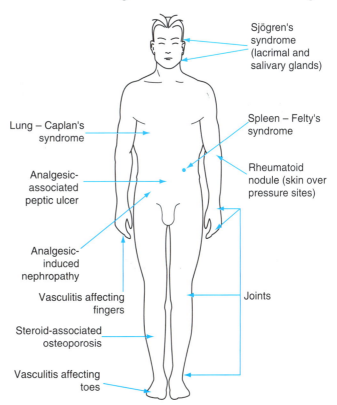

Fig. 7.19 Tissues and organs affected by rheumatoid disease.

ARTHRITIS

All patients show arthritis, although the severity and number of joints affected vary considerably. In general, rheumatoid disease results in intense chronic inflammation of the synovium of small joints in the hands and feet (Fig. 7.20). However, it can affect larger joints, particularly the knees and wrists.

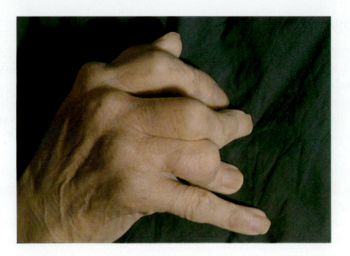

Fig. 7.20   Rheumatoid arthritis of the hands with 'swan-neck' deformity of the fingers and ulnar deviation.

The synovium of affected joints becomes hyperplastic and becomes villous with many folds. The inflammatory infiltrate is predominantly chronic, with many lymphocytes, plasma cells and often even germinal centres. In exacerbations, there is a fibrinous exudate into the swollen joints with many polymorphonuclear leukocytes also appearing in the synovial fluid. As the disease develops, these reversible changes give rise to the formation of **pannus**, a vascular form of granulation tissue which grows over the cartilaginous surfaces of the joint from the synovium at the edges and erodes them (Fig. 7.21). Subchondral **erosions** may be seen on radiography, and later the bone beneath the cartilage may be exposed to the mechanical forces within the joint.

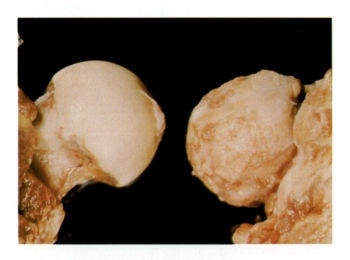

Fig. 7.21   Pannus destroying the cartilage overlying one femoral head, while the other is unaffected.

If the pannus persists, then eventually it may organize and give rise to ankylosis of the joint. More usually, the final effect is subluxation or dislocation of the joint with disuse atrophy of surrounding muscles.

Tendons may be involved in the inflammatory process and the bone adjacent to affected joints may show osteoporosis due in part to the hyperaemia associated with inflammation.

SKIN AND CONNECTIVE TISSUE

The most common lesion is the **rheumatoid nodule** (Fig. 7.22), which may occur in any organ but is most common in the subcutis. The lesion is distinctive, as shown in the figure, and tends to occur over pressure sites.

Nodules are present in some 20% of patients, usually those with more severe disease, and may be up to 2–3 mm diameter. In the lung, they may give rise to Caplan's syndrome in which they are associated with pneumoconiosis and there is rapidly progressive fibrotic lung disease. Nodules may also rarely cause cardiac problems when they interfere with the conducting system.

Fig. 7.22 Histology of a rheumatoid nodule. Note the palisading of macrophages around an area of fibrinoid collagen necrosis.

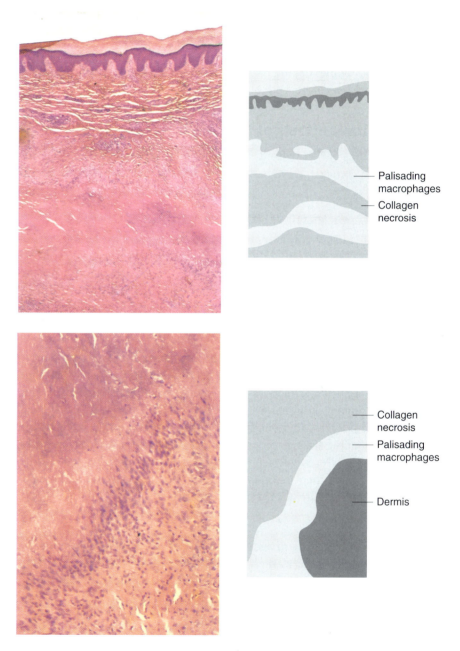

Palisading macrophages

Collagen necrosis

Collagen necrosis

Palisading macrophages

Dermis

VASCULITIS

Rheumatoid arteritis is rare, but severe and often difficult to control. There is fibrinoid necrosis of the vessel wall which is thought to be due to a type III hypersensitivity with immune complex deposition and complement activation within the vessel wall. Thrombosis and infarction of tissues with vulnerable blood supply may result: fingers and toes are especially at risk. There may also be a peripheral neuropathy. Nerve entrapment (as in the **carpal tunnel syndrome**) may occur.

SPLEEN AND LYMPH NODES

Rarely, reactive hyperplasia of lymphoid tissue may give rise to **Felty's syndrome** in which splenomegaly leads to anaemia and granulocytopenia with an increased risk of infection.

EYE AND MOUTH INVOLVEMENT

The term **Sjögren's syndrome** is usually applied to an organ-specific autoimmune disease affecting the lacrimal and salivary glands. However, a very similar secondary Sjögren's syndrome is present in many rheumatoid disease patients. Drying out of the cornea can lead to scarring and blindness, while drying of the mouth can cause serious dental problems. This is therefore a serious effect of the disease.

Complications: effects of treatment

The complications of rheumatoid disease are related in part to the effects of the disease on joints, but often to the effects of drugs given to try to alleviate the disease.

NON-STEROIDAL ANTI-INFLAMMATORY DRUGS

These are the mainstay of treatment for mild disease and act by interfering with arachidonic acid metabolism, inhibiting the production of prostaglandins and leukotrienes. Their most serious side effects are an increased risk of **peptic ulcer** and the risk of **analgesic-induced nephropathy** in patients who may be taking considerable quantities.

STEROID-RELATED SIDE EFFECTS

Immunosuppression appears to slow the course of the disease in more severe cases. Corticosteroids cause a long list of side effects, the most serious of which in patients with rheumatoid disease is probably **osteoporosis**. This results in a tendency to fracture long bones, which then heal poorly, and makes surgical joint replacement difficult. Since steroids are secreted by the adrenal as part of the stress response to injury or infection, and this may not occur in patients who have received steroids for many years, all should carry cards detailing their treatment to enable doctors to avoid addisonian crises should they require admission for any reason.

> **Side effects of steroids**
> - Osteoporosis
> - Poor healing
> - Risk of infection
> - Adrenal suppression

OTHER DRUGS

Other immunosuppressive drugs are sometimes used, including cytotoxic agents. These carry significant risks and are usually used only in very severe cases.

Systemic lupus erythematosus

Systemic lupus erythematosus (SLE) is an example of a group of diseases related to rheumatoid disease known as the connective tissue diseases. All have autoimmunity as part of their pathogenesis, and are diagnosed in part through the presence of autoantibodies in serum.

Aetiology

SLE is common – it affects 1 in 2000 in the USA. Patients are usually in their 20s or 30s and female (male:female ratio = 1:9). The cause is unknown, but genetic factors are important. At first glance, abnormal genes on chromosome 6 would seem to be implicated, since several HLA associations exist and deficiencies of C2 and C4 complement components are frequent in affected individuals. However, other complement deficiencies including C1q, C1r and C1s, which are coded on different chromosomes, are also associated with an increased incidence of SLE, and most SLE patients are not complement deficient. Monozygous twins have a 50% or more concordance for the disease. The female preponderance suggests that hormonal influences may exist, and the disease tends to get worse during and just after pregnancy. Environmental factors are also important – particularly drugs such as hydralazine, an antihypertensive drug which has now been largely superseded by safer agents. Luckily, the disease usually remits when the drug is stopped.

The pivotal problem appears to be autoimmunity. Antibodies to a variety of nuclear antigens have been described and are now the basis of diagnostic tests for the disease. Some are based on the patterns of nuclear immunofluorescence obtained after incubation of patient serum with frozen tissue sections (Fig. 7.23), while others use purified antigens in enzyme-linked immunosorbent assays (ELISAs).

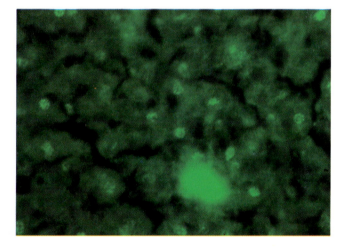

Fig. 7.23 Antinuclear antibody staining of a frozen section of patient's serum. Note the speckled pattern of nuclear staining.

Pathogenesis

Type III immune complex hypersensitivity is at the heart of SLE, as it is with rheumatoid disease. However, the results are considerably different as the immune complexes are laid down in different sites, predominantly in the arterioles of skin, kidney, joints and serosal membranes.

The vasculitis consists of **fibrinoid deposits** in vessel walls (Fig. 7.24). This leads in chronic cases to fibrous thickening of the walls with narrowing of the lumen. There is usually a dense perivascular infiltrate, which is particularly conspicuous in the skin. Immune complexes, DNA and complement can be demonstrated by immunofluorescence in cryostat sections of skin biopsies along the basement membrane and in the walls of small arterioles.

Lupus anticoagulant, an autoantibody cross-reactive with cardiolipin, is thought to be responsible for some of the haematological effects encountered in SLE because it neutralizes factor X of the coagulation cascade. Anti-cardiolipin antibodies are also associated with recurrent abortion in SLE patients.

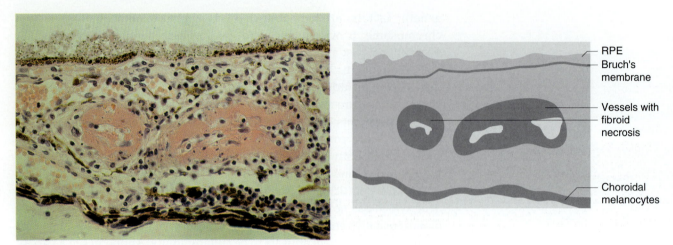

Fig. 7.24   Vasculitis in the choroidal vessels of a patient with systemic lupus erythomatosus showing extensive fibrin deposition. RPE, retinal pigment epithelium.

Effects

The most serious effects of SLE are usually in the kidney, which is involved in 60–70% of cases, but the clinical manifestations of SLE are very variable with a long list of possible problems. This makes it an important disease to think about in any patient (usually female) who presents with an odd constellation of signs and symptoms.

KIDNEY INVOLVEMENT

Five patterns of glomerulonephritis are recognized in SLE, the commonest being a diffuse proliferative form which is also the most serious. SLE is a significant cause of chronic renal failure (see Chapter 13).

SKIN INVOLVEMENT

The characteristic butterfly rash of SLE over the bridge of the nose and on to the cheeks is not the only problem. Other rashes also occur, and sunlight tends to exacerbate them. Histologically there is liquefaction of the basal layer of the epithelium with apoptotic bodies just beneath it.

HEART AND BLOOD VESSELS

The valves of the heart are affected in about half of patients, with endocardial vegetations (Libman–Sacks endocarditis) on the mitral and tricuspid valves. Normally these vegetations are small and composed mainly of platelets, but they may give rise to clinical signs.

OTHER ORGANS

The joints may also be affected, but unlike rheumatoid disease, the arthritis does not cause erosions and the synovitis is usually less severe. The central nervous system may be affected with a variety of focal neurological problems. These are also thought to be due to vascular disturbances which may also affect retinal vessels in the eye (see Fig. 7.24). Acute or chronic pleurisy and pericarditis are common and there may be sufficient inflammation for a fibrinous exudate to form, leading with organization to obliteration of the serosal cavity. Constrictive pericarditis may then require operative intervention.

Effects of treatment

At present the treatment of all autoimmune diseases is heavily dependent upon the use of steroids. SLE is no different, but other modalities such as renal dialysis are often also required.

Septicaemia and septic shock

The death rate from septicaemia has not altered appreciably since antibiotics were first introduced, despite considerable advances in intensive care. The problem seems to be a combination of widespread damage to endothelial cells in many tissues leading to loss of fluid with vasodilatation, resulting in profound hypotension – **shock**.

Aetiology

The organisms involved are usually Gram-negative bacteria such as *Escherichia coli* from the gut, but some Gram-positive pyogenic bacteria such as streptococci seem to be able to produce very similar effects.

Pathogenesis

In recent years, much attention has been focused on the role of **lipopolysaccharide** (**LPS**), a component of bacterial cell walls, in the pathogenesis of septic shock (Fig. 7.25). The hypothesis was that LPS triggered the release of toxic enzymes and free radicals from phagocytes within the circulation which then damaged the endothelium, leading to catastrophic endothelial cell damage. Unfortunately, anti-LPS antibodies were largely unable to protect patients against shock, despite initially encouraging results. Furthermore, normal healthy individuals (prisoners) injected in the 1960s with LPS did not die, suggesting that if LPS is

> **Definitions**
> - **Bacteraemia:** the presence of less than 10^5 bacteria /ml in the blood
> - **Septicaemia:** the presence of more than 10^5 bacteria/ml in the blood

Fig. 7.25 Pathogenesis of septic shock – a model.

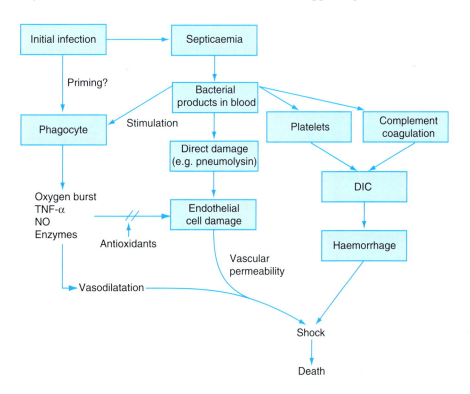

important, something about the patient makes them uniquely sensitive to it.

The role of various cytokines has also been studied in some detail. In particular, phagocyte production of TNF-α has been blamed, since levels are raised in many patients, but it now appears that this only occurs after the inciting event and its significance is uncertain. Anti-TNF-α antibodies are showing some promise in early treatment trials, but again the effects are not all that dramatic in most patients.

Since it is known that there is endothelial cell damage, and there is evidence that phagocytes are involved, suspicion has now fallen on the production of reactive oxygen species (ROS) and, more recently, **nitric oxide** by phagocytes. Production of nitric oxide explains the inappropriate vasodilatation observed in these patients, while the production of ROS and other products may be responsible for concomitant endothelial cell damage. The ability of patients to fight off such insults may be reduced as a result of the initial injury or infection, and cytokines produced during the early phase of the disease may prime phagocytes to produce ROS and other toxic substances inappropriately.

It remains to be seen whether this hypothesis is any more correct than those in vogue previously, but the story to date underlines the importance of understanding the timing of events in disease pathogenesis, as well as the complexity of such reactions.

Effects

The pathological features of septic shock suggest that multiple mechanisms result in damage. As well as pulmonary oedema, there may be multiple small haemorrhages into many tissues, including the skin. This may result from **disseminated intravascular coagulation (DIC)** in which components of the clotting and fibrinolytic systems are used up leading to a bleeding tendency, or to dissemination of bacteria to form focal colonies within tissues.

If death does not occur quickly, hypotension leads to a number of problems, including renal tubular ischaemia and consequent oliguric renal failure, and oedema of the brain. The adult respiratory distress syndrome (ARDS, see Chapter 9) may also develop as a result of lung damage.

Chapter 8   Cardiovascular disease

Learning objectives

To appreciate and understand:
- ❑ Various types of congenital abnormalities affecting the cardiovascular system
- ❑ Pathogenesis and effects of atherosclerosis
- ❑ Causes and effects of inflammation in vessels of differing size
- ❑ Diseases affecting the venous system
- ❑ Causes and effects of hypertension
- ❑ Factors involved in the various manifestations of ischaemic heart disease
- ❑ Causes and effects of heart failure
- ❑ Processes involved in valvular heart disease

Cardiovascular disease is the major cause of death in industrially developed countries and is increasing in the rest of the world as industrialization occurs. The most important disease, **atherosclerosis**, affects the arteries, especially the coronary and extracerebral cranial vessels, and this is reflected in the fact that 'heart attacks' and 'strokes' are the most common manifestations of cardiovascular disease.

Developmental abnormalities

Cardiac involvement is a frequent feature of most serious congenital abnormalities. Sometimes relatively minor abnormalities, such as anomalous coronary arteries or bicuspid aortic valve, may have serious consequences, particularly when age-related disease processes are superimposed.

Congenital abnormalities of the heart

The aetiology of many congenital cardiac abnormalities is obscure. However, viral infections such as rubella occurring during the first trimester of pregnancy appear to be particularly liable to produce cardiac defects. The heart develops first as a three-chambered structure (atrial and ventricular chambers, with an aortic bulb). Division of the aortic bulb leads to formation of the pulmonary artery and aorta. The septum dividing the aortic bulb then joins with another septum growing up from the base of the ventricular chamber and the vessels rotate to assume their correct position in relation to the ventricles. The atrial bulb is also divided by a septum.

Abnormalities tend to occur in the process of division leaving defects in the septum between either the two ventricles or the two atria. More complex abnormalities occur due to abnormal rotation of the vessels in relation to the ventricles, and lastly there are valvular abnormalities. The surgical treatment of congenital heart disease has improved dramatically over the last 20 years, and many of these defects are compatible with a normal life.

CYANOTIC CONGENITAL HEART DISEASE

Cyanotic congenital heart disease tends to present at birth or early in childhood. Major types include **Fallot's tetralogy** and **Eisenmenger's complex**, in both of which there is abnormal division of the aortic bulb with obstruction of right ventricular outflow through the pulmonary artery. Right ventricular hypertrophy results, with shunting of blood from right to left via a ventricular septal defect. Malrotation of the aortic bulb can lead to transposition of the aorta and pulmonary artery, compensated for by shunting of blood through an atrial or ventricular septal defect, or a patent ductus arteriosus.

ACYANOTIC DISORDERS

Acyanotic disorders may present quite late in life, due to the occurrence of some complication or intervening illness. The most important are valvular lesions, especially congenital **bicuspid aortic valve** (Fig 8.1), which predispose to infective endocarditis and calcific aortic stenosis. Sudden death or heart failure may result. Relatively minor degrees of atrial and even ventricular septal defects are relatively common. The foramen ovale remains probe-patent in up to one in four people.

Congenital abnormalities of the arteries and veins

Coarctation (narrowing) of the aorta between the left subclavian artery and the site where the ductus arteriosus joins the aorta is relatively common. It results in high blood pressure in the upper body, with low blood pressure in the legs, often with extensive collateral artery hypertrophy. Death may result from stroke, cardiac failure or aneurysm. The condition is curable by surgery if diagnosed.

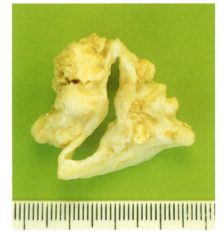

Fig. 8.1   Calcified stenotic congenitally bicuspid aortic valve surgically excised from a 55-year-old man.

Arterial disease

Atherosclerosis

Atherosclerosis and its complications are a major cause of morbidity and mortality in industrially developed countries, being responsible for 'heart attacks' and the majority of 'strokes'. The characteristic lesion is the **atherosclerotic plaque** (also known as atheroma) (Figs 8.2 and 8.3).

Pathogenesis

The original hypotheses of Virchow and of Rokitansky are still relevant to the pathogenesis of atherosclerosis, namely entry of lipid into the vessel wall versus organization of thrombus. Modern concepts view the disease as a response to injury where both processes may be of relevance. The

Atherosclerosis
A disease characterized by progressive narrowing of arteries by intimal plaques composed of smooth muscle cells, connective tissue, lipid deposits and macrophages, all in very variable proportions.

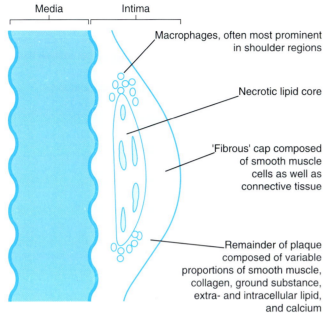

Media | Intima

Macrophages, often most prominent in shoulder regions

Necrotic lipid core

'Fibrous' cap composed of smooth muscle cells as well as connective tissue

Remainder of plaque composed of variable proportions of smooth muscle, collagen, ground substance, extra- and intracellular lipid, and calcium

Fig. 8.2   Components of an atherosclerotic plaque.

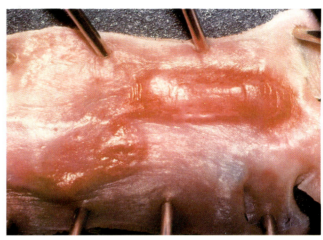

Fig. 8.3   Early atherosclerotic plaque in the left anterior descending coronary artery viewed from the intimal surface in a young adult. Lipid has been stained red with oil red O.

nature of the injury is not clear and indeed there may be a number of different injuries all of which may ultimately result in formation of atherosclerotic plaques.

Certain features are of relevance in considering the pathogenesis:

■ Any hypothesis must account for the main established risk factors:
- **hypertension**
- **hypercholesterolaemia**
- **smoking**
- **diabetes mellitus**.
■ Atherosclerosis has a focal distribution with a predilection for certain sites, such as abdominal aorta and proximal left anterior descending coronary artery. This implies that fluid dynamic and other mechanical factors are important. These could promote lipid entry or platelet adherence as either a primary event or part of a response to another injury.
■ The presence of T lymphocytes as well as macrophages in atherosclerotic plaques suggests that immunological events may be important in plaque evolution.
■ The possible role of lipid modification and in particular oxidation in the pathogenesis.

The main complications of atherosclerosis are:

■ **stenosis** (narrowing)
■ **aneurysm** (dilatation)
■ **thrombosis** of blood vessels.

STENOSIS

Atherosclerosis may involve part or all of the circumference of the vessel (eccentric or concentric atherosclerosis) and both of these may ultimately become significantly stenotic (Fig. 8.4). When considering a localized fixed stenosis it is usually suggested that, to be significant in terms of reducing flow, it has to be greater than 75% by cross-sectional area (that is, greater than 50% by diameter as seen in a two-dimensional angiogram). Since advanced atherosclerosis tends to be diffuse it is likely that longer

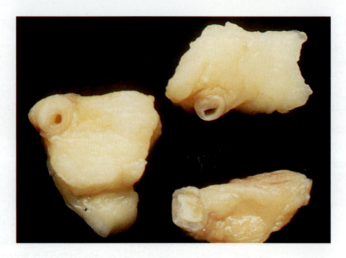

Fig. 8.4 Severe three-vessel coronary disease – disease involving the left circumflex, left anterior descending and right main coronaries. The vessels have been transversely sectioned to demonstrate degree of stenosis.

segments with a lesser degree of stenosis may also significantly impair flow. In clinical cardiology a cut-off point of 70% reduction in diameter by two-dimensional angiography has been selected as a benchmark for potential clinical significance.

However, the most important factor in terms of oxygen delivery to the tissues is the absolute luminal diameter. This is often forgotten in the clinical interpretation of angiograms. It is important to remember this point, as many arteries dilate progressively with age, possibly to a greater degree to accommodate potential atherosclerotic occlusion. Thus an artery apparently showing 75% occlusion by cross-sectional area may have a perfectly adequate absolute luminal diameter comparable to that in an undiseased vessel.

Stenotic atherosclerosis is associated with a number of clinical syndromes depending on the vascular bed affected. In the heart it may give rise to angina pectoris, whereas in the lower limb arteries it gives rise to intermittent claudication with different muscle groups affected depending on the location of stenosis.

THROMBOSIS AND THROMBOEMBOLISM

Thrombosis as a result of plaque rupture is recognized as one of the most important complications of atherosclerosis, being responsible for **unstable angina**, **sudden cardiac death** and **myocardial infarction** (see 'Ischaemic heart disease'). Embolization of atherosclerotic plaque material and thrombus from the extracranial cerebral arterial supply is responsible for most strokes.

ANEURYSM

Destruction of medial elastic tissue is one of the features of advanced atherosclerosis of the aorta and gives rise to aneurysmal dilatation (see below).

Aneurysms

Aneurysms are localized dilatation of arteries. It should be remembered that arteries dilate progressively with ageing.

Aneurysms may be:

- **fusiform**, involving whole circumference
- **saccular**, involving part of circumference ('blow-out')
- **dissecting**, where the media separate.

Thrombus
A solid or semi-solid mass formed in the living heart or vessels derived from the elements of blood. A **clot**, on the other hand, either forms outside the cardiovascular system or forms within it after death.
Thromboembolism
Migration of thrombotic material from its point of formation/origin to some other part of the cardiovascular system, e.g. from the leg veins to the pulmonary arterial system in pulmonary thromboembolism.

ATHEROSCLEROTIC ANEURYSMS

Atherosclerotic aneurysms occur most commonly in the abdominal aorta, usually below the level of the renal arteries, and are associated with severe complicated atherosclerosis (Fig. 8.5). They result from encroachment into the media of the aorta by atherosclerotic plaques with damage to and loss of elastic tissue. The aneurysm is usually filled by thrombus which may embolize to the lower limbs. Rupture is obviously life threatening and is a fairly common cause of sudden natural death.

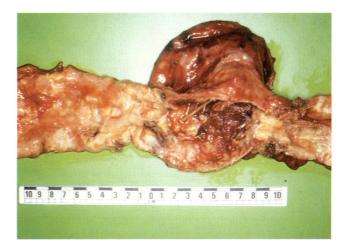

Fig. 8.5 Atherosclerotic aneurysm of the abdominal aorta. The sac is filled with thrombus.

Periadventitial inflammation is a frequent accompaniment to severe aortic atherosclerosis of the kind invariably present when aneurysm formation occurs. However, a number of patients are recognized clinically in whom periaortic inflammation and fibrosis are a conspicuous feature, in which case the term **inflammatory aneurysm** may be used. However, from a pathological point of view these cases probably represent one end of the spectrum of atherosclerotic aortic aneurysm.

CASE STUDY 8.1

A 67-year-old man is brought into Accident and Emergency in shock, having collapsed at home. He had complained of severe low back pain for some hours prior to his collapse. He had smoked 20–30 cigarettes per day since the age of 17. Relevant past history included a small inferior myocardial infarction five years previously from which he had made a good recovery. On examination the blood pressure was 80/40. While being assessed he suffered a cardiac arrest from which he was not resuscitated. It was noted that during resuscitation he had developed abdominal distension.

At postmortem examination there was about one litre of fluid and clotted blood free in the peritoneal cavity. There was about a further litre of haematoma in retroperitoneal tissues. The haemorrhage had originated from a ruptured atherosclerotic aortic aneurysm. Rupture had occurred at the inferior margin of the aneurysm which was filled with laminated thrombus. The remaining aorta showed severe complicated atherosclerosis with numerous ulcerated plaques, some showing mural thrombosis. Other findings of note were pallor of the kidneys consistent with haemorrhagic shock and an area of white fibrosis in the posterior wall of the left ventricle consistent with an area of healed myocardial infarction. There was severe three-vessel stenotic coronary atherosclerosis.

DISSECTING ANEURYSM

Dissecting aneurysms occur in the thoracic aorta, usually in middle age, and are associated with hypertension. Blood enters the media through an intimal tear and then tracks in any direction separating the media into two parts (Fig. 8.6). Histologically there is fragmentation of the elastic laminae and focal medial necrosis associated with accumulation of acid mucin. The underlying cause is not known in most cases.

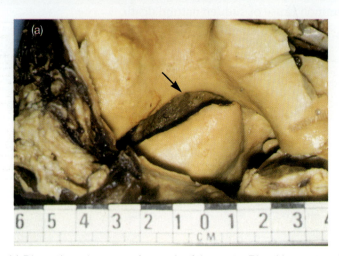

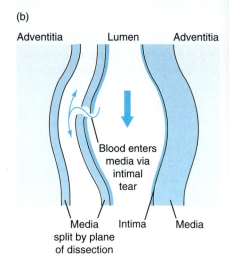

Fig. 8.6 (a) Dissecting aneurysm of an arch of the aorta. Blood has entered the media via an intimal tear (arrow). (b) Diagram of arterial layers showing track of blood in dissecting aneurysm.

People with **Marfan's syndrome** get dissecting aneurysm at an earlier age, and this appears to be the result of a defect in the gene for the connective tissue component fibrillin.

Blood entering the media of the aorta may track back and rupture into the pericardium producing **tamponade**, or may track distally compressing any side branches in the process. The latter scenario may lead to presentation with myocardial or cerebral ischaemia. Blood may rupture outwards through the adventitia anywhere along the length of the aorta with dramatic results or may rupture back into the lumen of the main vessel. Figure 8.7 illustrates the various scenarios.

SYPHILITIC ANEURYSMS

These affect the ascending aorta and arch, and are rare in industrialized countries. Dilatation of the ascending aorta may lead to aortic incompetence, there may be slow pressure atrophy of adjacent structures and the aneurysm may ultimately rupture.

Microscopically the essential features are chronic inflammation in the adventitia with prominent plasma cells, and **endarteritis obliterans** of the vasa vasorum. Endarteritis obliterans is characterized by partial or complete luminal occlusion due to intimal proliferation in these vessels which supply approximately the outer two-thirds of the media. The result is intimal and medial ischaemic fibrosis with loss of elastic tissue and dilatation of the affected portion of the aorta.

Vasculitis

Although most descriptions of the various types of vascular inflammation tend to describe involvement of arteries, veins and capillaries can also be

Fig. 8.7 Possible effects of dissection.

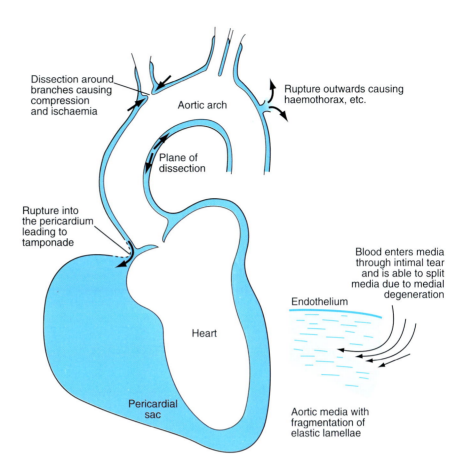

Dissection around branches causing compression and ischaemia

Aortic arch

Rupture outwards causing haemothorax, etc.

Plane of dissection

Rupture into the pericardium leading to tamponade

Blood enters media through intimal tear and is able to split media due to medial degeneration

Endothelium

Heart

Pericardial sac

Aortic media with fragmentation of elastic lamellae

affected. The common feature is one of inflammation and necrosis of the vessel wall. Some important examples of diseases are:

- **polyarteritis nodosa**
- **Wegener's granulomatosis**
- **temporal arteritis** (giant cell arteritis).

POLYARTERITIS NODOSA

In this necrotizing arteritis of small and medium-sized muscular arteries, all layers of the vessel wall are involved. In the acute stages there is fibrinoid necrosis with an inflammatory cell infiltrate of neutrophils, eosinophils and mononuclear cells. There is frequently thrombosis. Weakening of the wall may result in aneurysm formation and even rupture. Vessels in any organ may be affected. The kidneys and heart are most frequently involved. The disease appears to be related to deposition of immune complexes in the arterial wall and can thus occur in association with conditions such as systemic lupus and rheumatoid arthritis. It is thought that in some cases hepatitis B surface antigen–antibody complexes are involved.

WEGENER'S GRANULOMATOSIS

The essential features are necrotizing vasculitis involving both small arteries and veins with necrotizing **granulomatous inflammation** of tissues of the upper and lower respiratory tracts, and glomerulonephritis which is usually focal and necrotizing but may be diffuse and proliferative and become rapidly progressive with crescent formation. Vessels in any organ may become involved, most commonly those of the lungs and upper respiratory tracts. There may be granulomata present among the inflammatory infiltrate in vessel walls. This disease is associated with the presence of **anti-neutrophil cytoplasmic antibody (ANCA)**.

TEMPORAL ARTERITIS (GIANT CELL ARTERITIS)

This is a granulomatous inflammation in the walls of medium-sized and large arteries especially those of the head and neck, for example the temporal and ophthalmic arteries (Fig. 8.8). The disorder occurs mainly in old age, and has a large female preponderance. It is often associated with the muscular disorder known as **polymyalgia rheumatica**.

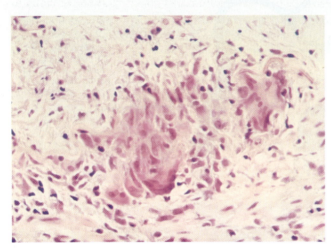
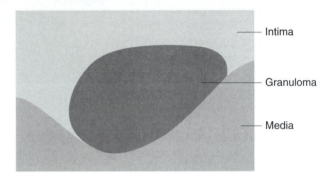

Fig. 8.8   Giant cell arteritis involving the temporal artery.

OTHER VASCULAR DISEASES

Rarer vasculitides include:

- **Takayashu's disease**
- **Raynaud's disease**
- **Buerger's disease**.

Takayashu's disease has similarities to giant cell arteritis, but affects the aorta; Raynaud's disease and Buerger's disease have more in common with polyarteritis nodosa.

Hypertension

Hypertension is the term used to describe an abnormally raised blood pressure in any vascular system, but when used alone the term relates to arterial blood pressure. There is a wide range of arterial blood pressure in the population and within individuals from hour to hour. Both systolic and diastolic blood pressure increase with age, but diastolic blood pressure measured on at least three occasions is the criterion most commonly used in clinical practice to decide whether a patient is hypertensive or not. Recently, the use of continuous ambulatory blood pressure monitoring has led to a wider appreciation of the variability in normal and abnormal pressures.

AETIOLOGY

In most cases (over 90%) there is no apparent cause – these patients are said to have **essential hypertension**, while the rest have **secondary hypertension**.

> **Hypertension**
> Raised blood pressure in any vascular bed, for example portal hypertension (liver), pulmonary hypertension (lung). If not otherwise specified it tends to be synonymous with raised systemic arterial blood pressure.

Causes of secondary hypertension

■ Renal disease
- Chronic pyelonephritis
- Glomerulonephritis
- Diabetes
- Polycystic kidneys
- Connective tissue diseases
- Renal artery stenosis
- Other diseases causing parenchymal loss

■ Adrenal disease
- Primary hyperaldosteronism
- Cushing's syndrome
- Phaeochromocytoma

■ Other endocrine disorders
- Hyper/hypothyroidism
- Acromegaly
- Hyperparathyroidism

■ Miscellaneous
- Coarctation of the aorta
- Pre-eclampsia
- Alcohol abuse
- Renin-secreting tumour

Essential hypertension has been related to a host of factors, with no one factor predominant. Familial and racial differences suggest that genetic influences are important, but environmental factors such as diet (salt intake, for example) and stress have also been implicated, though there is no consensus.

Causes for secondary hypertension are mainly due to renal or endocrine disease, owing to the importance of these organs in controlling blood pressure.

EFFECTS OF HYPERTENSION

Usually blood pressure rises slowly, without ill effects that are obvious to the patient. However, patients with benign hypertension are at increased risk of dying of strokes, myocardial infarcts and sudden cardiac death due to arrhythmias.

The term **malignant hypertension** is used to describe a rapidly progressive rise in blood pressure to high levels leading within weeks to eye damage (retinal exudates and haemorrhage), renal failure and even encephalopathy. In such patients, there may be a history of preceding benign hypertension or no evidence of previous disease.

PATHOLOGICAL CHANGES

Cardiac signs

It has been known for many years that systemic hypertension is associated with concentric **left ventricular hypertrophy (LVH)** (Fig. 8.9). However, this relationship is loose and in some cases relatively minor elevations of blood pressure may be associated with quite marked LVH whereas there may be relatively little LVH in quite severe hypertension. Furthermore, therapeutic agents to lower blood pressure vary quite widely in their ability to reverse left ventricular hypertrophy. One factor that is emerging as being of importance in cardiac remodelling and development of LVH is the **renin–angiotensin system**. It is now recognized that there is genetic polymorphism in relation to enzymes involved in this system and such polymorphisms may be important in the cardiac response to elevations of blood pressure. In relation to this angiotensin-converting enzyme, inhibitors may be effective not only in lowering blood pressure but also in reversing LVH. This is of importance because LVH caused by hypertension has long been recognized by pathologists as a potential cause of death in its own right due to cardiac arrhythmia.

Fig. 8.9 Concentric left ventricular hypertrophy in relation to hypertension. The heart has been sliced transversely approximately halfway between the base and the apex.

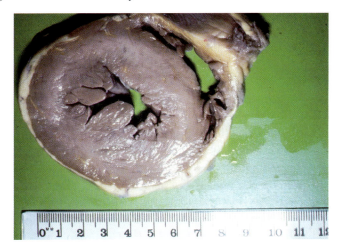

Vascular signs

In **benign hypertension** the primary finding is thickening of the media of small arteries and arterioles. This is most obvious in the kidney, liver and adrenal gland. Narrowing of the lumen results in increased resistance to the high arterial pressure.

Atherosclerosis is increased in the major blood vessels. Increased coronary artery atherosclerosis compounds the potential ischaemic effects of LVH discussed above.

Charcot–Bouchard microaneurysms form on small blood vessels deep in the brain substance. The walls of these aneurysms consist of collagen and elastin with little or no smooth muscle. They are prone to rupture, causing intracerebral haemorrhage, one of the causes of stroke particularly seen in hypertensives. Most strokes, however, result from embolization of atherosclerotic material from the extracranial vessels, especially the carotids.

Malignant hypertension produces similar changes, but there is no chance for arterioles to adapt and the key feature is **fibrinoid necrosis** of small arteries and arterioles, particularly in the kidney. The distinctive appearance is caused by exudation under pressure of plasma into the wall of the arteriole (**plasmatic vasculosis**) and death of the smooth muscle within it. Small haemorrhages may occur around such arterioles, resulting in a 'flea-bitten' appearance on the surface of the kidney and microscopic haematuria. The renal interlobular arteries may show **endarteritis** with intimal thickening, giving them an 'onion-skin' appearance. Coagulation within the damaged vascular bed, together with blood forced through at high pressure, may cause haemolysis leading to **microangiopathic haemolytic anaemia** in severe cases.

The heart

Ischaemic heart disease

Ischaemic heart disease is a major problem in industrialized countries, with Scotland having one of the highest incidences in the world. Clinically, ischaemic heart disease presents as recurrent chest pain (angina), acute myocardial infarction or sudden death. Angina can be classified as stable or unstable according to the predictability of the attacks. These clinical diagnoses reflect the pathological events taking place in the heart.

PATHOLOGY OF STABLE ANGINA

The angina is induced by a predictable increase in left ventricular work, such as might occur with mild exercise.

Coronary arteries

Almost all cases show areas of stenotic atherosclerosis, usually over 75% by cross-sectional area. About three-quarters of the stenotic segments have concentric plaques, the majority of which are fibrous. The other quarter are due to eccentric plaques which may be either fibrous or lipid-rich. Eccentric disease has the potential for contraction or 'spasm' of the normal uninvolved arterial wall opposite the plaque, leading to acute ischaemia of the area of heart muscle it supplies.

Most patients with stable angina show evidence of recanalized coronary thrombosis, even in the absence of evidence of old myocardial infarction.

> **Ischaemia**
> Lack of blood supplied to a tissue
> **Ischaemic heart disease (IHD)**
> Lack of blood supply to the heart via the coronary arteries
> **Angina**
> Pain resulting from ischaemia of cardiac muscle

Heart muscle

A variety of ischaemic changes may be seen either alone or in combination. There may be myocyte hypertrophy, diffuse fibrosis or more localized scarring suggestive of old healed myocardial infarction.

PATHOLOGY OF UNSTABLE ANGINA

This type of angina is much less predictable in onset and may occur at rest. Symptoms often increase in frequency and severity (crescendo angina) and ultimately sudden death or myocardial infarction may occur.

Coronary arteries

Angiographic studies both in life and at postmortem examination show that the degree and extent of arterial stenosis are similar to stable angina. The principal difference is that in stable angina the angiographic outline of stenosed segments is smooth, whereas in unstable angina it tends to be ragged. Detailed angiographic and histological correlation has shown that the ragged outline is due to non-occlusive mural thrombus overlying fissured atherosclerotic plaque (Fig. 8.10). This plaque fissuring tends to occur in the shoulder regions of plaques where progression occurs. These plaques are therefore undergoing rapid change in contrast to the 'static' plaques of stable angina.

Fig. 8.10 Plaque fissuring with associated mural thrombosis is the underlying pathology both in unstable angina and in most cases of sudden cardiac death.

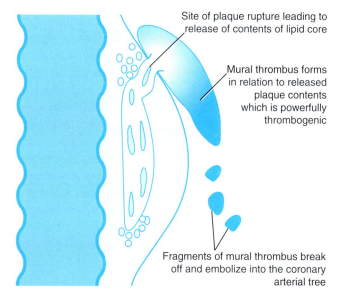

Site of plaque rupture leading to release of contents of lipid core

Mural thrombus forms in relation to released plaque contents which is powerfully thrombogenic

Fragments of mural thrombus break off and embolize into the coronary arterial tree

Heart muscle

Meticulous histological examination of the myocardium in fatal cases of unstable angina shows the presence of occlusive platelet emboli in small vessels in the downstream territory of segments showing mural thrombosis. This occurs in a background of changes similar to those in stable angina.

PATHOLOGY OF SUDDEN CARDIAC DEATH

This may arbitrarily be defined as death occurring within six hours of the onset of cardiac symptoms where the only cause of death apparent is stenotic coronary atherosclerosis.

Coronary arteries

There is a background of stenotic atherosclerosis. Only a proportion of cases (around 30%) show occlusive thrombus. Most of the remainder show non-occlusive mural thrombus associated with plaque fissuring and essentially similar to the lesions seen in unstable angina. This may be easily missed at postmortem examination.

Heart muscle

As in unstable angina, careful examination may reveal the presence of small occlusive platelet thrombi in intramyocardial vessels. In some cases there may be tiny foci of myocardial necrosis as a result. Again there is a background of changes similar to stable angina. Interestingly, only about a quarter of victims successfully resuscitated from what would otherwise constitute a sudden cardiac death go on to develop evidence of myocardial infarction.

This mode of death therefore does not generally represent early acute myocardial infarction. Rather, it is the result of a fatal arrhythmia, usually ventricular fibrillation, developing as a consequence of plaque fissuring and associated mural thrombosis with downstream showering of platelet emboli. Pathologically it is similar to unstable angina, the only difference being that sudden death is precipitated by development of an arrhythmia.

CASE STUDY 8.2

The body of a 60-year-old man is brought into the public mortuary from his home address. The coroner's officer provides the following history elicited from the deceased's wife: the deceased had been reasonably healthy all his life without any episodes of serious illness. He had smoked 20 cigarettes per day until five years previously. On the morning of his death he had woken up as usual but shortly after breakfast he complained to his wife that he felt generally unwell with pain in the chest and in the left arm. About 20 minutes after that he collapsed and his wife could not find a palpable pulse. She immediately called an ambulance which arrived within 10 minutes. The ambulance crew attempted cardiopulmonary resuscitation without success. Some time later the deceased's general practitioner arrived and confirmed that death had occurred. Not having seen the deceased recently, that is during his last illness, she referred the case to the coroner who ordered a postmortem examination to establish the cause of death.

At postmortem examination the heart was mildly enlarged owing to left ventricular hypertrophy, suggesting hypertension. Sectioning of the myocardium showed no focal abnormality. The coronary arteries showed moderate atherosclerosis. The only area of significant stenosis was in the proximal left anterior descending coronary artery which was about 75% stenosed by cross-sectional area. In addition there appeared to be some recent haemorrhage into this area of stenotic atherosclerotic plaque associated with some non-occlusive mural thrombus. Death was recorded as being due to ischaemic heart disease.

PATHOLOGY OF MYOCARDIAL INFARCTION

Myocardial necrosis develops as a result of an acute reduction in myocardial blood supply.

Infarction
Necrosis due to lack of blood supply

Coronary arteries

At postmortem examination only a proportion of cases show occlusive thrombus (Fig. 8.11) and this has led to confusion. This finding is now presumed to be the result of rapid fibrinolysis. In fact angiographic studies

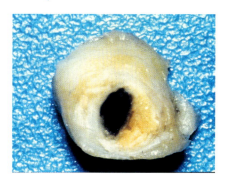

Fig. 8.11 Left anterior descending coronary artery seen in transverse section. It is completely occluded by thrombus which has developed in a background of atherosclerosis in a case of fatal myocardial infarction.

in the early phase of acute myocardial infarction have demonstrated occlusive thrombosis in the vast majority of cases, supporting the case for early fibrinolytic therapy.

Angiographic studies in life or careful postmortem histological examination shows that, as in unstable angina and sudden cardiac death, the precipitating event appears to be one of fissuring of a rapidly transforming plaque.

Heart muscle

The extent of myocardial necrosis is very variable. It may be transmural or partial thickness. Clearly factors such as the location of the fissured plaque and the degree of stenotic atherosclerosis elsewhere will influence this. If the fissured plaque develops in a heart which otherwise shows only non-stenotic disease elsewhere then infarction may develop in a background of otherwise normal myocardium. However, ischaemic changes elsewhere are common, owing to the widespread nature of advanced coronary atherosclerosis.

CASE STUDY 8.3

A 50-year-old male smoker was brought into Accident and Emergency with severe crushing pain in the chest radiating into the left arm. The pain started quite suddenly about two hours prior to his admission. He had previously suffered from angina pectoris for about two years for which he took sublingual glyceryl trinitrate tablets. This pain, although similar in nature to his angina, was more severe and had failed to respond to his medication. Electocardiography suggested an extensive anterior myocardial infarct. He was immediately started on thrombolytic therapy. His initial 24 hours was complicated by short periods of ventricular tachycardia which settled without therapy. On the second day following admission he suffered a cardiac arrest associated with ventricular fibrillation. He remained in intractable ventricular fibrillation and could not be resuscitated. At postmotem examination there was quite extensive myocardial infarction of the anterior septal region characterized by softening and pallor of the myocardium. Microscopy showed the characteristic early changes of myocardial infarction with increased eosinophilia of myocytes, loss of nuclei and, mainly towards the edges of the infarct, conspicuous infiltration by neutrophil polymorphs. The proximal left anterior descending coronary artery showed occlusive thrombosis in a background of stenotic atherosclerosis which was 80% stenotic. The other coronary arteries showed moderate atherosclerosis with areas of up to about 60% occlusion. The cause of death was recorded as myocardial infarction due to coronary thrombosis resulting from coronary atherosclerosis.

TIME COURSE OF MYOCARDIAL INFARCTION

- **Early**: macroscopic changes are difficult to detect until about 24 hours have elapsed (Fig. 8.12). Microscopically the earliest change is seen after a few hours and tends to be an increase in **eosinophilia** of affected myocytes. Thereafter **neutrophil polymorphs** tend to infiltrate, particularly at the edges of the infarct where there is still a blood supply (Fig. 8.13). Myocyte nuclei start to degenerate with **pyknosis, karyorrhexis** and **karyolysis**.
- **Intermediate**: a few days after myocardial infarction the changes in the affected muscle are obvious with a difference in colour, usually lighter

and more yellow than the adjacent myocardium. Microscopically there is a **mixed inflammatory infiltrate** with less conspicuous neutrophils and numerous macrophages which start to organize the area of infarction (Fig. 8.14).

- **Late**: organization of the infarct leads to scarring (Fig. 8.15) with a progressive reduction in inflammatory infiltration.

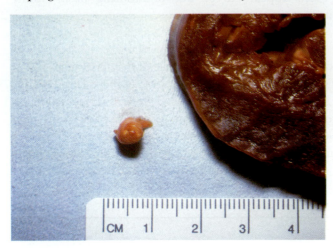

Fig. 8.12 Early myocardial infarction involving the inner half of the wall of the left ventricle and characterized by slight pallor of the myocardium.

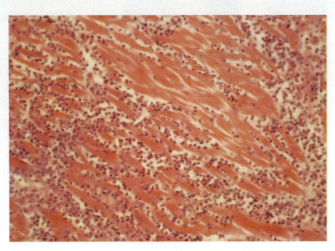

Fig. 8.13 Photomicrograph to show neutrophil polymorph infiltration around the edge of an area of acute myocardial infarction.

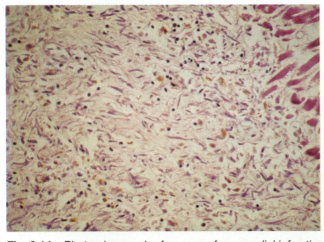

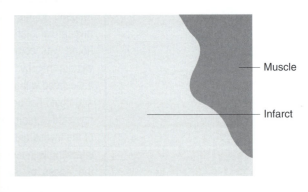

— Muscle

— Infarct

Fig. 8.14 Photomicrograph of an area of myocardial infarction several days old. Many of the infiltrating cells are macrophages.

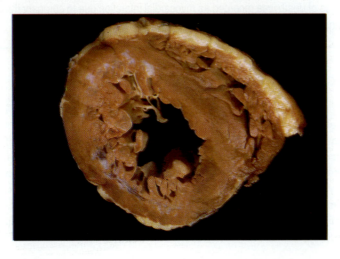

Fig. 8.15 Heart failure due to extensive fibrosis resulting from healed myocardial infarction.

COMPLICATIONS OF MYOCARDIAL INFARCTION

- **Early**: death may result from acute arrhythmia, particularly in the first 24 hours. Alternatively there may be a progressive downhill course in cardiogenic shock, a state of poor cardiac output resulting from extensive loss of functional myocardium. Occasionally death results from rupture of a myocardial infarct and in these circumstances demise is often rapid due to tamponade (see 'Pericardium'). Acute mitral incompetence due to **papillary muscle rupture** and ventricular septal defect, due to infarction involving the interventricular septum, are complications that can potentially be treated surgically and should always be considered in a patient who suddenly deteriorates after an infarct.
- **Late**: extensive areas of fibrosis usually resulting from full thickness myocardial infarction may progressively dilate to produce a **cardiac aneurysm**. Apart from severely impairing cardiac function, these may fill with thrombus and be a source of emboli to the brain and elsewhere.

Heart failure

Oxygen deprivation may affect strength of contraction and/or coordination of contraction either directly or indirectly due to arrhythmias. Heart failure may develop in the face of new acute ischaemia, or old diffuse fibrosis or healed infarction. Heart failure is also one of the manifestations of heart muscle and valvular heart disease.

CASE STUDY 8.4

An 80-year-old woman was admitted to the geriatric ward with shortness of breath. She had been looked after in her own home by her general practitioner and had been increasingly breathless over the past six months. She was on diuretic tables for congestive cardiac failure. Past history included a myocardial infarct several years previously. On examination there was gross pitting oedema of the lower legs and sacrum and there were changes in the chest indicative of pulmonary oedema. In spite of being given further diuretics following admission, her breathlessness continued and she died in her sleep two days after admission. Resuscitation was felt to be inappropriate. Death was certified as being due to congestive cardiac failure. It was the consultant geriatrician's practice to request a postmortem examination on all his patients and with the consent of the relative this was carried out in the hospital. This showed moderate cardiac enlargement (400 g) due to left ventricular hypertrophy. All cardiac chambers were dilated and the left ventricle showed a localized area of fibrosis in the anteroseptal region consistent with an old healed infarct in a background of more diffuse fibrosis due to chronic ischaemia. Coronary arteries showed stenotic three-vessel disease, i.e. left anterior descending, left circumflex and right coronary arteries. The lungs were congested and moderately oedematous. The left lung weighed 500 g and the right 650 g. The liver showed conspicuous nutmeg change with dilated intrahepatic veins. Postmortem histology confirmed the presence of pulmonary oedema and in addition showed evidence of more chronic heart failure with haemosiderin-laden alveolar macrophages.

EFFECTS OF FORWARD FAILURE

Forward failure, reduced cardiac output produces stagnant hypoxia, predominantly reflecting poor left ventricular output.

Brain

Circulation is preferentially maintained. An acute sudden and marked fall in cardiac output leads to unconsciousness, for example in a large coronary thrombosis and in massive pulmonary embolism, or transiently during an episode of complete heart block.

Heart

Coronary circulation is also preferentially maintained. Severe arrhythmias, such as ventricular tachycardia or systemic hypertension, may lead to a reduced coronary flow potentially exacerbating heart failure.

Kidneys

Acute severe reduction in cardiac output, for instance in cardiogenic shock, may precipitate acute tubular necrosis resulting in acute renal failure. More chronic heart failure produces little in the way of structural changes.

Liver

Hypoxic effects are most marked at the periphery of the acinus (furthest from the hepatic artery branch), which is at the centre of the lobule, and here there is hepatocyte loss. Closer to the centre of the acinus, hypoxia may produce fatty change.

BACK PRESSURE EFFECTS

These may reflect left or right ventricular failure.

Acute left ventricular failure

Acute left ventricular failure results in pulmonary venous engorgement and pulmonary oedema.

Chronic left ventricular failure

Chronic left ventricular failure (and mitral stenosis) result in pulmonary venous engorgement, but there is resistance to pulmonary oedema. Small haemorrhages give rise to haemosiderin-laden macrophages, eventually producing brown induration of the lung.

Right ventricular failure

Right ventricular failure produces peripheral oedema with or without ascites and enlargement and tenderness of the liver. Microscopically the engorgement of the central veins, together with the surrounding loss of hepatocytes due to hypoxic effects, with or without more peripheral fatty change, combine to produce '**nutmeg liver**'.

Heart muscle disease

MYOCARDITIS

Inflammation of the myocardium (myocarditis) is rare. Diagnosis may be made on purely clinical grounds, but there is considerable overlap with dilated cardiomyopathy which may present quite acutely with heart failure. The essential histological feature is one of inflammatory infiltration associated with myocardial damage. The degree of inflammation and damage must be appropriate to the degree of heart failure present – the presence of scattered areas of inflammation does not equal acute

---

Mechanisms in heart failure

Potential factors as a cellular basis for contractile failure include:

- Loss of myocytes
- Reduced adrenergic drive
- Reduced β-adrenergic receptor density
- Reduced calcium availability (excitation–contraction coupling)
- Impaired mitochondrial function
- Reduced ATPase function
- Microcirculatory spasm

myocarditis. This may be diagnosed on endomyocardial biopsies or on postmortem examination.

The causes include:

- **bacterial or fungal infection** as part of generalized sepsis in susceptible groups
- **protozoal disease** (such as toxoplasmosis, mainly confined to immunosuppressed patients)
- **viral infection** (for example, Coxsackie B).

Myocarditis may also be 'idiopathic'. **Sarcoidosis** can involve the heart. The granulomatous inflammation and resultant fibrosis predispose to cardiac arrhythmias which can be fatal (Fig. 8.16).

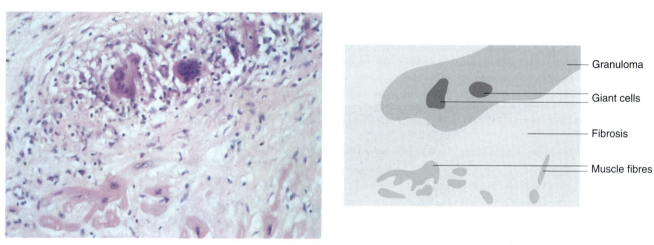

Fig. 8.16 Granulomatous myocarditis in a fatal case of sarcoidosis.

CARDIOMYOPATHY

Cardiomyopathies are the result of abnormal myocardial cell function in the face of normal or insignificantly diseased coronary arteries. There are two main types, **idiopathic dilated** and **hypertrophic**.

Idiopathic dilated cardiomyopathy

This is rare clinically, although mild asymptomatic disease may be more common. The essential pathological features are cardiomegaly and ventricular dilatation (Fig 8.17). Hypertrophy is accompanied by ventricular dilatation, so there may be little increase in wall thickness.

Fig. 8.17 Transverse slice through the heart in a case of idiopathic dilated cardiomyopathy. Note biventricular hypertrophy and cavity dilatation.

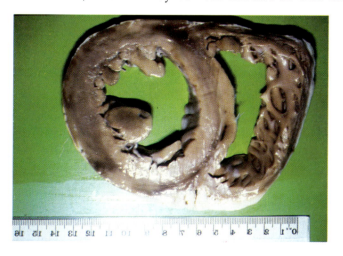

Myocyte volume increases both as a result of hypertrophy seen microscopically in cross-section and as a result of elongation which is more difficult to assess microscopically. There is also myocyte degeneration with variable degrees of interstitial fibrosis. Subendocardial fibrosis is often prominent. Scattered inflammatory cell infiltrates may be seen and lead to difficulties in differentiation from myocarditis. Indeed it is likely that many cases are actually the end-stage of healed myocarditis.

Hypertrophic cardiomyopathy

This disease is also rare, but many cases are familial. The essential pathological abnormality is cardiomegaly often with left ventricular outflow tract obstruction (Fig. 8.18). Various patterns of left ventricular hypertrophy may be seen, including the most well-known and frequent pattern, asymmetrical septal hypertrophy. Microscopically there is myocyte hypertrophy, conspicuous myocyte disarray (Fig. 8.19) and patchy interstitial fibrosis. The myocardial contractility is normal or enhanced. Sudden death may occur due to arrhythmias.

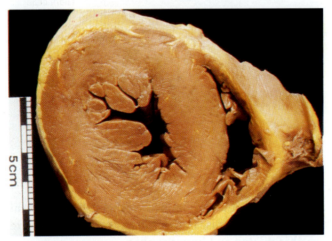

Fig. 8.18   Transverse slice through the heart is a case of hypertrophic cardiomyopathy of the less common concentric type. Note concentric left ventricular hypertrophy

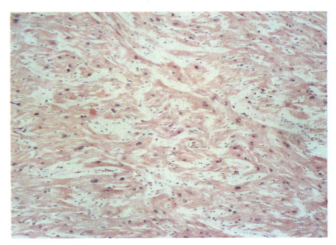

Fig. 8.19   Photomicrograph showing myocyte disarray in a case of hypertrophic cardiomyopathy.

The disease appears to be inherited as an autosomal dominant trait with variable degrees of penetrance and phenotypic expression. There appear to be several genetic abnormalities which may be associated with this syndrome, such as defects in the myosin heavy chain gene. Sporadic cases may occur, possibly as the result of new mutations.

Myocardial infiltrations or depositions

ENDOMYOCARDIAL FIBROSIS

Predominantly endocardial and subendocardial fibrosis produces a restrictive pattern of cardiac function. In the active phase there may be intense inflammatory infiltration, mainly by eosinophils associated with a generalized eosinophilia (**Loeffler's syndrome**).

AMYLOIDOSIS

A general account of amyloidosis is given in Chapter 6. Cardiac involvement may be seen in both AA type (secondary to chronic

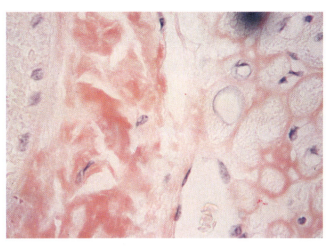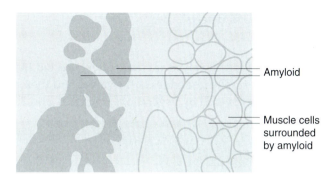

Fig. 8.20 Photomicrograph of cardiac amyloidosis, AL type (Congo red stain). The pink-staining areas showed characteristic apple-green birefringence.

inflammatory diseases) and AL type (secondary to immunocyte dyscrasias) (Fig. 8.20). The myocardial stiffening tends to produce a predominantly restrictive picture. Senile cardiac amyloidosis may be a cause of abnormal cardiac function in elderly people.

HAEMOCHROMATOSIS

This causes cardiac dysfunction due to massive deposition of myocardial haemosiderin and associated fibrosis.

Valvular heart disease

INFECTIVE ENDOCARDITIS

This is an inflammation of the heart valves due to infection, chiefly bacterial. In some groups, such as the immunosuppressed, fungal infections may be seen.

Aetiology

This is most commonly caused by low-grade pathogens such as *Streptococcus viridans* and coagulase-negative staphylococci. Occasionally more virulent organisms such as *Staphylococcus aureus* may be involved.

Pathogenesis

For endocarditis to develop, micro-organisms must enter the body and cause bacteraemia. *Streptococcus viridans* bacteraemia may occur during dental extraction, and hence antibiotic cover is given to patients undergoing this procedure who are known to have abnormal valves. Staphylococci may enter the body by a variety of routes – in heroin addicts injections and abscesses are a common problem. Gram-negative bacteria may enter the bloodstream during operations on the genitourinary tract.

Immunosuppression aids the survival of organisms in the bloodstream and their growth on the valves. It may occur as a result of diseases themselves, as in lymphoma, or it may occur as a result of necessary treatments, such as cytotoxic chemotherapy in malignancy or immunosuppressant regimens following solid organ transplants.

Often, the affected valves were previously abnormal, due to a congenital or acquired abnormality of the heart or great vessels (such as congenital bicuspid aortic valve, scarring by previous rheumatic endocarditis, degeneration associated with old age, grafted or prosthetic valves, ventricular septal defects).

Pathology

The aortic and mitral valves are more often affected than those on the right side of the heart. The free edges of the valves and their areas of contact with each other are covered by vegetations (Figs 8.21 and 8.22).

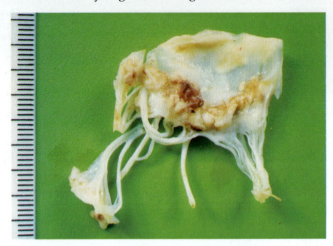

Fig. 8.21   Vegetations on the mitral valve in a case of infective endocarditis.

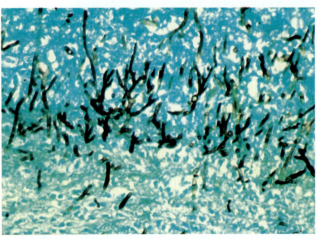

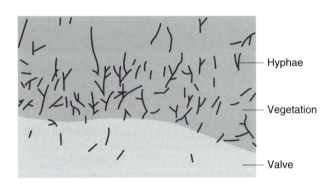

Hyphae

Vegetation

Valve

Fig. 8.22   Photomicrograph of the mitral valve in a heart transplant recipient dying of invasive aspergillosis. The fungal hyphae stain black in this silver stain and show acute angle branching characteristic of *Aspergillus* spp.

Vegetations consist of a superficial layer of fibrin and platelets, a middle layer in which colonies of micro-organisms are seen, and a deeper layer of organizing inflammatory exudate. The latter becomes progressively organized owing to growth of capillaries and fibroblasts from the base of the valve.

Complications

The main complications are:

- perforation or rupture of the valve leading to heart failure
- embolism leading to major cerebral damage
- septic embolism with formation of mycotic aneurysms
- a combination of immune-complex/microembolism-mediated disease leading to Ostler's nodes, myocardial damage, renal damage (focal, segmental glomerulonephritis), cerebral damage, etc.

Laboratory diagnosis

This is by repeated blood culture before antibiotic treatment starts.

RHEUMATIC HEART DISEASE

Rheumatic fever is a systemic disease affecting the heart, joints and other organs, now extremely rare in Britain. It follows 2–3 weeks after an upper respiratory tract infection.

Aetiology

The disease usually occurs after tonsillitis due to a β-haemolytic group A streptococcal infection.

Pathogenesis

No organisms are isolated from the heart and joints, and damage resulting from hypersensitivity mechanisms has been postulated. Hypersensitivity could be due to common antigens shared by streptococci and connective tissues (antibodies against streptococcal antigens are found in the serum, but are not proven to cause damage), deposition of immune complexes or other mechanisms.

Pathology

The pathology is that of a pancarditis – in other words there are changes affecting endocardium, myocardium and pericardium. The mitral and aortic valves are more commonly affected than other heart valves, but the aortic valve is usually only affected if the mitral valve is involved as well.

Aschoff's nodules form the characteristic histological lesion (Fig. 8.23). These microscopic fusiform granulomata are composed of macrophages, large cells with prominent nucleoli (some of which may be derived from damaged heart muscle fibres) and plasma cells. They occur mainly in the interstitium of the heart and may occur in other tissues such as joints and subcutaneous tissue. There may be glycoproteins ('fibrin') in the middle. In the valves they also damage the elastic tissue, and small vegetations form on the inflamed areas.

Fig. 8.23   An Aschoff's nodule.

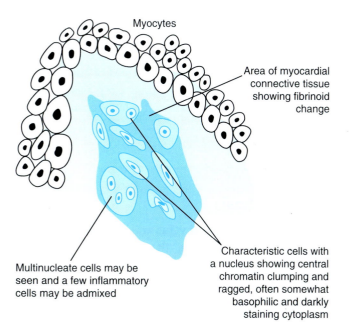

Myocytes

Area of myocardial connective tissue showing fibrinoid change

Multinucleate cells may be seen and a few inflammatory cells may be admixed

Characteristic cells with a nucleus showing central chromatin clumping and ragged, often somewhat basophilic and darkly staining cytoplasm

Complications

The most important early complications are death due to heart failure or arrhythmia in the acute stage, but both are rare. However, later complications are common. Lesions in the heart heal by fibrosis ultimately leading to stenosis and/or incompetence of the valves which ultimately tend to calcify. Mitral stenosis and aortic stenosis are the most common results and are often seen today in patients who had rheumatic fever in their childhood (Fig. 8.24). Many surgically excised heart valves show evidence of past inflammation in the form of neovascularization, and this is taken to be presumptive evidence of past inflammation of rheumatic type.

The basal ganglia of the brain may be damaged acutely (**Sydenham's chorea**), but inflammation of joints and other organs usually resolves without untoward effects.

CALCIFIC AORTIC VALVE DISEASE

Severe calcification of the aortic valve leading to stenosis is often seen in old people without prior history of infective endocarditis.

Possible causes include:

- rheumatic valve disease, unlikely in the absence of coexistent mitral disease
- end result of a silent endocarditis (brucellosis has been suggested)
- congenital valve disease, most commonly bicuspid aortic valve
- **degenerative valve disease**.

Of these, degenerative calcific disease of the aortic valve is clinically the most important, accounting for most aortic valves surgically excised for valve replacement (Fig. 8.25). It is distinguished from postinflammatory causes by the tendency of calcification to spare the free edges and by the lack of commissural fusion and neovascularization.

MYXOID MITRAL DEGENERATION

The mitral valve may undergo myxoid degeneration of the cusps, with resultant incompetence. The cause of this is not clear. In younger people it is associated with disorders of collagen and elastin metabolism, such as Marfan's syndrome, where there is also a tendency to develop dissecting aortic aneurysms.

The principal features include thinning/rupture of chordae tendineae with ballooning of valve cusps (Fig. 8.26). Areas of cusp thickening due to friction lesions may result from redundant cusp tissue. Microscopically there is myxoid degeneration of valvular connective tissue with accumulation of acid mucins.

Venous disease

Deep vein thrombosis

Formation of thrombus in the calf veins and more proximally in the lower limbs is probably more common than is realized clinically. Venous obstruction generally leads to oedema of the limb involved. Cellulitis may develop. However, by far the most important complication is thromboembolism where part or all of the venous thrombus breaks off, ultimately becoming lodged in the pulmonary circulation. The effect of this

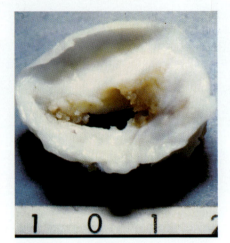

Fig. 8.24 Surgically excised stenotic mitral valve from a patient aged 60 years who had had rheumatic fever in childhood.

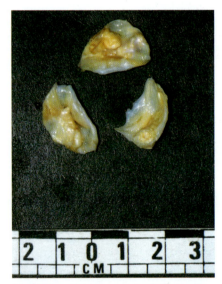

Fig. 8.25 Degenerative calcific aortic stenosis. The three cusps have been surgically excised separately. Note calcification is mainly central, sparing the free edges.

Fig. 8.26 Ballooning of the mitral valve leaflets in a case of severe mucinous degeneration.

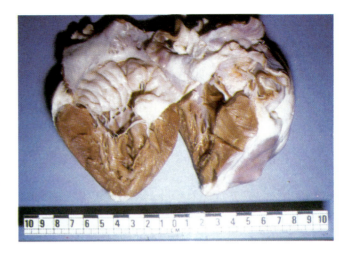

is very variable and clearly depends on the size and amount of thrombus released into the circulation. Fatal pulmonary embolism is, however, a relatively common cause of sudden death, particularly in those with risk factors for venous thrombosis, such as immobility, and trauma including surgical trauma (Fig. 8.27). Hence the tendency for it to occur in hospital inpatients, and the increasing efforts to prevent it by prophylactic anticoagulation, support stockings, etc.

Fig. 8.27 Fatal pulmonary thromboembolism. Both left and right pulmonary arteries were occluded by a mass of thrombus originating in the legs.

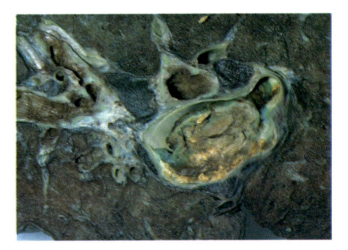

Thrombophlebitis

Thrombophlebitis results from inflammation of veins with superimposed thrombosis. This may be infective and occur in relation to a nidus of infection, for example in the uterus following septic abortion, in the central vein following facial or sinus infection. Recurrent thrombophlebitis of superficial veins is often a paraneoplastic syndrome and may be the first sign that the patient has a carcinoma somewhere. It is often associated with pancreatic cancer, but may occur in relation to breast, stomach, ovarian or bronchial malignancy.

Varicose veins

Varicose veins may occur in response to gravitational stress or obstruction of venous outflow. Predispositions to saphenous varicosity in the legs include obesity, child bearing and poor fitness. Haemorrhoids in the anus form in response to prolonged straining at stool and may bleed or prolapse through the anus. Obstruction of veins by tumours or in the liver by cirrhosis is common. In portal hypertension, which often accompanies cirrhosis, the high portal venous pressure gives rise to dilated varicose veins in areas where portosystemic shunting can occur, such as in the lower oesophagus (Fig. 8.28) where erosion and rupture can cause torrential haemorrhage.

Pericardium

The pericardium forms a potential space around the heart. Free movement of the visceral and parietal surfaces over one another is facilitated by a small amount of pericardial fluid. Normally this is clear and serous, but in pericarditis the quantity may increase dramatically and it may become purulent.

Release of blood into the pericardium due to rupture of the heart following myocardial infarction or trauma (haemopericardium) may restrict cardiac contraction severely (**cardiac tamponade**) (Fig. 8.29). Low-output cardiogenic shock and death rapidly supervene if the pressure of fluid is not released. Occasionally, rapid accumulation of pericardial effusions can also cause tamponade.

The most common cause of a non-inflammation pericarditis is spread of malignant disease, usually metastatic carcinoma.

Cardiac tumours

Primary cardiac tumours are very rare; most tumours involving the heart are metastatic in origin with the pericardium being the most commonly involved part. The **atrial myxoma** is the most frequently encountered primary cardiac tumour. This forms a glistening friable mass (Fig. 8.30), usually in the left atrium where it may behave like a ball-valve and obstruct the mitral valve. These tumours are derived from pluripotential mesenchymal cells. Tumour haemorrhage and degeneration are common, and fragments may break off and embolize. Systemic symptoms may occur due to production of cytokines, including interleukin-6.

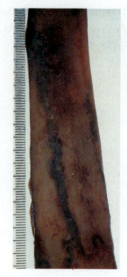

Fig. 8.28 Varices at the lower end of the oesophagus in a case of portal hypertension. The oesophagus has been turned inside out to facilitate demonstration of the varices.

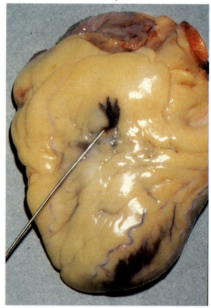

Fig. 8.29 Accidental puncture of the right ventricle during sternal marrow puncture precipitated rapid death due to cardiac tamponade.

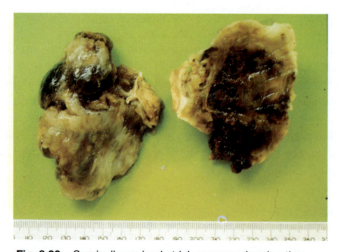

Fig. 8.30 Surgically excised atrial myxoma showing the friability and tendency to haemorrhage in these tumours.

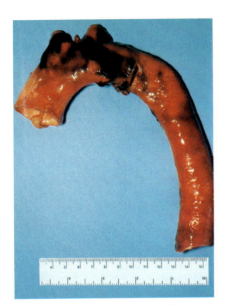

Fig. 8.31 Traumatic rupture of the aorta in a fatal road traffic accident (front seat passenger in a high-speed collision).

Cardiovascular trauma

Haemorrhage due to vascular injury is a frequent manifestation of trauma to any part of the body. The heart may be contused in crushing injuries, or it may be injured directly in stabbing of the chest or gunshot wounds. Apart from the direct functional consequences of cardiac injury and haemorrhage, there may also be indirect results of cardiac perforation such as tamponade. The aorta may rupture in high-speed road traffic accidents (Fig. 8.31). Rupture usually occurs close to the isthmus adjacent to the ligamentum arteriosus where the ductus arteriosus was inserted. The injury is quite clean cut and transverse often with a number of further partial thickness transverse tears inferior to it. In the past this was thought to be a pure deceleration injury. This is partially correct, but it is now thought that tearing results from direct crushing of the aorta between the left clavicle and chest wall anteriorly and the spine posteriorly during severe deceleration. The crushing is typically the result of chest compression against seat belt restraint or the steering wheel.

Chapter 9 Respiratory disease

Learning objectives

To appreciate and understand:
- ❏ Normal structure and development of the respiratory tract, and how this relates to disease
- ❏ Main diseases affecting the nose, larynx and upper airways
- ❏ Importance of respiratory infections
- ❏ Pathogenesis of pneumonia
- ❏ Aetiology and pathology of chronic obstructive and other inflammatory lung disease
- ❏ Main types of lung tumour, their likely methods of spread and presentation

The respiratory tract

The respiratory tract includes the nose, sinuses, larynx, trachea, bronchi and lungs (Fig. 9.1). Diseases of the pleura will also be considered in this chapter.

The basic function of the respiratory tract is **gas exchange**. This requires conduction of air from the nose to the site of gas exchange in lung alveoli which are lined by a thin layer of cells which is easily damaged. The dry air must therefore be humidified in the nose and the airways must be defended against microbial invasion. The basic morphology – an epithelial cell layer composed of ciliary cells, goblet cells, basal cells capable of regeneration, neurosecretory cells, separated by a basal membrane from the submucosal cells – ensures an effective defence mechanism by mucus secretion and ciliary movements

In order to transport the air in both directions in this one-way tubular system, air must be inhaled and exhaled rhythmically, and its volume has to be minimal compared with the volume in which peripheral exchange takes place. This basic morphology is closely associated with normal and abnormal lung function.

The nasal passages

The nose is the entrance to the air-conducting system. It is a symmetrical hollow organ composed of bone, cartilage, muscle, connective tissue and epithelium. In the entrance to the nose (the nares), this epithelium is of stratified squamous type, like the skin, while in the posterior nasal space it is of pseudostratified ciliated columnar type with interspersed goblet cells

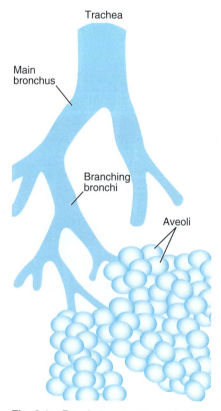

Fig. 9.1 Respiratory tract morphology from trachea to alveolus.

Fig. 9.2 Nasal mucosa. Note the ciliated epithelium with interspersed goblet cells and the submucosal glands.

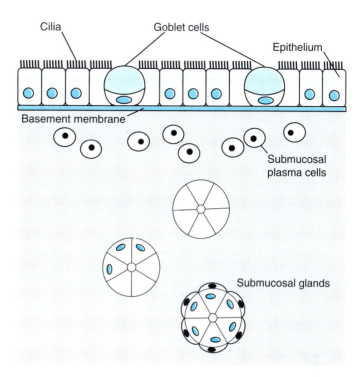

(Fig. 9.2). Mixed mucous glands are present in the submucosa. The mucus produced traps particles and the cilia transport them towards the pharynx. This system is 'activated' by various agents such as tobacco smoke, cold air or dust. The frontal, maxillary, ethmoidal and sphenoidal sinuses connect with the nasal cavity, and are also covered by pseudostratified ciliated epithelium.

RHINITIS

The nose is exposed to a wide variety of external agents and inflammation (acute or chronic rhinitis) is common. **Acute rhinitis** is usually due to viral infection or type I hypersensitivity reactions (hay fever). Common allergens are pollens of blooming grasses, dusts and animal proteins. The reaction induced is not limited to the nose, but may involve the conjunctivae and lungs, in which case asthma is the result. Repeated infection or allergy may lead to chronic rhinitis which can be classified into three main types (see box).

Wegener's granulomatosis is a specific granulomatous entity in which necrotizing granulomatous inflammation coexists with inflammation of small blood vessels (vasculitis). This appears to be an autoimmune disease, with antibodies to neutrophil cytoplasmic antigens (ANCA) in serum. Starting in the upper respiratory tract, it eventually affects the lungs. It is often combined with glomerulonephritis, and a generalized vasculitis similar to polyarteritis nodosa.

TUMOURS

These can be divided into those which arise on the skin covering the nose, and those which arise inside the nose. External benign tumours include basal cell and squamous papillomas, while malignant tumours include **basal cell carcinomas** and **squamous cell carcinomas**. Inside the nose, squamous cell carcinomas and adenoid cystic carcinomas occur, as well as the T-lymphocyte-derived lymphoma known confusingly as **lethal**

Types of chronic rhinitis
- **Hyperplastic rhinitis**, in which chronic hypersensitivity reaction leads to the formation of nasal polyps with epithelial metaplasia to a stratified squamous form
- **Chronic atrophic rhinitis**, a disease of young people induced by infection with *Klebsiella ozoneae* or endocrine/neural disorders
- **Chronic granulomatous rhinitis**, caused by *Klebsiella rhinoscleromatis*, tuberculosis, syphilis or leprosy

midline granuloma, which can completely destroy the nose. Exposure to nickel and other toxic agents can lead to the development of benign or malignant nasal tumours. In certain parts of the world, particularly eastern Asia, **nasopharyngeal carcinoma** related to Epstein–Barr virus infection is a particular problem. This tumour arises within the posterior nasal space and is often detected only at an advanced stage.

The larynx

The larynx connects the pharynx with the trachea and is closed during swallowing by the epiglottis. It is composed of a cartilaginous framework connected by intrinsic and extrinsic muscles which change the shape of the larynx during phonation. The proximal part of the larynx is covered by squamous epithelium, while the basal part is covered by ciliated columnar epithelium similar to that lining the trachea. Disorders of the larynx usually present with choking or hoarseness.

Inflammation of the larynx (**laryngitis**) is similar in principle to that seen in the nose, but acute reactions with oedema may be life-threatening. Acute laryngeal oedema can be caused by:

- bacterial toxins (such as diphtheria)
- physical and chemical agents (such as heat, smoke or smog)
- allergic (type 1) reactions (from bee stings, food or drugs, for example).

Angioneurotic oedema is a congenital disorder based on a defect of the complement C1-inhibitor system, which induces recurrent activation of C1 and separation of C-kinin from complement component C2, leading to acute oedema. Acute oedema of the larynx, lips, skin, neck and genitalia may be seen. **Bacterial laryngitis** may produce membranes or pseudomembranes which can detach from the mucosa and block the air passage. This is a particular danger with diphtheria, but parainfluenza viruses may cause a similar syndrome (**croup**) in children. **Chronic laryngitis** is usually related to smoking and results in pseudopolyp formation on the vocal folds (vocal cords).

True neoplasms include **squamous papillomas**, which are associated with papilloma virus infection (types 6 and 11). Malignant tumours are usually **squamous cell carcinomas** in which smoking and alcohol play a role. The sex ratio is heavily male-oriented (male:female = 10:1) and about 50% of all laryngeal carcinomas develop on the vocal folds.

The trachea and bronchi

Disturbances of the conducting airways relate to increased cellular turnover, chronic inflammation, narrowing of the bronchial lumen and collapse or expansion of the alveoli.

Irritation of the bronchial mucosa by infection, inflammation or inhalation of toxins (as in smoking) leads to an increase of goblet cells, and an increased turnover and number of basal cells. Severe disturbance may cause ulcerative inflammation and squamous metaplasia, which are often combined with signs of cellular dysplasia. These alterations are normally limited to specific areas such as the carina. There may be a focal narrowing of the lumen, leading to an increase in conduction resistance, as occurs in asthma and chronic bronchitis.

The stability of the bronchi is maintained as long as the cartilage and the smooth muscle cells are not endangered by fibrosis, chronic destructive inflammation and infection.

BRONCHIAL OCCLUSION

Complete **acute bronchial occlusion** of the upper airways is usually caused by aspiration of solid objects (such as peanuts), or acute allergic reactions. **Partial bronchial occlusion** is more common: it is the reason for wheezing in asthma caused by bronchospasm (contraction of bronchial muscle) which may be acute or chronic. Bronchial narrowing increases the conduction resistance, and hence diminishes the volume of transported air. Patients compensate for this by breathing faster and using the voluntary muscles of the chest to increase the volumes transported. Some forms of bronchial narrowing may affect expiration more than inspiration, or vice versa. Diminished inspiration, as seen in focal bronchial narrowing, results in areas of collapsed peripheral lung parenchyma (atelectasis); diminished expiration causes over-expansion of the peripheral lung parenchyma and may result in emphysema.

Some tumours prefer to grow into the bronchus (carcinoid tumours, for example) (Fig. 9.3). These can clinically simulate bronchial asthma and lead to collapse of the lung behind the obstruction. The collapsed tissue may become infected or filled by lipid-containing macrophages (lipid pneumonia).

BRONCHIECTASIS

Focal or diffuse enlargement of the bronchial lumen is associated with severe disturbance of the bronchial defences and, consequently, with chronic pulmonary infections which affect the stability of the bronchial wall and lead to further damage (Fig. 9.4).

Pulmonary arteries and veins

The pulmonary arteries and veins are the main blood transport vessels in the lung. The pulmonary arteries transport deoxygenated blood from the right heart to the peripheral lung zones; the pulmonary veins transport

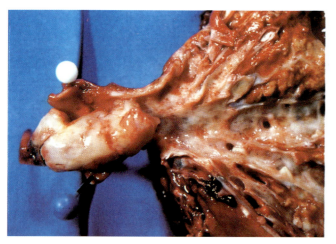

Fig. 9.3   Macroscopic appearance of a tumour causing bronchial obstruction and distal dilatation (localized bronchiectasis).

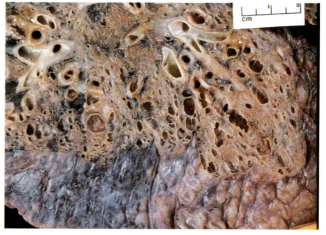

Fig. 9.4   Diffuse bronchiectasis (dilatation of bronchi), shown here in cross-section, is caused by damage to the bronchial walls, often as the result of infections such as whooping cough.

oxygenated blood from the lung parenchyma to the left heart. The arteries have to transport blood at a pressure of 20 mmHg to the peripheral capillary system, and have a distinct external and internal elastic lamina in their proximal parts.

Disturbances of the pulmonary arteries may be acute or chronic. Focal narrowing is usually not caused by atherosclerotic changes, but by external compression of the lumen due to fibrotic inflammation or, more frequently, by malignant neoplasms. Small thrombotic lesions are often reactive to inflammation or infection.

DILATATION

Dilatation may be induced by inborn alterations of the arterial walls (Ehlers–Danlos syndrome) or may be related to a focal narrowing downstream. The amount of transported blood is often only minimally altered owing to an adaptive increase in blood pressure from the right ventricle of the heart. Several inflammatory disorders such as sarcoidosis, tuberculosis or autoimmune disease can also destroy the arterial walls, leading to haemorrhage into bronchioles or bronchi.

OCCLUSION

Acute occlusion is commonly caused by emboli from the right side of the heart or femoral–tibial veins (deep venous thrombosis), and is often lethal. Acute occlusion of medium-sized arteries in patients with chronic left heart insufficiency can induce **haemorrhagic lung infarction**. Non-lethal thrombotic lesions can be completely or partially reabsorbed, with no long-term damage to the lung, or reorganized to form a fibrous scar.

Chronically increased pulmonary arterial pressure causes a proliferation of the smooth muscle cells in the small to medium-sized arterial walls and, secondarily, thrombotic lesions. Narrowing of the arterial lumen due to this atherosclerosis-like process further diminishes blood flow and causes further increase in arterial pressure. This cycle is only broken when the heart can no longer compensate for the increased resistance and right heart failure ensues.

Narrowing of the venous lumen is usually caused by external compression of the walls; chronic occlusive narrowing induces severe **pulmonary hypertension**, and may be fatal (**veno-occlusive disease**). This occlusion, which can be associated with various agents, is attended by organized thrombotic lesions and spreading fibrosis.

BRONCHIAL ARTERIES AND VEINS

Bronchial arteries are of systemic origin, originating from the aorta. They supply the conducting airways and the related structures, but have numerous anastomoses to their pulmonary counterparts. Their clinical importance is related mainly to thoracic surgery.

The bronchial veins enter the systemic venous system by way of the azygos or hemiazygos vein. They have thin valves, in contrast to the pulmonary veins. Between pulmonary arteries and veins and bronchial arteries and veins there are numerous anastomoses of muscular arterioles and venules. These may be responsible for clinically important shunting of blood from the systemic to the pulmonary circulation. Despite congenital abnormalities, thoracic surgery is the major cause of stenosis or occlusion of bronchial arteries and veins, and no severe atherosclerotic lesions are reported. Artificial occlusion or narrowing of bronchial arteries can induce infarct-like lesions of the bronchial walls with severe secondary bacterial infections.

Lymphatic system

The lymphatic vessels follow the bronchi along the submucosa and the pulmonary arteries along the adventitia. They start around the terminal bronchioles and are not present in the interalveolar septa. The lymphatic system can be hyperplastic, hypoplastic, associated respectively with ectasia or obliteration of the conducting vessels and lymph nodes. **Focal lymphoid hyperplasia** is a frequent harmless lesion (circumscribed 'pseudolymph nodes' in the peripheral lung parenchyma). It is indistinguishable from malignancy (usually metastases) on radiographs and is therefore of major clinical importance. **Ectasia of the lymphatic vessels** is usually a fatal congenital disorder (due to associated severe cardiovascular malformations) and affects mainly the subpleural vessels. Obliteration of central localized intrapulmonary lymph nodes is mainly caused by fibrosis and scarring, often associated with infections (tuberculosis) or inhalation of toxic particles (such as silicosis). Involvement of the lymphatic system and intrapulmonary lymph nodes in primary lung cancer usually determines the prognosis of the patient.

Lung parenchyma

Most of the lung is composed of tightly packed alveoli, which provide a total area for gas exchange similar in size to a tennis court. The main function of the peripheral lung parenchyma is the exchange by diffusion of oxygen and carbon dioxide between the inhaled air and the blood of the interstitial capillaries. The alveoli (Fig. 9.5) have a thin lining of type I pneumocytes which permit gas diffusion and are derived from larger type II pneumocytes which secrete surfactant, a protein important in maintaining lung aeration. Type II pneumocytes respond to injury by proliferation. Severe disturbances are usually caused by diffuse thickening or destruction of the interstitial

Fig. 9.5 Normal alveoli showing the flat type I pneumocytes and the larger type II pneumocytes responsible for surfactant production. Note the proximity of the alveolar lumen to the interstitial capillaries which is important for gas exchange.

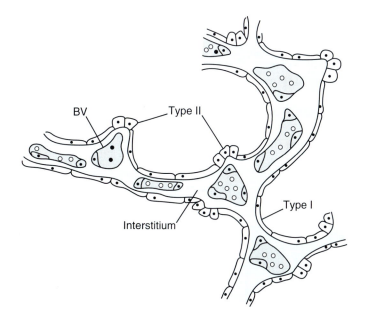

barrier. Destructive agents can attack from the airspaces or from the blood barrier side. Those attacking from the alveoli are usually infectious agents (anaerobic bacteria, viruses, rickettsia, fungi), fibres passing the clearance of the conducting airways (asbestos) or airborne toxins. The most important exogenous source of toxins is cigarette smoking, which causes damage to the surface of the conducting airways and the cellular defence mechanisms of the peripheral lung. Those attacking from the inner side of the capillaries are usually abnormal components of the immune system (autoantibodies, cytokines, phagocytes), blood-borne infectious agents (septicaemia) or cancer cells (metastasis). In addition, disturbances in nutrition can induce focal tissue breakdown as seen in infarction.

RESPONSE TO INJURY

The possible **tissue reactions** of the lung to airborne attack (Fig. 9.6) include **pulmonary oedema, acute inflammation, haemorrhage**, and isolation of the inciting agents by **granuloma** or **abscess formation**. These reactions are followed by either resolution or organization of damaged area with fibrosis (Fig. 9.7). Airborne infectious attacks usually have an acute onset and trigger an acute inflammatory response in which the stage of the defence reaction can be recognized morphologically.

The inciting inhaled agent may modify the nature of the parenchymal reaction. Slowly growing fungi or bacteria such as *Mycobacterium tuberculosis* or exogenous agents induce immunological hypersensitivity resulting in epithelioid granuloma formation, while viral agents need to grow within cells to survive and may induce nuclear inclusions and other morphological abnormalities in pneumocytes or macrophages.

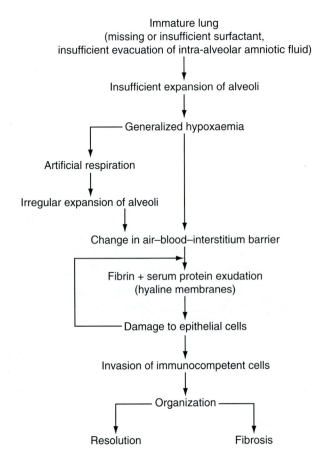

Fig. 9.6 Response to infectious attack in the lung.

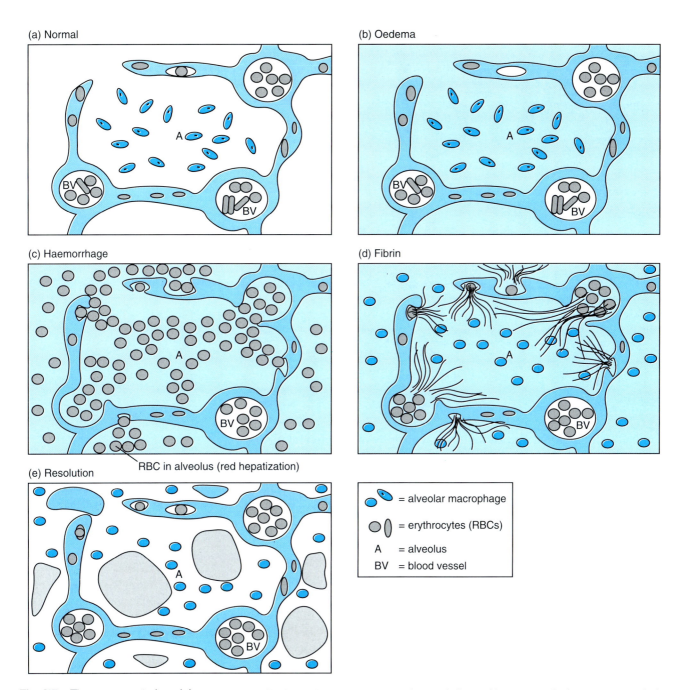

(a) Normal

(b) Oedema

(c) Haemorrhage

(d) Fibrin

RBC in alveolus (red hepatization)

(e) Resolution

= alveolar macrophage

= erythrocytes (RBCs)

A   = alveolus
BV = blood vessel

Fig. 9.7   The response to lung injury follows the pattern of acute inflammation and (usually) resolution as discussed in Chapter 6, but the anatomy of the alveolus creates special features. The alveoli (a) become filled with oedema fluid (b). This is followed by inflammatory cell migration (c) and there may be some haemorrhage into the alveoli at this stage. Fibrin formation may be followed by organization (d), but often resolution (e) is complete.

All disturbances can result in diffuse fibrosis and destruction of the alveolar architecture of the lung (honeycomb lung), which is the end stage of all chronic active inflammatory diseases. The function of such lungs is severely impaired and affected patients usually die from respiratory failure.

Pleura

The pleura lines the thoracic cavity and covers the external surface of the lung. Its function is to provide a leakproof container for the gas exchange membrane and to permit lung movement. The pleura (Fig. 9.8) consists of a layer of mesothelial cells on a layer of loose connective tissue resting on a thick elastic membrane. **Pneumothorax** (leakage of air into the pleural space) is usually seen in the upper parts of the pleura or lungs and is often

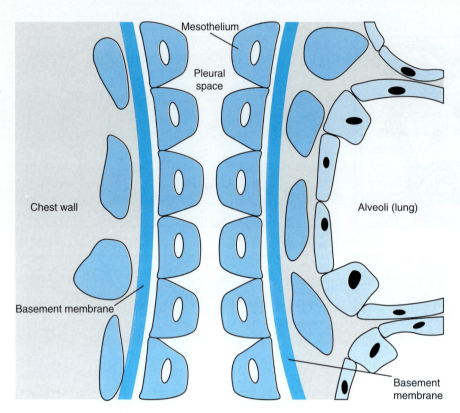

Fig. 9.8   Pleura showing the double layers of mesothelium which slide over each other. In disease, the potential space between them may be filled with air (pneumothorax) or fluid (pleural effusion).

combined with a partial fibrosis and partial atrophy of the visceral pleura. It is associated with chronic obstructive airway disease, asthma, subpleural postpneumonic scars, or rare disorders such as histiocytosis X or *Pneumocystis carinii* infection. It induces acute collapse of the affected lung. **Haemothorax** results from bleeding into the pleural space. **Pleural effusion** is usually caused by diseases which interfere with normal fluid transport across the mesothelium.

Pleural fibrosis is often induced by pneumonia, especially if recurrent, and any scarring that occurs during their resolution. Some inhaled fibres can induce severe pleural fibrosis, including asbestos which induces pleural plaques with a histologically distinctive basket-weave appearance. Acute and chronic (bacterial) infections are difficult to treat and arise as complications of thoracic surgery or pneumonia. Inflammatory pleural diseases often progress to severe pleural fibrosis which can induce irreversible damage to the lung due to chronic constriction. Recurrent inflammation induces a dramatic proliferation of the mesothelial cells, usually combined with severe cellular atypia, making the histological appearance difficult to distinguish from malignant mesothelioma.

Diseases of the lung

Lung diseases and other organs

The function of the lungs is strongly bound to that of the heart in both health and disease. Failure of lung function affects the heart and the central nervous system, and induces a feed-forward mechanism, often with fatal outcome. Increasing pulmonary blood resistance increases the pressure in the right heart and vice versa, as well as exacerbating insufficiency of the left side of the heart. **Pulmonary hypertension** is, in addition, associated

---

Causes of pleural effusion

■ **Increased fluid entry**: this may occur as the result of pleural inflammation owing to
  ● infection of the underlying lung (pneumonia, tuberculosis)
  ● connective tissue disease
  ● pulmonary infarction
  ● malignancy
  ● subphrenic abscess
  ● acute pancreatitis.

■ Inflammatory pleural effusions may be serous, fibrinous, haemorrhagic or purulent (causing empyema if localized). In addition, right heart failure, hypoproteinaemia or increased blood volume leads to increased fluid entry and may cause an effusion.

■ **Reduced fluid output**, usually as a result of lymphatic obstruction due to malignancy. This may be situated locally (lymphangitis carcinomatosa, for example) or at the hilar lymph nodes.

with liver cirrhosis, congenital malformations, and some parasitic infections (schistosomiasis).

Similarities between the lungs and the kidneys can be seen in their capillary system: both organs are often involved simultaneously in immunological disorders. Precursors of angiotensin-converting enzyme are altered into their active form in the lungs, and lipoid substances are altered by the intrapulmonary macrophages. Abnormal molecular components may be shared with other organs, cystic fibrosis being the prime example.

The lungs are the target organ for metastases of malignancies from many other organs, especially carcinoma of the breast, colon–rectum, thyroid, testis, kidneys and various childhood tumours. Metastatic tumour growth can occur via the lymphatic or vascular system, and is not necessarily associated with metastatic spread into the liver.

Congenital and developmental diseases

Severe malformations of the lung include complete or partial absence of bronchial, peripheral lung, arterial, venous or lymphatic structures, and are usually incompatible with life. Most are associated with coexistent malformations of other organs. The lungs are formed in the fourth week of gestation, when the right and left stem bronchi and lung buds become recognizable (Fig. 9.9). Isolated or bilateral absence of the lung have been reported rarely, but absence of one or several lobes is more common. Mild

Fig. 9.9 Fetal and neonatal lung development: (a) embryonal period (weeks 4–7); (b) pseudoglandular period (weeks 8–16); (c) canalicular period (weeks 16–25; (d) terminal period (week 24–birth): (e) early alveolar period in the newborn.

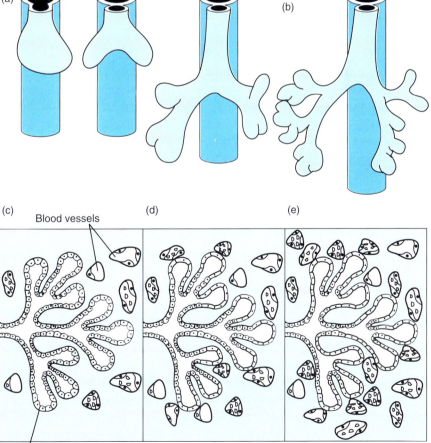

abnormalities may be clinically silent or result in chronic or recurrent pulmonary infections. Maturity of the lung parenchyma is closely associated with the birth weight; clinically severe disorders associated with immature lung parenchyma are the **infant respiratory distress syndrome** (hyaline membrane disease) and **bronchopulmonary dysplasia**.

Of clinical importance are those abnormalities which decrease the bronchopulmonary defence mechanism and proceed to chronic pulmonary infections. Abnormal connection of the airway system with the peripheral lung parenchyma (and of the blood supply with the systemic vessels) is called **sequestration**.

- In **intralobular sequestration**, the disconnected part is within a pulmonary lobe – the sequestrated lobe is surrounded by the pleura covering the normal and abnormal lung parenchyma.
- In **extralobular sequestration**, there is a separated pleura covering the (accessory) sequestrated lobe.

Intralobular sequestration can become clinically important as a result of recurrent infections in both young children and adults, and is usually discovered as a circumscribed intrapulmonary mass. Infection of extralobular sequestrated lungs is less common, and the malformation can be clinically silent or is discovered due to coexisting abnormalities such as diaphragmatic hernia or pectus excavatum, or arteriovenous shunts.

Malformations of the peripheral lung parenchyma include **pulmonary hypoplasia**, which is defined as abnormal reduction of one or both lungs in weight or volume with normal macroscopic arrangement. It can be associated with various factors including Down's syndrome, scoliosis, diaphragmatic hernia, polycystic kidneys, amniotic fluid deficit (renal agenesis), metabolic defects (rhesus incompatibility), or decreased blood flow as seen in congenital pulmonary valve stenosis. Congenital intrapulmonary cysts and heterotopic tissue are usually of minor clinical importance, but congenital overinflation (lobar infantile emphysema) is usually associated with bronchial obstruction caused by inborn stenosis or external bronchial compression due to abnormal vessels.

Malformations of the vascular system include:

- alveolar capillary dysplasia
- abnormal origin of the pulmonary arteries from the aorta or its branches
- origin of the left pulmonary artery from the right and indentation by the trachea
- absent or hypoplastic arteries of one or both sides
- anomalous return of the pulmonary veins.

Congenital abnormalities of the lymphatic tissue are usually ectatic lesions, induced mechanically or by hamartomatous lesions (multiple lymphangiomas). A separate disorder which includes features of a hamartomatous lesion and dysplastic growth of the peripheral lung parenchyma is called **adenomatoid cystic malformation of the lung**. It is seen in young children and usually affects one lobe. This disorder is characterized by lack of major bronchi and dysplastic lung parenchyma which communicates with the adjacent normal lung parenchyma.

Classification of congenital abnormalities of the bronchi

- Increased or decreased number of bronchi either on one or both sides (bronchial isomerism syndrome, i.e. bilateral right or left formation of bronchi, often associated with anisosplenia, polysplenia, cardiac malformation)
- Supernumerary bronchi, accessory cardiac bronchus (arising from the intermediate bronchus), abnormal connections between the right and left bronchi (bridging), abnormal connection with other organs (broncho-oesophageal, bronchobiliary fistula)
- Abnormalities of the composition of the bronchial wall and epithelial cells

Infant respiratory distress syndrome

The events at birth, when the lungs are needed within seconds of delivery, are of special clinical importance. The maturity of the lung is closely associated with the weight of the newborn, and the production and composition of the surfactant which is needed for the normal expansion of the lungs. Insufficient expansion of the lungs induces severe disturbances of the gas exchange and leads to the infant respiratory distress syndrome (see Chapter 16) which may require prolonged artificial respiration.

The primary feature of this disease on microscopy is the presence of hyaline membranes within the terminal bronchioles and alveoli. Hyaline membranes are a mixture of exuded fibrin and serum proteins which stain positively with the periodic acid–Schiff (PAS) stain. Degenerating epithelial cells, macrophages and histiocytes are also present. The alveoli are collapsed and the lumen of the bronchioles and smaller bronchi may be expanded. Hyaline membranes may resolve, or may undergo organization to produce the changes known as **bronchopulmonary dysplasia**, which may be related to oxygen toxicity. Histologically this condition shows marked proliferation of fibroblasts intermingled with mononuclear inflammatory infiltrates and squamous metaplasia of the epithelial lining. In its later stages, there is formation of broad bundles of collagen fibres and proliferating smooth muscle cells. The end result is **honeycomb lung**. The prognosis of children with bronchopulmonary dysplasia is poor: 50% will die within the first week and the survivors develop severe disturbances in lung function and progressive respiratory failure.

Infection of the lung

BACTERIAL INFECTION

Infective agents of the lung are usually inhaled, but can reach the lung via the blood and lymphatic vessels. Community-acquired pneumonias affect healthy and pre-damaged lungs, while opportunistic infections are seen in hospitalized or immunocompromised patients. Pneumonias often appear in elderly or hospitalized people a few days prior to death from other causes. Infections of previously damaged areas of the lung usually result in scarring and further damage, often with focal honeycomb change. Pneumonia has a high mortality rate: community-acquired pneumonia is a common cause of death and can affect the young as well as the old or those with predisposing lung disease.

Bacterial infections of the lung are usually acquired via the conducting airways, in other words by inhaled agents. The second pathway is the metastatic spread of infectious agents through the blood, rarely, by invasion from adjacent tissues, such as liver abscess or skin injuries. Although they are clinically common, bacterial infections of the bronchial system are less of a threat to life.

Two major pathological types of pneumonia are recognized: **bronchopneumonia** and **lobar pneumonia**. In bronchopneumonia, there is focal inflammation around small bronchi which may coalesce to involve large areas of the lung. Lobar pneumonia shows diffuse inflammation of large areas of lung, usually based on segments or lobes (Fig. 9.10). Similar aetiological agents are involved in both types, although pneumococci are the classic cause of lobar pneumonia.

Aetiological classification of bacterial lung infections
- Infectious agent
- Clinical presentation (acute, subacute or chronic)
- Intrapulmonary manifestation (lobar pneumonia, bronchopneumonia, suppurative pneumonia)
- Relationship to the environment (community-acquired and opportunistic infections)
- Condition of affected lung (infection of pre-damaged or healthy lung areas)

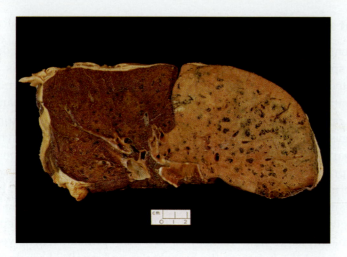

Fig. 9.10 The macroscopic appearance of lobar pneumonia showing red hepatization in the lower lobe and grey hepatization above.

The classic morphological presentations of lobar bacterial pneumonias include four stages, according to their macroscopic and microscopic appearance. These stages are related to the time difference between onset of infection and date of tissue examination. Rapid bacterial growth inside the lungs is accompanied by a relatively slow host response, starting with disturbance of the air–blood barrier, release of cytokines and infiltration by inflammatory cells, followed later by the elimination of bacteria and resolution (see box below).

Complete resolution is usually not seen in pre-damaged lung areas which will heal with scarring and focal emphysema. The classic morphological course of bacterial pneumonias is associated with their aetiology: community-acquired (outside the hospital) infections are often of the lobar pattern. They are caused mainly by the following organisms:

- *Streptococcus pneumoniae* (pneumococcus)
- *Klebsiella* sp.
- *Legionella* sp.
- *Staphylococcus aureus*
- *Haemophilus influenzae.*

Infections with streptococci and staphylococci have an acute onset with high fever, and are severe in young children with possible abscess formation and pyopneumothorax. Infections with *Klebsiella* and

---

Stages of lobar pneumonia

- The wet, hyperaemic, dark-red areas of the lung correspond microscopically to a **congestive stage** which is seen 1–2 days after infection. It is characterized by intra-alveolar oedema, beginning with extravasation of erythrocytes and granulocytes into the airspaces, enlarged and blood-filled capillaries (vascular engorgement).
- Increased and brittle consistency and dark-red colour of the involved areas demonstrate the stage of **red hepatization**, which is seen after 3–4 days and microscopically displays additional deposits of fibrin, beginning destruction of the interalveolar septula, release of haemoglobin and fibrinous pleural deposits.
- The third stage, called the **grey hepatization** stage, can be recognized by days 4–6 macroscopically by greyish, brittle areas of the lung, which compress the adjacent healthy lung parts, and microscopically by dense agglutinations of neutrophilic and eosinophilic granulocytes, macrophages and, to a lesser degree, lymphocytes and plasma cells, destroyed interalveolar septulas and air–blood barrier.
- The **resolution** or **yellow hepatization** stage starts after the sixth day and displays macroscopically greyish-yellowish lung areas or microscopically restoration of the interalveolar septulas and air–blood barrier, loss of the intra-alveolar macrophages, and disappearance of the cellular debris and inflammatory infiltrates.

Haemophilus spp. are seen in immunocompromised patients (alcoholics, for example): the mortality rate is high for people infected with *Klebsiella* sp. and relatively good for those infected with *Haemophilus* sp. Infections with *Legionella* sp. occur as a sporadic or endemic disease (people working in air-conditioned rooms), have a subacute onset with complaints of fever, malaise and myalgia several days before pulmonary manifestation, and a long stage of resolution. A large number of legionella patients develop a progressive respiratory failure which is often fatal.

All bacterial pneumonias may have **bacteraemia**. This can cause meningitis, renal failure and myocarditis. It is thought to be an important precursor of fatal pneumonia.

Opportunistic infections usually manifest in hospitalized or immunocompromised patients. The most important pathogenic organisms are Gram negative and include:

- *Bacteroides* sp.
- *Escherichia coli*
- *Pseudomonas aeruginosa*
- *Serratia marcescens*
- *Klebsiella* sp.
- *Legionella* sp.

Infections with *Escherichia coli*, *Klebsiella* and *Serratia* spp. have a poor prognosis in immunocompromised patients and premature infants. The mortality of pseudomonas infections has remained unchanged since 1960, and still amounts to 70–80%. All opportunistic infections usually present with abscess formation and malodorous expectoration.

Subacute and **chronic bacterial infections** are normally caused by *Actinomyces israelii*, *Nocardia asteroides* and *Pseudomonas pseudomallei*, and manifest in patients with constitutional abnormalities. Pseudomonas infections may have, in addition, an acute onset. Infection with actinomycetes can proceed with therapy-resistant destruction of the lung parenchyma and involve the pleura, pericardium and chest wall by invasive progression. They can be microscopically recognized by their characteristic sulphur granules, which consist of a granular basophilic centre corresponding to the bacterial colony, and radiating eosinophilic, hyaline clubs.

Of specific clinical importance are pneumonias seen in primarily healthy people who have close contact with infected animals, especially sheep, goats and rodents. The infectious agents (*Yersinia pestis*, *Bacillus anthracis*, *Francisella tularensis*) cause severe rapidly progressive pneumonias with a mortality rate of 5–10%. (This relatively low mortality is due to modern antibiotic therapy: before antibiotics were available, it was 80–90%.)

Rarely, bacterial infections of the upper respiratory tract spread to the peripheral lung parenchyma. Before inoculation against whooping cough was introduced, acute infections with *Bordetella pertussis* could extend into the terminal bronchioles, which became filled with yellowish mucus and contained dense mononuclear inflammatory infiltrates within the submucosa. Aspiration can induce acute pneumonic infections with infective organisms not usually seen in the peripheral lung. Nearly all chronic diseases with severe insufficiency of the corresponding organ (heart, kidneys, liver, immune system, central nervous system) weaken the defence mechanisms of the lung, and thus induce bacterial infections, often with fatal outcome.

Mycobacterial lung diseases, including **tuberculosis** and infections with atypical mycobacteria (*Mycobacterium avium-intercellulare, Mycobacterium kansasii*), are discussed in Chapter 7.

VIRAL INFECTION

Viral infections of the lung are common and usually self-limited, but may be life-threatening in immunocompromised patients. They have an acute onset and various morphological images (see box). Bacterial superinfection is common, especially in respiratory syncytial viral infections.

Viral infections of the lung belong to the so-called atypical pneumonias and, although they are common infections, they are rarely seen by the pathologist. These cases are limited to the newborn, infants, children and those with defects in their pulmonary defence mechanism. The most common infectious viral organisms are RNA and DNA viruses and include cytomegalovirus, herpesvirus, measles virus and adenovirus. Usually, all infectious agents enter the body via the terminal airspaces; however, not all of them induce infections of the lung. The clinical symptoms include high fever, headache, malaise, cough and dyspnoea, and are often abrupt. The prognosis is usually good unless the patient is immunocompromised.

The basic morphological findings of pneumonia may be present to various degrees, resulting in a very variable histological appearance. Additional findings include eosinophilic inflammatory infiltrates, thrombotic obliteration of the small arteries and hyaline membranes. Haemorrhage is predominant in adenovirus, herpes, measles and influenza virus infections, while chronic interstitial pneumonia is prominent in cytomegalovirus infection, which also has large nuclear inclusion bodies. Focal necrosis and diffuse alveolar damage are commonly present in all viral pneumonias; bronchiolitis obliterans is often associated with beginning fibrosis and moderate-to-severe disturbances in lung function.

In contrast to bacterial pneumonias, those induced by viruses tend to resolve and to re-infect in different lung areas at the same time, so the lung parenchyma may display areas with acute exudation and fibrinous organization simultaneously. In addition, viral pneumonias can be superinfected by bacteria, especially after infection with influenza virus. These types of bronchopneumonia are characterized by necrotic damage to the bronchial epithelial cells due to viral infection, and additional bacterial (staphylococcus) infection of the peripheral lung parenchyma. Macroscopically, red (haemorrhagic) areas, greyish (fibrinous) areas and yellowish (necrotic) areas are present simultaneously. **Reye's syndrome** (acute hepatocerebral syndrome) is an uncommon complication of respiratory infections in children, and is thought to be related to the use of non-steroidal anti-inflammatory drugs (NSAIDs). Serological identification is successful in most viral respiratory infections, but newer methods such as the polymerase chain reaction which detect viral DNA may also be useful.

FUNGAL DISEASES

Fungal infections can be classified into community-acquired and opportunistic disorders, and have both acute and chronic forms.

Morphological images of viral infection
- Acute bronchitis
- Haemorrhage
- Diffuse alveolar damage
- Mononuclear interstitial pneumonia
- Focal necrosis
- Atypia of the cells of the alveolar lining
- Bronchiolitis obliterans
- All stages of honeycombing

Light microscopic characteristics of fungi

Genus	Characteristic findings
Aspergillus	Hyphae, dichotomous rectangular branching
Blastomyces	Uniform, round yeast, 'double-contoured' wall
Candida	Yeast-like organisms; pseudohyphae
Coccidioides	Large (30–300 μm) spherules, thick capsule
Cryptococcus	Small, yeast-like cells with mucinous capsule
Fusarium	Branched septate hyphae, similar to *Aspergillus*
Geotrichum	Hyphae (non-rectangular branching), spores
Histoplasma	Uniform, yeast-like cells (buds, in macrophages)
Mucor	Pleomorphic hyphae (larger than *Aspergillus*)
Paracoccidioides	Oval, yeast-like cells, 5–40 μm in diameter
Penicillium	Oval yeast-like cells (no buds)
Pseudallescheria	Small, multibranched hyphae
Rhinosporidium	Large (10–200 μm) sporangia with spores
Sporotrichum	Oval, cigar-shaped buds
Torulopsis	Small round yeast; single buds (histoplasma)
Trichosporon	Pleomorphic yeast, septate hyphae

Opportunistic fungal infections are of great importance because of the increasing number of immunocompromised patients, particularly those with HIV infection. Community-acquired fungal infections used to be limited to certain geographical areas, but can be noted today in all countries because of the increased incidence of international travel. In the lung, non-invasive and invasive infections occur. Non-invasive fungus grows in previously damaged, usually ectatic airways or cavities, and can induce allergic reactions and severe asthmatic attacks.

All fungal organisms may form circumscribed necrotic masses in the bronchi or peripheral lung parenchyma, often with characteristic radiological findings (cavities with intracavitary masses separated from the boundary by crescents of air). Miliary, tuberculosis-like spread is seen less frequently, and diffuse lobular infection almost never occurs. The visualization of the fungal organisms by light microscopy is difficult in general, and needs the application of specific stains, such as PAS or silver–reticulin (Grocott) (Fig. 9.11). Fungi infecting the lung and other tissues can be recognized by their characteristic hyphae or spherules. Histologically, the fungal organisms can be separated into those with

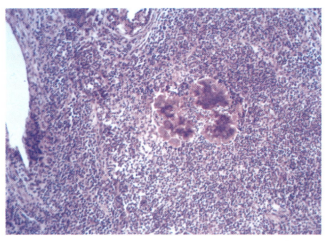
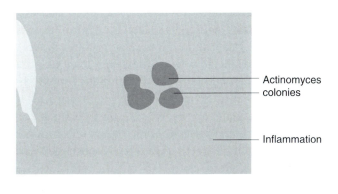

Fig. 9.11   Actinomyces infection of the lung with colonies surrounded by a dense chronic inflammatory reaction.

limited invasive growth and granulomatous reaction of the host tissue, such as non-invasive *Aspergillus*, *Blastomyces*, *Coccidioides*, *Cryptococcus*, *Histoplasma*, *Paracoccidioides* spp., and those with diffuse invasive growth, which include invasive *Aspergillus* sp., *Candida albicans*, *Torulopsis* and *Mucor* spp.

Moderate to dense eosinophilic infiltrates can be seen in patients with IgE or IgG antibodies that are associated with hypersensitivity pneumonitis in patients with non-invasive aspergillosis. The granulomata consist of a central caseous zone containing the fungal organisms, and an outer zone built from mononuclear inflammatory infiltrates, scattered multinucleated giant cells and a varying number of eosinophils. These appearances vary according to the age of the infection and the immunogenic potency of the host. Fibrosis and calcification may be present.

Invasive fungal diseases are almost always seen in immuno-compromised patients and are characterized by a serofibrinous exudate and dense granulomatous infiltrates. Eosinophils may not be prominent.

In contrast to tuberculosis, fungal infections, even associated with granulomatous tissue reaction, do not induce a lifelong immunity to the organisms; thus, primary or secondary infections cannot be distinguished. However, 'encapsulation' of the infective organisms by fibrotic bundles (**mycetomas**) and final calcification of the lesion demonstrate focal long-lasting immunity as seen with *Histoplasma* or *Coccidioides* spp.

IMMUNOSUPPRESSION AND LUNG INFECTION

Mycoplasmal, rickettsial, chlamydial and protozoal diseases are of growing importance as a result of HIV infection and their prevalence in developing countries. The clinical course is usually good except in patients with generalized infections or severe immunosuppression. The histological image varies widely: usually mild-to-moderate mononuclear inflammatory infiltrates are present.

PROTOZOAL INFECTIONS

Pneumocystis is the most important protozoal lung disease, although systemic protozoal infections such as **trypanosomiasis** (Chagas' disease), **leishmaniasis**, **malaria**, **toxoplasmosis**, **amoebiasis**, **cryptosporidiosis** and **trichomoniasis** may also involve the lungs. Pneumocystis infection is almost always seen in immunocompromised patients, especially in those infected with HIV, and less often in patients undergoing heart, liver or bone marrow transplantations. *Pneumocystis carinii* infections are limited to the lung and induce a broad variety of clinical presentations with either subacute, mild onset and minimum symptoms, or a rapid course with high fever, hypoxaemia and severe illness, and even pneumothorax. Most of the other infectious organisms are transmitted by blood-sucking mosquitoes and occur in healthy people. The main natural reservoirs for many protozoal infections are rodents. Lung infections of the other protozoal organisms are usually secondary to the manifestation in liver, spleen, brain or gastrointestinal tract, and often associated with a severe course. Congenital infections can occur in all protozoal diseases, and are often fatal, especially in trypanosome infections.

The histological reaction varies broadly. *Pneumocystis carinii* usually induces a mild mononuclear interstitial inflammation and a serous

Diseases caused by rickettsial infective organisms

- Typhus (worldwide)
- Rocky Mountain spotted fever (America, North Asia, Africa, India)
- Tsutsugamushi's disease (south Asia, Pacific)
- Q fever (worldwide)
- Trench fever (Europe, former USSR, Mexico)

exudation of intercellular fluid into the airspaces, which is indistinguishable from that seen in alveolar proteinosis. However, epithelioid granulomata may be seen, as well as abscess formation or virtually normal lung tissue. A similar foamy or fibrinous exudate can occur in infections with trypanosomes, *Leishmania* and *Plasmodium* spp. and trichomonads. An increased number of macrophages, often seen with ingested protozoans, are more common in infections with *Toxoplasma*, *Acanthamoeba* and *Cryptosporidium* spp. Entamoebae usually induce abscess formation. The organisms are difficult to demonstrate in ordinary slides stained with haematoxylin and eosin, and specific staining techniques such as silver-reticulin (Grocott) or Giemsa stains are needed.

CHLAMYDIAL AND RICKETTSIAL INFECTIONS

Human chlamydial infections are caused by *Chlamydia psittaci* (psittacosis) or *Chlamydia trachomatis* (infantile pneumonia). The infections occur via the upper respiratory tract, usually after contamination by an infected bird (usually of the parrot family). Immunocompromised people are at specific risk for infection with *Chlamydia trachomatis*. The clinical course includes headache, fever and cough after an incubation time of 14 days, and the prognosis is good. Histology shows a dense mononuclear inflammatory infiltrate predominant in the bronchioles and small bronchi. Hyaline membranes and mild diffuse alveolar damage can occur.

Rickettsial infective organisms are responsible for several diseases, some of which are found worldwide and some restricted to certain geographical areas. Rickettsiae are common parasites of arthropods and are considered to be bacterial with DNA and RNA. However, they lack certain enzymes and cannot live outside the cell. The clinical picture usually mimics that of a common cold after an incubation time of approximately three weeks, followed by skin rash, headache and high fever. The prognosis is usually good. Multifocal, partly necrotic foci of granulocytic inflammation and moderate histiocytic inflammatory infiltrates are the common findings in the lung. The lesions usually heal without residual damage.

MYCOPLASMA INFECTIONS

Mycoplasma pneumoniae infections are common community-acquired disorders which may cause epidemics within institutions such as military camps. The clinical picture is characterized by a subacute onset and a self-healing pneumonia. Histologically, the lungs show dense inflammatory infiltrates (lymphocytes, plasma cells, macrophages) in the bronchioles and small bronchi, often associated with a marked hyperplasia and dysplasia of the cells lining the alveoli. Ill-defined epithelioid granulomata may occur.

Higher organisms that can settle into the lung

- Arthropods, usually inhaled (mites, leeches), or transmitted by mosquitoes (*Linguatula rhinaria* larvae)
- Cestodes (causing cysticercosis, for example), usually transmitted by ingestion
- Nematodes (causing ascariasis, filariasis, toxocariasis, for example), usually transmitted in undercooked food
- Trematodes (causing schistosomiasis, for example)

PARASITIC INFECTIONS

Parasitic infections are common in developing countries and still seen in industrialized countries. Well-adapted organisms seldom cause severe pulmonary symptoms and are often detected accidentally. Poorly adapted parasites often appear as degenerate necrotic masses which are hard to identify. Most parasites are ingested (faecal–oral spread), although some invade through the skin and settle in the lung, while others are inhaled. Larger parasites such as nematodes and trematodes are a severe health problem in the developing countries. Even in Europe, parasitic infections, for example with cestodes, can cause severe clinical problems, particularly if their presence is not suspected.

Pulmonary infection is usually quite rare in many of these diseases and often represents an aberrance, but it may define the clinical course, which is usually determined by the severity of infections and the species. In general, well-adapted species such as schistosomes or *Paragonimus* sp. seldom induce severe symptoms and can remain undetected until the death of the host. Others, usually poorly adapted parasites such as dipteran larvae or filaria such as *Wuchereria bancrofti* can induce severe reactive inflammation and granulomatous reaction of the host tissue.

Most intrapulmonary parasites have been found in the pulmonary arteries. Some can induce chronic pulmonary hypertension (schistosomes). Infection with *Echinococcus* sp. (hydatid disease) usually presents with large circumscribed cysts, which are often also present in the liver. Commonly, clinical symptoms are absent, and the lesions are detected accidentally on chest radiographs. However, ruptured cysts can cause severe anaphylactic shock. The cystic wall is embedded in a ring of fibrous tissue with some scattered mononuclear inflammatory cells. The attached inner germinal layer contains multiple invaginated scolices of about 100 μm maximum diameter. Intrapulmonary cestodes are usually living organisms at the time of clinical detection; nematodes and trematodes have often been killed by the pulmonary defence system and present as radiographic shadows.

Environmental (occupational) disease and pneumoconiosis

Inhaled natural and synthetic mineral substances can be divided into inert and harmful fibres. Dependent upon their physical and chemical properties, harmful fibres induce focal or diffuse interstitial fibrosis, epithelioid granulomata, bronchiolitis obliterans, pulmonary oedema or emphysema (see box).

Smoking induces chronic bronchitis, damage of the epithelial cells including squamous metaplasia and dysplasia, emphysematous changes and lung cancer.

Although the lungs are equipped with an effective clearance and defence mechanism, the burden of inhaled dust particles can exceed its capacity and cause considerable damage to the peripheral lung parenchyma. An increasing number of dust particles is deposited with increasing age, particularly for people living in a modern industrialized environment. The amount of deposited dust particles depends significantly upon two factors: the size and shape of the particles, and their concentration in the air. Fibres measuring less than 1 μm in diameter and 10 μm in length can usually

Occupational lung diseases and their sources	
Quartz (silica)	Focal fibrosis (silicosis)
Asbestos	Diffuse fibrosis (asbestosis)
Beryllium	Epithelioid granulomata (berylliosis)
Irritative gases	Pulmonary oedema (intoxication)
Hard metal fumes	Bronchiolitis obliterans (hard metal disease)
Organic fibres	Emphysema (byssinosis)

Definition of pneumoconiosis
- Cause: inhaled dust
- Inorganic/organic reaction: inert, fibrous, allergic or neoplastic
- Risk of other coexisting disease

Reaction of the lungs to inhaled particles

- Storage of the particles in the alveoli and terminal bronchioles with or without mild reactive inflammatory response
- Creation of fibrotic hard nodules, often in an onion-shaped form
- Massive fibrotic lesions, measuring several centimetres in maximum diameter with surrounding bullous emphysema and bacterial superinfection (tuberculosis)
- Non-caseating epithelioid granulomata with and without fibrosis diffuse interstitial fibrosis, often with consecutive honeycombing and metaplasia of the cells of the alveolar lining
- Acute pulmonary oedema
- Fibrin exudation and plugs, usually intermingled with histiocytes in the terminal bronchioles (bronchiolitis obliterans)

penetrate into the distant airways. Two categories of inhaled fibres have to be distinguished: those that are harmless (inert) to the lung parenchyma, and those that induce progressive lung damage, usually in terms of active interstitial fibrosis. The classification holds true for different particle/air mixtures. such as:

- aerosols (stable suspensions of liquid or solid particles in the air)
- fumes (condensates of smallest solid particles from the gaseous stage)
- dust (dispersion of solid particles in the air).

Environmentally important inert materials include carbon or coal, titanium, iron, tin, antimony, zirconium, barium and cerium. Inert particles or fibres are often contaminated with silica which can induce circumscribed fibrotic lesions; therefore, the distinction between inert and harmful fibres is often difficult or impossible and miners of these inert materials risk silicosis (nodular fibrosis).

SILICOSIS

The most important agent inducing focal or massive fibrosis is free silica or quartz, which is the main dust component in metalliferous and coal mining, quarrying for sandstone, tunnelling, metal grinding and 'flour' foundries using crystalline respirable material as an abrasive cleaner. Macroscopically the lung contains circumscribed, hard, greyish-black, fibrous nodules which characteristically exhibit three different zones at the light microscopic level:

- a central zone of whorled hyaline connective tissue
- a midzone of similar material with intermingled histiocytes
- an outer zone with dust-laden macrophages.

In severe cases with massive fibrosis, the multiple fibrotic nodules are fused by intervening fibrosis leading to a shrunken fibrotic end stage (Fig. 9.12). Complicated silicosis exhibits, in addition, epithelioid caseous granulomata which are the morphological equivalent of tuberculous infection.

Fig. 9.12 The end result of silicosis: a grey contracted lung with an irregular fibrotic surface.

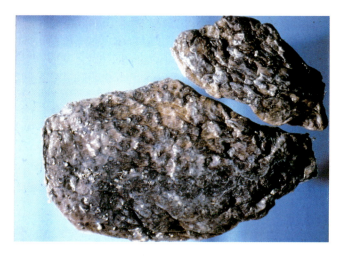

BERYLLIOSIS

Inhaled beryllium particles can induce a characteristic granulomatous reaction indistinguishable from that seen in sarcoidosis: non-caseating epithelioid granulomata with multinucleated giant cells.

ASBESTOSIS

Asbestos is the most important inhaled cause of pneumoconiosis. In addition, it is one of the environmental substances with the highest carcinogenic potency, and nearly all malignant tumours of the pleura develop as a result of (even minimal) exposure to asbestos. The asbestos fibres are commonly ingested by pulmonary macrophages which fail to digest or transport the fibres. As a result, about 30% of the inhaled fibres become coated by haemosiderin-containing proteins and acid mucopolysaccharides, and are called **ferruginous bodies** because of their positive reaction to colloidal iron stains (Fig. 9.13). The coated and non-coated birefringent fibres are deposited in the alveoli and respiratory bronchioles. Their concentration can be measured by digestion of a defined part of the lung parenchyma using 40% potassium hydroxide solution, and counting the fibres in the solution. The pathophysiology of the fibrosis and the asbestos-related malignancies is still unknown, although recently the anti-oncogene p53 has been implicated.

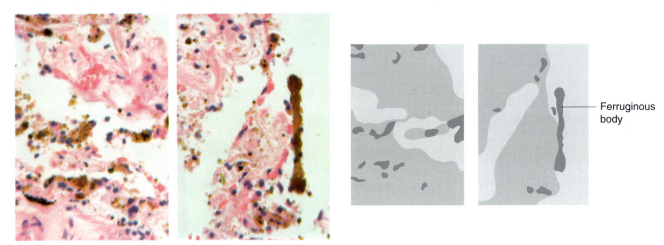

Ferruginous body

Fig. 9.13   Asbestos fibres become coated with haemosiderin and form distinctive 'ferruginous' bodies.

OTHER DUSTS AND THE LUNG

Other important substances inducing fibrous changes of the lung parenchyma include aluminium and substances used in the machine tool industry (hard metals). The induced disorder is called **hard metal disease**; associated substances are tungsten carbide, nickel and chromium. Organic material such as cotton fibres (flax workers, **byssinosis**) irritate the bronchioles, and severe emphysematous changes are noted after decades of exposure. **Uranium mining** in Schneeberg (in the Erzgebirge, Germany) provided the first evidence that the inhalation of radioactive particles is harmful to the lungs in terms of an increased risk for lung cancer and progressive fibrosis.

ACUTE EXPOSURE TO TOXINS

Acute pulmonary toxicity results in pulmonary oedema or **pulmonary alveolar proteinosis**, and has been reported from those exposed to high concentrations of silica (acute silicosis), and irritating gases such as chlorine, phosgene, nitrous oxide and ammonia. Long-lasting intoxication or lower concentrations of these gases can induce fibrinous plugs in the terminal bronchioles (bronchiolitis obliterans) and severe disturbances of the gas exchange, followed by progressive respiratory failure. Similar changes have been reported after exposure to resin fumes. Atmospheric pollutants, for example released by dense traffic or volcanic eruptions, normally irritate the conducting airways, and those exposed suffer from chronic bronchitis, although children often develop a hypersensitivity reaction and chronic asthma.

SMOKING

Smoking is associated with chronic inflammatory alterations of the conducting airways, dust-laden macrophages in the distant airways, deposits of black coal particles in the lymphatic vessels and disturbances of the mucociliary system. The chronic inflammation induces significant changes of the composition of the bronchial epithelial cells; the turnover of the basal cells is increased, and squamous metaplasia with various degrees of cellular atypia can be noted. The alteration of the clearance mechanism and the protease–antiprotease system effects an increased mucus production, and atrophic changes occur in the interalveolar interstitium resulting in emphysema. The risk of lung cancer is closely associated with the numbers of cigarettes smoked per day, the age of beginning to smoke and the number of years smoking is practised.

Chronic obstructive airway disease (COAD)

Chronic obstructive airway disease – chronic bronchitis and emphysema, often abbreviated to COAD – is a common disorder associated with prolonged exposure to environmental toxins. It is closely associated with focal or diffuse degenerative changes of the distal lung parenchyma (emphysema), as well as with chronic inflammation of the bronchial wall (chronic bronchitis). Degenerative changes of the lung can affect all of its structures: the airways, vessels, nerves and peripheral lung parenchyma. In addition, chronic inflammation of these compartments can induce secondary degeneration of one or several of the others.

CHRONIC BRONCHITIS

Chronic bronchitis is a common disorder seen with increasing frequency in all age groups of the population in developed countries. In clinical terms, it is defined as chronic cough with increased mucus production for at least three consecutive months observed in two consecutive years at minimum. Chronic bronchitis affects both the larger and smaller bronchi. Functionally, the chronic bronchitis may present with increased mucus production (catarrhal bronchitis), or – at a later stage – atrophy of the epithelial cells and squamous metaplasia. Deformation of the bronchial walls and enlargement of the bronchial lumen is common (bronchiectasis). Chronic bronchitis is often associated with bronchospasm (contraction of the bronchial smooth muscle).

EMPHYSEMA

Emphysema is the term given to chronic dilatation of the respiratory bronchioles and/or alveoli as a result of destructive changes within their walls due to inflammation and loss of elastin. The disease may vary in severity between different lobes of the lung. Several types of emphysema may be present in the same patient (Fig. 9.14).

Aetiological factors for COAD

- Congenital abnormalities
  - Cystic fibrosis
  - IgA deficiency
- Exogenous factors
  - Smoking (including passive smoking)
  - Sulphur dioxide
  - Metallic fumes (industry)
  - Heat exposure
  - Mist or humid, cold air
- Bacterial infections

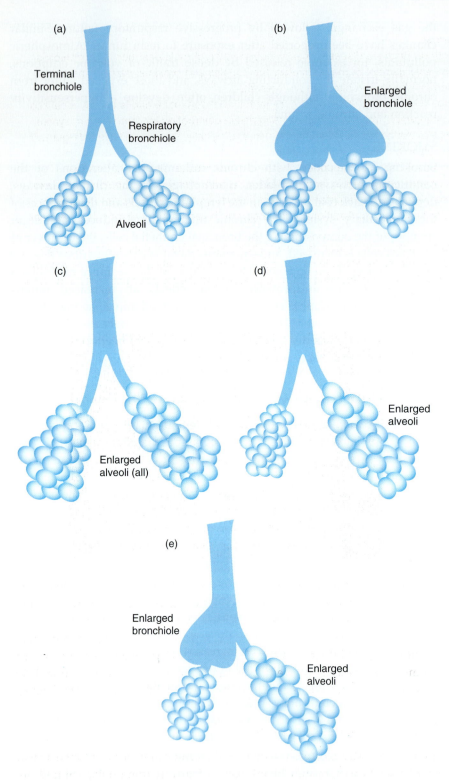

(a)

Terminal
bronchiole

Respiratory
bronchiole

Alveoli

(b)

Enlarged
bronchiole

(c)

Enlarged
alveoli (all)

(d)

Enlarged
alveoli

(e)

Enlarged
bronchiole

Enlarged
alveoli

Fig. 9.14 Diagrammatic representation of the different types of emphysema in comparison with: (a) normal architecture; (b) proximal or centrilobular type with dilatation of respiratory bronchioles; (c) panacinar type with dilatation of alveoli and alveolar ducts (not shown); (d) paraseptal with patchy alveolar enlargement; and (e) irregular affecting various parts of the bronchiole or alveolus.

Clinically, centrilobular emphysema is associated with the so-called 'blue bloater', an obese patient with productive cough, cyanosis and insufficiency of the right heart, while the panlobular emphysema is associated with the 'pink puffer', a slim non-cyanotic patient suffering from severe dyspnoea and respiratory insufficiency.

Additional emphysematous disorders include **primary atrophic emphysema** (associated with the age of the patients) and **interstitial emphysema**, in which forced inspiration induces increased content of air in

Anatomical classification of emphysema

- **Centrilobular emphysema** is a slowly progressive disease, usually induced by a chronic destructive bronchiolitis due to smoking. It is characterized by enlargement of the respiratory bronchioles and proximal parts of the acini, thus alveolar wall destruction and normal alveolar architecture are present.
- **Panlobular emphysema** is associated with α_1-antitrypsin deficiency (autosomal dominant) and is usually localized in the lower parts of the lungs. α_1-Antitrypsin is important in preventing tissue destruction by proteolytic enzymes, especially those derived from neutrophils during acute inflammation. Morphologically, there is uniform enlargement of the respiratory bronchioles and the alveoli.
- **Paraseptal (bullous) emphysema** is usually seen in the upper lobes and a progressive disorder of younger patients. The interalveolar septa are completely absent in large (usually subpleural parts) of the lung and may lead to the formation of bullae – air spaces over 1 cm in diameter. Recurrent pneumothorax due to rupture of bullae is commonly associated with this form of emphysema. Additional obstruction of the conducting airways is a frequent finding.
- **Irregular emphysema** (scar emphysema) observed in association with healed postinflammatory lesions is a non-progressive disorder. Its manifestation is frequently noted in healed post-tuberculous scars. The proteolytic activity of the inflammation has been transferred to the neighbouring tissue and destroyed the interalveolar septa and walls of the corresponding bronchioles and bronchi.

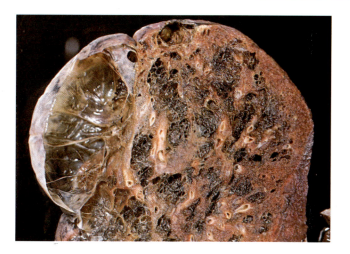

Fig. 9.15 An emphysematous bulla at the apex of the lung. Such bullae may rupture spontaneously releasing air into the pleural space (pneumothorax).

the interstitial lung tissue and that of the mediastinum or neighbouring skin. All emphysematous changes are associated with an altered ratio of the protease–antiprotease enzymes which are released by granulocytes and macrophages. The released enzymes degrade elastin which is important in maintaining the integrity of the alveolar wall. Degenerative changes of the pulmonary arteries or veins are extremely rare diseases noted in generalized connective tissue disorders (such as Ehlers–Danlos syndrome).

Immunological disorders

Immunologically mediated disease in the lung can be induced by extrinsic or intrinsic factors, or may be idiopathic. Extrinsic immunological diseases affect either the conducting airways as observed in asthma or the peripheral lung parenchyma as observed in exogenous allergic alveolitis, or both.

ASTHMA

Asthma leads to recurrent acute attacks of dyspnoea caused by generalized obstruction of the bronchi resulting from contraction of smooth muscle within their walls (**bronchospasm**). Both allergic and non-allergic forms are recognized, with different predisposing factors.

Major categories of extrinsic allergic alveolitis
- Inhaled **thermophilic actinomycetes** usually presenting with non-caseous granulomata and seen in a variety of occupational exposures (farmers' lung, bagassosis, mushroom workers' lung, etc.)
- Inhaled **moulds** often seen with diffuse mononuclear and eosinophilic infiltrates (maple bark strippers' lung, sequoiosis, etc.)
- Inhaled **animal products** presenting with granulomata or diffuse eosinophilic and mononuclear inflammatory infiltrates (bird fanciers' disease, bat lung, fish meal workers' lung, etc.)
- **Unknown inhaled agents** (sauna takers' lung, etc.)
- **Drug toxicity** induced either by oxidant injury or direct toxic alteration of the lung parenchyma (cytotoxic drugs) or by a hypersensitivity reaction, usually with acute onset after a latent period

Allergic (**exogenous** or **atopic**) **asthma** is usually caused by a type I IgE-mediated hypersensitivity reaction. Reaginic antibody on mast cell membranes combines with antigen resulting in the release of leukotrienes and other factors which attract eosinophils, lymphocytes and other cells into the bronchial mucosa. The antigen varies – often faecal material from house dust mites is to blame, but pollens, dusts and animal fur are also important. Occupational asthma is due to agents inhaled at work, but has a similar pathogenesis. Over time, the mucosa may become thickened with mucous gland hypertrophy, an increase in diameter of the epithelial basement membrane and smooth muscle hyperplasia. Large numbers of eosinophils are present within the mucosa, leading to the formation of Charcot–Leyden crystals. Thickened mucus plugs bronchioles leading to local overinflation or collapse of alveoli. Sputum cytology shows large numbers of eosinophils and desquamated epithelium in characteristic Curshmann's spirals. Patients may have other atopic conditions such as eczema or perennial rhinitis.

Non-allergic (**intrinsic**) asthma may be induced by drugs including non-steroidal anti-inflammatory drugs (NSAIDs), inhalation of toxic substances, cold, exercise, or psychosomatic factors such as anxiety. It may also be associated with recurrent respiratory tract infection. Allergen testing is negative.

EXTRINSIC ALLERGIC ALVEOLITIS

Extrinsic allergic alveolitis can be induced by a broad variety of substances reaching the lung either by the airways or via the blood system.

The granulomata seen in allergic extrinsic alveolitis are small and similar to those seen in **sarcoidosis** (see Chapter 7). Extrinsic allergic pneumonitis can be distinguished from sarcoidosis by the ratio of T-helper (CD4+) to T-cytotoxic (CD8+) cells in the lavage fluid, which is decreased in allergic pneumonitis patients and increased in sarcoidosis patients. The granulomata seen in allergic alveolitis or sarcoidosis measure several millimetres in maximum diameter and can become larger lesions by fusion and fibrosis of neighbouring small granulomata. Allergic extrinsic pneumonia is related to type III (immune complex) and type IV (granulomatous) hypersensitivity. Cytotoxic antibody-mediated hypersensitivity reactions (type II) also affect the lung and are important in the antiglomerular basement membrane disease (**Goodpasture's syndrome**), in which there is diffuse intrapulmonary haemorrhage and glomerulonephritis.

PULMONARY ANGIITIS AND GRANULOMATOSIS

A second granulomatous entity of lung diseases related to abnormalities of the immune system is the **pulmonary angiitis and granulomatosis** group.

Pulmonary angiitis and granulomatosis group of disease
- Wegener's granulomatosis
- Allergic angiitis and granulomatosis (Churg–Strauss syndrome)
- Necrotizing sarcoid-like granulomatosis
- Lymphomatoid granulomatosis
- Bronchocentric granulomatosis (often associated with asthma)

This group of diseases is characterized by caseous or necrotizing large (several centimetres) granulomata with central localized arteries and/or bronchi. Eosinophilic inflammatory infiltrates are often present and prove the association with abnormalities of the immune system.

SYSTEMIC IMMUNOLOGICAL DISEASE AND THE LUNG

The diseases described above usually show themselves clinically in the lung before other organs. On the other hand, the lung is involved in a variety of immunological diseases with predominantly extrapulmonary manifestations. These include most connective tissue diseases.

About 40% of patients with **rheumatoid disease** have pulmonary symptoms; however, involvement of the pleura is more common than that of the lung. The histological findings again include a broad variety of alterations, most commonly chronic interstitial inflammatory infiltrates (usual interstitial pneumonia), bronchiolitis obliterans, constrictive bronchiolitis and, less often, the formation of rheumatoid nodules. Diffuse interstitial fibrosis is observed in collagenous diseases, especially in dermatomyositis or polymyositis. Emphysematous alterations in both upper lobes are sometimes associated with **ankylosing spondylitis**.

Interstitial lung disease

PULMONARY OEDEMA AND INTOXICATION

Pulmonary oedema is by definition an increased content of fluid in the interstitial tissue (interstitial oedema) and/or the alveoli (alveolar oedema). It induces severe disturbance of the blood–air barrier and of gas exchange, and is life threatening. Pulmonary oedema is caused by disturbances of the relationship of hydrostatic pressure, osmotic pressure, the resistance (permeability) of the alveolar–capillary membrane and the resistance in the lymph drainage – just like peripheral oedema. Diminished flow of blood to the left heart (left heart insufficiency) induces an increase of the hydrostatic pressure and cardiac pulmonary oedema results. This can be of acute onset and develop into a chronic stage.

Macroscopically, postmortem examination shows oedema fluid oozing from the cut surface of the lung, which is heavy and does not collapse on removal from the chest. Histologically there is protein-containing fluid in the alveoli (Fig. 9.16) and interalveolar septa with some scattered

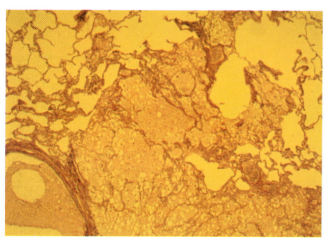 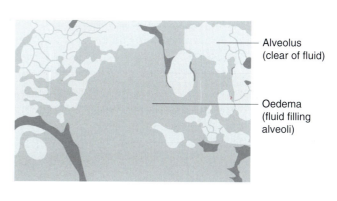

Alveolus (clear of fluid)

Oedema (fluid filling alveoli)

Fig. 9.16 Chronic pulmonary oedema. Proteinaceous fluid fills the alveoli and can be observed in formalin-fixed tissue.

mononuclear cells (alveolar macrophages) and granulocytes close to the cells of the alveolar lining. Some extravasated erythrocytes may be present. The fluid can become organized by macrophages which also ingest fragments of haemosiderin and erythrocytes (heart failure cells). Eventually, diffuse fibrosis of the interalveolar septa develops.

Chronic pulmonary oedema produces induration of the lungs known as **red induration** or **brown induration**, in which the lungs become firmer than usual and fail to collapse on removal from the chest cavity, owing to interstitial fibrosis and long-standing oedema. Brown induration is usually seen in patients with long-standing left heart insufficiency (heart failure) or in children with malformations of the heart such as stenosis of the mitral valve.

Other causes of pulmonary oedema mainly affect the resistance at the blood–air barrier, the basal membrane of the intra-alveolar capillary system. Disturbances at this interface can be induced by immune complexes or antibodies against the basal membrane (Goodpasture's syndrome). Chronic oedematous changes result.

ADULT RESPIRATORY DISTRESS SYNDROME (ARDS)

The basement membrane can, in addition, become altered by abnormalities of the cells lining the alveoli. These cells can be the target of inhaled toxic fumes or smoke, infectious agents, radiation or ischaemia as part of shock. The reaction pattern of the lung tissue is similar for all these agents. It is enhanced by the release of lysosomal enzymes of activated polymorphonuclear leukocytes and by the generation of reactive oxygen species during their respiratory burst. Two different stages of the **adult respiratory distress syndrome** (Fig. 9.17) can be distinguished clinically and pathologically.

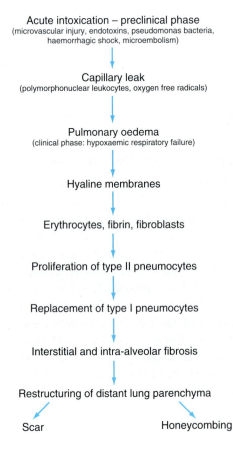

Acute intoxication – preclinical phase
(microvascular injury, endotoxins, pseudomonas bacteria, haemorrhagic shock, microembolism)

Capillary leak
(polymorphonuclear leukocytes, oxygen free radicals)

Pulmonary oedema
(clinical phase: hypoxaemic respiratory failure)

Hyaline membranes

Erythrocytes, fibrin, fibroblasts

Proliferation of type II pneumocytes

Replacement of type I pneumocytes

Interstitial and intra-alveolar fibrosis

Restructuring of distant lung parenchyma

Scar   Honeycombing

Fig. 9.17 The pathogenesis of ARDS.

Causes of ARDS
- Infectious agents such as bacterial toxins, virus, malaria, mycoplasmae
- Toxic fumes such as nitrogen dioxide, cadmium, manganese, smoke, resin smoke, sulphur dioxide, oxygen
- Aspiration of fresh or sea water (drowning)
- Radiation

- Within 24 hours of exposure there is an oedematous (exudative) stage forming hyaline membranes. In addition, numerous granulocytes, cellular debris and an intra-alveolar oedema are present.
- After 3–7 days the organization develops, characterized by an invasion of macrophages and by partial digestion of the cellular debris, with proliferation of type II pneumocytes. Fragments of collagen replace the cellular debris. Proliferation of pneumocytes remains prominent so that after 10–14 days the airspaces are filled with collagenous fibres, numerous macrophages and pneumocytes. Fibrinous thrombi are present in the capillaries and smaller arteries. If resolution does not occur, the end stage is a fatal severe fibrosis with complete alteration of the original architecture of the lung.

FIBROSING ALVEOLITIS

This idiopathic group of conditions leads to lung fibrosis and may present as an acute or chronic illness. In the acute form (**usual interstitial pneumonia**), there is hyperplasia of type II pneumocytes, while in **chronic interstitial pneumonia** (**desquamative interstitial pneumonia**) the histological appearance is of intra-alveolar macrophage accumulation. A related condition in which the bronchioles become filled with granulation tissue is known as **bronchiolitis obliterans**. The long-term effects are due to fibrosis with progressive pulmonary hypertension and cor pulmonale with respiratory failure.

SARCOIDOSIS

This idiopathic granulomatous condition also leads to pulmonary fibrosis. Respiratory failure is the eventual cause of death in about 15% of these patients (see Chapter 7).

OTHERS

Diffuse involvement of the interstitial lung parenchyma is also seem in **histiocytosis X** caused by proliferation of Langerhans' cells, alveolar lipoproteinosis, and diffuse malignancies due to spread of tumour through lung lymphatics (lymphangitis carcinomatosa).

Pulmonary hypertension and embolus

Pulmonary hypertension is defined as an increased systolic arterial intrapulmonary pressure above 30 mmHg. **Chronic pulmonary hypertension** induces vascular changes of the arterial walls, particularly in the larger, more muscular vessels. The size and the number of smooth muscle cells in the media increases, and secondary smooth muscle cell proliferation occurs in the intima. The increased pressure is often combined with a (focally) low flow state, and usually resistance exceeds the pressure necessary for normal flow conditions. Thrombotic lesions of the arterial walls are a consequence of low flow rates in such vessels.

A broad variety of diseases can be combined with pulmonary hypertension. In early childhood, malformations of the heart such as pre-tricuspid shunts, post-tricuspid shunts and mitral stenosis are common associated diseases. In later life, other causes include chronic hypoxaemia (associated with emphysema, chronic obstructive bronchitis, kyphoscoliosis, pickwickian syndrome or high altitude), pulmonary fibrosis, parasites (schistosomes), recurrent pulmonary embolism and idiopathic pulmonary hypertension.

The vascular changes start with a proliferation of the smooth muscle fibres of the arterioles and small arteries followed by an intimal proliferation and concentric laminar fibrosis with, finally, complete obliteration of the vessel. Other vessels may become ectatic and display dilated vein-like branches simulating angiomatoid alterations. The development of the morphological changes until obliterative changes occur takes only a few weeks.

PULMONARY EMBOLISM

Acute pulmonary embolism (Fig. 9.18) is usually associated with thrombosis of the deep peripheral veins of the body (legs), usually seen in immobilized patients or patients at a specific risk because of an increased tendency to clotting. This is associated with smoking, oestrogen therapy and surgery (especially if pelvic). Massive acute pulmonary thrombosis is often fatal (especially if the output from the right heart is decreased by 75% or more). It is quite common for the source of the **emboli** (femoral, calf, iliac veins) not to be demonstrated afterwards. Small emboli may not cause clinical symptoms, and are removed from the lobar arteries by thrombolysis within four weeks. Emboli from extravascular sources comprise air emboli (trauma, head and neck surgery, intrauterine manipulation, etc.), amniotic fluid emboli and tissue emboli, especially fat and bone marrow emboli (trauma). Severe amniotic fluid emboli are rare, in contrast with insignificant emboli which are seen in almost every delivery.

PULMONARY INFARCTION

Pulmonary infarction leads to haemorrhage into the alveoli and subsequent death of the alveolar and interstitial cells. Macroscopically, this is seen as a wedge-shaped area of solid, dusky purple lung tissue. Thrombi

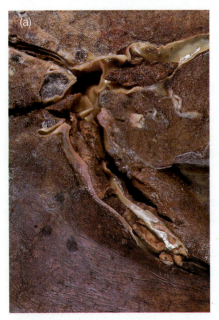 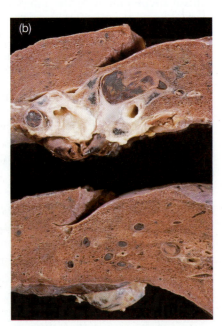 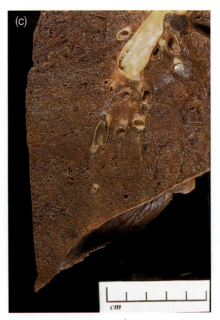

Fig. 9.18   Pulmonary emboli can often be found within the pulmonary arteries at postmortem examination (a). Examination of the leg veins may show deep venous thrombosis (b). Those who survive for some time with smaller emboli may develop pulmonary infarction (c).

may be seen within the pulmonary arteries serving the affected area. If the patient survives, there is an acute inflammatory response which starts at the edge of the infarct leading to its liquefaction. Much of the dead tissue and blood clot is removed by phagocytes, but haemoptysis is common. The area will eventually heal by fibrosis, although ventilation–perfusion abnormalities may persist.

BENIGN TUMOURS AND BORDERLINE LESIONS

The incidence of malignant lung tumours far exceeds that of tumours of benign or borderline behaviour. Nevertheless, benign lung tumours are important since they can easily be confused with malignancy on radiographs. As usual, benign tumours can be classified according to their histogenesis, and epithelial and mesenchymal tumours are of importance. Epithelial benign tumours comprise adenomatous tumours (adenomas, papillomas) and tumours of submucosal bronchial gland origin (mucous gland adenomas, pleomorphic adenomas, low-grade mucoepidermoid carcinomas, acinic cell tumours, bronchial oncocytomas). Small collections of glomus cells associated with the pulmonary vasculature may give rise to pulmonary chemodectomas, which are usually incidental findings in lung biopsies or at postmortem examination. All these tumours are of benign biological behaviour, and curative resection is usually possible. Most have solid, adenoid (tubular) growth patterns.

PAPILLOMA

Bronchial papillomas are probably virus-associated and form epidermoid lesions with intrabronchial polypoid growth. The basic cellular features are a uniform distribution of nuclear size and chromatin, abundant cytoplasm, and a weak or non-existent inflammatory response of the host tissue corresponding to slow tumour growth. The common central localization of these tumours induces an obstruction of the corresponding bronchus and clinical symptoms such as cough, expectoration or sometimes asthma attacks.

EPITHELIAL BORDERLINE TUMOURS

There are three major types of epithelial borderline tumour:

- **carcinoids** (Fig. 9.19), which are tumours originating from the neuroendocrine system with infrequent metastatic behaviour; they usually grow with an adenoid histological pattern, with many blood capillaries which may lead to severe bleeding if the tumour is biopsied.
- **mucoepidermoid carcinomas of medium grade**
- **adenoid cystic carcinoma** which grows in large, mucus-filled tubules with a lining of cuboidal, relatively small cells. These tumours tend to invade the submucosa not detectable by bronchoscopic techniques. Recurrences are frequent and often not curable.

MESENCHYMAL LUNG TUMOURS

Mesenchymal benign lung tumours are most frequently **hamartomatous lesions** located in the peripheral lung parenchyma and often detected by accidental chest radiographs. Two main types have to be mentioned:

- **hamartomas** (fibrochondrolipomas), tumorous lesions consisting of fatty and chondromatous tissue surrounded by bronchial epithelial cells

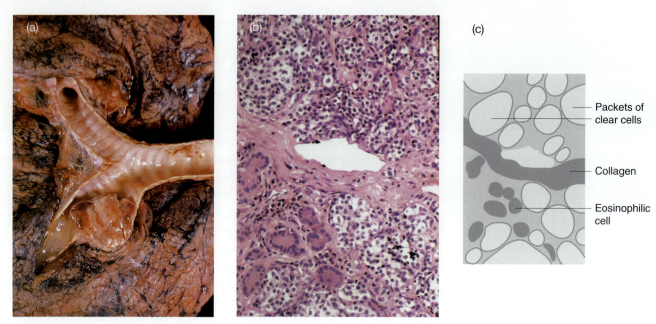

Fig. 9.19   A bronchial carcinoid showing (a) the tumour sitting within the bronchi and (b, c) the typical histological appearance of a tumour with packets of cells containing uniform small round nuclei and clear cytoplasm.

- **granular cell tumours** consisting of large tumour cells with small condensed nuclei and abundant granular eosinophilic cytoplasm.

Other benign mesenchymal lesions are extremely rare and include all forms of mesenchymal tissues – lipoma, fibroma, chondroma, etc. The **sclerosing haemangioma** is usually a solitary, peripherally localized mass of uncertain origin. It presents with numerous sclerotic blood vessels surrounded by numerous, quite uniform and small cells – a texture giving the tumour a characteristic histological appearance.

Other entities of benign or borderline behaviour are mild lymphoproliferative disorders, including low-grade **B-cell lymphoma** derived from bronchus-associated lymphoid tissue (**BALT**) and **idiopathic inflammation with fibrosis**. BALT lymphoma in the lung presents radiologically as a solid circumscribed mass which is histologically formed by mature lymphocytes and plasma cells, sometimes with remaining germinal centres. The lesions are usually localized and few have spread outside the lung at presentation. Idiopathic inflammation with fibrosis is the most common tumour-like lesion in children under 16 years of age and composed of plasma cells and a varying number of histiocytes and fibroblasts, often mimicking Hodgkin's lymphoma.

Tumour-like diffuse alterations of the lung are sometimes seen in women during their reproductive years and are characterized by an enormous proliferation of smooth muscle cells resulting in bronchiolar obstruction. The lesion called **lymphangioleiomyomatosis** is usually progressive, but may respond to antioestrogen therapeutic regimens in some cases. A non-neoplastic, proliferative disorder affecting either the lung in isolation or multiple organs (skin, liver, bone marrow, spleen), histiocytosis X or eosinophilic granuloma is characterized by an enormous eosinophilic infiltrate which is replaced by macrophages and finally fibrotic nodules at a later stage. The aetiology of the disease is not known, but nearly all patients are heavy smokers.

Malignant tumours

Malignant lung tumours, again, can derive from epithelial or mesenchymal tissue. In contrast to the relatively uncommon benign lung tumours, they contribute to 10–20% of all human malignancies. Carcinomas comprise more than 90% of all lung tumours. This was an almost unknown disorder at the beginning of the twentieth century. The associated risk factors include smoking (the main carcinogenic agent) and exposure to various (occupational) toxins such as asbestos, aluminium, cadmium, radioactive substances, nickel and chromium. Many bronchial carcinomas arise from areas of squamous metaplasia via a dysplastic process similar to that seen in other epithelia.

LUNG CARCINOMA

The classification of lung carcinomas is defined by WHO and comprises four major types, based on the constituent cell type:

- **squamous cell carcinoma**, usually a central localized tumour with epidermoid growth pattern, production of keratin and formation of intercellular junctions
- **adenocarcinoma** (Fig. 9.20), a centrally or peripherally localized tumour with papillomatous or tubular growth pattern and the production of various amounts of mucus
- **small cell anaplastic carcinoma**, usually a centrally localized tumour of neuroendocrine origin formed by small cells with a scarce cytoplasm and a mosaic-like pattern of the nuclei (moulding), large areas of necrosis and absent inflammatory infiltrates
- **large cell anaplastic carcinoma** (Fig. 9.21), a group of carcinomas which cannot be classified into one of the above three categories.

A specific subentity of adenocarcinoma is the **bronchioloalveolar carcinoma** which is either a diffuse multilocular growing tumour or a circumscribed tumour mass associated with scars and typical intra-alveolar growth along the interalveolar septa. The diffuse growing type often presents with enormous mucus production and involvement of all parts of both lungs.

Clinically, lung tumours are staged according to the TNM categories, i.e. according to their size, location, extent, lymph node involvement and distant metastases. Localized tumours can be resected, sometimes with

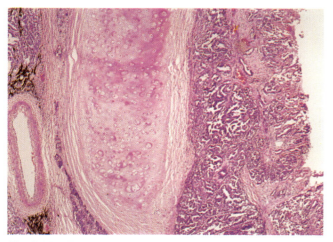
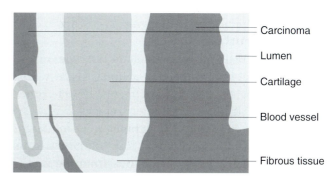

Carcinoma

Lumen

Cartilage

Blood vessel

Fibrous tissue

Fig. 9.20   The microscopic appearance of an adenocarcinoma of the bronchus showing replacement of the mucosa and invasion around the cartilage of bronchial wall.

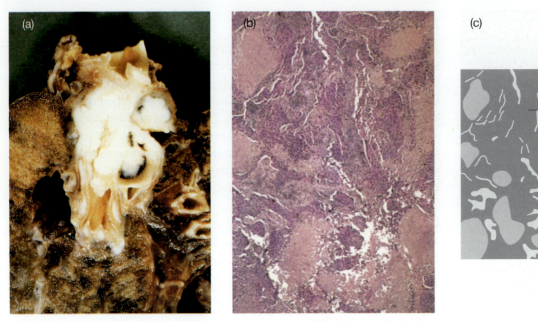

Fig. 9.21 (a) An anaplastic lung carcinoma with a white cut surface. Note the extension down one of the bronchi. (b, c) Microscopy shows the tumour to consist of solid sheets of malignant cells with large areas of necrosis.

good outcome. Liver, bone and brain are favourite sites of metastasis for lung carcinomas and patients may present with these before the primary tumour becomes symptomatic.

The cell type and the TNM stage are the fundamental requirements for estimation of the patient's prognosis and for planning treatment. Clinically, two different cell types are of major importance, the small cell carcinomas versus the non-small cell carcinomas. Patients suffering from small cell carcinoma are treated with cytotoxic drug regimens, and surgical resection is performed only in those with small tumours. Patients with other carcinomas are primarily candidates for surgical treatment or radiotherapy, as chemotherapy is rarely helpful.

Besides the classic histological tumour features, biological characteristics become more and more important, especially the expression of oncogenes (*ras*, *myc*, *erb*, *p53*), chromosomal abnormalities (chromosome 7; 13 in small cell carcinoma), blood group antigen expression, the percentage of proliferating cells measurable by specific antibodies or analysis of the DNA content (flow cytometry), and the presence of neuroendocrine differentiation detectable by monoclonal antibodies.

MESENCHYMAL TUMOURS

The mesenchymal group of malignant lung tumours is rare and comprises about 5% of all lung tumours. **Sarcomas** usually arise from the vascular walls or mesenchymal compartments of the bronchi, manifesting as fibrosarcoma, leiomyosarcoma, chrondrosarcoma, rhabdomyosarcoma, liposarcoma, fibrous histiocytoma, etc. Intrapulmonary sarcoma metastases are far more common than primary sarcomas.

Lymphomas are thought to derive from the BALT, comparable to the mucosa-associated lymphatic tissue (MALT) of the intestinal tract, and are most frequently B-cell lymphomas. Other leukaemic infiltrates include **Hodgkin's disease**, **plasmacytoma** and **Waldenström's macro-globulinaemia**. All these entities are rare.

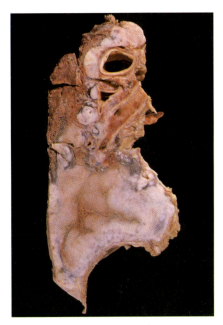

Fig. 9.22 The macroscopic appearance of a mesothelioma which has invaded around the lower lobe and replaced much of it. Note the enlarged hilar lymph nodes.

METASTASIS FROM OTHER SITES

Similar to the liver, the lung is host to a variety of extrapulmonary malignancies, most frequently breast carcinoma, adenocarcinoma of the kidneys (hypernephroma), colorectal carcinoma, carcinoma of the prostate and seminoma of the testis. All of these tumours can appear in the lungs prior to metastatic growth in other organs such as liver or bone marrow, and about 20% of hypernephromas are primarily detected by their intrapulmonary metastases.

MESOTHELIOMA

Malignant tumours of the pleura derive from the mesothelial cells and can be diffuse (most frequently) or localized (seldom). Most patients with these mesotheliomas have a history of asbestos or glass fibre exposure, and the tumours arise 10–15 years after the initial exposure. Histologically, the tumours are composed of epithelial cells mimicking adenocarcinomas and mesenchymal cells mimicking fibrosarcomas; the proportion of both components can vary to a large extent (Fig 9.22). The prognosis of patients suffering from mesotheliomas is poor, and no adequate curative treatment is known.

Chapter 10   Oral pathology

Learning objectives

To appreciate and understand:
- ❏ The range and scope of oral pathology
- ❏ Oral manifestations of systemic disease
- ❏ Correlation of clinical features in the mouth with histopathological changes

The tissues of the oral cavity are subject to the same basic pathological process as other parts of the body. However, as a consequence of the presence of structures peculiar to the oral cavity these processes often show distinctive features. In addition there are a number of important diseases which are specifically related to teeth and their supporting structures. The teeth consist of calcified tissues, the enamel, dentine and cementum, and non-calcified pulp. A complex periodontal fibrous ligament supports and attaches the tooth to investing alveolar bone. The oral epithelium is stratified squamous in type and shows regional variation in the degree of keratinization. Oral epithelium has a high rate of cell turnover whereas the supporting connective tissues vary from the loose corium of lining mucosa to the dense mucoperiosteum of the hard palate.

Salivary secretions contain mucin, electrolytes, secretory IgA and lactoferrin, and the oral cavity contains a rich microflora. The oral cavity may be the primary site for systemic diseases especially those which also affect the gastrointestinal tract, bone and skin.

The teeth and periodontium

Normal structure

The crown of a tooth comprises a hard outer layer called **enamel** which is non-cellular, consisting of calcium apatite crystals with a delicate organic matrix. The bulk of the tooth is made up of **dentine** which consists of a thick layer of calcified collagenous tissue surrounding the soft tissues of the **pulp**. A similar, thinner layer of **cementum** invests the dentine in the root portion of the tooth. At the apex of each root is an apical foramen through which vessels and nerves enter the pulp. Tooth development and eruption of the primary (deciduous) dentition and then secondary (permanent) dentition begin at about 3 months of intrauterine life and continue through adolescence. The early development of teeth is heralded by projections from the primitive oral epithelium and morphogenesis is determined by the continued proliferation of these cells. Specialized cells – the **ameloblasts** – form enamel which is ectodermal in origin whilst mesenchymal cells, the **odontoblasts** and **cementoblasts** contribute to dentine and cementum formation. When tooth formation is complete, remnants of epithelium may remain within bone and become the site of pathology in later life.

Disorders of tooth development

Developmental disorders of teeth may be prenatal or postnatal in origin and may be inherited or acquired. Clearly, their recognition and evaluation require a thorough knowledge of the normal chronology of the human dentition, and of normal development and structure of the teeth. It is of value to distinguish between abnormalities of **morphodifferentiation** and those of **histodifferentiation**. The former occur due to disorders in the dental lamina and tooth germ and result in abnormalities in the number, size and form of teeth. The latter, arising from abnormalities in the formation of the dental hard tissues, give rise to structural defects.

The congenital absence of teeth may be referred to as **hypodontia**, **anodontia** or **oligodontia**, and may be partial or total. Hypodontia or partial anodontia is common, occurring in about 3–7% of the population. Total anodontia is rare and in most cases is associated with other defects, such as hereditary hypohidrotic ectodermal dysplasia, a disorder usually inherited as an X-linked recessive trait.

Enamel hypoplasia is relatively common and may follow infection or trauma during tooth development. Any serious nutritional deficiency or systemic disease occurring during the time of tooth formation is capable of giving rise to enamel hypoplasia. Examples of genetically determined enamel lesions include amelogenesis imperfecta, ectodermal dysplasia syndromes, epidermolysis bullosa and Down's syndrome (trisomy 21). A dominant, autosomal hereditary disease with variable expressivity which affects dentine is **dentinogenesis imperfecta**. In this condition, dentine has reduced mineral content, pulp chambers are obliterated and root formation is arrested.

Thus genetic and environmental factors play a role in dental abnormalities. The administration of some tetracyclines during tooth development may lead to permanent staining of calcified tissues and is a good example of iatrogenic disease.

Dental caries

Dental caries may be defined as a bacterial disease of the calcified tissues of the teeth characterized by the demineralization of the inorganic and destruction of the organic substance of the tooth. It is a complex and dynamic process involving physiochemical processes associated with the movements of ions across the interface between the tooth and the external environment. Biological processes associated with the interaction of bacteria in **dental plaque** with host defence mechanisms are also involved. The prevalence and severity of dental caries vary in different populations and are associated with urbanization and the increased availability of refined carbohydrates.

With regard to aetiology, the acidogenic theory, which proposes that acid formed from the fermentation of dietary carbohydrate by oral bacteria leads to the progressive decalcification of tooth substance and subsequent disintegration of the organic matrix, is universally accepted. Experiments with germ-free animals have shown that bacteria are essential for the development of dental caries. Bacteria are present in dental plaque and acid is generated within its substance to such an extent that enamel may be dissolved. Diffusion of dietary sugars through plaque leads to acid production, mainly lactic acid but also acetic and proprionic acids, by bacterial metabolism. The pH of plaque may fall by 2 units within minutes of sugar ingestion and at the critical pH (5.5) mineral ions are liberated from hydroxapatite crystals of the surface enamel. It should be noted that reprecipitation of mineral, facilitated by fluoride ions which can substitute for hydroxyl ions leading to deposition of fluoroapatite, may take place at neutral pH. Thus, at the plaque–enamel interface ion exchange occurs as the chemical environment within plaque changes. Acid production is a general product of bacterial metabolism. Members of the *Streptococcus mutans* group of bacteria are the most efficient cariogenic organisms.

As the carious lesion develops, lactobacilli appear to play an increasingly important role. Numerous epidemiological studies have demonstrated a direct relationship between fermentable carbohydrate in the diet and dental caries. Other factors which influence site attack and rate of progression in individual teeth or subjects can be either intrinsic or extrinsic to teeth.

Dental caries usually starts in two principal areas of the tooth: the fissures on the occlusal surfaces of posterior teeth, and the areas between teeth – **interproximal caries**. Bacteria do not enter enamel until decalcification has led to cavity formation. Thereafter, bacterial invasion through enamel and dentine leads to proteolytic breakdown of the collagen matrix. Carious dentine is yellowish in colour because of absorption of pigment from bacterial metabolic products. As the **pulp tissue** – a highly vascular connective tissue confined within a rigid pulp chamber in dentine – is approached, inflammatory changes occur giving rise to the clinical symptom of **pulpitis** which may be acute or chronic. Ultimately the carious process will lead to necrosis of the pulp, rendering the tooth non-vital. Spread of infection from pulpitis through the apical foramina reaches the periodontal membrane, and may give rise to an acute periapical abscess. This painful condition is usually accompanied by cervical lymphadenopathy, fever and malaise. More often low-grade pulpitis leads to periapical granuloma formation from which an inflammatory odontogenic cyst may develop.

Factors influencing development of caries
- Intrinsic factors
  - Enamel composition and structure
  - Tooth morphology
  - Tooth position
- Extrinsic factors
  - Salivary flow rate and composition
  - Diet
  - Immunity

CASE STUDY 10.1

A 35-year-old man presented with facial pain and swelling of several weeks' duration. He had not attended for routine dental care in the past. Immediately prior to presentation he complained of acute, throbbing dental pain in the incisor and premolar region of the right maxillary alveolus together with palatal swelling, unpleasant taste and halitosis. On clinical grounds (Fig. 10.1) the diagnosis of dental caries and acute alveolar abscess was made. Radiographic evidence suggested spread of infection to the periapical area of the right lateral incisor and first premolar teeth. These were extracted and an abscess associated with the incisor tooth was surgically drained. Both ground sections and decalcified sections of the extracted teeth showed variously smooth surface caries, pulpitis and dentine caries (Figs 10.2–10.4).

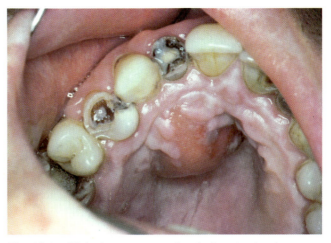

Fig. 10.1   Clinical appearance of typical acute alveolar abscess affecting the anterior maxilla. Gross dental caries is present in the lateral incisor and first premolar teeth.

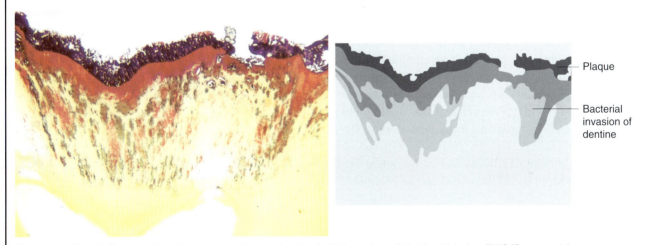

Fig. 10.2   Decalcified section of incisor tooth showing bacterial invasion of dentinal tubules (PAS/Gram stain).

Fig. 10.3   Ground section of carious lesion in enamel mounted in Canada balsam and viewed by transmitted polarized light. Various coloured zones represent varying degrees of mineral loss.

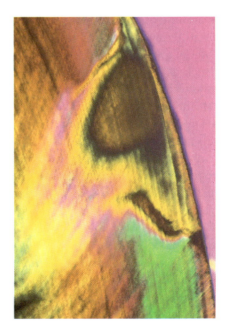

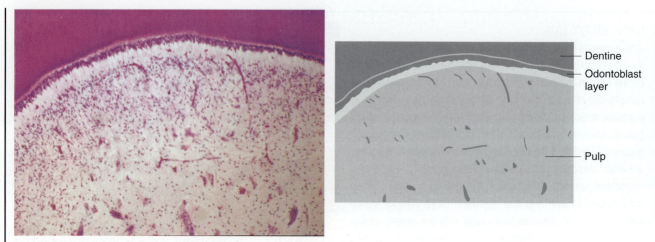

Fig. 10.4 Decalcified section of pulp chamber showing vasodilatation and mild non-specific inflammatory cell infiltrate.

Periodontal disease

Periodontal disease is a major clinical problem which results from the accumulation of dental plaque at the marginal gingivae leading to inflammation of the periodontal tissues. The disease is prevalent in most human populations and may lead to premature tooth loss in severely affected individuals. It is convenient to recognize the conditions of **gingivitis** and **periodontitis** depending upon whether destruction of the periodontal attachment has occurred and to distinguish between acute and chronic conditions. In most instances periodontal disease is chronic and persistent.

On the basis of current clinical and pathological evidence, the forms of destructive periodontal disease which can be identified are

- **adult periodontitis**
- **localized juvenile periodontitis**
- **rapidly progressive periodontitis**
- **prepubertal periodontitis**.

The primary cause is accumulation of **dental plaque** which is made up of bacterial aggregations adhering to teeth or mucosa. Plaque is complex and consists of matrix material and embedded bacteria. The matrix is derived from host products such as salivary glycoprotein, dead cells and serum proteins. Bacterial polysaccharides also contribute to the matrix.

Both supragingival and subgingival plaque may mineralize to form **calculus**. Saliva is supersaturated with calcium phosphate and in susceptible individuals nuclei of mineralization form in new plaque within 3 weeks. Plaque activates both inflammatory and immune host defences and both are active together in an integrated host response.

A distinctive condition known as **acute necrotizing ulcerative gingivitis** (ANUG, Vincent's infection) is characterized by painful necrotic ulcers at the gingival margins. Young adults are most commonly affected though the prevalence of the disease appears to be declining. The microflora associated with this condition include spirochaetes and anaerobic bacteria. A characteristic form of periodontal disease, clinically resembling a chronic form of ANUG, is now recognized in patients with HIV infection.

Microbial species commonly isolated from plaque
- *Streptococcus* spp.
- *Staphylococcus* spp.
- *Actinomyces* spp.
- *Lactobacillus* spp.
- *Neisseria* spp.
- *Veillonella* spp.

Cysts of the jaws

ODONTOGENIC CYSTS

Cysts of the jaws are more common than in any other bone and the majority are lined wholly or in part by epithelium. The majority (90%) are **odontogenic cysts**, the epithelial lining being derived from the epithelial residues of the tooth-forming organ. They can be divided into developmental and inflammatory types depending on their aetiology. The non-odontogenic cysts have epithelial linings derived from sources other than the tooth-forming organ. Recent studies on the distribution of cytokeratins in cyst epithelium tend to support this division because all derivatives of odontogenic epithelium are similar in their cytoplasmic filament content.

Inflammatory odontogenic cysts are by far the most common of all jaw cysts and originate from epithelial remnants (cell rests of Malazzez). They develop in periapical granulomata and are lined by non-keratinized stratified squamous epithelium supported by a connective tissue capsule. Epithelial hyperplasia is common and metaplastic changes such as mucous cells, respiratory type epithelium and hyaline bodies may be observed. Deposits of cholesterol crystals are common within the capsules. Mural cholesterol clefts are associated with a foreign body giant cell reaction. The cholesterol is probably derived from the breakdown of red blood cells as a result of haemorrhage into the cyst capsule, and deposits of haemosiderin are commonly associated with clefts. Cyst expansion and growth are governed by the rate of local bone resorption and hydrostatic pressure of the contents causes cyst enlargement. Prostaglandins, especially PGE_2, PGF_2 and PGI_1, together with collagenase derived from fibroblasts in the cyst capsule are important bone-resorbing factors which stimulate osteoclastic activity. The production of these factors is increased by the action of cytokines released by the inflammatory cell infiltrate and interleukin-1 may be especially important. Osmotically active molecules in cyst fluid result in cyst contents being hypertonic compared with serum. Thus, high osmolarity of cyst contents and the semipermeable nature of the cyst wall lead to the movement of fluid into the cyst along the osmotic gradient.

The relatively common developmental odontogenic cysts are the **dentigerous**, **eruption** and **primordial** cysts. A dentigerous cyst is one which arises in the follicular tissues covering the fully formed crown of the unerupted tooth. It encloses all or part of the crown and commonly involves teeth which are impacted or erupt late. The majority are associated with a mandibular third molar.

Eruption cysts involve both the deciduous and permanent dentitions and, since they arise from epithelium in an extra-alveolar location, they present clinically as fluctuant swellings on the alveolar mucosa. Typically the lining of developmental cysts is thin, regular and non-keratinized. Mucous cell metaplasia is common and increases with age. These cysts must be differentiated from the primordial cyst (or **odontogenic keratocyst**) which has a distinctive keratinized stratified squamous epithelial lining. This lesion has aroused much interest because of its unusual growth pattern and tendency to recur. It arises from remnants of the dental lamina and may replace a missing tooth in the dental arch, especially in the mandibular third molar region extending into the ramus.

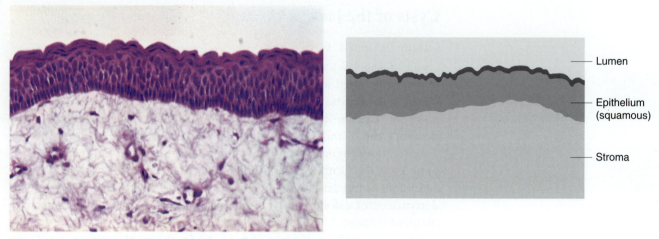

Fig. 10.5   Classic histological appearance of an odontogenic keratocyst.

They tend to enlarge in an anteroposterior direction and reach large size without causing bony expansion. Rarely multiple keratocysts are associated with the **basal cell naevus syndrome** (Gorlin–Goltz syndrome), inherited as an autosomal dominant trait with marked penetrance and variable expressivity. Histopathologically, the cyst wall is thin and often folded and is lined by a regular layer of stratified squamous epithelium some 5–10 cells thick (Fig. 10.5). Parakeratosis and orthokeratinization are features of note, and mitotic activity is higher than in other odontogenic cysts. The capsule may contain small satellite or daughter cysts whilst the lumen contents comprise keratin and low-soluble proteins making aspiration biopsy a useful diagnostic tool.

NON-ODONTOGENIC CYSTS

Among the non-odontogenic cysts, the most important is the **nasopalatine duct** (incisive canal) **cyst**. It is a distinct clinicopathological entity, being developmental in origin and arising from epithelial remnants of the nasopalatine duct. The cysts may be lined by a variety of different types of epithelium. Thus, alone or in combination, stratified squamous, cuboidal or pseudostratified ciliated columnar epithelium may be noted.

Neurovascular bundles are prominent in the connective tissue capsule. Other rare cysts in this category are the **globulomaxillary**, **nasolabial** and **median palatal**. These cysts were thought to be fissural but current embryogenesis does not support this concept and it is probable that they are odontogenic in origin.

It is worth noting that non-epithelialized bone cysts which occur in long bones may occasionally be observed in the jaws. They include the solitary bone cyst and the aneurysmal bone cyst. With the exception of salivary mucoceles including the ranula, soft tissue cysts of the oral tissues are rare. However, dermoid, lymphoepithelial and thyroglossal cysts may require to be included in the differential diagnosis of orofacial swellings.

Odontogenic tumours

Odontomes and odontogenic tumours are lesions derived from the dental formative tissues. Some of these lesions are neoplasms; others are developmental anomalies or malformations and are best thought of as dental hamartomas.

Odontomes are hamartomatous, non-neoplastic lesions containing the calcified dental tissues. A **complex odontome** consists of a disorganized mass of dental tissues whereas a **compound odontome** contains numerous small teeth or **denticles**. However, all gradations between the two may be encountered. Microscopically the complex odontome consists of a mass of enamel, dentine and cementum, surrounded by a fibrous capsule. The bulk of the lesion comprises dentine and in decalcified sections the participation of enamel is indicated by clear spaces or remnants of fibrillar enamel matrix.

The most important of the odontogenic neoplasms is the **ameloblastoma**. It is a benign but locally invasive neoplasm derived from odontogenic epithelium. Ameloblastomas are most frequent in the molar region of the mandible. They are slow growing and non-tender, and gradually lead to facial deformity and jawbone expansion. They are usually diagnosed in the fourth or fifth decade of life.

Depending upon the arrangement of the neoplastic epithelium, two histopathological patterns are recognized – follicular and plexiform – though there appears to be no difference in the clinical behaviour of the various types. A layer of cuboidal or columnar cells resembling ameloblasts lines a central mass of loosely arranged elongated cells similar to stellate reticulum. Within the stellate reticulum areas, cystic change, squamous metaplasia and granular cell change may be observed. The lesions lack a peripheral condensation of connective tissue.

Malignant lesions of the odontogenic apparatus are exceedingly rare, but ameloblastomas showing true malignant behaviour with metastases have been described. Similarly, occasional convincing reports of primary intraosseous carcinoma, malignant change in odontogenic cysts and odontogenic sarcoma have appeared in the literature.

Two tumours of debatable origin are worthy of mention. The **melanotic neuroectodermal tumour of infancy** occurs between the ages of one and three months, usually in the maxilla. Histologically the tumour comprises epithelium-like cells containing melanin together with small, dark, round cells in a fibrous stroma. The lesion is thought to be derived from cells of neural crest origin. The **congenital epulis** (congenital gingival granular cell tumour) occurs in the newborn, usually in the incisor region of the maxilla. Female infants are affected about ten times more frequently than male. It comprises closely packed granular cells and is benign, probably reactive rather than neoplastic.

Finally, the diagnosis of odontogenic cysts, tumours and neoplasms should take account, where possible, of radiographic evidence. Unilocular radiolucencies characterize odontogenic cysts whilst multilocular lesions are typical of ameloblastoma and some keratocysts.

Rare benign odontogenic tumours
- Calcifying epithelial odontogenic tumour
- Ameloblastic fibroma
- Adenomatoid odontogenic tumour
- Benign cementoblastoma
- Cementifying fibroma

CASE STUDY 10.2

A 26-year-old man attended for a routine dental examination. An asymptomatic firm swelling in the mandibular molar region was radiographed by the lateral oblique view. A multilocular radiolucency was noted (Fig. 10.6) and the differential diagnosis included an odontogenic cyst, a keratocyst or ameloblastoma. A biopsy showed the typical appearance of an ameloblastoma (Fig. 10.7).

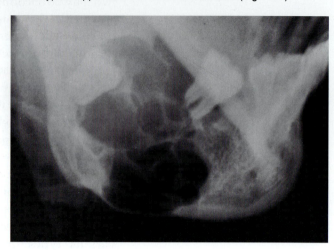

Fig. 10.6 Lateral oblique radiograph showing multilocular lesion at angle of jaw.

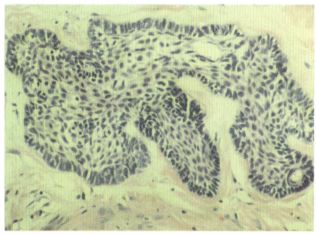

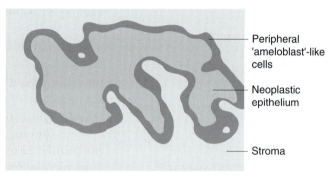

Peripheral 'ameloblast'-like cells

Neoplastic epithelium

Stroma

Fig. 10.7 Ameloblastoma. The island of neoplastic epithelium shows a central area of stellate reticulum-like cells. The peripheral, darkly staining cells are ameloblast-like.

The oral mucosa

Oral ulceration

The oral epithelium may be divided into three structural varieties:

- Non-keratinized **lining mucosa** is loose and mobile and covers the cheeks, lips, floor of mouth, ventral surface of tongue and the soft palate.
- **Masticatory mucosa** is keratinized and covers the hard palate, alveolus and gingiva.
- Specialized **gustatory epithelium** covers the dorsal tongue surface and is keratinized.

Ulceration is the most common lesion of the oral mucosa and is a manifestation of many local and systemic disorders. Oral ulceration may be traumatic and follow mechanical or chemical injury. The ulceration of recurrent aphthous stomatitis is essentially idiopathic, though a number of predisposing factors are implicated. Ulceration associated with dermatological disease includes erosive lichen planus and the vesiculobullous disorders. Squamous cell carcinoma often presents as a deep, indurated ulcer.

A traumatic ulcer shows the histological features of chronic non-specific ulceration.

The aetiology of **recurrent aphthous stomatitis** remains to be fully elucidated but there is increasing evidence that damaging immune responses to oral mucosal antigens or to cross-reacting microbial antigens are involved. Other aetiological factors include hereditary predisposition, trauma, stress, nutritional deficiency and hormonal disturbance.

In clinical practice a distinction is made between minor, major and herpetiform aphthous ulceration. In addition, any form may be associated with **Behçet's syndrome** which displays a range of signs including mucocutaneous ulceration, arthritis, central nervous system involvement and uveitis. There is a strong association with histocompatibility antigen HLA-B5. Aphthous ulcers tend to occur in crops, each ulcer being about 5 mm in diameter, having a grey–yellow base with an erythematous margin. Histopathologically, the ulcers are chronic and non-specific. They heal within 10 days but recur at variable intervals. Recurrent aphthous ulceration and angular cheilitis together with lip and oral mucosal swelling are oral features of **Crohn's disease** (Figs 10.8 and 10.9). Nutritional deficiency and

Fig. 10.8 Markedly swollen lips with angular cheilitis: oral Crohn's disease.

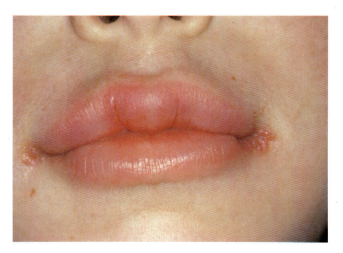

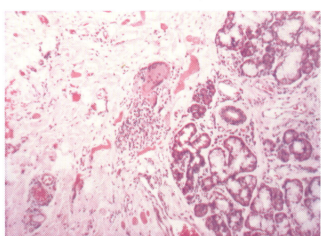

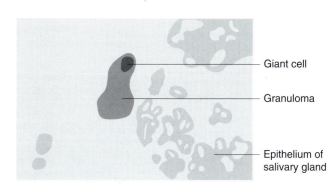

Giant cell

Granuloma

Epithelium of salivary gland

Fig. 10.9 Crohn's disease. Note the non-caseating granulomata containing Langhans' giant cells.

hypersensitivity may be factors common to this condition and other gastrointestinal disorders such as coeliac disease and ulcerative colitis.

Oral ulceration is a common presenting feature of the **vesiculobullous disorders**, as the vesicles or bullae tend to rupture very soon after their appearance in the oral cavity (see also Chapter 19). These diseases may be divided into **intraepithelial** or **subepithelial** vesiculobullous diseases, depending on the histological location of the lesion (see box).

Immunopathological investigations involving direct immunofluorescence studies of fresh, unfixed biopsy material to detect tissue-bound immune products and indirect immunofluorescent techniques to detect circulating autoantibodies in patients' sera are essential to establish and differentiate between pemphigus and pemphigoid.

> **Intraepithelial and subepithelial vesiculobullous diseases**
> ■ Intraepithelial lesions
>   - Acantholytic (pemphigus vulgaris)
>   - Non-acantholytic (viral diseases)
> ■ Subepithelial lesions
>   - Erythema multiforme
>   - Benign mucous membrane pemphigoid
>   - Dermatitis herpetiformis
>   - Epidermolysis bullosa

CASE STUDY 10.3

A 45-year-old woman presented with a 3-month history of recurrent blisters affecting the oral mucosa generally. She reported occasional vesicular eruptions on the skin. Clinically (Fig. 10.10) lesions were noted on the posterior hard palate and soft palate. The vesicles broke down to form shallow sloughing ulcers. The differential diagnosis included atypical viral disease, mucous membrane pemphigoid and pemphigus vegetans. A biopsy of an intact vesicle (Fig. 10.11) showed intraepithelial bulla formation together with acantholysis. An indirect immunofluorescent test revealed positive staining (Fig. 10.12) around prickle cells of the stratified epithelium. A diagnosis of pemphigus was established.

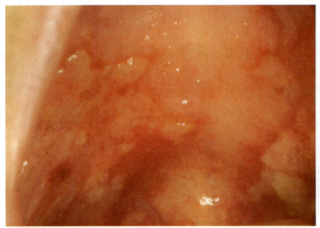

Fig. 10.10   Vesicular eruption at junction of hard and soft palate. Note the sloughing areas which remain after rupture of vesicles.

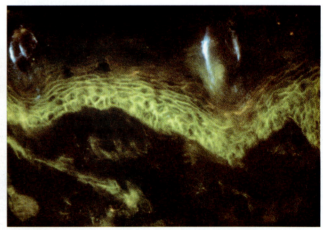

Fig. 10.12   Positive immunofluorescent staining of intercellular matrix around prickle cells: pemphigus vulgaris.

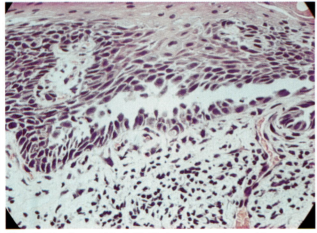

Fig. 10.11   Intraepithelial bulla in a case of pemphigus vulgaris. Note acantholytic cells being shed into the bulla.

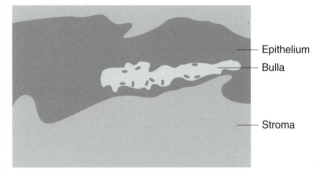

Epithelium

Bulla

Stroma

Factors predisposing to candida infection

- Trauma (especially from ill-fitting dentures)
- Long-term antibiotics
- Steroid or immunosuppressive therapy
- Xerostomia
- Iron deficiency
- Diabetes mellitus
- HIV infection

Infections

BACTERIAL INFECTIONS

Specific bacterial infections of the oral cavity are extremely rare. The intact oral mucosa acts as a barrier to infection. Saliva has a mechanical cleansing effect and contains non-specific and specific antibacterial substances, such as lysozyme and immunoglobulins. **Secretory IgA** is present in gingival crevicular fluid. Neutrophil leukocytes are continually released into the oral cavity and their phagocytic function is enhanced by complement activation. However, acute ulcerative gingivitis, actinomycosis, syphilis, tuberculosis and gonorrhoea may affect the oral cavity as primary or secondary disease.

FUNGAL INFECTIONS

Candida albicans is the main species associated with fungal infections of the oral mucosa, but others such as *Candida glabrata* and *Candida tropicalis* are also pathogenic. Most *Candida* species are dimorphic and exist as ovoid yeast forms or hyphae. It should be noted that over half the population harbour oral candida as a commensal organism.

Acute pseudomembranous candidiasis (**thrush**) is a condition found most often in children or debilitated adults and is characterized by detachable white fungal plaques on the epithelium

Chronic atrophic candidiasis (denture sore mouth) is found under ill-fitting dentures. The mucosa is markedly red and may have a granular or nodular appearance. The condition is often accompanied by angular cheilitis characterized by soreness, erythema and fissuring at the corners of the mouth. *Candida albicans* together with *Staphylococcus aureus* or, less frequently, β-haemolytic streptococci are implicated in the troublesome condition. Nutritional deficiencies, especially iron deficiency though also those of riboflavin, folic acid and vitamin B_{12}, are predisposing factors in some cases. Candida hyphae may be found in adherent hyperkeratotic localized lesions, especially on the buccal mucosa at the angle of the mouth, as **chronic hyperplastic candidiasis** (candidal leukoplakia). There is evidence to suggest that this condition may predispose to oral cancer.

Rare manifestations of candidal infection are represented by **acute erythematous candidiasis** (antibiotic stomatitis) and chronic mucocutaneous candidiasis in which nails and skin are also involved. Oral swabs and smears will demonstrate Gram-positive candidal organisms whilst tissue biopsy shows hyphae in the superficial layer of hyperplastic epithelium. Special staining with periodic acid–Schiff (PAS) is especially helpful.

Specific antibodies to *Candida* spp. are present in the sera of most individuals and increased titres of humoral antibodies against *Candida* species are found in infected patients when compared with control subjects. There is considerable evidence to suggest that cell-mediated immune responses are impaired in patients with chronic mucocutaneous conditions.

VIRAL INFECTIONS

The main viral diseases of the oral cavity are herpetic stomatitis, herpes zoster, herpangina, infectious mononucleosis, measles and viral warts. HIV, mumps and influenza may be also associated with oral mucosal lesions.

The **herpes simplex virus** (HSV) is a DNA virus and is the most frequent cause of viral infection in the mouth. Primary infection with HSV type 1 often occurs via the oral mucosa and lips, presenting as primary herpetic gingivostomatitis, characterized by extensive painful ulceration and systemic upset. Secondary or recurrent herpetic lesions are more frequent, especially at the mucocutaneous junction around the lip. A vesicular eruption is followed by ulceration and crusting. Histological examination of an intact herpetic vesicle is rarely performed, but shows the vesicle to be intraepithelial. Infected cells become swollen, and have an eosinophilic cytoplasm and large, pale vesicular nuclei with chromatin distributed as a thin rim round the periphery. Giant cells containing many nuclei form as a result of fusion of cytoplasm of infected cells. Smears stained with monoclonal immunofluorescent antiserum to HSV give specific results which are useful in rapid diagnosis. Primary herpetic stomatitis is associated with local replication of HSV at the sites of clinical infection. However, the virus is capable of migration to the sensory ganglion of the trigeminal nerve where it remains in a latent state. Various stimuli, such as ultraviolet light or trauma, may alter the latency state and cause the virus to migrate towards the nerve endings and thus give rise to recurrent herpes.

Both **chickenpox** and **herpes zoster** are caused by the same DNA virus, zoster being the manifestation of recurrent infection following a primary attack of chickenpox. In herpes zoster, oral lesions are localized to the distribution of one or more sensory nerves as a characteristic unilateral vesicular eruption.

Herpangina is caused by Coxsackie virus A, an RNA virus. The disease is common in children, and vesicles affect the tonsils, palate and uvula.

Infectious mononucleosis is caused by **Epstein–Barr virus (EBV)**, a member of the herpes group. Lymph node enlargement, fever and inflammation are the hallmarks of the disease, which may last for several months. Diagnosis may be confirmed by testing acute serum for IgM antibodies to EBV capsid antigen or by a specific monospot slide test.

Measles virus produces vesicles which rupture giving rise to the classic **Koplik's spots**. HIV infection may give rise to an unusual oral lesion called **hairy leukoplakia** in which a stratified white patch affects the tongue bilaterally. It appears highly probable that hairy leukoplakia results from the opportunistic infection of the oral epithelium by Epstein–Barr virus. Kaposi's sarcoma associated with HIV may affect the mouth, especially in the palate.

Keratoses

A lesion appearing as a white area on the oral mucosa is usually due to abnormal or increased keratin production. The colour of normal oral mucosa results from a balance between vascularity, melanin pigmentation, epithelial thickness and keratinization. The term **leukoplakia** has been defined as 'a whitish patch or plaque which cannot be characterized clinically or pathologically as any other disease, and is not associated with any chemical or physical agent except the use of tobacco'. It is a clinical term decided by exclusion. White patch lesions are extremely common in the oral cavity. They may be classified according to aetiology as hereditary, traumatic, infective, idiopathic, dermatological or neoplastic.

Oral epithelial naevus (familial white folded gingivostomatitis) is a hereditary disorder which appears in infancy or early childhood. Histologically, the epithelium is acantholytic and markedly oedematous. The lesion is benign. Traumatic keratosis is common and may affect any part of the oral mucosa and is due to mechanical, chemical or thermal irritation. The histological features are those of hyperkeratosis and acanthosis. Inflammatory change tends to be minimal and the lesion regresses when the stimulus is removed.

Candidal infections may give rise to adherent white patch lesions, as in chronic hyperplastic candidiasis, whereas syphilis and HIV infections may result in characteristic lesions.

Idiopathic leukoplakia may occur in any part of the oral mucosa, though the palate (in pipe-smokers), buccal mucosa and ventral surface of the tongue are common sites. The latter condition, **sublingual keratosis**, has a high malignant potential. At the edge of such white patches a reddened area may be noted. This appearance of **erythroplakia** may be defined as a bright red velvety plaque which cannot be categorized as being due to any other condition. The combination of leukoplakia and erythroplakia – so-called **speckled leukoplakia** – is an important clinical sign which may herald the onset of pre-malignant or malignant change.

The striated white patch lesions of **lichen planus** may affect the oral mucosa, especially the buccal mucosa (Fig. 10.13) and lateral border of the

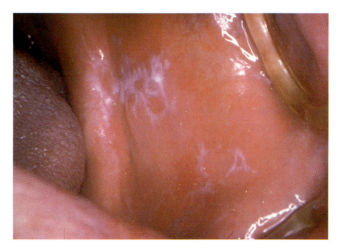

Fig. 10.13 Striated white patch lesions on the buccal mucosa, typical of lichen planus.

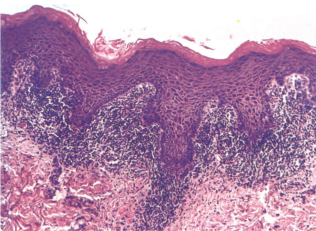

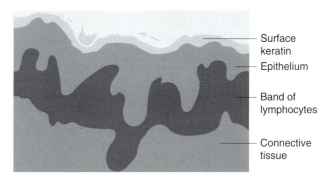

Surface keratin

Epithelium

Band of lymphocytes

Connective tissue

Fig. 10.14 Lichen planus. Note the main histological features: hyperkeratosis, acanthosis and broad band of lymphocytes at the epithelium–connective tissue interface.

tongue. The epithelial hyperplasia and predominantly broad-banded lymphocytes infiltrate and the epithelium–connective tissue interface is pathognomonic (Fig. 10.14). Similar lesions of lupus erythematosus may occasionally be seen and basal lamina thickening and perivascular lymphocytic infiltration will be noted.

Neoplasms

Tumours arise from any of the tissues of the oral mucosa, but the most frequent neoplasms are epithelial: the squamous cell papilloma and squamous cell carcinoma.

The **squamous cell papilloma** is common and occurs usually as a solitary lesion and may be pedunculated or sessile. Histologically, finger-like processes of proliferating stratified squamous epithelium are supported by a thin vascular connective tissue core. The lesion is benign, though a variety of virally induced hyperplasias of oral mucosa may simulate the papilloma clinically.

The most frequent malignant tumour is **squamous cell carcinoma**, which accounts for more than 90% of oral malignancies. The incidence of oral cancer varies enormously around the world. In the UK, oral cancer accounts for 1–2% of all malignant tumours, but in India it accounts for 30–40%. In the UK there are about 1900 new cases and 960 deaths per year from oral cancer. Early recognition should be possible, but despite this fact many oral cancers have a poor prognosis because of failure to recognize and treat early lesions.

Squamous cell carcinoma can occur at any site, though almost half involve the lower lip or lateral border of the tongue. Histologically, most oral cancers are well differentiated and show invasion and destruction of local tissues. Keratin pearls are often seen surrounded by prickle cells showing varying degrees of cellular atypia.

Immunohistochemical markers to demonstrate cytokeratins (intermediate filament proteins) are valuable to demonstrate epithelia in anaplastic tumours. Lymph nodes are involved relatively late. Carcinomas may be graded on a scale of 1–4 ranging from well-differentiated to undifferentiated tumours as in Broder's classification. The TNM clinical staging system is useful and incorporates those factors thought to influence prognosis. Recent refinements to the technique of exfoliative cytology offer hope for a screening test for oral cancer and the early recognition of precancer. A lesion may be called premalignant if it precedes or coexists with a tumour more frequently than would be expected by chance alone.

Other tumours occuring in the mouth include lymphoma, lipoma, neurofibroma and minor salivary gland tumours.

Aetiological factors in oral cancer
- Tobacco
- Alcohol
- Nutritional deficiency
- Ultraviolet light
- Viruses
- Betel chewing
- Immunosuppression

Oral premalignant conditions
- Leukoplakia
- Erythroplakia
- Epithelial atrophy
- Submucous fibrosis
- Hyperplastic candidiasis
- Atrophic lichen planus

CASE STUDY 10.4

A 60-year-old man presented with a long-standing white patch on the lateral border of the tongue (Fig. 10.15). The lateral margin of the white patch showed areas of erythroplakia and erosion. The patient admitted to both a smoking habit and an alcohol habit. The differential diagnosis included frictional keratosis, chronic hyperplastic candidiasis and oral carcinoma. An incisional biopsy revealed a varied histological picture. At one level the features were those of atrophic lichen planus (Fig. 10.16) and, at another, hyperkeratosis, acanthosis and mild cellular atypia were noted (Fig. 10.17). At this level, PAS staining revealed candidal hyphae (Fig. 10.18). However, deeper levels showed the typical cellular features of an early invasive squamous cell carcinoma (Fig. 10.19).

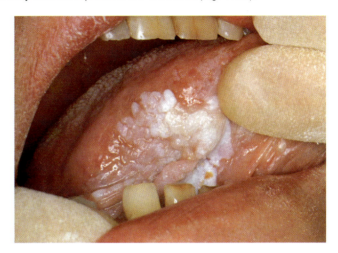

Fig. 10.15 Extensive white patch on lateral border of tongue. Patchy areas of erythroplakia give the lesion a speckled appearance.

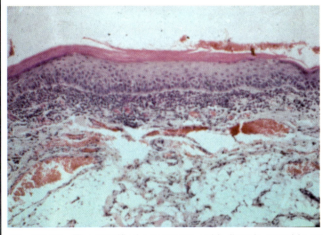

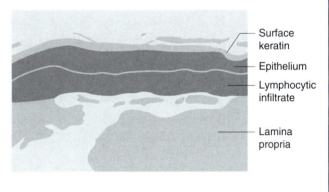

Fig. 10.16 The stratified squamous epithelium is atrophic and dense; predominantly lymphocytic infiltration affects the upper lamina propria. These features suggest a lichenoid reaction.

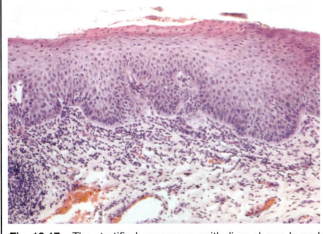

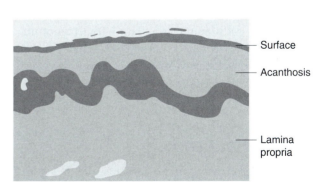

Fig. 10.17 The stratified squamous epithelium shows hyperkeratosis and irregular acanthosis with basal cell hyperplasia.

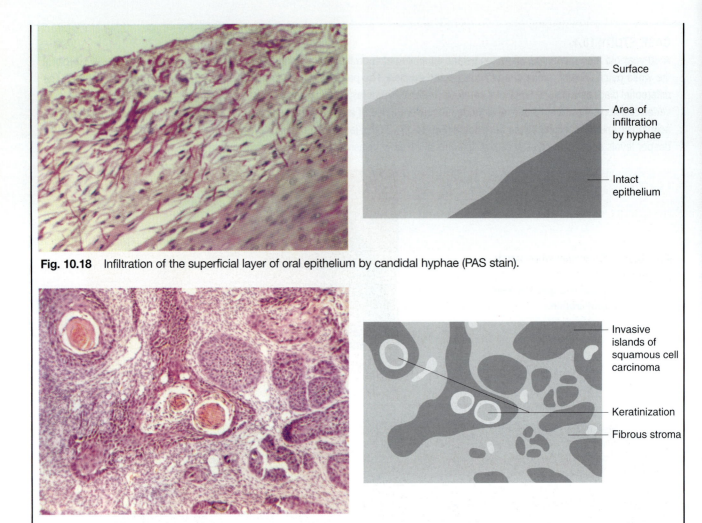

Fig. 10.18   Infiltration of the superficial layer of oral epithelium by candidal hyphae (PAS stain).

Fig. 10.19   Squamous cell carcinoma. Premature keratinization: cellular atypia including hyperchromatism are features of note.

Connective tissue hyperplasia is common in the oral cavity, resulting as a response to chronic inflammation. Fibroepithelial polyps, denture irritation hyperplasia and papillary hyperplasia of the palate are all well recognized. Localized swellings of the gingiva (**epulides**) are common and include, the fibrous epulis, pyogenic granuloma and the giant cell epulis. The latter has a distinctive histology comprising focal collections of multinucleated osteoclast-like giant cells lying in a rich vascular and cellular stroma. The hamartomatous haemangioma and lymphangioma are also common, especially on the lips and tongue. **Sturge–Weber syndrome**, a congenital disorder, involves haemangiomatous lesions on the face and mouth over the branches of the trigeminal nerve.

The salivary glands

There are three pairs of major salivary glands – **parotid**, **submandibular** and **sublingual** – and numerous intraoral minor salivary glands. The secretion of saliva is essential for normal oral function, and disorders of the salivary glands predispose to oral disease.

CASE STUDY 10.5

A 20-year-old woman presented with a reddish-purple swelling on the gingival margin between the mandibular canine and premolar on the right-hand side. The swelling was painless and had been slowly growing for 2 years. Occasional trauma had led to mild bleeding. The lesion was firm to palpation and radiographs showed no evidence of alveolar bone involvement. On clinical grounds (Fig. 10.20) the differential diagnosis included pyogenic granuloma, haemangioma and giant cell epulis. An excision biopsy revealed the typical histopathological features of the last entity (Fig. 10.21).

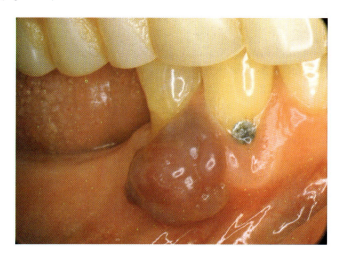

Fig. 10.20 Giant cell epulis affecting the gingiva.

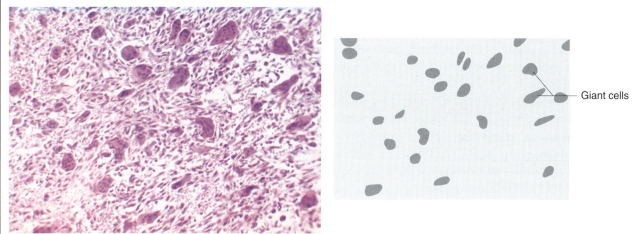

Giant cells

Fig. 10.21 Main body of an excised epulis. Note the marked giant cells diffusely distributed throughout a highly cellular connective tissue stroma.

Infections

Bacterial sialadenitis may present as an acute or chronic infection, and the main organisms involved are *Streptococcus pyogenes* and *Staphylococcus aureus*. There is usually pain, swelling and redness of the overlying skin. Bacterial infections tend to be recalcitrant, and recurrent low-grade chronic sialadenitis is a common outcome. Duct obstruction leads to acinar atrophy and interstitial fibrosis. Viral sialadenitis caused by paramyxovirus (mumps) is an acute, contagious infection which occurs in minor epidemics. The diagnosis is made on clinical grounds though detection of IgM class antibodies may be useful in atypical cases.

Obstruction

Obstructive and traumatic diseases of the salivary glands are relatively common. **Salivary calculi** cause obstruction within the duct lumen, affecting the submandibular gland in 70–90% of cases. The aetiology and pathogenesis of salivary calculi are poorly understood. Mucus plugging may provide an organic nidus into which inorganic material is deposited in a circumferential fashion.

The most frequent lesion of minor salivary glands is the **mucocele**. It is observed especially in the lower lip, presenting as a bluish swelling with a cyst-like appearance. Trauma to the excretory duct(s) leads to extravasation of saliva which becomes localized by a condensation of connective and granulation tissue. Some mucoceles result from obstruction leading to duct dilatation. The ranula in the floor of the mouth is a good example of these mucus retention cysts, associated with the sublingual salivary ducts.

Sjögren's syndrome

Sjögren's syndrome and related disorders are important conditions which involve both the major and the minor salivary glands. **Benign lymphoepithelial lesion** (or **Mikulicz's disease**) refers to a bilateral salivary gland swelling, the histopathological features of which are similar to Sjögren's syndrome. However, the widespread systemic involvement associated with the latter is absent. **Mikulicz's syndrome** is a term used to describe bilateral swelling of the salivary glands which occurs as part of a diagnosed generalized disease such as tuberculosis, sarcoidosis or malignant lymphoma.

Sjögren's syndrome is a chronic inflammatory disease characterized by focal lymphocytic infiltration and acinar destruction of the salivary and lacrimal glands. The association of xerostomia and xerophthalmia is referred to as **primary Sjögren's syndrome** (or **sicca syndrome**) whereas these features associated additionally with a connective tissue disorder, usually rheumatoid arthritis, denote **secondary Sjögren's syndrome**. Other autoimmune connective tissue disorders which may replace rheumatoid arthritis in the triad are systemic lupus erythematosus, systemic sclerosis, primary biliary cirrhosis and dermatomyositis. Sjögren's syndrome predominantly affects middle-aged women.

Primary Sjögren's syndrome may be complicated by lymphoma in 10% of cases, highlighting the association of autoimmune disease and lymphoreticular neoplasia. Histopathological features include focal lymphocytic sialadenitis which tends to be periductal in distribution, acinar atrophy and fibrosis. Occasionally, epimyoepithelial cell islands are observed. The lymphoid infiltrate includes both B and T lymphocytes, plasma cells and macrophages. These changes are reflected in the intraoral minor glands and their biopsy is a useful investigative technique. Other salivary gland investigations include flow rate estimation, sialography, radioisotope scintigraphy and saliva biochemistry. Although the immunological and histopathological findings in Sjögren's syndrome support an autoimmune pathogenesis, characterized by hyperactivity of B lymphocytes and the production of a wide range of autoantibodies, little is known of the underlying defect in immunoregulation.

The term **sialosis** is applied to a non-inflammatory non-neoplastic, painless swelling of the salivary glands. Hormonal disturbances (diabetes mellitus), liver cirrhosis, malnutrition, starch ingestion and drugs, such as isoprenaline hydrochloride and iodide-containing medications, have been implicated. The histological features are those of acinar hypertrophy and hyperplasia.

Tumours

Salivary gland tumours are not common, but their varied histological appearances give rise to diagnostic problems. The parotid gland is by far the commonest site. Intraorally, about 55% of minor gland tumours arise in the palate and 20% in the upper lip. Although the minority of salivary tumours occur in the mouth, the proportion of carcinomas is higher than in the major glands. The adenomas include **pleomorphic adenoma**, adenolymphoma and oxyphilic adenoma. The carcinomas comprise mucoepidermoid, acinic cell, **adenoid cystic** and adenocarcinoma types. Only very rarely do connective tissue neoplasms affect the salivary glands.

The **pleomorphic salivary adenoma** (PSA) is a slow-growing, encapsulated tumour comprising clumps and crops of neoplastic epithelial cells derived from ductal epithelium (Fig. 10.22). Marked change in the connective tissue stroma includes mucoid, hyaline and cartilaginous metaplasia. Rarely, frank carcinoma arises in the PSA.

Adenolymphoma, a monomorphic lesion, is fundamentally a papillary cystadenoma with a characteristic double-layered epithelium and with lymphoid tissue providing the bulk of the stroma (Fig. 10.23). The lesion may be multiple and bilateral. Acinic cell tumours are usually well circumscribed but tend to invade locally. The mucoepidermoid tumour is of variable grade ranging from histologically benign to malignant.

The commonest malignant tumour is the **adenoid cystic carcinoma**. Approximately 25% of all intraoral salivary gland neoplasms are of the type. The lesion is slow growing and metastasizes late. It comprises small, darkly stained, basophilic duct cells which enclose stromal tissue to give a cyst-like, cribriform pattern. The neoplasm has a tendency to infiltrate along nerves (Fig. 10.24).

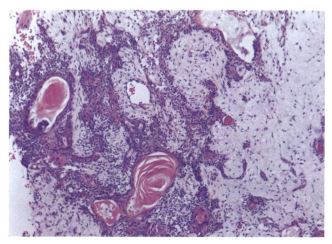
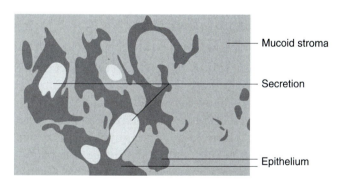

Mucoid stroma

Secretion

Epithelium

Fig. 10.22 Pleomorphic adenoma. Tumour cells derived from salivary duct epithelium form strands and clumps infiltrating a delicate, mucoid stroma.

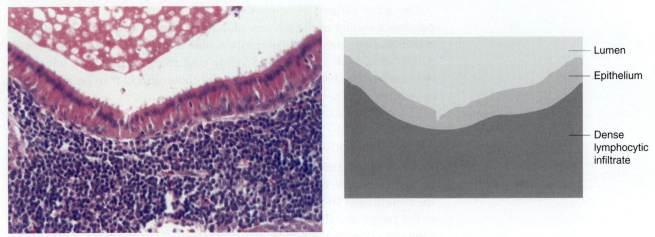

Fig. 10.23   Adenolymphoma. Typical histological appearance of this 'monomorphic' salivary gland tumour. Columnar duct-like cells are supported by a diffuse lymphocytic hyperplasia.

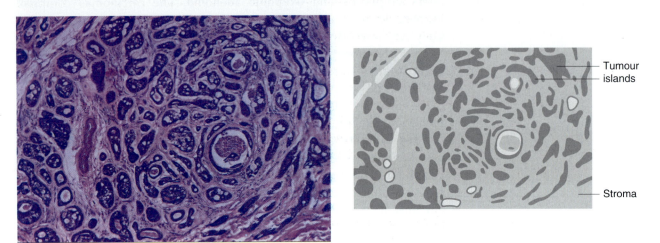

Fig. 10.24   Adenoid cystic carcinoma. Darkly staining tumour cells form a cribriform pattern and spread along nerve sheaths.

Bone and joint disorders

The diagnosis of bone disorders is made by a combination of clinical radiological, histological, biochemical and haematological investigations.

Developmental disorders

Inherited and developmental disorders of bone which have orofacial manifestations include osteogenesis imperfecta, cleidocranial dysplasia, fibrous dysplasia and cherubism.

Osteogenesis imperfecta is often associated with defects of dentine, especially in the deciduous dentition. The basic defect appears to be one of collagen synthesis involving type I collagen. In **cleidocranial dysplasia**, the maxilla is underdeveloped, the palatal vault is high, tooth eruption is delayed and impaction of teeth is common. **Fibrous dysplasia**, especially the monostotic variety, may affect the jaw bones; painless swelling with increasing facial asymmetry are features of note. The roots of teeth in the involved area may be separated and teeth may be displaced.

Inflammatory and metabolic disorders

Inflammatory disease of the jaw bones is now a rare condition, though acute and chronic suppurative osteomyelitis may follow severe injury or as a complication of extensive oral surgery. A localized alveolar osteitis (**dry socket**) is a not uncommon complication of tooth extraction, especially if the blood clot is disturbed.

Metabolic and endocrine disorders of the jaw bones include primary hyperparathyroidism, rickets and acromegaly.

In **primary hyperparathyroidism** both the radiological and histopathological features in the jaw bones require differentiation from other more common lesions. The multicystic radiolucencies are similar to those seen in ameloblastoma or keratocysts, whilst the vascular, multinucleate giant cell histological picture is identical with the giant cell tumour of bone. Biochemical changes – elevated parathyroid hormone, raised serum calcium and reduced serum phosphate levels – will establish the diagnosis.

In **rickets**, dental abnormalities include enamel hypoplasia and deficient growth of the condylar cartilage may lead to lack of mandibular growth. In **acromegaly**, the facial features are coarsened, the jaws enlarged and the teeth spaced.

Paget's disease of bone may affect the maxilla, and teeth are spaced. An interesting dental change is marked hypercementosis around the root of the teeth. This cementum, like bone, undergoes extensive and disorganized remodelling and may show the characteristic mosaic pattern.

Tumours

Bony exostoses – **torus palatinus** and **torus mandibularis** – occur in the jaw bones.

Primary tumours of bone are uncommon lesions in the jaws, although osteosarcoma, giant cell tumours, myeloma and fibrosarcoma do occur. Metastatic tumours to jaw bones, especially the mandible, account for about 1% of malignant tumours in the oral cavity. Although functional disorders of the temporomandibular joint are common, intrinsic disease is rarely encountered in clinical practice.

Chapter 11   Gastrointestinal disease

> ### Learning objectives
>
> To appreciate and understand diseases which affect the following organs:
>
> ❏ Oesophagus
> ❏ Stomach
> ❏ Duodenum
> ❏ Jejunum
> ❏ Ileum
> ❏ Colon
> ❏ Rectum
> ❏ Anus
> ❏ Peritoneum

The structure of the alimentary tract from the oesophagus to the anus is remarkably uniform considering the great variety of functions in the different parts of the gut.

- The luminal lining, the **mucosa**, shows the greatest diversity and, as a general rule, most inflammatory and neoplastic pathology arises in the mucosa.
- The underlying **submucosa** is composed of connective tissue containing blood vessels, nerves and ganglia.
- The **muscularis propria** consists of two layers – an inner circular muscle layer and an outer longitudinal muscle layer.
- Finally, the outer **adventitial** or **subserosal** layer is predominantly a connective tissue layer often containing much adipose tissue.

The mucosa of the oesophagus and anus is of stratified squamous type and is largely protective whereas the stomach, small intestine and large intestine all possess highly specialized glandular mucosa embedded in a fine connective tissue, the **lamina propria**. All produce mucin, of various forms, and again this is mainly protective. The stomach's more specialized cells produce acid, proteolytic enzymes and other proteins. The small intestinal mucosa is largely absorptive and this is reflected in the predominance of absorptive secretory cells in the mucosa which is characterized by finger-like processes, **villi**, which greatly increase the total mucosal surface area for enhanced absorption. The large intestinal mucosa is also absorptive, primarily for water, but the ratio of mucin-secreting goblet cells to absorptive cells is much higher than in the small bowel. Both stratified squamous and glandular mucosa in the gut show a propensity to change, in response to noxious agents, to an epithelium more able to resist the effects of that agent. This phenomenon, **metaplasia**, is a significant feature in the pathogenesis of many important conditions in the gut.

Oesophagus

The oesophagus is a muscular tube, some 25 cm long, extending from the pharynx to the stomach. It is lined by stratified squamous mucosa. Although there are submucosal mucous glands, these are seldom the cause of pathology; mucosal disease and occasional muscular abnormalities account for most of the pathology that occurs in the oesophagus.

Congenital and mechanical disorders

Congenital abnormalities include oesophageal webs, rings, diaphragms, diverticula, atresias and fistulae, particularly into the trachea. Atresias and fistulae most usually present perinatally and are potentially life threatening. **Hiatus hernia** is probably the commonest acquired mechanical disorder of the oesophagus (Fig. 11.1). In this disorder, part of the stomach becomes

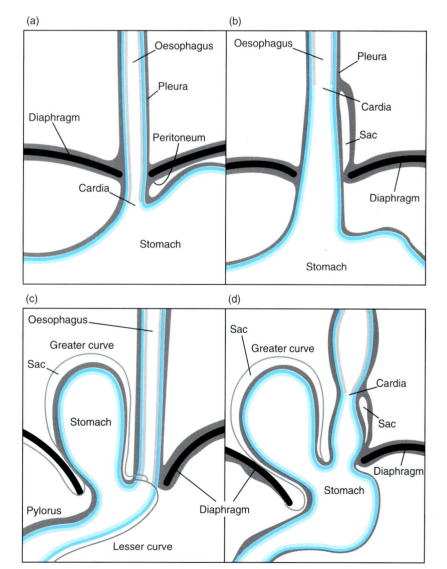

Fig. 11.1 Types of hiatus hernia: (a) normal (note intra-abdominal portion of oesophagus); (b) sliding hiatus hernia (85% of cases); (c) rolling hiatus hernia (10% of cases); (d) mixed or transitional type (5% of cases)

intrathoracic as a result of either sliding or rolling mechanisms. The pathogenesis is related to laxity or fibrosis of ligamentous membranes that fix the cardia of the stomach to the crura of the diaphragm, often in association with raised intra-abdominal pressure and shortening of the oesophagus. Complications include reflux oesophagitis and stricture formation.

Achalasia is the commonest disorder of motility of the oesophagus. It is characterized by a neuromuscular abnormality in which the myenteric plexus ganglia are reduced, the muscular wall thickened and the lower oesophageal sphincter hypertonic. The oesophagus becomes progressively more dilated and yet the muscle wall remains hypertrophic creating a grossly thickened and enlarged oesophagus. Recognized complications include stasis with potential for aspiration into the lungs and carcinoma (particularly of squamous cell type) and reflux oesophagitis, the latter as a result of therapeutic manoeuvres such as endoscopic balloon dilatation or surgery to the lower oesophageal sphincter.

Much more rarely the oesophagus may be affected by other motility disorders. **Progressive systemic sclerosis (scleroderma)** causes motor abnormalities in about 60% of patients with associated reflux of gastric contents. The disorder is caused by fibrosis of the submucosa and muscularis propria. Other much rarer causes of oesophageal dysmotility include South American trypanosomiasis (Chagas' disease), visceral myopathy and amyloidosis.

Inflammatory disorders

REFLUX OESOPHAGITIS

Inflammatory disorders of the oesophagus are almost universally centred on the mucosa and **reflux** of the gastroduodenal contents is over-whelmingly the most common form of acute oesophagitis. Reflux is a normal phenomenon, and pathology is only apparent in patients with abnormal reflux of acid, pepsin, bile and alkali of the duodenum. In contrast to most other inflammatory processes, the pathological appearances in mild to moderate disease relate primarily to reparative processes and there is relatively little inflammatory infiltrate or exudate. Thus, histologically, basal hyperplasia and papillary elongation of the squamous mucosa are the characteristic features whilst in more severe disease active inflammatory infiltrate with ulceration may supervene. Chronic ulceration, with pathological similarities to peptic ulceration of the stomach and duodenum, may lead to stricture formation in the oesophagus. In general, there is relatively poor correlation between histopathological features and symptoms: clinicians more often rely on endoscopic appearances for an accurate assessment of the disease process.

BARRETT'S OESOPHAGUS

When reflux is recurrent, prolonged and severe, the squamous mucosa becomes eroded. Probably as a protective response, the mucosa undergoes glandular metaplasia (Fig. 11.2). This phenomenon, known as Barrett's oesophagus or **columnar-lined oesophagus** (CLO), is seen in about one in six patients with reflux disease. The glandular mucosa is of three varieties:

- gastric cardiac type (secreting mucins only)
- gastric fundic type (secreting acid and pepsin)
- small intestinal type.

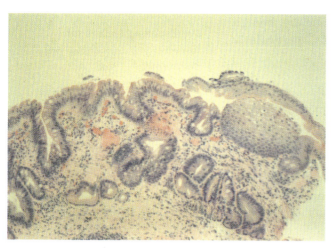
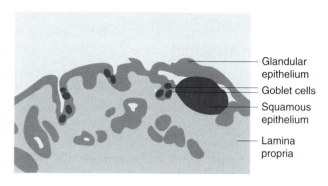

Glandular epithelium
Goblet cells
Squamous epithelium
Lamina propria

Fig. 11.2 Barrett's oesophagus: this is composed of glandular epithelium in which goblet cells are recognizable indicating intestinal-type Barrett's mucosa. There is an island of squamous mucosa (right).

The presence of acid-producing fundic-type mucosa reinforces the pathological effects of acid and pepsin on the mucosa whilst unstable, intestinal-type mucosa predisposes to an increased incidence of adenocarcinoma in the oesophagus. The latter accounts for about 40% of all oesophageal malignancies and appears to be increasing in incidence, perhaps because of increased recognition. It is clear that successful therapy for Barrett's oesophagus demands effective acid eradication from the oesophagus and recent work with omeprazole, a proton pump inhibitor, suggests that partial reversion to squamous-type mucosa may occur in time.

INFECTIVE OESOPHAGITIS

Most infective oesophagitides occur in immunocompromised patients. **Candidiasis** is by far the most common infection of the oesophagus and may occasionally be seen in otherwise normal patients. It is a common early accompaniment of AIDS. The macroscopic appearances are characteristic and the diagnosis is often made at the time of endoscopy. The oesophageal mucosa is lined by creamy, friable plaques with evidence of inflammation and ulceration in the intervening areas. When the condition is severe, a pseudo-membrane or polyps may be seen. Histology demonstrates the characteristic yeast and hyphal forms of *Candida albicans*. Herpes simplex oesophagitis occurs in the immuno-compromised, especially AIDS patients. It is characterized by rather shallow discrete ulcers, and biopsies show the characteristic multinucleate cells and cytopathic effects of the virus. Bacterial oesophagitis is very rare; tuberculous and syphilitic oesophagitis are now extremely uncommon.

OTHER OESOPHAGITIDES

There are various forms of chemical and physical oesophagitis, the former most often caused by drugs and the swallowing of acid or alkali. Other forms of chronic oesophagitis are shown in the box.

Tumours

BENIGN TUMOURS

These are surprisingly rare in the oesophagus. Squamous papilloma is common in cows and papilloma virus has been implicated in its aetiology.

Chronic oesophagitides
- Involvement by Crohn's disease (very rare)
- Associations with various skin diseases (including pemphigus, pemphigoid, lichen planus and tylosis)
- Radiation oesophagitis

The human equivalent is extremely rare. Very occasionally benign connective tissue tumours are seen in the oesophagus, particularly leiomyoma, but these are again rare.

MALIGNANT TUMOURS

Squamous cell carcinoma is currently the most common malignant tumour of the oesophagus. It accounts for about 50% of all primary oesophageal malignancies. In the UK, oesophageal cancer is the tenth most common fatal malignancy. There is a striking geographical variation, the tumour being especially common in northern China, among the black population of South Africa and in central Asia. Men are more commonly affected than women and this is especially so with tumours of the lower two-thirds of the oesophagus.

Most squamous cell carcinomas of the oesophagus present with dysphagia due to stricturing, obstructing lesions (Fig. 11.3). Unfortunately the tumour is often advanced at presentation and prognosis is relatively poor. Local spread outwith the wall involves local structures such as the respiratory tree, mediastinal tissues, pleura and lungs, and spread to mediastinal lymph nodes is an early feature. The optimal treatment depends primarily on the stage of the tumour. For advanced carcinomas, radiotherapy and surgery result in similar palliation and survival rates. Surgery is generally reserved for early potentially curative cases.

Histologically, squamous cell carcinoma of the oesophagus shows histological similarities to such tumours arising elsewhere (e.g. cervix) although differentiation is often poor with little evidence of keratinization. Variants described include spindle cell carcinoma and small cell undifferentiated carcinoma, the latter showing histological identity with its bronchial counterpart (see Chapter 9).

Adenocarcinoma of the oesophagus was formerly thought to be unusual; most such tumours were considered to be primary gastric cancers with spread into the oesophagus. It is now accepted that adenocarcinoma accounts for about 40% of primary oesophageal cancers and that most of these arise on a basis of Barrett's oesophagus. As a result of screening of Barrett's patients, many adenocarcinomas are detected at a relatively early stage and are amenable to curative surgery. Tumours of the submucosal oesophageal glands are distinctly rare, mucoepidermoid carcinoma being

> **Predisposing factors for oesophageal squamous cell carcinoma**
> - Alcohol
> - Smoking
> - Vitamin deficiencies
> - Achalasia
> - Patterson–Brown–Kelly syndrome (in association with iron deficiency anaemia, upper oesophageal webs and koilonychia)

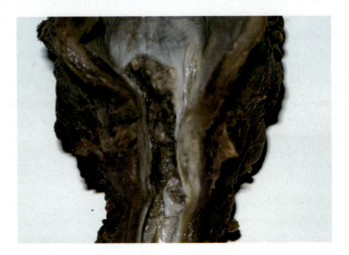

Fig. 11.3 Carcinoma of the oesophagus. There is a large deeply ulcerating tumour of the upper oesophagus. Histologically it was a squamous cell carcinoma.

the most often seen. Primary malignant melanoma is a recognized tumour of the oesophagus but is very rare and has an appalling prognosis. Primary sarcoma and lymphoma are also described although very rare. Metastatic carcinoma does occur in the oesophagus but is not often of clinical significance.

Stomach

The stomach's chief functions are to act as a reservoir for ingested food and to secrete various digestive substances, particularly acid. Many pathological conditions of the stomach are the result of complex interactions between ingested materials, these secretions and the mucosa, which is highly specialized.

Congenital abnormalities

These include atresia and stenosis, the latter particularly at the pylorus. **Congenital hypertrophic pyloric stenosis**, commonly seen in first-born males, presents with projectile vomiting and is characterized by gross enlargement of the circular muscle layer at the pylorus. It is probably a primary neurogenic problem, there being a deficiency of ganglion cells of the myenteric plexus at this site. Much more unusual congenital anomalies include duplications and abnormalities of position such as malrotation. Acquired mechanical conditions include volvulus which is distinctly rare in the stomach, acute dilatation (seen after surgery and trauma) and diverticula.

Inflammatory disorders

Gastritis is by no means a specific term and includes any condition in which inflammatory mechanisms are at play in the mucosa of the stomach. It is very much a pathological diagnosis. Endoscopy is notoriously poor at identifying gastritis, particularly when there is no evidence of significant active inflammation and erosion or ulceration. Traditionally, gastritis has been divided into acute and chronic forms, but many types of gastritis are chronic and show fluctuating activity. The entire concept of gastritis has undergone radical revision in recent years and it is becoming increasingly clear that there are three main forms. The three major forms of gastritis are autoimmune, bacterial and chemical – giving the convenient mnemonic **ABC** (Fig. 11.4).

AUTOIMMUNE GASTRITIS

Of the three forms, this is undoubtedly the rarest. **Chronic atrophic gastritis** predominantly affects the body mucosa and correlates with the clinical condition of pernicious anaemia. Thus, it can be considered an autoimmune gastritis with inflammatory processes directed against the chief cells and parietal cells, resulting in the presence of parietal cell antibodies in the blood (which can be measured by immunological means) and atrophy of the specialized glands of the gastric mucosa. This is accompanied by a predominant chronic inflammation, particularly lymphocytes and plasma cells, in all layers of the mucosa and **intestinal metaplasia**, in which a switch to intestinal-type mucosa is seen. Pernicious

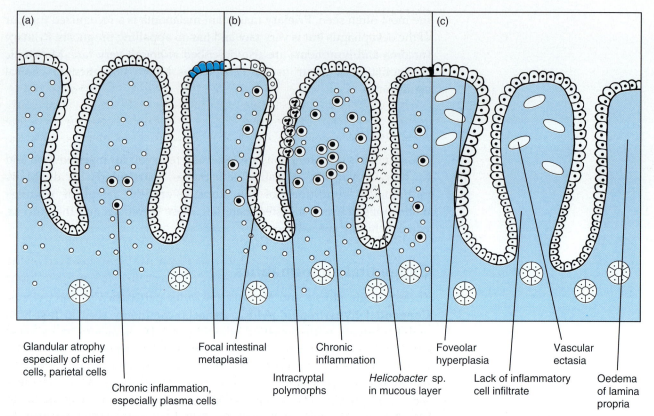

Fig. 11.4 Comparison of the three major forms of gastritis: (a) autoimmune (especially body); (b) bacterial (especially antrum; (c) chemical.

anaemia results from a lack of intrinsic factor normally produced by parietal cells and required for the absorption of vitamin B_{12}. It should be emphasized that chronic atrophic gastritis may be seen in the absence of clinical evidence of pernicious anaemia. Long-term gastritis from many causes will eventually result in atrophic changes.

BACTERIAL GASTRITIS

The high acid load in the stomach ensures that classic bacterial infection of the stomach is very rare, but despite this the association between chronic 'environmental' gastritis and the bacterium *Helicobacter pylori* has become clearly established. These small curved or spiral Gram-negative bacteria selectively colonize the mucous layer of the mucosa, thus being protected from the contents of the stomach. They can be detected in a high proportion of asymptomatic individuals and in patients presenting both with non-ulcer dyspepsia and with peptic ulcer disease. There is now convincing data that the bacteria can induce a characteristic chronic active gastritis of the antrum, in which chronic inflammatory changes are associated with a variable polymorph infiltrate, indicating activity, closely associated with the bacteria. The pathogenesis primarily relates to the production by the bacteria of urease, an enzyme which produces ammonium ions from urea. These ions protect the bacterium from the harmful effects of acid but also induce the inflammatory changes in the gastric mucosa. There is now good evidence that the bacteria are closely associated with the pathogenesis of chronic peptic ulcers of the stomach and duodenum. *Helicobacter* sp. selectively colonizes the antrum; they may also involve the whole stomach, resulting in a pangastric *Helicobacter*-associated chronic active gastritis.

CHEMICAL GASTRITIS

The presence of substances toxic to the gastric mucosa in the stomach may, not surprisingly, induce acute gastritis. Pathologically, a characteristic appearance of the mucosa, now termed **reactive gastritis**, is seen in which foveolar epithelial hyperplasia, oedema and small blood vessel dilatation occur with/without superficial erosion and ulceration. Drugs, particularly aspirin and NSAIDs, excessive alcohol and bile alkali (due to reflux particularly after stomach surgery) may all induce these changes. When the condition is very acute, there is associated erosion or ulceration and terms such as 'acute erosive gastritis' and 'acute stress ulceration' are used. The latter is the result of the effect of acid on a mucosa whose defences (particularly mucus) are weakened after acute stress.

OTHER FORMS OF GASTRITIS

Gastritis is a complex subject and its complexity has been enhanced by the use of many and varied terminologies. Pathologically, there are conditions in addition to those already described. **Lymphocytic gastritis** is characterized by a heavy intraepithelial lymphocytic infiltrate and appears to represent a specific pathological appearance with varied clinical significance: it may represent an unusual response to intraluminal antigens, particularly *Helicobacter*. Other forms of gastritis are associated with mucosal hypertrophy, including Ménétrièr's disease, in which there is also hypersecretion of mucus. Granulomatous gastritis may occur in Crohn's disease but may also be due to a histiocytic reaction to intraluminal material.

Peptic ulceration

This common disorder of the stomach and duodenum causes considerable morbidity: about 10% of the population will be affected in their lifetime. Although the endoscopic and pathological features of gastric and duodenal peptic ulcers are relatively uniform, the diseases cannot be considered homogeneous for they differ in clinical associations and pathogenic mechanisms. An **ulcer** is essentially a breach in the mucosa to a level of at least the submucosa. Similar pathogenic mechanisms occur in more superficial disease, particularly acute erosive gastritis. Ulcers are considered acute when they are superficial and heal quickly, and chronic if they are deep and have failed to heal over a considerable period of time.

CHRONIC GASTRIC ULCERS

These are most common on the lesser curve of the stomach, particularly in the antrum. There is a slight male preponderance for gastric peptic ulcer. Most gastric ulcers are less than 3 cm in diameter. Although usually single, multiple gastric ulcers may occur, particularly when acute. Peptic ulcers in general are lined by a fibrinous exudate and granulation tissue. In chronic ulceration, the base is composed of densely fibrotic connective tissue often replacing the muscularis propria (Fig. 11.5). These features explain the chronicity of untreated ulcers: the scarring and ulceration make it difficult for the mucosal continuity to be restored. The pathogenesis of gastric peptic ulcers is complex: there is a close association with chronic gastritis, particularly *Helicobacter*-associated, and with drugs, alcohol and other chemicals toxic to the gastric mucosa. The amount of acid present is often

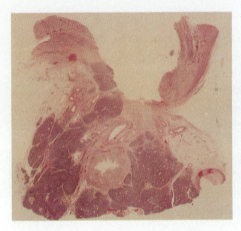

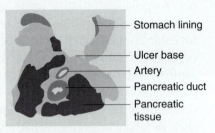

- Stomach lining
- Ulcer base
- Artery
- Pancreatic duct
- Pancreatic tissue

Fig. 11.5 Chronic peptic ulcer of the antrum of the stomach from a patient who died of gastrointestinal haemorrhage.

normal or reduced. Nevertheless acid is still a major factor in the pathogenesis of ulcers as the host defence mechanisms are damaged, particularly by *Helicobacter* spp. which may also be a factor in the reduced acid because of pangastric chronic active gastritis causing atrophy of acid-producing cells in the gastric body mucosa.

CHRONIC DUODENAL ULCERS

These are usually found in the cap or first part of the duodenum. They are much more common in men: pathogenic factors include stress, excessive acid and environmental factors, particularly the bacterium *Helicobacter pylori*. As with gastric ulcers, they are associated with chronic active inflammation of the duodenal mucosa. One plausible theory for the pathogenesis is that excessive acid (induced by helicobacters in the antrum increasing gastrin secretion) induces gastric metaplasia in the duodenal mucosa. *Helicobacter* spp., already resident in antral mucosa, colonize this metaplastic mucosa (it is notable that *Helicobacter* spp. are unable to colonize intestinal-type mucosa) and induce inflammation and superficial erosions and, in a complex interaction with excessive intestinal acid, produce ulceration. The relationship between acid and duodenal ulceration is evidenced by the **Zollinger–Ellison syndrome** in which a gastrin-secreting tumour, usually of the pancreas, induces excessive acid secretion in the stomach and hence multiple ulcers in the duodenum in association with gastric metaplasia of the mucosa. Duodenal ulcers show similar pathological features to gastric ulcers.

COMPLICATIONS OF PEPTIC ULCER

Some complications are common to both peptic and gastic ulcers (see box). Carcinoma is a recognized complication of gastric ulcer but not of duodenal ulcer. Nevertheless, the prevalence of carcinoma arising in gastric ulcers is probably overstated. Many such 'ulcer–cancers' represent carcinomas *de novo* which have become secondarily ulcerated. Current evidence indicates that the incidence of malignancy arising in a gastric ulcer is low. Nevertheless, at the time of endoscopy, multiple biopsies are usually taken from all gastric ulcers to rule out the presence of malignancy.

MANAGEMENT OF PEPTIC ULCER

The management and epidemiology of peptic ulceration have undergone considerable changes in recent years. This is largely related to the advent of acid-controlling drugs, particularly H_2-receptor antagonists which have

Recognized complications of gastric and duodenal ulcers
- Haemorrhage from blood vessels in the base of the ulcer (see Fig. 11.5)
- Penetration and inflammation of adjacent organs, especially the pancreas (see Fig. 11.5)
- Perforation and associated peritonitis
- Scarring leading to visceral stenosis, particularly of the pylorus

become one of the mainstays of treatment and have considerably reduced recurrence and complications of peptic ulceration. More recently proton pump inhibitors, such as omeprazole, which induce a more efficient acid control, have further modified the disease process. These drugs have now almost entirely taken over from surgical treatment, such as partial gastrectomy and vagotomy, in the primary therapy of peptic ulcer disease.

BENIGN TUMOURS OF THE STOMACH

Most **gastric polyps** are non-neoplastic: they are the result of regenerative and hyperplastic mechanisms subsequent to mucosal inflammation. These **hyperplastic** or **regenerative polyps** account for about 80% of all gastric polyps. Polyps may be rarely seen as part of hereditary polyposis syndromes, although gastric adenomas are unusual in familial adenomatous polyposis, which usually affects the colon: most gastric lesions in this condition are benign fundic gland polyps. The stomach may be involved in **Peutz–Jeghers polyposis** and in **juvenile polyposis**, which is dealt with in the section on colon later in this chapter.

Adenomas are seen in the stomach but in Western populations they are not as common as their large intestinal equivalent. They are more common in countries with a high incidence of gastric cancer such as Japan. They share similar macroscopic and microscopic features of their colorectal equivalent. Rarer polyp types in the stomach include stromal lesions such as **inflammatory fibroid polyps** and **smooth muscle tumours (leiomyoma)**. Apart from adenomas, most other benign neoplasms of the stomach are stromal in origin. **Leiomyoma** presents endoscopically as a polypoid mass, often with central ulceration, protruding into the lumen. They are usually asymptomatic but may present with gastrointestinal haemorrhage. Pathologically, it may be difficult to assess the likely behaviour of such a tumour: generally an assessment of proliferation (such as mitotic rate) gives a guide to likely prognosis. Other stromal tumours are rare; these include neurofibromas, lipomas and vascular malformations.

Carcinoma of the stomach

In industrialized societies, carcinoma of the stomach is a leading cause of cancer death and in terms of mortality is only surpassed by those of the lung and large intestine. Changes in diagnosis and management have affected the poor prognosis of this tumour little. Although the incidence of the tumour appears to be declining, it remains a major cause of mortality, little modified by medical intervention. There are striking geographical differences in incidence rates, Japan and South America showing the highest incidence. The tumour is unequivocally more common in men.

AETIOLOGY

Although the cause of gastric cancer is not fully understood, many predisposing factors and conditions have been identified. There are genetic factors, the tumour being more common in blood group A patients, and examples of gastric cancer families are described. Social factors, probably dietary, are responsible for differences in gastric cancer prevalence between social groups. There is little doubt that diet has a major influence. A diet rich in salt and carbohydrate and high in nitrates (as in Japan) may induce the production of carcinogens such as nitrosamines in the lumen of the stomach. High intake of fresh fruit is a protective factor (probably from an effect of vitamin C) .

There is a complex interaction of the many intraluminal factors which produce the milieu in which gastric carcinoma arises. As with other tumours, there is little doubt that many steps are required for the development of gastric cancer. Thus, pathologically, predisposing gastric lesions are readily recognized. The concept of gastritis has already been fully described but there is evidence for an association between chronic gastritis (and *Helicobacter* spp.) and carcinoma. Gastritis is associated with **intestinal metaplasia**, an unstable epithelial alteration to mucosa producing small and large intestinal-type mucins. There is also close correlation between intestinal metaplasia and the development of **dysplasia** in which neoplastic change is identified in the gastric mucosa but without evidence of infiltration. Low-grade dysplasia is regarded as a marker of neoplastic change requiring close endoscopic and histological surveillance, but high-grade dysplasia is considered an indication for gastric surgery before invasive tumour has arisen. Other predisposing factors to gastric cancer include chronic atrophic gastritis and pernicious anaemia, gastric peptic ulcers and previous operative surgery. Whilst much is known of all these predisposing factors and conditions, little is known of the molecular basis for the development of gastric cancer. Certain molecular biological changes are described (*p53* mutation, various oncogene amplifications and overexpressions) but none of these is entirely consistent.

PATHOLOGICAL FEATURES

Gastric cancers are commoner adjacent to mucosal junctions especially in the antrum, cardia and the lesser curvature. Macroscopically they are irregular, often ulcerating, polypoid plaques or masses (Fig. 11.6). Endoscopically it may not always be possible to differentiate benign ulcers from ulcerated cancers, but nodularity and irregularity with raised edges are helpful features in favour of malignancy. **Linitis plastica** describes a particular type of cancer in which diffuse infiltration of much of the stomach wall results in rigidity of the gastric wall (a lack of inflatability endoscopically).

Histologically, most gastric cancers are **adenocarcinomas**. There are two main types, according to the Lauren classification: intestinal and diffuse types (Fig. 11.7). The latter accounts for most cases of linitis plastica and has the worse prognosis. Individual cells, with morphology akin to signet rings, diffusely infiltrate the wall of the stomach. The intestinal type shows

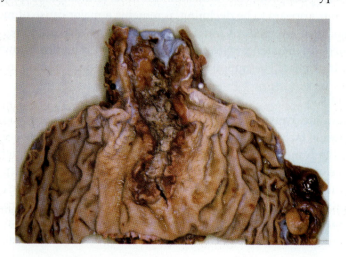

Fig. 11.6 Partial gastrectomy for carcinoma of the stomach. There is a large ulcerating tumour, arising at the cardia and involving the lower oesophagus (above). The tumour has typical raised rolled edges and appears irregular.

Fig. 11.7 Lauren classification of the histological types of gastric carcinoma: (a) intestinal type (50–60% of cases); (b) diffuse type (35–45%).

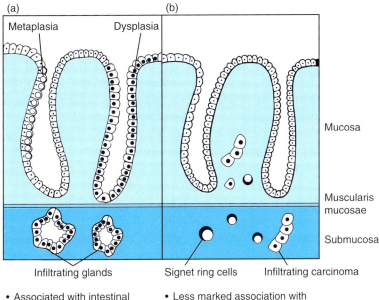

(a)   (b)

Metaplasia   Dysplasia

Mucosa

Muscularis mucosae

Submucosa

Infiltrating glands   Signet ring cells   Infiltrating carcinoma

- Associated with intestinal metaplasia and dysplasia
- Well-formed glandular structures with mucin secretion

- Less marked association with intestinal metaplasia
- Diffuse infiltration of poorly defined epithelial structures and signet ring cells

analogy to colorectal carcinomas and is associated with intestinal metaplasia. Differentiation is variable; the prognosis is better than that of diffuse tumours but is still not good. Five-year survival rates after curative surgery are still only 35%. These two carcinoma types are occasionally intermixed, producing a heterogeneous tumour. Together, they account for about 90% of all gastric carcinoma: rarer forms include adenosquamous carcinoma, parietal cell carcinoma, pyloroglandular carcinoma and small cell carcinoma.

Spread of tumour and staging

Gastric carcinoma may spread into all layers of the gastric wall. Submucosal extension beneath normal mucosa is a common feature. If the tumour has spread through the muscularis propria to involve subserosal tissues, serosal involvement may lead to transperitoneal spread and secondary deposits especially in the omentum, mesentery and ovary (**Krukenberg's tumour**). Lymphatic and venous spread is an early feature. Local lymph nodes (especially cardiac and subpyloric) become involved and ultimately tumour spreads more widely to coeliac axis, para-aortic and paraoesophageal lymph nodes. Blood-borne metastases are seen most often in the liver but lung, bone and bone marrow may also be involved.

Although histological parameters (such as differentiation and type) give a guide to prognosis, staging gives the most accurate prognostic information. TNM-type staging classifications are most often used. Because the prognosis of established gastric cancer is so poor, stress has been put on the early detection of gastric cancer, particularly in Japan. Thus the concept of 'early gastric cancer', when the tumour involves only mucosa, with or without involvement of the submucosa, has developed. Such tumours have an excellent prognosis (5-year survival rate in excess of 80%) and screening has been instituted in Japan to detect such lesions.

ENDOCRINE CELL TUMOURS

Endocrine cells are diffusely scattered throughout the mucosa of the gut and are particularly concentrated in the gastric glands. Hyperplasia (often diffuse) of enterochromaffin (EC) cells of the stomach is seen in hypergastrinaemic states such as Zollinger–Ellison syndrome and in the chronic atrophic gastritis associated with pernicious anaemia. Such hyperplasia may eventually result in an anatomical tumour, the carcinoid. Whilst both of these lesions usually behave in a benign way, some may be malignant and it may be difficult pathologically to identify such cases. Generally the treatment of such lesions, especially when multiple, is conservative unless there is strong evidence of malignancy.

LYMPHOMAS

Malignant lymphoma in an extranodal site is most commonly seen subsequent to spread of a nodal lymphoma, and 50% of patients with widespread primary nodal disease will show gastrointestinal involvement *post mortem*. However, **primary gastrointestinal lymphoma** accounts for 20% of all cases of lymphoma and, in Western industrialized populations, the stomach is the most common site (50–60% of all primary gastrointestinal lymphomas but only 4% of all primary gastric malignancies). It is now clear that most primary lymphomas of the stomach derive from a gut-specific lymphoid cell in the mucosa-associated lymphoid tissue (MALT). These lymphomas are of B-cell type, frequently localized and have a relatively good prognosis. They may be multiple. They are often associated with chronic active gastritis and helicobacter infection, suggesting that this bacterium may also be involved in the pathogenesis of primary gastric lymphoma. Recently, it has been suggested that early gastric lymphoma may regress after antibiotic treatment for *Heliobacter* spp. Histologically there is often a heterogeneous infiltrate of lymphoid cells with a predominance of small angulated cells which show involvement of the epithelium producing the characteristic 'lymphoepithelial lesion'. Prognostic factors include stage, grade and involvement of adjacent structures.

OTHER MALIGNANT TUMOURS

Carcinomas, lymphomas and malignant carcinoid tumours make up the great majority of primary gastric malignancies. Clinically significant metastasis to the stomach is distinctly rare. Stromal malignancies include **leiomyosarcomas** and rarely other types of sarcoma. Kaposi's sarcoma is seen increasingly, as the tumour may involve the gut in patients with AIDS.

Small intestine

In terms of volume and certainly in terms of surface area, the small intestine is the largest part of the gastrointestinal tract. It is perhaps surprising, therefore, that significant pathological conditions are relatively rarer than in other parts of the gut. This is particularly so with epithelial neoplasia, both adenomas and carcinomas being distinctly uncommon in the small bowel despite the amount of epithelium present and its high level of proliferation. On the other hand, inflammatory conditions of the small bowel do cause much more morbidity, especially infective gastroenteritis, inflammatory bowel disease and the malabsorption syndromes.

Congenital defects

Abnormalities include malrotation, malpositions, atresias and stenoses. **Meckel's diverticulum** (persistence of the distal portion of the embryonic vitellointestinal duct) is common, occurring in about 2% of the population. Histologically, it is lined by small bowel-type mucosa although the presence of heterotopic acid-secreting gastric mucosa may lead to peptic ulceration in and around the diverticulum. Meckel's diverticulum may also cause obstruction, volvulus and occasionally intussusception (see below).

Mechanical disorders

The small bowel is some 5 m long and is suspended throughout its length by a mesentery, so mechanical disorders leading to obstruction are not uncommon.

- **Intussusception** is the invagination of a length of bowel into the succeeding bowel segment. It is usually a disease of very young children (particularly under the age of 3) and viral infection, especially with adenovirus, leads to **Peyer's patch hyperplasia** and subsequent propagation of the lymphoid mass distally. Occasionally, intussusception may occur in adults: it is usually then due to an intraluminal tumour such as lymphoma, smooth muscle tumour, Meckel's diverticulum or polyp.
- **Volvulus** is a twist of a loop of bowel resulting in compromise of blood supply and subsequent ischaemia or gangrene. Initial presentation is with small bowel obstruction but infarction of the loop of bowel leads to peritonitis and an 'acute abdomen'.
- **Hernias** also cause luminal restriction and obstruction of blood supply and may present in a similar way.

All of these conditions cause small intestinal obstruction by mechanical means.

Acute paralytic ileus is an example of 'pseudo-obstruction' in which peristalsis of the small bowel fails due to acute peritonitis, trauma or abdominal surgery. Similarly, **chronic pseudo-obstruction** may result from the loss of neurogenic stimuli (for instance in diabetes mellitus, visceral neuropathy and due to some drugs) or by muscle anomalies (congenital visceral myopathy, progressive systemic sclerosis).

Inflammatory disorders

INFECTIVE ENTERITIS

This is common – it is caused predominantly by viruses and bacteria – but most patients recover without need for surgery or pathological assessment. Most viral enteritides (especially those due to rotavirus and adenovirus) are self-limiting and are particularly seen in children. **Acute bacterial enterocolitis** primarily affects the mucosa and leads to profound diarrhoea with/without ulceration (and subsequent bleeding). It is the more chronic infective enteritides that are more likely to come to the attention of the pathologist.

Tuberculous enteritis is less common than formerly and is now usually seen as secondary gut involvement subsequent to pulmonary infection with *Mycobacterium tuberculosis*. Characteristically, the small bowel shows transverse ulceration with bowel wall thickening: histologically the characteristic caseating granulomata with multinucleate Langhans-type

---

Bacteria causing acute enterocolitis
- *Salmonella* sp.
- *Campylobacter* sp.
- Enterotoxigenic *Escherichia coli*
- *Shigella* sp. (causing dysentery)
- *Vibrio* sp. (causing cholera)

giant cells are seen. Acid-fast bacilli are demonstrated in the tissues in only about 50% of cases, and it may be difficult to differentiate tuberculosis from Crohn's disease (see below). Most cases of tuberculous enterocolitis in this country are seen in immigrants from southern Asia.

Yersiniosis may also stimulate Crohn's disease pathologically with bowel wall thickening and histologically necrotizing granulomata. It is primarily a disease of the terminal ileum and colon in children. Often serological studies are required to make the appropriate diagnosis. Other bacteria may cause severe acute enteritis in certain situations – for instance, necrotizing enterocolitis due to clostridia and *Escherichia coli* in neonates.

PROTOZOAL AND METAZOAL DISEASE

Protozoa may infect the small intestines and cause diarrhoea or malabsorption. **Giardiasis**, caused by *Giardia lamblia*, causes mucosal enteritis, diarrhoea and malabsorption. Giardiasis may be diagnosed by small bowel biopsy, the flagellated protozoa being easily recognizable in the lumen adjacent to the inflamed small intestinal mucosa (Fig. 11.8). Giardiasis and other opportunistic protozoan infections (microsporidiosis, cryptosporidiosis, isosporiasis) are characteristically seen complicating immunosuppression, particularly AIDS.

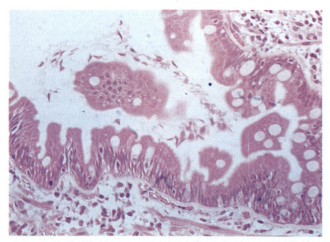
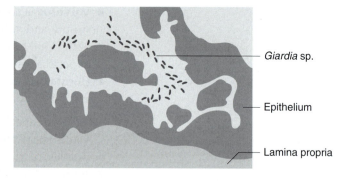

Giardia sp.

Epithelium

Lamina propria

Fig. 11.8   Giardiasis in the small intestine. This is a high-power view of the mucosa of the small bowel. Within the lumen of the small bowel adjacent to the mucosa are multiple comma-shaped protozoa typical of giardiasis.

Helminthic infections may affect the small bowel in several ways. Large worms such as ascaris and tapeworms lead to poor nutrition, but may also cause bowel obstruction. Hookworms (*Necator* and *Ankylostoma* spp.) cause iron deficiency anaemia by inducing chronic bleeding from the small bowel mucosa. Other metazoal infections are most common in the immuno-suppressed or immunocompromised. Recurrence of intestinal strongyloidiasis may be fatal in such patients. Schistosomiasis may affect the small bowel, but clinically significant effects are more common in the colon.

CROHN'S DISEASE

In the UK, Crohn's disease is perhaps the most common chronic inflammatory condition of the small bowel. It may affect any part of the gut, but is most common in the terminal ileum. Although undoubtedly originally described by a Scottish surgeon, Dalziel, in 1913, it is the description by Crohn and his colleagues of 'regional ileitis' in 1932 which holds sway. Crohn's disease is a chronic inflammatory disorder of unknown aetiology which causes bowel wall inflammation, ulceration and thickening together with obstruction.

Aetiology

Pathologically, the disease shows a spectrum of appearances and this has led some to suggest a heterogeneous aetiology. Aetiological factors include heredity (it is much commoner in siblings and other close relatives of affected patients), environmental factors (particularly dietary products) and smoking (there is a strong link between the disease and smokers). For many years researchers have attempted to identify evidence of an infective aetiology, particularly as the disease is characterized by a granulomatous infiltrate with similarities to tuberculosis. Variable results have accrued in searches for mycobacteria, particularly *Mycobacterium paratuberculosis*: DNA of this bacterium has been detected by various techniques in Crohn's disease tissue. Similarly, viral particles (including a measles-like virus) have also been demonstrated. Although much is known of the immunological mechanisms at play in Crohn's disease, the actual cause of the disease remains obscure.

Pathology

Although primarily a disease of the intestines, Crohn's disease may occur at any site from the mouth to the anus. Indeed, involvement of sites outside the gut including the genital tract and skin has been described. Only 5% of patients will have evidence of gastroduodenal involvement whilst 25% have anal involvement and this is of importance in the initial diagnosis of the disease. Complex fistulae of the anal region are most usually caused by Crohn's disease.

There is evidence of a sequential sequence in the development of Crohn's disease. Mucosal inflammation and ulceration occurs over lymphoid follicles in both small and large bowel and causes the characteristic 'aphthous ulcer' seen at endoscopy (see Case study 11.1). Subsequently, the ulceration becomes more extensive with transmural inflammation and deep fissuring ulceration and ultimately fistulae (these are three of the hallmarks of the disease). Transmural inflammation leads to fibrosis, stricturing and bowel obstruction (Fig. 11.9a). Granulomata are found in 50% of cases and are a useful diagnostic feature. The diagnosis is usually attained by a combination of clinical features, endoscopy and/or radiography and confirmed by biopsy appearances. Perhaps its most characteristic feature is the focality of disease: this is seen radiologically, endoscopically, surgically and pathologically. **Skip lesions** – segments of disease with intervening normal areas – are highly distinctive (see Case study 11.1).

Crohn's disease confined to the small bowel (in about 60% of all cases) may present to the surgeon and a diagnosis may be made at the time of laparotomy. The patient may also present with complications of the disease, particularly small or large bowel obstruction, fistulae and localized intra-abdominal sepsis, acute dilatation (particularly of the colon) and malabsorption. Malignant transformation is well described in both small and large bowel Crohn's disease although it is not as common as in the second major form of chronic inflammatory bowel disease, ulcerative colitis. Pathologically, it may be difficult to differentiate these two conditions (see

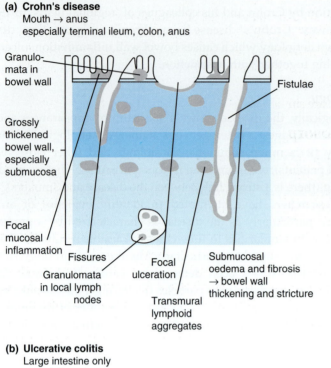

(a) Crohn's disease
Mouth → anus
especially terminal ileum, colon, anus

Granulomata in bowel wall

Fistulae

Grossly thickened bowel wall, especially submucosa

Focal mucosal inflammation

Fissures

Granulomata in local lymph nodes

Focal ulceration

Transmural lymphoid aggregates

Submucosal oedema and fibrosis → bowel wall thickening and stricture

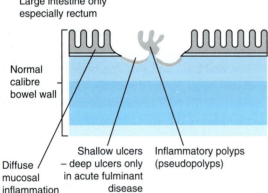

(b) Ulcerative colitis
Large intestine only
especially rectum

Normal calibre bowel wall

Diffuse mucosal inflammation

Shallow ulcers – deep ulcers only in acute fulminant disease

Inflammatory polyps (pseudopolyps)

Fig. 11.9 A comparison of the pathology of (a) Crohn's disease and (b) ulcerative colitis (see page 271). Crohn's disease may be found anywhere from the mouth to the anus, especially in the terminal ileum, colon and anus; ulcerative colitis is restricted to the large intestine, especially the rectum.

Fig. 11.9) when there is only colonic pathology (seen in about 20% of Crohn's disease patients) and often the diagnosis of non-specific chronic inflammatory bowel disease is retained until subsequent events clarify the diagnosis.

OTHER CHRONIC INFLAMMATORY CONDITIONS OF THE SMALL BOWEL

These may present with small bowel ulceration and obstruction and/or malabsorption.

- **Ischaemia** and **infarction** may be caused mechanically (by volvulus, intussusception or hernias, for example) or by atheromatous and/or embolic stenosis of mesenteric arteries. Infarction may result in acute abdomen, or alternatively chronic strictures may occur.
- **Radiotherapy** (particularly for carcinoma of the cervix) causes similar pathological changes to those of chronic ischaemic enteritis and such radiation enteritis is characterized by stricture formation.
- **Drugs**, particularly potassium supplements and NSAIDs, cause mucosal ulceration and subsequently stricturing with small intestinal obstruction.
- **Surgery** in the small bowel may lead to various acute-on-chronic inflammatory conditions. Surgical defunctioning of the small bowel causes

mucosal inflammation. Similar inflammatory changes are seen in the pelvic ileal reservoir in which a pouch is constructed from ileum and anastomosed to the anus after total proctocolectomy (usually for ulcerative colitis or familial adenomatous polyposis). This inflammatory condition of the reservoir (known as **pouchitis**) causes considerable morbidity and there are similarities to chronic inflammatory bowel disease.

Malabsorption

The major function of the small bowel is the digestion and absorption of nutrients. Various pathological conditions of the small bowel lead to failure of this function and **malabsorption**. Most patients present with steatorrhoea (excessive fatty constituents in the stool) and anaemia. Transient

---

CASE STUDY 11.1

A 25-year-old woman presented with a 2-week history of abdominal pain, diarrhoea and weight loss. She was a smoker, and a sister suffered from Crohn's disease. She had a history of a perianal abscess 6 months before. On clinical examination she was anaemic with a mass in the right iliac fossa. Investigations showed a haemoglobin of 9.2 and platelets of 520. Viscosity (1.9) and C-reactive protein (95) were raised. Albumin (29) was low. All other routine investigations were normal.

Colonoscopy (Fig. 11.10a) demonstrated small aphthous ulcers in the sigmoid colon typical of Crohn's disease. Colonic biopsy (Fig. 11.10c, d) showed patchy chronic inflammation and a single well-formed granuloma with normal crypt architecture, again typical of Crohn's disease.

A small bowel barium meal showed a stricturing, fissuring pathology in the ileum. She subsequently developed more severe abdominal pain with distension and vomiting. Laparotomy showed an ileal stricture which was resected (Fig. 11.10b). This segment of bowel reveals the typical focal longitudinal ulceration with mucosal cobblestoning of Crohn's disease and a central stricture.

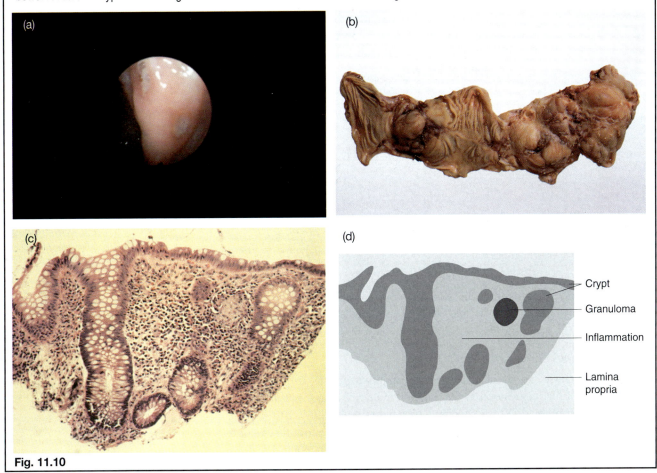

Fig. 11.10

malabsorption may be caused by infective enteritis, particularly giardiasis. Histopathological assessment of the small bowel mucosa, either by biopsy of the distal duodenum at oesophagogastroduodenoscopy or by capsule biopsy of the jejunal mucosa, is an essential part of the diagnosis. Dietary insufficiency (particularly of protein) and intolerance to various constituents of the diet (for example cows' milk protein sensitivity in children) may cause anomalies of the small bowel mucosa but the principal function of a small bowel biopsy is to establish a definitive diagnosis of **coeliac disease**.

COELIAC DISEASE

This disorder is due to an increased sensitivity of the small intestinal mucosa to gluten. It is alternatively known as **gluten enteropathy**. The jejunum is primarily affected, the duodenum patchily so and the disease becomes less severe distally in the ileum. Pathologically there is loss of the normal villous architecture of the mucosa and thus the mucosa often becomes completely flat (subtotal villous atrophy) with a striking chronic inflammatory cell component (particularly within the surface epithelium) and hyperplasia of crypts (Fig. 11.11). Withdrawal of gluten from the diet results in an improvement of the pathological changes and the mucosa may revert to normal. Despite the advent of serological tests (such as anti-gliadin antibody), small intestinal mucosal biopsy remains the mainstay of diagnosis. Whilst malabsorption and anaemia are usually the presenting features of the disease, there are complications which result from poor control of the disease. The development of a T-cell malignant lymphoma (enteropathy-associated T-cell lymphoma) is a sinister complication. Coeliac disease is also associated with an increased risk of pharyngeal, oesophageal and small intestinal carcinoma. Finally, there is a recognized associated between coeliac disease and dermatitis herpetiformis (see Chapter 19).

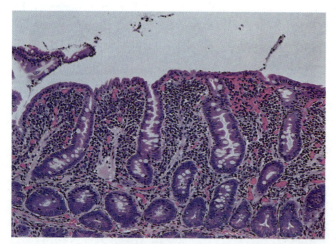
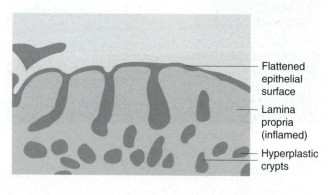

Flattened epithelial surface

Lamina propria (inflamed)

Hyperplastic crypts

Fig. 11.11   Jejunal biopsy of coeliac disease. There is subtotal villous atrophy, crypt hyperplasia and chronic inflammation in the lamina propria.

OTHER CAUSES OF MALABSORPTION

Whipple's disease is a rare cause of malabsorption. Intramucosal accumulation of histiocytes occurs and current evidence suggests that this is an infective condition due to a specific Gram-negative bacillus. **Blind loop syndrome**, **jejunal diverticulosis**, drugs and various pseudo-obstructive states all cause malabsorption mainly due to alteration in bacterial flora within the small bowel. Finally, chronic obstruction and short bowel syndrome (after previous surgery, particularly for Crohn's disease) may also lead to malabsorption.

Tumours

Most benign tumours of the small intestine present as polyps. These are relatively unusual, but multiple polyps may be seen as part of polyposis syndromes, e.g. **Peutz–Jeghers syndrome**. In **familial adenomatous polyposis (FAP)**, polyps are not uncommon around the ampulla in the duodenum. Adenocarcinoma of the duodenum is the second most common cause of death in FAP patients. Outside FAP patients, adenocarcinomas of the small intestine are very rare compared with those in the stomach and large intestine: they account for less than 1% of all gastrointestinal carcinomas. The ampulla of Vater is the most common site but many of these tumours actually derive from bile duct epithelium rather than intestinal mucosa. Small intestinal adenocarcinomas show macroscopic, histological staging and prognostic features similar to those of large intestinal carcinomas. They may complicate various conditions of the small bowel including Crohn's disease, coeliac disease and defunctioning intestine.

Tumours of neuroendocrine cells (carcinoids) are just as common as adenocarcinomas in the small bowel. They occur in the jejunum and ileum and often present because of hormonal secretion. Most will secrete **serotonin** (5-hydroxytryptamine, 5HT) and, when liver metastases are present, manifest as the carcinoid syndrome in which flushing, diarrhoea and right-sided heart valve lesions are all a direct effect of 5HT secretion. Alternatively, like carcinoma, they may present as obstructing lesions. Unlike carcinoids elsewhere in the gut, small bowel carcinoids have a distinctly malignant behaviour.

The small intestine contains plentiful lymphoid tissue, and hyperplasia of Peyer's patches may cause tumour-like lesions. Such **nodular lymphoid hyperplasia** is seen in various congenital immune deficiency syndromes. In Western populations, the most common type of malignant lymphoma in the small bowel is of B-cell type and shows pathological similarities to those seen elsewhere in the gut (compare gastric lymphoma). Two further lymphoma types deserve special mention.

- **High-grade T-cell tumours** are relatively common in the small bowel perhaps reflecting the amount of lymphoid tissue normally present here and only a proportion of these arise as a complication of coeliac disease (Fig. 11.12). In general, these are aggressive tumours with a poor prognosis.
- **α-Chain disease** (immunoproliferative small intestinal disease, IPSID) is a B-cell lymphoma characterized by massive plasmacytic infiltrate producing abnormal immunoglobulins (α heavy chain). It is most common in the Middle East and Mediterranean, and unusually for lymphoma, shows a dramatic response, in early cases, to antibiotic therapy. This suggests that bacterial infection may be involved in the genesis of this lymphoma, in a similar fashion to *Heliobacter* and gastric lymphoma.

Tumours of the connective tissues in the small bowel include smooth muscle tumours, like those in the stomach, lipomas, neurogenic tumours and haemangiomas. They are all rare. Secondary spread to the small bowel occurs from intraperitoneal extension particularly from primary tumours in the stomach, colon and ovary. Malignant melanoma has a predilection to spread to the gut and may cause obstruction or multiple subserosal polypoid masses.

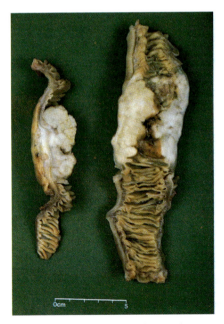

Fig. 11.12   A small bowel resection specimen demonstrating a malignant lymphoma. The opened bowel right shows a stricturing ulcerating tumour mass whilst the cross-section left demonstrates the diffuse, 'fish-flesh' nature of the tumour.

Large intestine

Appendix

The **vermiform appendix** is a vestigial organ in the human. Despite its small size (it averages just 7 cm in length in the adult), it contributes much morbidity. This is largely because of acute appendicitis, clinically significant tumours being relatively uncommon.

ACUTE APPENDICITIS

Acute 'non-specific' appendicitis is the most common cause of acute abdomen in children and young adults. Although predisposing factors, including faecoliths, foreign materials, tumours and even worms are recognized, the cause is undetermined in most cases. Lymphoid hyperplasia is often evident and this is one factor that may contribute to luminal obstruction and subsequent inflammation.

Pathology

Acute inflammation is seen first in the mucosa but in most cases the disease is usually advanced and inflammatory changes are seen throughout the wall and in the peritoneal membrane of the appendix. Generalized peritonitis is an accompaniment of advanced appendicitis especially if there is associated mural necrosis and perforation. The inflammation may be localized to the region of the appendix with development of local abscesses.

All of these complications, particularly in the very young and very old, increase the morbidity and mortality: early operative intervention is the single most important factor which determines successful outcome in acute appendicitis.

The concept of **chronic appendicitis** is controversial. The appendix may be blamed for cases of recurrent right iliac fossa pain but there is little correlation between 'grumbling appendix' cases and significant chronic inflammatory pathology of the appendix. There are clinically significant chronic appendicitides; tuberculosis and Crohn's disease may be seen in the appendix and other infections, especially actinomycosis and schistosomiasis, may be centred on it.

TUMOURS

Carcinoid tumours account for about 90% of all primary appendiceal neoplasms. Most often they are discovered incidentally at the time of appendicectomy and have an entirely benign natural history. They are usually found at the tip of the appendix with no propensity to metastatic disease, despite their histological similarities to the much more aggressive small intestinal carcinoids (see above). They seldom secrete hormones. Only very occasionally are these tumours more aggressive and this is usually with a rare variant, the goblet cell carcinoid.

Adenomas are seen in the appendix but not as commonly as in the colon and rectum (see below). **Cystadenoma** and **cystadenocarcinoma** are mucin-secreting tumours and it may be difficult on pathological grounds to demonstrate overt evidence of malignancy. It is now generally accepted that low-grade cystadenocarcinoma, particularly of the appendix and ovary, is the major cause of **pseudomyxoma peritonei**

in which mucus-secreting tumour diffusely involves the peritoneal cavity resulting in bowel obstruction, progressive disease and death.

Colon and rectum

The large intestine extends from the caecum to the anus. It is the source of much important pathology, including the relatively common inflammatory bowel disease and tumours, colorectal cancer being the second most common cause of cancer death in the UK.

CONGENITAL DEFECTS

Abnormality of the proximal colon is relatively unusual; atresia, stenosis and malrotation are all recognized anomalies. The anorectal region shows a variety of congenital abnormality from complete agenesis through congenital fistulae to relatively minor stenoses. Congenital diverticula, cysts and duplications all occur, especially in the rectal area.

Hirschsprung's disease is caused by a disturbance of innervation of the rectum and lower colon. It occurs mainly in male infants and presents with constipation. There is an aganglionic distal segment of bowel with gross proximal dilatation of normally innervated colon. Deep biopsy of the rectum demonstrates the characteristic absence of ganglia and hypertrophy of nerve trunks. Resection of the aganglionic segment with subsequent restorative surgery is usually curative.

MECHANICAL DISORDERS

Diverticular disease

This is a common condition, particularly in developed countries. The presence of multiple sac-like outpouchings of mucosa, **diverticulosis**, is not in itself an important cause of morbidity. However, when diverticula are the source of inflammation, **diverticulitis** supervenes and this may have more serious complications (Fig. 11.13). Although diverticula may be found elsewhere in the colon and indeed in the small intestine, diverticular disease is most common in the sigmoid colon. The disease is prevalent in the aged population of industrialized societies and diet, particularly a lack of fibre, is the most significant causative factor. The lack of fibre alters the intraluminal pressure and the result is a marked

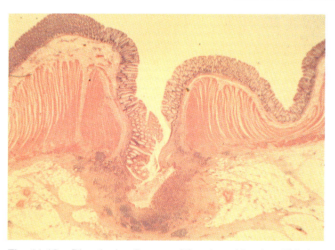
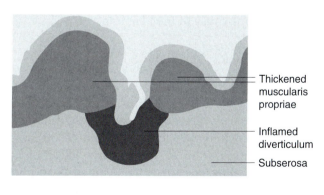

Thickened muscularis propriae

Inflamed diverticulum

Subserosa

Fig. 11.13 Diverticular disease of the sigmoid colon. This low-power photomicrograph shows a diverticulum with associated thickening of the muscularis propria and diverticulitis.

thickening of the muscularis propria with secondary out-pouching of mucosal pockets through anatomical defects in the muscle layer. The exact mechanisms of the muscular changes are still uncertain but it is clear that this is the primary event in the development of the disease.

The sigmoid colon affected by diverticulosis shows gross thickening of both muscle layers with formation of mucosal sacs outwith the muscle and a characteristic excess of mucosa within the lumen. This mucosal redundancy accounts in part for luminal obstruction in diverticulosis. Strictures may form as a result of previous inflammation and these also contribute to luminal stenosis. Other complications of diverticular disease are recurrent diverticulitis, abscess formation and perforation of inflamed diverticula with peritonitis, haemorrhage and fistula. Complications of right-sided diverticulosis, usually in the ascending colon, are similar to those of the sigmoid disease. The jejunum may also be the site of diverticulosis. Jejunal diverticula are antimesenteric and wide mouthed. Complications relate to malabsorption due to changes in bacterial flora rather than to the inflammatory and obstructive pathology seen in colonic diverticular disease.

Other mechanical disorders

- **Volvulus** in the large bowel usually involves the sigmoid colon and leads to obstruction, dilatation and ultimately perforation.
- **Intussusception** is most often seen in the small intestine although the caecum may be the site of the intussuscipiens.
- **Mucosal prolapse** is a pathological phenomenon with characteristic histological appearances seen in several situations. It characterizes the defaecatory abnormality known as the **solitary ulcer syndrome** of the rectum but may be seen at other sites (at a colostomy, for example).
- **Idiopathic megacolon and constipation** describe syndromes, often in women, where there is gross peristaltic failure in the absence of currently recognized pathological abnormality.
- **Pseudo-obstruction** may be seen in the large as well as the small intestine. Collagen diseases (especially progressive systemic sclerosis), drugs, inherited abnormalities (such as visceral myopathy) and infections (especially Chagas' disease) are all recognized causes of pseudo-obstruction.
- **Angiodysplasia** is a condition afflicting elderly people, leading to severe bleeding *per ano*. It is characterized by dilated blood vessels in the mucosa and submucosa, particularly in the proximal colon, which are the cause of the bleeding.

INFLAMMATORY DISORDERS

Infections

Many of the acute infective colitides, such as salmonellosis, shigellosis and campylobacter infection, also afflict the small bowel and have been considered previously. Sexually transmitted diseases and opportunistic infections complicating AIDS are more likely to be seen in the large bowel. Viral colitis, such as cytomegalovirus and herpes simplex virus, is also common in the immunosuppressed.

Amoebic colitis is caused by the protozoan *Entamoeba histolytica*, which causes bloody diarrhoea and may masquerade to the clinician as acute chronic inflammatory bowel disease; it is diagnosed by identifying the protozoa in hot stools or in colorectal biopsies. Complications include acute fulminating colitis (which may cause extensive colonic ulceration, perforation and death) and liver involvement with amoebic abscesses.

Helminthic infections of the colon include schistosomiasis (*Schistosoma mansoni* and *Schistosoma japonicum*) which causes acute proctitis and more chronic disease with characteristic multiple polyp formation, trichuriasis and strongyloidiasis. These are usually seen in tropical countries and are rare in industrialized societies.

Inflammatory bowel disease

Both Crohn's disease and ulcerative colitis may involve the large intestine. Crohn's disease has already been considered in the section on the small intestine, but it should be appreciated that the distinction between these disorders may not be easy clinically or pathologically.

Ulcerative colitis is a chronic inflammatory condition of the large intestine; it is primarily a rectal disease (despite its name) but may extend proximally in a continuous way to involve the more proximal colon. It is essentially a mucosal disease (unlike Crohn's disease – see Fig. 11.9). The cause is still unknown. Current evidence favours an abnormal immunological response to colonic infection, particularly Gram-negative bacteria, such as *Escherichia coli,* or to mucins and other intraluminal agents. The disease has certain psychological associations and there is an inverse relationship with smoking. Familial factors have also been identified.

Ulcerative colitis is characterized macroscopically by superficial mucosal ulceration with congestion of the adjacent intact mucosa. Microscopically there is diffuse inflammation (paralleling the diffuse involvement macroscopically) of the mucosa with intraepithelial acute inflammation and crypt abscesses (see Fig. 11.9b). The latter are a characteristic feature and are usually disruptive resulting in crypt architectural distortion, a characteristic chronic sequela of the disease. Although an acute toxic phase may occur, the disease is usually characterized by relapses and remissions which may well be documented histologically.

Complications of acute ulcerative colitis include haemorrhage (and anaemia) and disturbances of water and electrolyte physiology. The most severe acute complication is **toxic dilatation** when fulminant active inflammation involves the whole bowel wall (especially in the transverse colon) and, if not treated surgically, results in perforation and a high mortality. Inflammatory polyps are a characteristic feature of chronic ulcerative colitis.

The chronic and recurrent inflammation in ulcerative colitis may eventually cause proliferative abnormalities in the colorectal mucosa and the pre-neoplastic lesion known as **dysplasia**. This may in turn lead to the development of cancer in colitic patients. The incidence of colorectal cancer in ulcerative colitis is about 10% in patients with extensive disease (to at least the hepatic flexure) with a 20-year history. Surveillance programmes have been established for such patients (i.e. extensive disease for greater than 10 years) to enable the premalignant phase of dysplasia to be detected by colonoscopy and pathological assessment of multiple biopsies. High-grade dysplasia is generally considered an indication for colectomy in such patients.

Systemic complications of ulcerative colitis
- Liver (primary sclerosing cholangitis, chronic pericholangitis)
- Eyes (iridocyclitis)
- Joints (arthritis)
- Skin (especially erythema nodosum and pyoderma gangrenosum)

CASE STUDY 11.2

A 30-year-old woman presented with diarrhoea (with blood and mucus), nocturnal diarrhoea and lower abdominal pain. She had been a smoker but had recently given up. Clinical examination was normal and investigations revealed only a marginally elevated C-reactive protein (15). A plain abdominal radiograph showed no abnormality. Rigid sigmoidoscopy revealed a granular, friable mucosa with spontaneous haemorrhage and loss of vascular pattern. There was no upper limit discernible. Rectal biopsy (Fig. 11.14a, b) showed diffuse chronic inflammation, crypt abscesses and crypt architectural abnormalities typical of active ulcerative colitis. She was treated with systemic steroids but failed to improve and developed fever, tachycardia and falling haemoglobin and albumin. Surgery was indicated and she underwent total colectomy with ileostomy and mucus fistula (i.e. the rectum was left but its proximal margin closed). Figure 11.14c shows the total colectomy specimen. There is diffuse abnormality of the colon from the splenic flexure to the sigmoid colon (right). The mucosa is granular, congested and friable with focal but quite extensive ulceration. There is a dramatic cut-off at the splenic flexure, the proximal colon appearing entirely normal. This diffuse involvement with distal colonic predominance is absolutely typical of active chronic ulcerative colitis.

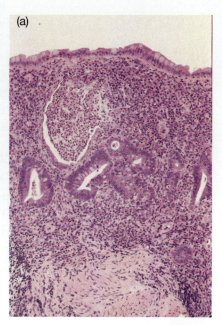
(a)

(b)

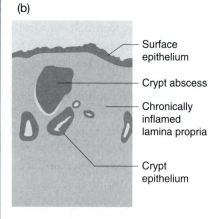

- Surface epithelium
- Crypt abscess
- Chronically inflamed lamina propria
- Crypt epithelium

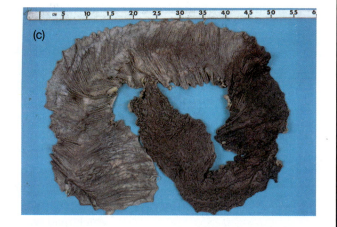
(c)

Fig. 11.14

Other forms of colitis include **pseudomembranous colitis**, an iatrogenic disorder of the colon with characteristic endoscopic and macroscopic features. It is caused by antibiotic therapy. The yellow plaque-like pseudomembranes line the focally ulcerated bowel mucosa with histological features characterized by an eruption of pus from disruptive crypt abscesses, producing the pathognomonic 'summit' or 'volcano' lesions. *Clostridium difficile* toxin is the usual cause and many antibiotics are implicated in the elaboration of the toxin. Less severe antibiotic-associated diarrhoea may occur in the absence of pseudomembranes.

Acute ischaemic colitis shows histological similarities to its small intestinal equivalent and particularly affects the splenic flexure, an area with a blood supply most easily compromised, particularly in hypotension. Radiation and surgical diversion also cause forms of chronic colitis.

Fig. 11.15 Tubulovillous adenoma (TVA) of sigmoid colon. This pedunculated polyp shows both tubular and villous configuration. There is normal colonic mucosa in the stalk.

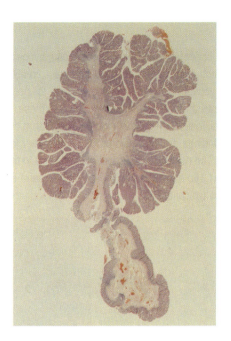

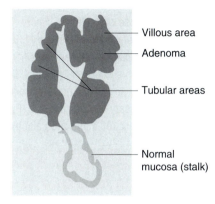

Villous area
Adenoma
Tubular areas
Normal mucosa (stalk)

TUMOURS
Adenomas

The **adenoma** is a benign neoplasm of the colorectal epithelium. They are of three types – tubular, tubulovillous and villous – depending on their histological morphology (Fig. 11.15). Their macroscopic appearances vary from small pedunculated lobulated nodules to large, sessile lesions carpeting the mucosa. By definition they are dysplastic and premalignant. It is now well established that the normal mucosa–adenoma–carcinoma sequence is the single most important pathway for the genesis of colorectal cancer. Size, villous type and high grades of dysplasia are all associated with increased cancer risk in adenomas. Nevertheless, adenomas are relatively common (20% of the population over the age of 60 will have an adenoma) and certainly few will develop into cancers. Thus, although adenomas themselves are seldom of clinical significance (only large polyps cause haemorrhage, anaemia, and water and electrolyte disturbances), their importance lies in their premalignant potential.

Sporadic adenomas may be multiple, but FAP (see Case study 11.3) is an inherited (autosomal dominant) condition characterized by in excess of 100 adenomatous polyps in the colon and rectum. These develop in the second and third decade and cancer will inevitably occur in one or more of the polyps. Prophylactic colectomy is therefore performed in the second and third decade of life to prevent this. The genetic defect that causes the susceptibility to adenoma has now been identified on the long arm of chromosome 5. This genetic defect is also a prevalent accompaniment of sporadic colorectal cancer. Thus, familial adenomatous polyposis has become a useful model for the morphological and molecular biological study of the adenoma–carcinoma sequence and large intestinal carcinogenesis. In keeping with a constitutional chromosomal abnormality, FAP is associated with abnormalities in other systems including adenomas of the duodenum, stomach and ileum, fibromatosis (desmoid) especially of the peritoneal tissues, odontomas of the jaw and epidermal cysts (Gardner's syndrome) and various malignancies including thyroid cancer and hepatoblastoma.

CASE STUDY 11.3

The father of a 15-year-old boy was known to suffer from familial adenomatous polyposis (FAP) and two of his four older sisters also had the disease. This is a typical familial distribution of an autosomal dominant condition. He underwent routine screening for the disease because of the family history. This involved rigid sigmoidoscopy to look for polyps in the rectum and sigmoid colon. Twenty polyps were demonstrated. Figure 11.16a shows an area from a biopsy of one of these. At left there is a crypt showing adenomatous change with enlarged, dark and stratified nuclei, indicating the presence of dysplasia, in comparison to a normal crypt at right. In a child of this age with such a family history, these findings are indicative of FAP and a year later he underwent total proctocolectomy with construction of an ileoanal pouch or reservoir. The risk of development of carcinoma in the colon or rectum is such that removal of the colon is necessary in these patients. Figure 11.16b shows part of the descending and sigmoid colon demonstrating the presence of multiple (at least 100 in this area alone) polyps typical of FAP.

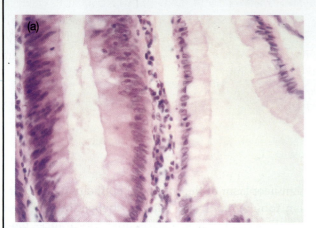 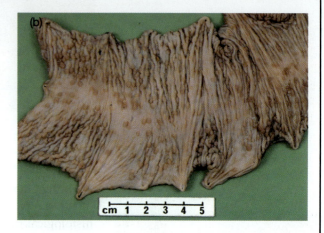

Fig. 11.16

Other benign tumour and polyps

Polyps are defined as lesions rising above the level of any mucosa and thus may be the result of various pathological mechanisms.

- **Metaplastic (hyperplastic) polyps** are numerically the most common and are a non-neoplastic abnormality of maturation of the colorectal mucosa. These polyps are usually small. They are most commonly found in the rectum of elderly patients, and their only significance lies in their endoscopic and macroscopic mimicry of adenomas.
- **Hamartomatous polyps** are usually solitary (as in **juvenile polyp**, a lesion of the young occurring in the rectum) but may be multiple, as seen in the hereditary **juvenile polyposis** and **Peutz–Jeghers polyposis syndromes**.
- **Inflammatory polyps** are relatively common and are the result of chronic inflammatory bowel disease, especially ulcerative colitis and Crohn's disease, and occasionally diverticular disease and schistosomiasis.

Finally, both benign and malignant stromal and lymphoid tumours may be polypoid; these include lipomas, haemangiomas, leiomyomas and a variety of rare sarcomas including Kaposi's sarcoma. Equally, adeno-carcinoma can occasionally be polypoid.

Colorectal cancer

AETIOLOGY AND PATHOGENESIS. In the UK colorectal cancer is the second most common cause of death from malignancy. The tumour is almost universally an **adenocarcinoma** and most of these tumours arise in pre-

Pathogenic factors in colorectal cancer

- Diet (low fibre, high protein and fat)
- Bacterial degradation of bile salts
- Hereditary factors (especially FAP, family cancer syndromes)

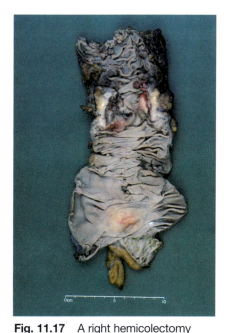

Fig. 11.17 A right hemicolectomy resection with the appendix (bottom) and terminal ileum (bottom right). In the ascending colon is an ulcerating circumferential tumour mass typical of colorectal adenocarcinoma.

existing adenomas. The pathogenesis of colorectal cancer is complex (see box). The high-fat diet results in increased bile salts which are degraded by bacteria to produce potentially carcinogenic substances in the colon. Low-fibre diet prolongs intestinal transit times and this also potentiates the effects of intraluminal carcinogens. Ulcerative colitis, Crohn's disease, uretero-sigmoidostomy and radiation are all conditions associated with an increased colorectal neoplastic potential. Of all human cancers, our knowledge of the molecular changes that underlie the development of tumours is perhaps most advanced for colorectal cancer. This is due partly to the availability of tissue for molecular biological study. Many and varied genetic changes have been described and many of these appear to occur at specific points in the adenoma–carcinoma sequence. For instance, the FAP gene (known as *APC*) mutation is an early feature, whilst various oncogene mutations and amplifications occur later. Mutation of the *p53* tumour suppressor gene is also a late feature.

PATHOLOGY. In the UK the rectum is the most common site (about 40%) although a quarter occur in the sigmoid colon. The caecum accounts for about 10% of tumours. Most rectal cancers are large ulcerating lesions which present with haemorrhage or anaemia. More proximal tumours may present with stricturing, frank obstruction or occult bleeding (Fig. 11.17). The diagnosis is usually established at sigmoidoscopy, colonoscopy or barium enema with subsequent histological confirmation. Most tumours are adenocarcinomas of varying degrees of differentiation. Mucinous tumours are relatively common in the right colon but the distinction is of little practical value. After surgery, the single most important determinant of survival is the extend of spread. This includes an assessment of local spread and lymph node involvement: these two parameters form the basis of the **Dukes' classification** (Fig. 11.18). The relationship of rectal cancer to the deep (mesorectal) resection margin may predict local recurrence. The presence of extramural venous spread and the proximity of colonic tumours to the closest peritoneal surface are also important assessments. Spread may occur by local extension to adjacent organs, by transcoelomic spread across the peritoneum, by lymphatic spread to lymph nodes and blood-borne spread, especially to the liver, but also to lung and bone.

Other tumours

Carcinoid tumours are distinctly rare in the colorectum; the rectum is the usual site, and most tumours are benign. Equally, secondary lymphomatous/leukaemic involvement of the colorectum is unusual. Primary malignant lymphomas of the large intestine show similarities to their gastric and small bowel counterparts, being typical B-cell lymphomas of mucosa-associated lymphoid tissue (MALT) type. Smooth muscle tumours, both benign and malignant, are uncommon in the colorectum.

Anus

VASCULAR DISORDERS

Haemorrhoids (piles) are the most most common cause of anorectal bleeding. They are caused by dilatation of vascular spaces in the

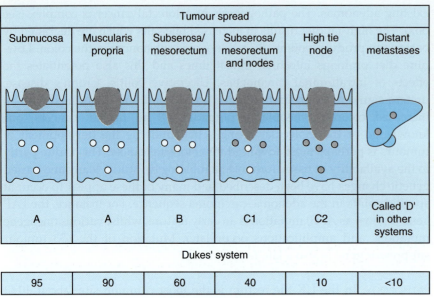

Tumour spread					
Submucosa	Muscularis propria	Subserosa/ mesorectum	Subserosa/ mesorectum and nodes	High tie node	Distant metastases
A	A	B	C1	C2	Called 'D' in other systems

Dukes' system

95	90	60	40	10	<10

Prognosis (%)*

Fig. 11.18 Staging of colorectal carcinoma: the Dukes' classification. The prognosis is for approximate 5-year cumulative survival.

submucosa of the anal canal. They show consistent positioning in the right anterior, right posterior and left lateral quadrants of the anus. Histological examination reveals thick-walled vascular spaces with abundant smooth muscle in their walls. Complications include haemorrhage and thrombosis, ischaemic necrosis, prolapse and secondary infection.

INFLAMMATORY DISORDERS

- **Anal fissures** are the most common form of ulceration in the anus and are most often seen in the posterior midline. Recognized predisposing factors include constipation and the passing of hard stool with anal mucosal trauma. There is associated spasm of the anal sphincter. Only occasionally are fissures associated with Crohn's disease.
- **Fistulae** of the anal region are divided into high and low types. The less complex low type is secondary to localized sepsis, particularly of anal glands. High fistulae, on the other hand, are often a complication of Crohn's disease. Thus tissues from anal fissures and fistulae are submitted for histological assessment to confirm or refute a diagnosis of Crohn's disease.
- Many inflammatory conditions of the skin may also be seen in the anal region but these are usually not of clinical significance. Nevertheless, there are conditions more specific to the anus which are important. **Hidradenitis suppurativa** is a chronic suppurating and scarring inflammatory condition and is probably a primary folliculitis. Syphilis, tuberculosis, herpes simplex infection (especially in AIDS) and lymphogranuloma inguinale may all involve the anal region.

TUMOURS

Many of the tumorous lesions that afflict the anal region are closely associated with **human papilloma virus** (HPV, wart virus) infection. In fact there is a spectrum of pathological changes from the benign condylomata acuminata through precancerous conditions to overtly malignant squamous cell carcinoma, all of which are linked with HPV infection (Fig. 11.19). These lesions show epidemiological and pathological similarities to

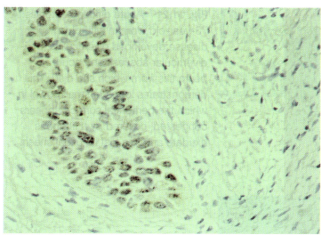
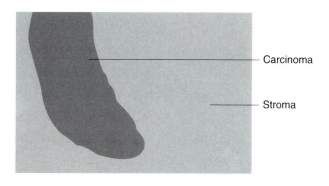

Carcinoma

Stroma

Fig. 11.19 HPV16 in situ hybridization in anal squamous cell carcinoma. An island of malignant epithelium is demonstrated and the nuclei stain positively (brown) for HPV16 DNA. In situ hybridization allows the presence of specific DNA to be demonstrated in histological sections.

Some rare malignant tumours of the anal region
- Malignant melanoma
- Adenocarcinoma of anal glands
- Paget's disease of the anus
- Basal cell carcinoma
- Lymphoma/leukaemia

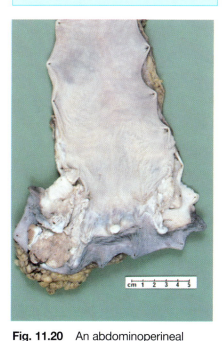

Fig. 11.20 An abdominoperineal resection for anal carcinoma. There is a protuberant tumour mass (lower left) arising in the anal canal. This was in a 55-year-old woman with a previous history of treated uterine cervical carcinoma (there is an association between HPV infection and anogenital neoplasia).

genital and uterine cervical neoplasia (see Chapter 15). These anal lesions are associated with anal sexual intercourse, although there are also associations with poor hygiene and poverty, particularly in countries such as Brazil and India where anogenital malignancy is common.

Carcinoma of the anus

Most cancers of the anus are of **squamous cell** type although there is a variety of histological appearances depending on the site of the tumour. Basaloid carcinoma characteristically occurs in the upper anal canal (Fig. 11.20). Spread of tumour depends upon the site of the primary cancer. Local spread is often upwards into the rectum whilst lymphatic spread is to both inguinal and haemorrhoidal lymph nodes. Prognosis is largely dependent upon stage. Primary treatment is now either local resection or radiotherapy and/or chemotherapy rather than major resection. It should be emphasized that, although mucinous carcinoma is a recognized complication of anal fistulae, adenocarcinoma in the anus is most usually due to direct spread from a primary rectal carcinoma.

Peritoneum

INFLAMMATORY DISORDERS

Acute infection of the peritoneum may be localized or diffuse depending on the cause of the infection and the local anatomy of the peritoneal serosal folds and viscera in the region of the primary infective focus. Acute generalized peritonitis (Fig. 11.21) is usually caused by perforation of a hollow viscus, especially in acute appendicitis, perforated peptic ulcers and sigmoid colon diverticulitis. In these situations, Gram-negative organisms, especially *Escherichia coli*, are usually the infecting organisms although often the infection is mixed. Acute diffuse peritonitis is a serious condition associated with a high mortality. The most serious complications are paralytic ileus and toxaemia. Paralytic ileus results in gross fluid and electrolyte disturbances while toxaemia contributes to hypotension and circulatory failure. Peritonitis may remain localized in which case localized abscess formation supervenes particularly in the subphrenic space or in the pelvis.

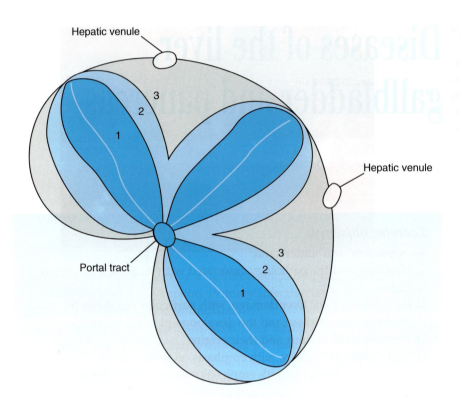

Fig. 12.1 The supposed acinar structure of the liver. Zone 1 hepatocytes are closest to the oxygen supply whereas zone 3 is adjacent to the terminal hepatic venule.

arboviruses (causing yellow fever) may at times be responsible for liver dysfunction. By convention, hepatitis is used to refer to diffuse liver injury although the severity of the injury may be heterogeneous.

HISTOLOGY

Morphologically there is very little difference between the acute effects of the different hepatitis viruses.

Many hepatocytes show sublethal injury in the form of cloudy swelling, or hydropic hepatocytes, characteristically by programmed cell deletion (apoptosis). These shrunken, pyknotic cells are clearly visible in biopsies. In severe cases there may be bridging necrosis linking adjacent portal tracts and even massive widespread necrosis. This is associated clinically with fulminant liver failure. Associated with this there is a lymphoid infiltrate in both sinusoids and portal tracts. Sinusoidal Kupffer's cells are activated and are prominent; many contain ceroid pigment. In infection caused by hepatitis A, virus plasma cells may be prominent in portal areas. **Cholestasis** (reduced bile flow) is common, with bile visible in sections of liver.

Since the liver can rapidly regenerate, evidence of hepatocyte proliferation such as mitotic figures and binucleate cells can be seen. Resolution results in structurally normal liver with no fibrosis, although a mild increase in chronic inflammatory cells may persist in portal areas for more than 6 months. However, sometimes the viral hepatitis enters a chronic stage and may even progress to cirrhosis.

HEPATITIS VIRUSES

These viruses primarily attack the liver but are not related to one another.

- **Hepatitis A virus** characteristically produces a mild illness, and full recovery occurs.

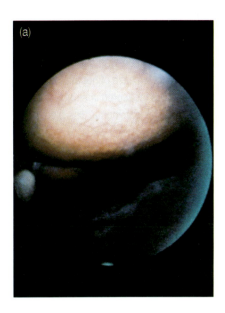
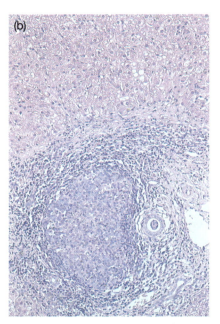
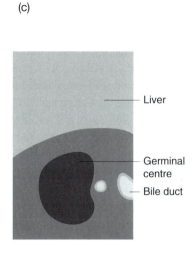

Liver

Germinal
centre

Bile duct

Fig. 12.2   (a) View of the liver at laparoscopy in a case of hepatitis C virus infection. The liver is inflamed and the surface vessels are congested. (Courtesy Dr R. Jalan.) (b, c) Histology reveals a large lymphoid aggregate with a prominent germinal centre in the biopsy specimen.

- **Hepatitis B and C viruses** frequently produce chronic hepatitis (Fig. 12.2) leading to cirrhosis and even hepatocellular carcinoma.
- **Hepatitis D** synergizes with hepatitis B to produce more severe disease.
- **Hepatitis E** generally resolves after a mild illness but pregnant women sometimes develop life-threatening liver failure.

A summary of the viruses is provided in Table 12.1.

Table 12.1   Characteristics of viruses which primarily cause hepatitis

	A	B	C	D	E
Virus	RNA	DNA	RNA	Defective RNA	RNA
Spread	Faecal–oral	Blood	Sexual	Blood. Probably as for B	?Sexually Faecal–oral
Incubation period	15–40 days	50–180 days	40–75 days	Co-infection with B or subsequent infection	30–50 days
Pathogenesis	Direct cytopathic	Triggers immune	?Immune	Synergizes with B	?Direct destruction
Chronicity	No	Yes	Yes	Yes	Uncommon
Geography	Worldwide	Worldwide	Worldwide	?	Predominantly Asia
Diagnosis	IgM to virus	e antigen = infective IgG to s antigen indicates previous infection	Antibody to HCV HCV RNA detected by polymerase chain reaction	Protein present in hepatocyte nuclei	Antibody to HEV

CASE STUDY 12.1

A 34-year-old man presented with **haematemesis** due to **bleeding oesophageal varices**. His biochemistry and haematology on admission showed a low serum albumin and a raised prothrombin ratio indicating that liver synthetic function was diminished. An ultrasound scan showed changes consistent with cirrhosis. Further investigation revealed that he was a known case of hepatitis B virus infection, acquired some years previously when he was an intravenous drug abuser. His α-fetoprotein was measured in serum. It was 1720 ng/ml (upper limit of normal 20 ng/ml) raising the strong possibility of an associated hepatocellular carcinoma. His bleeding varices were injected and, at a later stage, he underwent laparoscopic liver biopsy.

This showed a nodular, cirrhotic liver and confirmed the presence of varices and portal hypertension (Fig. 12.3). In view of his age, liver transplantation was undertaken. The removed liver was dissected and confirmed the presence of cirrhosis (Fig. 12.4). In addition, there were several larger nodules which were discoloured by bile, suspicious of hepatocellular carcinoma. Sections of the liver (Fig. 12.5a) were examined by immunohistochemistry for the presence of hepatitis B surface antigen (Fig. 12.5b). When the larger nodules were examined histologically, they were noted to be hepatocellular carcinoma and to have a much less developed reticulin framework than the adjacent smaller cirrhotic nodules (Fig. 12.6a). The tumour cells expressed α-fetoprotein which was detected by immunohistochemistry (Fig. 12.6b).

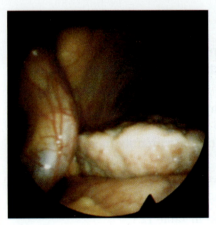

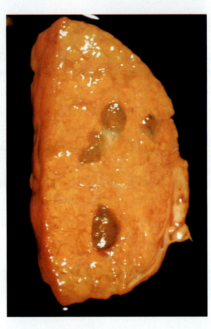

Fig. 12.4 Slice of resected liver confirming cirrhosis but also showing several large nodular hepatocellular carcinomas.

Fig. 12.3 Laparoscopic view of liver prior to biopsy. The liver edge is rough and nodular and, on the left, dilated variceal vessels can be clearly identified. (Courtesy Dr R. Jalan.)

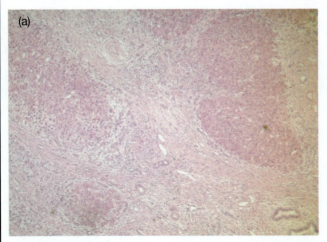

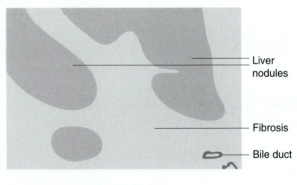

Liver nodules

Fibrosis

Bile duct

Fig. 12.5 (a) Histological appearance of typical cirrhotic nodules separated by broad, inflamed fibrous septa. (b) Demonstration of hepatitis B virus surface gantigen by immunohistochemistry. No positivity was seen in neoplastic cells (not shown).

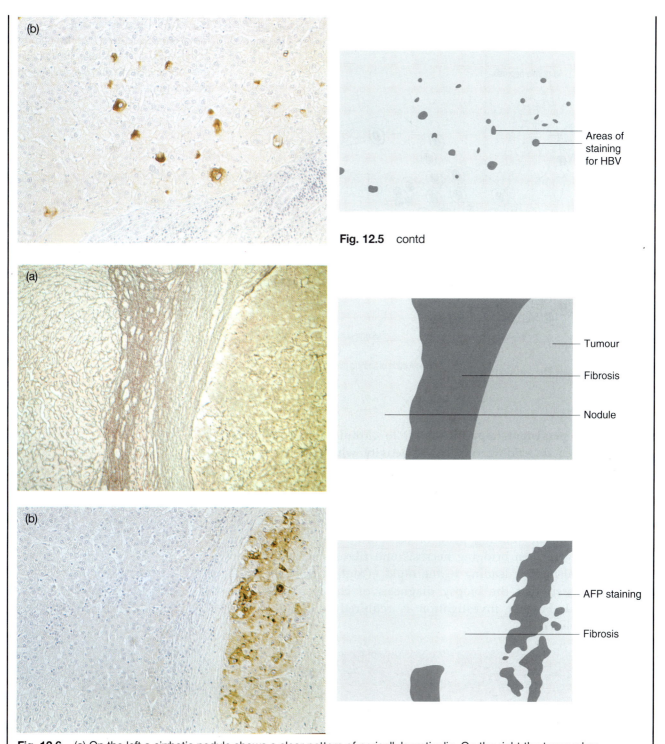

Fig. 12.5   contd

Labels for top right diagram: Areas of staining for HBV

Labels for middle right diagram: Tumour, Fibrosis, Nodule

Labels for bottom right diagram: AFP staining, Fibrosis

Fig. 12.6   (a) On the left a cirrhotic nodule shows a clear pattern of pericellular reticulin. On the right the tumour has reduced reticulin staining. This can be a useful diagnostic help in tumours that are very well differentiated. (b) AFP was present in only the neoplastic cells.

Chronic hepatitis

Liver inflammation persisting for more than 6 months without sustained improvement is defined as chronic hepatitis. However, the disease may have a fluctuating course in terms of injury as assessed biochemically or by liver biopsy. A spectrum of biopsy changes ranging

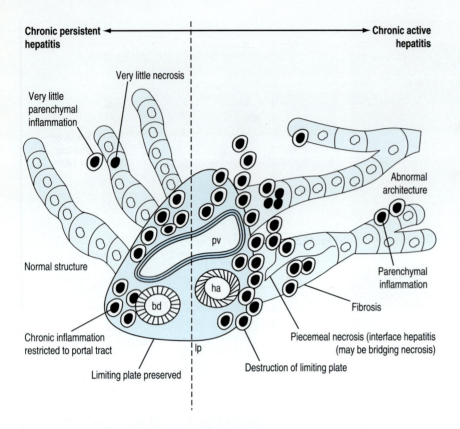

Fig. 12.7 The spectrum of morphological features seen in chronic hepatitis. pv, portal venule; ha, hepatic arteriole; bd, biliary ductule; lp, limiting plate of portal tract.

from **chronic persistent hepatitis** (mild) to **chronic active hepatitis** (severe) is seen depending on disease activity which itself may be modulated by immunosuppressive drugs. The pathological features are summarized in Fig. 12.7. The hallmark of chronic active hepatitis is the presence of **piecemeal necrosis** or **interface hepatitis** (Fig. 12.8). This is a process of chronic inflammation leading to necrosis and fibrosis, which occurs at the limiting plate of the portal tract. If piecemeal necrosis is severe then bridging necrosis and fibrosis occur between adjacent portal regions leading to the rapid evolution of cirrhosis. It must be stressed that the biopsy diagnosis of chronic hepatitis is morphological. Further investigation is required to establish the aetiology (Table 12.2).

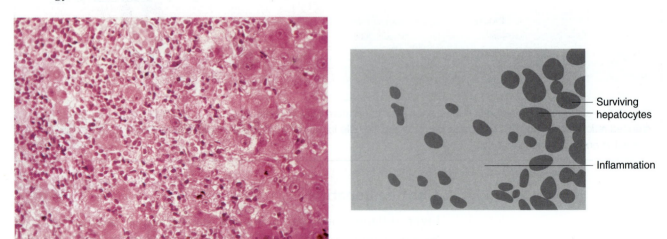

Fig. 12.8 Piecemeal necrosis in a case of autoimmune chronic active hepatitis. Lymphocytes are spilling over from the portal tract into the hepatic parenchyma obscuring the limiting plate.

Table 12.2 The aetiology and diagnosis of chronic active hepatitis

Aetiology	Clinical	Biochemical	Immunological	Additional biopsy features
Autoimmune	F>M Peak 15–20 and 45–55 years Other autoimmune diseases	–	Antinuclear antibodies Antismooth muscle antibodies	May have frequent plasma cells
Hepatitis B	M>F Any age More severe if HDV present	–	HBe and HBs antigens present	HBs antigen detected in hepatocytes by immuno-histochemistry
Hepatitis C	Any age Often post-transfusion, homosexual or drug abuser	–	Anti-HCV antibodies HCV RNA present	Steatosis and multinucleate hepatocytes by immuno-histochemistry Lymphoid aggregates in portal tracts
Idiopathic and drug-induced	Methyldopa Isoniazid	–	Often have autoantibodies	Like autoimmune
α_1-Antitrypsin deficiency	Late childhood/ young adult presentation May have emphysema	Defect in α_1-AT secretion Homozygous ZZ phenotype causes disease Low serum α_1-AT abnormal phenotype	–	Accumulation of α_1-AT and PAS-positive globules in hepatocytes
Wilson's disease	Childhood Kayser–Fleischer rings in cornea Lenticular degeneration in brain	Low serum ceruloplasmin	–	Excess copper in liver

Biliary disease

One function of the liver is to conjugate and excrete toxic substances in bile. It follows therefore that failure of this pathway leads to cholestasis, which in turn causes secondary damage to the hepatocytes themselves. If prolonged cholestasis occurs then cirrhosis may ensue. Biliary disease is summarized in Table 12.3.

Table 12.3   A summary of biliary disease

Disease	Clinical	Biochemistry	Immunology	Biopsy	Other
Primary biliary cirrhosis	F>M 9:1 Itch Xanthelasma	Very high alkaline phosphatase	Anti-mito-chondrial antibodies (AMA)	Granulomata Small bile duct destruction Chronic inflammation Cirrhosis	–
Primary sclerosing cholangitis	M>F 3:1. Two-thirds have ulcerative colitis	Very high alkaline phosphatase	Antibodies to neutrophil cytoplasmic antigens (ANCA) (Fig. 12.9)	Fibrous obliteration of larger ducts. Chronic inflammation	Risk of cholangio-carcinoma
Obstruction (secondary)	Any age Gallstones Tumours Scarring	High alkaline phosphatase Very high bilirubin	–	Bile lakes Acute inflammation	Risk of ascending infection

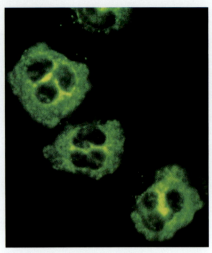

Fig. 12.9   Demonstration of antibodies against neutrophil cytoplasmic antigens (ANCA) in a case of primary sclerosing cholangitis. The patient had a history of inflammatory bowel disease. The presence of ANCA is not specific for this disease, nor is it always present.

PRIMARY DISEASE

In primary biliary disease there is destruction of bile ducts by immunological mechanisms. Damage to hepatocytes and subsequent fibrosis and hepatocyte regeneration lead to cirrhosis. In **primary biliary cirrhosis** there is a chronic inflammatory infiltrate in portal tracts, and lymphocytes can be seen migrating into the biliary epithelium which becomes degenerative. Fibrosis and obliteration then occur. This disease primarily affects small bile ducts. Approximately one-quarter of biopsies contain epithelioid **granulomata**, sometimes in the hepatic parenchyma but often close to bile ducts (Fig. 12.10).

Primary sclerosing cholangitis is usually associated with ulcerative colitis. In this condition there is fibrous obliteration of bile ducts. Larger ducts and even extrahepatic bile ducts may be affected. These patients are at risk of developing cholangiocarcinoma. In both conditions periportal

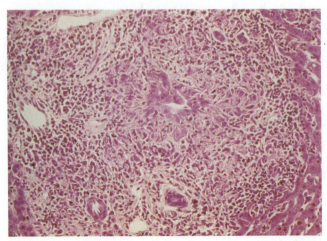

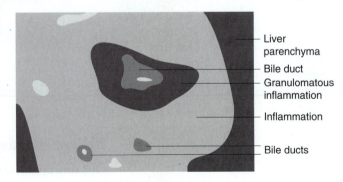

Liver parenchyma
Bile duct
Granulomatous inflammation
Inflammation
Bile ducts

Fig. 12.10   Portal tract in a liver biopsy from a 59-year-old woman with primary biliary cirrhosis. The central bile duct is disrupted by inflammatory cells and it is surrounded by a loose granuloma.

hepatocyte injury occurs and there is often proliferation of poorly formed ductular structures – so-called 'biliary reduplication' or 'ductal metaplasia'. This is probably a regenerative phenomenon.

SECONDARY DISEASE

This is usually the result of bile outflow obstruction caused by gallstones. However, bile duct carcinoma, pancreatic carcinoma, extrinsic compression of the bile duct by porta hepatis lymph nodes, or post-traumatic stricture may also cause obstruction.

Bile accumulates in canaliculi between hepatocytes, and in Kupffer's cells. It may extravasate to form bile lakes. These are more common in zone 3, the perivenular hepatocytes. There is an inflammatory response, predominantly of acute inflammatory cells, which is most notable in the portal tracts. Oedema in portal tracts is often marked and there may be very extensive biliary reduplication. Prolonged obstruction leads to bridging between adjacent portal areas and eventual cirrhosis.

Alcoholic liver disease

Alcohol is one of the commonest causes of liver disease in so-called developed countries. It can produce acute reversible injury (**steatosis** or fatty change) or irreversible changes characterized by hepatocyte death and fibrosis (**alcoholic hepatitis** and **cirrhosis**).

CASE STUDY 12.2

A 54-year-old woman with a long history of alcohol abuse presented with abdominal discomfort and epigastric pain. This was due to a peptic ulcer. General examination, however, showed features of chronic liver disease such as spider naevi and palmar erythema. She was referred for assessment of her liver function and possible biopsy.

Laparoscopy showed a large pale liver (Fig. 12.11) in keeping with steatosis. There was no evidence of cirrhosis, nor of portal hypertension. Histology showed features typical of alcoholic liver disease, macro- and microvesicular **steatosis** (Fig. 12.12a, b), **lipogranuloma** (Fig. 12.12c, d), **spotty necrosis** and **Mallory's hyaline** (Fig. 12.12e, f), **giant mitochondria** (Fig. 12.12g, h) and **perivenular fibrosis** (Fig. 12.12i, j). None of these features is absolutely specific for alcoholic liver disease, and must be interpreted with caution in the absence of a clinical history that supports the diagnosis.

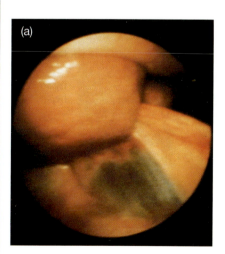

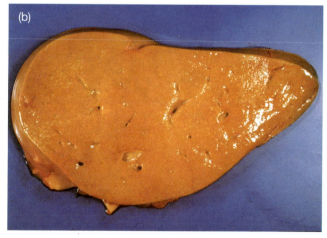

Fig. 12.11   (a) Pale fatty liver at laparoscopy. (Courtesy Dr R. Jalan.) (b) Macroscopic specimen showing marked steatosis.

CASE STUDY 12.2   contd.

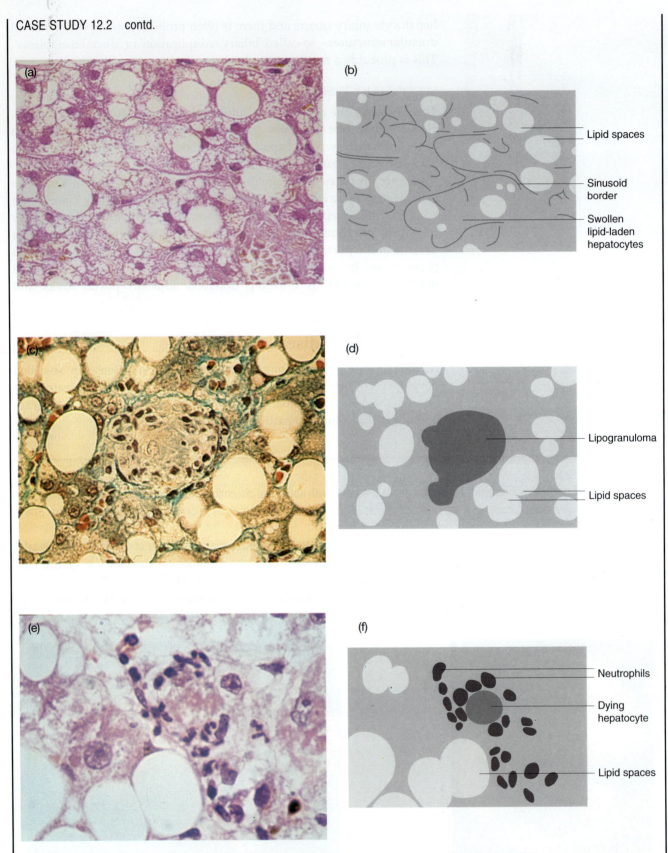

Fig. 12.12   (a, b) Macro- and microvesicular steatosis in hepatocytes. (c, d) A small lipogranuloma. The Masson trichrome stain also highlights the pericellular fibrosis green. (e, f) Spotty necrosis. Neutrophils are gathered round a dying hepatocyte which contains Mallory's hyaline, a phenomenon sometimes referred to as 'satellitosis'. (g, h) A large pink 'giant' mitochondrion in a hepatocyte. (i, j) A van Gieson's stain demonstrates fibrosis around terminal venules and zone 3 hepatocytes.

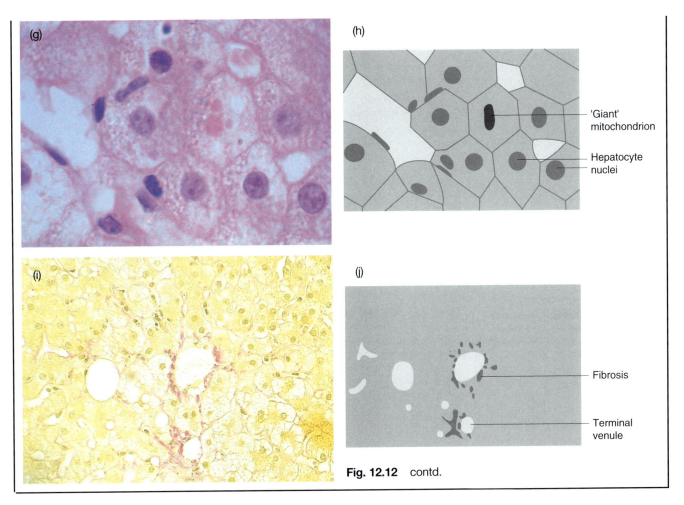

Fig. 12.12 contd.

PATHOGENESIS

Habitual alcohol intake induces the microsomal ethanol oxidizing system (particularly the cytochrome P450, CYP2E1). This, in addition to alcohol dehydrogenases, produces acetaldehyde and depletes the cell of NADPH. These changes directly cause triglyceride accumulation leading to fatty change as well as cell death (Fig. 12.13). The inflammatory response to cell death includes cytokine production which triggers perisinusoidal Ito cells to synthesize collagen.

Steatosis

Hepatocytes become swollen as cytoplasm accumulates globules of fat, particularly evident in zone 3 where alcohol-metabolizing enzymes predominate. Steatosis is not specific to alcohol injury; it is also seen in obesity, diabetes, malabsorption syndromes and malnutrition. It is reversible.

Alcoholic hepatitis

Hepatocytes lose osmotic control and become ballooned and hydropic. Occasional cells undergo necrosis and elicit a focal neutrophil response (**'spotty necrosis'**). The cytoskeleton of cells is damaged and aggregates of prekeratin intermediate filaments are visible as Mallory's hyaline. Although not specific, this is a useful diagnostic clue.

Cirrhosis

Progressive injury and fibrosis lead to fibrous septa which join adjacent perivenular acinar zone 3 regions. Portovenous bridging also occurs.

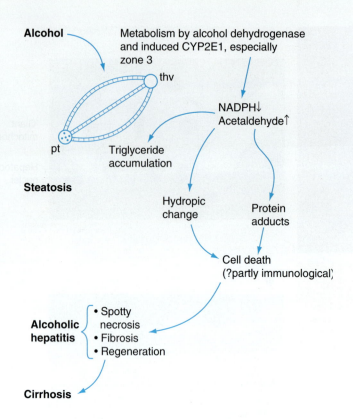

Alcohol — Metabolism by alcohol dehydrogenase and induced CYP2E1, especially zone 3

thv

pt

Triglyceride accumulation

Steatosis

NADPH↓
Acetaldehyde↑

Hydropic change

Protein adducts

Cell death
(?partly immunological)

Alcoholic hepatitis
- Spotty necrosis
- Fibrosis
- Regeneration

Cirrhosis

Fig. 12.13   Pathogenesis of alcohol-induced injury in the liver. pt, partial triad; thv, terminal hepatic venule.

Within these small delineated regions regenerative hepatocytes form nodules (**micronodular cirrhosis**).

Liver injury caused by drugs

This may be a predictable, dose-related, toxic injury (caused by paracetamol, for example) or an idiosyncratic, unpredictable reaction (such as the immunological injury present in halothane hepatitis). The injury may be primarily **hepatotoxic**, as with paracetamol (Fig. 12.14) or halothane, or **cholestatic**, as with chlorpromazine. The possibility of an adverse drug reaction should always be considered in patients taking medication who have abnormal liver function biochemistry.

Storage diseases

α_1-Antitrypsin deficiency (Fig. 12.15) and Wilson's disease have already been mentioned under chronic hepatitis (see Fig. 12.7 and Table 12.2).

Many other **lipid** and **glycogen storage diseases** affect the liver, but their precise description is beyond the scope of this book.

HAEMOCHROMATOSIS

Haemochromatosis is an inherited condition resulting in enhanced absorption of iron from the gut and a gross excess of iron stored in the liver (more than 10 times normal). The gene responsible for this defect is on chromosome 6 and is in linkage disequilibrium with HLA-A3.

The excess iron is found in hepatocytes, but as the severity of iron overload increases it is also found in the Kupffer's cells and biliary epithelium (Fig. 12.16). The presence of iron is directly fibrogenic and periportal fibrosis eventually leads to a predominantly macronodular

Fig. 12.14 Fulminant liver failure following ingestion of paracetamol in an attempt to commit suicide. Histologically, 90% of the liver parenchyma was necrotic.

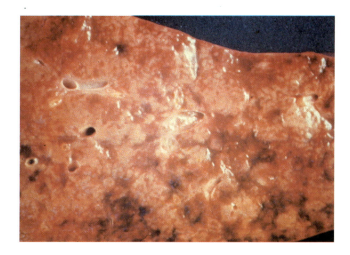

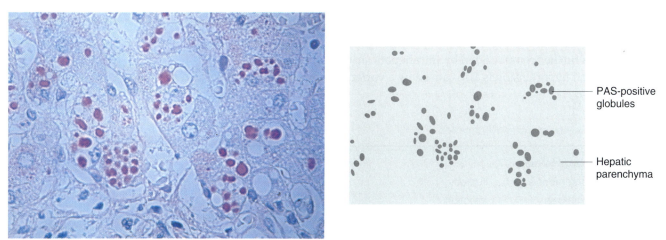

PAS-positive globules

Hepatic parenchyma

Fig. 12.15 Accumulation of α_1-antitrypsin globules in hepatocytes stained with periodic acid–Schiff after diastase treatment. The patient also had emphysema.

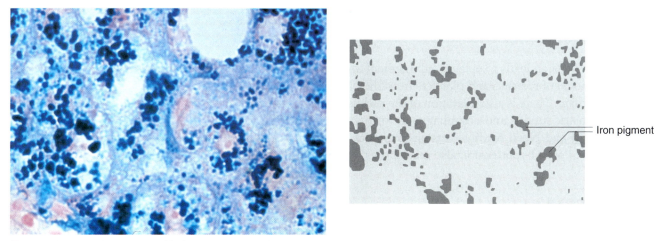

Iron pigment

Fig. 12.16 Iron demonstrated in hepatocytes by the Prussian blue reaction in a case of primary haemochromatosis.

cirrhosis. Treatment by venesection or with iron-chelating drugs such as desferrioxamine prevents disease progression. This is a multisystem disease, and iron is deposited in other organs. Excess accumulation in islets can lead to diabetes; other endocrine effects include excess melanin production resulting in skin pigmentation – the syndrome of **bronze diabetes**.

Secondary iron overload (**secondary haemosiderosis**) can occur in alcoholics, haemoglobinopathies and multiply transfused patients. Iron is particularly prominent in Kupffer's cells. Differentiation from primary genetic haemochromatosis may be impossible from a liver biopsy alone.

Cirrhosis

This is the end stage of many forms of liver injury and is defined as the presence of regenerative nodules separated by fibrous tissue septa, affecting the whole liver. Many clues to the aetiology of cirrhosis are not apparent in biopsies taken at this 'end stage'. If serological or biochemical evidence fails to reveal a cause then the cirrhosis is said to be **cryptogenic**.

PORTAL HYPERTENSION

This increased blood pressure in the portal vein, above 1 kPa (7 mmHg), reflects the resistance to blood flow through grossly disturbed liver structure. It is further compounded by intrahepatic arteriovenous shunting of blood. Portal hypertension is also caused by a variety of other conditions (Table 12.4).

Table 12.4   Causes of portal hypertension

Presinusoidal hypertension	
Portal vein thrombosis	Tumour
Postal tract fibrosis	Infection
Sinusoidal hypertension	Nodular regenerative hyperplasia
	Cirrhosis
	Sinusoidal fibrosis (some drugs)
Postsinusoidal hypertension	Veno-occlusive disease (hepatic veins)
	Budd–Chiari syndrome (hepatic vein thrombosis)

Portal hypertension leads to splenic enlargement and this may result in excessive removal of red cells and platelets from the blood – the syndrome of **hypersplenism**. There is also dilatation of the plexus of venous channels around the gastric fundus and oesophagus to form **varices**. These varices are thin-walled and bleed readily, causing torrential and life-threatening haematemesis. Portal hypertension also contributes to the development of **ascites**.

COMPLICATIONS

Liver excretory and synthetic failure

If hepatocytes continue to die (as in alcoholic cirrhosis) or if bile excretion is irreparably impaired (as in primary biliary cirrhosis), liver function may fail to cope adequately with the metabolic requirements of the body, a state known as **decompensation**. Decreased synthesis of albumin reduces colloid osmotic pressure causing peripheral oedema and exacerbating ascites. Decreased clotting factors potentiate the bleeding tendency following from hypersplenism. Failure to excrete nitrogenous waste and bile pigments leads to **encephalopathy** and jaundice (Fig. 12.17).

Fig. 12.17 Complications of cirrhosis.

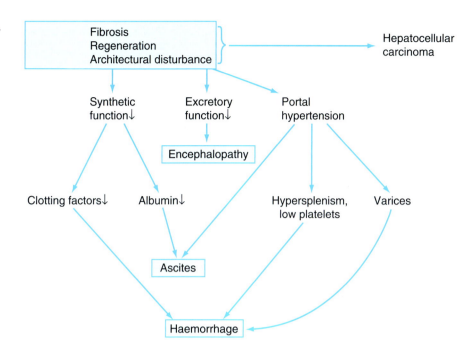

Hepatocellular carcinoma

All forms of cirrhosis predispose to hepatocellular carcinoma, but patients with cirrhosis related to hepatitis B and C virus are at particularly high risk.

Congenital malformations

- **Biliary atresia** presents in neonates with signs of biliary obstruction. It may be partial or complete.
- **Solitary cysts** and **multiple cysts** in association with some forms of renal cystic disease and congenital hepatic fibrosis are part of a spectrum of abnormal duct development.
- **Von Meyenberg's complexes** are small nodules, often capsular, formed by groups of bile duct-like structures in a fibrous stroma.
- **Focal nodular hyperplasia** is a rare hamartoma sometimes associated with the oral contraceptive pill.

Benign tumours

- **Cavernous haemangiomas** are found incidentally in about 2% of postmortem examinations (Fig. 12.18).
- **Liver cell adenomas** are associated particularly with oral contraceptive pill and anabolic steroid use. They are well-defined nodules, vascular and well differentiated (Fig. 12.19). They lack biliary elements.

Malignant tumours

The commonest malignant tumour is **metastatic carcinoma** of the lung, breast, gastrointestinal tract or pancreas (Fig. 12.20).

About four-fifths of primary tumours are **hepatocellular carcinomas**. The majority of cases arise in cirrhotic livers and may be multifocal.

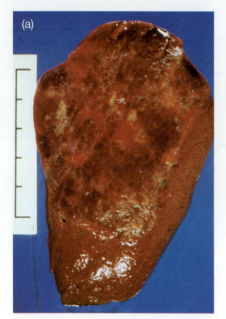
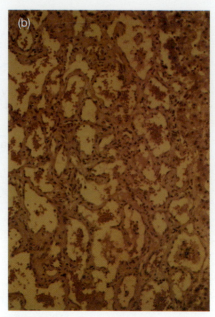
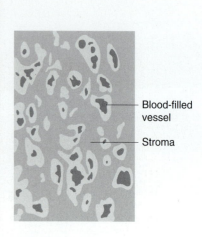

Blood-filled vessel

Stroma

Fig. 12.18   (a) An unusually large haemangioma removed from a young woman presenting with right upper quadrant pain and discomfort. (b, c) Microscopy shows dilated, blood-filled channels with thin walls.

However, a small number arise in non-cirrhotic livers, including the **fibrolamellar variant** in young women which has a slightly better prognosis than the usual hepatocellular carcinoma.

Histologically the tumours vary from well to poorly differentiated, but the cells often resemble hepatocytes. There may be evidence of bile secretion in well-differentiated tumours. Many less well-differentiated tumours produce and release α-**fetoprotein** (**AFP**), a useful serum marker for diagnosis and follow-up.

Worldwide, the commonest aetiological factors are hepatitis B virus acting synergistically with **aflatoxin B₁**, a mycotoxin product of *Aspergillus flavus*. Hepatitis C is probably also important, and alcohol may have a promoter function. All forms of cirrhosis increase the risk of hepatocellular carcinoma.

CHOLANGIOCARCINOMA

This tumour comprises about one-sixth of primary liver cancers. It is an adenocarcinoma which often spreads by ramification of portal tracts through the liver. Its incidence is high in patients with primary sclerosing cholangitis and in south-east Asia where liver flukes are prevalent.

OTHER TUMOURS

- **Angiosarcomas** are rare but important since they may be related to occupational exposure to vinyl chloride.
- **Hepatoblastomas** are very rare tumours of infancy.
- **Small cell undifferentiated carcinoma** and **lymphoma** arising in the liver have been described.

Liver transplantation

Increasingly, **liver transplantation** is being used to treat patients with end-stage liver disease. The commonest preceding illness is primary biliary

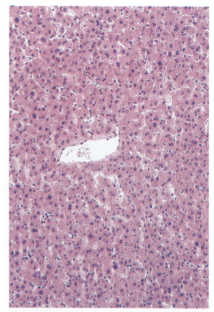

Fig. 12.19   Histology of an adenoma showing regular, well-differentiated hepatocytes arranged in almost normal plates. Biliary development was not seen.

cirrhosis but many other conditions including fulminant failure due to drugs or infection, viral hepatitis and even alcoholic liver disease have also been transplanted. The overall survival is good, although patients with malignancy or viral hepatitis do less well.

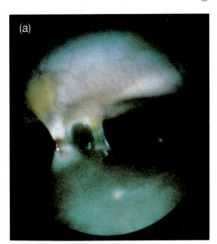
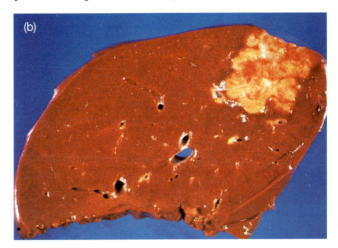

Fig. 12.20   (a) Laparoscopic view of adhesions between a metastasis at the liver surface and the overlying diaphragm. (Courtesy Dr R. Jalan.) (b) Resection shows that the metastasis, from the pancreas, is more extensive than was apparent externally.

CASE STUDY 12.3

Fourteen days after liver transplantation for end-stage primary biliary cirrhosis, a 62-year-old woman presented with fevers, rigors and deteriorating liver function. A presumptive diagnosis of **rejection** was made and liver biopsy performed. This showed a marked mixed acute and chronic inflammatory cell infiltrate in portal tracts (Fig. 12.21a, b), associated with venulitis, destruction of the bile ducts and necrosis of hepatocytes around terminal venules (Fig. 12.21c, d). A diagnosis of severe acute rejection was made and the patient was treated with high-dose prednisolone to suppress the immune response. Several weeks later she again deteriorated, having apparently made a slow recovery from the episode of rejection. Biopsy was again performed and this time showed little evidence of rejection. Within hepatocytes there were large eosinophilic inclusions which prompted the diagnosis of **cytomegalovirus infection** (Fig. 12.22). This was subsequently proved by immunohistochemistry and demonstration of the virus directly.

Her poor health continued and some time later she presented again with rigors and fever. Blood cultures grew *Candida* sp. and a streptococcus. The liver would have looked like that shown in Fig. 12.23 with discrete, multiple abscesses on the capsular surface. Histology showed small, ill-defined abscesses in the hepatic parenchyma, although no micro-organisms were demonstrated (Fig. 12.24).

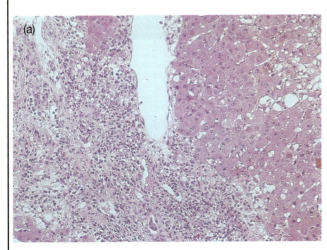
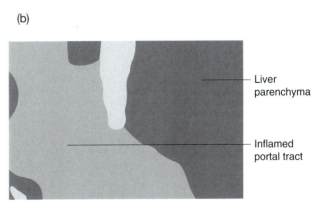

Liver parenchyma

Inflamed portal tract

Fig. 12.21   (a, b) Inflamed portal tract with evidence of immune destruction of both venules and bile ducts in the portal tract. (c, d) Necrosis and collapse around the terminal venule in acute rejection.

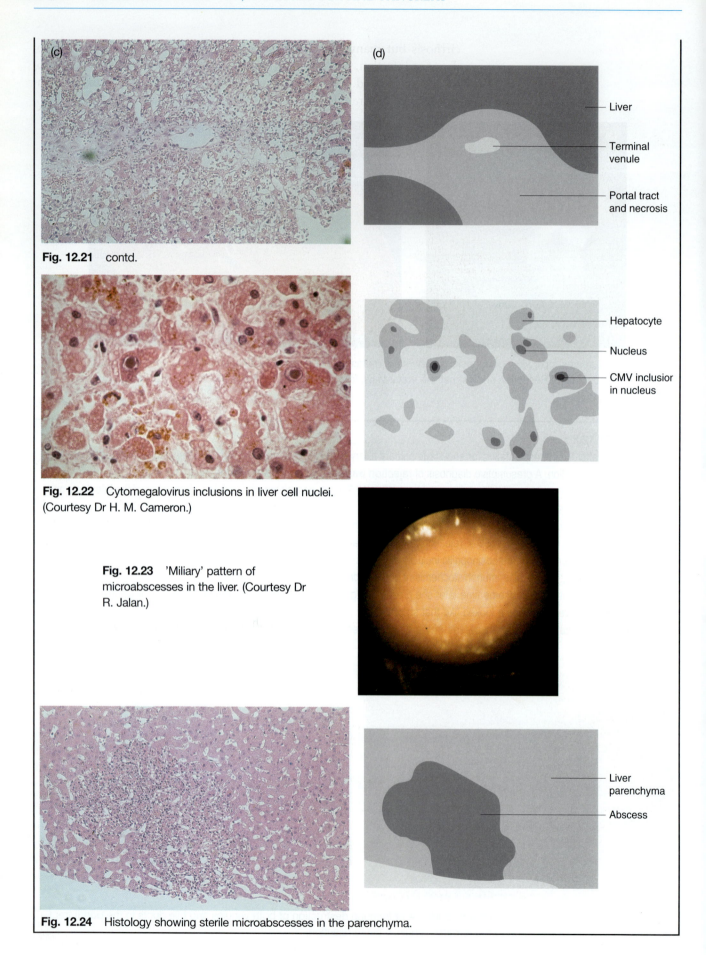

(c)

(d) — Liver

— Terminal venule

— Portal tract and necrosis

Fig. 12.21   contd.

— Hepatocyte

— Nucleus

— CMV inclusion in nucleus

Fig. 12.22   Cytomegalovirus inclusions in liver cell nuclei. (Courtesy Dr H. M. Cameron.)

Fig. 12.23   'Miliary' pattern of microabscesses in the liver. (Courtesy Dr R. Jalan.)

— Liver parenchyma

— Abscess

Fig. 12.24   Histology showing sterile microabscesses in the parenchyma.

The liver in systemic disease

The liver often shows non-specific reactive changes when intercurrent disease is present elsewhere, including mild inflammation and steatosis.

Other more specific abnormalities include:

- **amyloidosis**
- **sarcoidosis**, where granulomata may be found
- malignant infiltration by **metastatic carcinoma** or **leukaemia**
- **tuberculosis**, in miliary cases
- **fungal infection**, in cases of immunodeficiency such as **AIDS** or immunosuppressive therapy
- **cardiac failure**, where perivenous congestion and atrophy may occur
- **graft versus host disease** following bone marrow transplantation
- **fatty liver of pregnancy**.

Gallbladder

Normal function

The gallbladder is connected to the intrahepatic and extrahepatic bile ducts by the cystic duct. It stores and concentrates bile from the liver and increases its viscosity by releasing mucus from the lining epithelium. The release of bile from the gallbladder is stimulated by food, especially fatty food, in the duodenum under the influence of cholecystokinin.

Gallstones

Although rare in developing countries, **gallstones** (**cholelithiasis**) (Fig. 12.25) are extremely common in industrialized countries. In many cases cholelithiasis remains undetected clinically and may be an incidental finding at postmortem examination.

The primary problem is supersaturation of bile. Bile normally contains a suspension of cholesterol, held in suspension by phospholipid micelles containing lecithin, as well as bile acids and pigments derived from bilirubin. Nucleation occurs in the supersaturated, lithogenic bile and stones then enlarge (Fig. 12.26). Stones may be single or multiple, small or large.

In some gallbladders excess cholesterol is phagocytosed by macrophages in the lamina propria. These aggregates of foamy macrophages produce yellow stippling and protrusion of the gallbladder mucosa, and appearance known as **cholesterolosis** or 'strawberry' gallbladder. This is of no clinical significance.

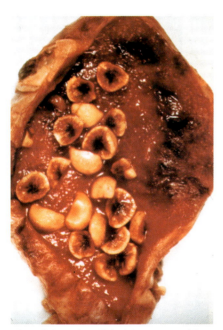

Fig. 12.25   A gallbladder removed for acute inflammation opened to demonstrate large numbers of calculi. (Courtesy Dr H. M. Cameron.)

Cholecystitis

ACUTE CHOLECYSTITIS

Initially, acute cholecystitis is usually the result of an injury to the gallbladder mucosa caused by gallstones, perhaps by obstruction of the cystic duct. However, in developed cases there is often superimposed infection by bowel commensal bacterial which further amplifies the acute inflammatory response.

Histologically there is ulceration of mucosa with vascular congestion, oedema and exudation. The neutrophil polymorph infiltrate may extend

Alport's disease

Alport's disease is an inherited autosomal dominant disorder. Its manifestations are:

- Renal disease in the form of haematuria, usually presenting in the first decade, with progression to chronic renal failure.
- Men appear to be more severely affected than women.
- High-tone deafness of variable severity.
- Ocular disorders – cataracts, lens dislocation.

Diagnosis is confirmed by renal biopsy and electron microscopy, showing abnormal capillary basement membranes.

Renal dysplasia

This term refers to abnormal renal development, and in this context does not imply premalignancy. The abnormally formed kidney may present as a large multicystic mass, to be differentiated from a malignant tumour.

Cystic disease

Renal cystic disease is manifested by a diverse group of conditions, both hereditary and acquired. Some of these conditions are genetically transmitted, so accurate diagnosis is important for counselling purposes.

SIMPLE CYSTS

Simple cysts are very common, and have no effect on renal function. They can be single or multiple, often several centimetres in diameter.

Multiple secondary simple cysts are often found in kidneys of patients on long-term renal dialysis.

CASE STUDY 13.1

A 48-year-old man presented to his general practitioner with a six-month history of abdominal 'fullness' and general lethargy. Abdominal examination suggested a large mass and the blood pressure was 195/120. Preliminary blood tests showed normochromic anaemia and high serum levels of urea and creatinine. Ultrasound examination of the abdomen showed markedly enlarged cystic kidneys and also liver cysts. The patient was referred to hospital for further investigation. However, prior to hospital admission he developed sudden severe headache and subsequent loss of consciousness. He was admitted as an emergency with a preliminary diagnosis of cerebrovascular accident. Despite resuscitative measures his condition rapidly deteriorated and he died three hours after admission. A postmortem examination was carried out and relevant findings were:

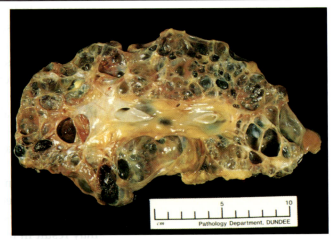

Fig. 13.1 Adult polycystic disease: the normal renal architecture is totally effaced by innumerable cysts.

- bilateral massive renal enlargement with innumerable cysts of varying size (Fig. 13.1)
- cardiomegaly with left ventricular hypertrophy
- extensive subarachnoid haemorrhage and aneurysm formation in vessels of the circle of Willis
- scattered liver cysts.

ADULT POLYCYSTIC DISEASE

The case study on page 304 highlights important features of adult polycystic disease:

- Presentation usually occurs in middle age but occasionally in younger adults.
- Patients may present with features of chronic renal failure, an abdominal mass or subarachnoid haemorrhage due to rupture of a berry aneurysm in the circle of Willis, a well-recognized associated feature.
- Left ventricular hypertrophy is related to systemic hypertension as a result of chronic renal failure.
- Cysts may be present in other organs, namely liver, lung and pancreas. Function of these organs is not usually impaired.
- After more detailed clinical history it was apparent that other family members of previous generations died in chronic renal failure.

Adult polycystic disease is transmitted genetically as an autosomal dominant trait. The degree of penetrance is high. Recent genetic studies show that the defect is related to abnormalities in chromosomes 4 or 16. This condition is found in up to 10% of all adult patients on renal dialysis in Europe. Clearly, genetic counselling has an important role in the management of affected families.

CHILDHOOD POLYCYSTIC DISEASE

In contrast to the adult variant, this disorder is transmitted as an autosomal recessive disorder (Fig 13.2). Most cases occur in the perinatal period, but there is a gradation of severity. Neonatal, infantile and juvenile subgroups are recognized and are associated with less severe disease.

Fig. 13.2 Infantile polycystic disease: note marked dilatation of tubules and ducts.

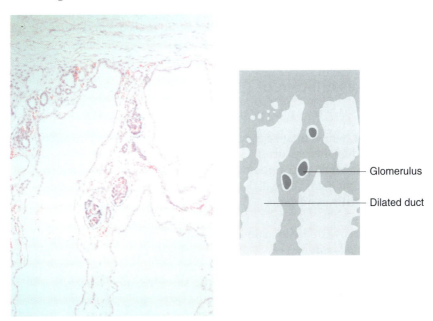

Glomerulus

Dilated duct

Renal failure

Acute renal failure

There is a wide variety of causes of acute renal failure, which are described in detail later in this chapter.

Chronic renal failure

Chronic renal failure can follow a wide variety of conditions which cause progressive and often irreversible renal damage. Clinical manifestations of chronic renal failure include:

- general lethargy
- polyuria due to osmotic diuresis
- polydipsia
- dyspnoea
- nausea and vomiting.

There is usually systemic hypertension. Waste products cannot be eliminated, and this is reflected in high serum urea and creatinine levels.

Pathological findings in advanced chronic renal failure include:

- bone disease (renal osteodystrophy)
- anaemia
- gastrointestinal bleeding
- immune deficiency
- neurological disorders such as peripheral neuropathy and myopathy.

Glomerulonephritis and glomerular disease

Glomerular disorders are an important cause of both acute and chronic renal failure. They constitute a widely varied group of conditions, some of which are primary renal disorders, while others are glomerular manifestations of systemic disease.

Several primary glomerulopathies are known to have an immunological basis, but in others the aetiology remains uncertain. A detailed knowledge of the pathological changes of glomerular disorders is beyond the scope of undergraduate teaching, and a simplified account is given here.

Clinical presentation of glomerular disease

Glomerular disease may present clinically in one of five ways:

- **Haematuria**, which may be macroscopic or microscopic, is usually painless and is often recurrent.
- **Proteinuria**, which may be asymptomatic and is often only detected during routine medical investigation.
- **Acute nephritic syndrome**:
  - oliguria
  - haematuria with dusky coloured urine
  - mild (facial) oedema
  - hypertension.
- **Nephrotic syndrome**: heavy proteinuria resulting in hypoalbuminaemia and extensive pitting oedema. Hypercholesterolaemia is also a feature.
- **Renal failure**, which may be acute or chronic. Patients in chronic renal failure may present clinically with systemic hypertension.

It must be emphasized that the clinical presentation of glomerulopathies is extremely variable, and there is a significant degree of overlap. Some conditions may usually present with one of the above syndromes, but some entities may give rise to any of them. For example, minimal change disease

---

Classification of acute renal failure

- **Prerenal failure**: a condition resulting in severe shock or circulatory failure. Severely reduced renal blood flow results in the formation of low volumes of concentrated urine.
- **Renal parenchymal failure**: causes include acute tubular necrosis, severe forms of glomerulonephritis, interstitial nephritis, and vascular disorders including cortical and papillary necrosis.
- **Postrenal (obstructive) failure**: complete bilateral obstruction of the lower urinary tract is usually due to prostatic disease obstructing the bladder outlet, or malignancy. Extensive bladder carcinoma or advanced carcinoma of the cervix may result in bilateral lower ureteric obstruction.

Common causes of chronic renal failure

- Chronic pyelonephritis
- Chronic glomerulonephritis
- Diabetic glomerulosclerosis
- Chronic obstruction of the urinary tract
- Hypertensive disease (severe)
- Congenital disorders, especially adult polycystic disease
- Drugs and toxins (for example analgesic nephropathy)

Fig. 1
prepa
mesa

> ### Glomerular reactions to injury
>
> The glomerulus reacts to injury in a limited number of ways.
>
> - **Cellular proliferation:** hypercellular glomeruli may result from proliferation of glomerular cells or infiltration by inflammatory cells.
> - **Changes in glomerular capillary buds:** this is usually seen histologically as mural thickening. It may occur in association with cellular proliferation, as seen in mesangiocapillary glomerulonephritis.
> - **Epithelial crescent formation:** this is a manifestation of severe glomerular damage. Proliferation of the epithelial cells in Bowman's capsule results in compression and distortion of the glomerular tuft.

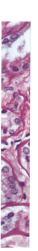

Fig. 1:

presents only as the nephrotic syndrome, but in mesangiocapillary glomerulonephritis, the clinical presentation is much more variable.

The extent of glomerular damage in the glomerulopathies is variable. The term **diffuse** means that all glomeruli show histological changes, whereas **focal** means that some are affected, but others appear normal. Any individual glomerulus may show **global** change, where the entire tuft is affected, or **segmental** change involving only part of the glomerulus.

Immune mechanisms in glomerular disease

In most glomerulopathies there is an immunological basis for glomerular damage. This may be due to antibody-mediated damage or deposition of immune complexes.

ANTIBODY-MEDIATED DAMAGE

Antibody-mediated damage takes the form of an IgG autoantibody acting against constituents of the glomerular capillary basement membrane. A typical linear pattern of IgG deposition is seen on capillary loops by immunofluorescence. Severe glomerular damage ensues due to complement activation and infiltration by inflammatory cells. This pattern of injury occurs in anti-glomerular basement membrane antibody disease.

DEPOSITION OF IMMUNE COMPLEXES

Antigen–antibody complexes in the peripheral circulation may be deposited in the kidney, activate the complement cascade and attract inflammatory cells, resulting in glomerular damage. Factors favouring deposition of circulating complexes in the glomerular tuft include the large renal blood flow and high glomerular intracapillary pressure. The site of deposition depends partly on the size and charge of the complexes. Cationic charge favours passage across the anionic basement membrane. Larger complexes often lodge in the subendothelial location without passing across the basement membrane, but smaller complexes may reach the subepithelial area.

Alternatively, immune complexes may form in the glomerulus itself. Circulating antibodies react with trapped or 'planted' antigens and form complexes particularly in the capillary basement membranes. Immune complex deposition in the glomerulus is recognized by granular staining for immunoglobulins by immunofluorescence, both in capillary loops and in the mesangium.

Glomerular diseases

The term **glomerulonephritis** is traditionally given to glomerular diseases with an immunological basis, but it is rather misleading. Some types of glomerulonephritis show little if any evidence of inflammation. For convenience, the variants of glomerulonephritis and other important glomerular diseases will be described together in this section. As the clinical presentation of glomerular disease is variable, percutaneous renal biopsy is frequently used for accurate diagnosis as prognosis and treatment differ from type to type. Tissue from the renal cortex is examined by:

- conventional histology and special stains
- immunofluorescence or immunohistochemistry

as hyperkalaemia) are an important cause of mortality. Early clinical recognition of this condition is important, since prolonged supportive therapy and effective treatment of the predisposing disease may result in complete recovery of renal function. Following the oliguric phase a period of diuresis often occurs, due to defective concentration of urine by the regenerating tubular epithelium.

In the early stages of acute tubular necrosis, histological changes may be subtle, but eventually dilatation of tubules, epithelial cell necrosis, tubular cast formation and regenerative changes are seen. There are two causes of acute tubular necrosis: **ischaemia** and **nephrotoxic injury**.

ISCHAEMIA

Any clinical condition resulting in profound shock may result in acute renal failure due to acute tubular necrosis. Examples are:

- severe blood loss
- extensive burns
- cardiogenic shock
- multiple injury
- obstetric disorders such as pre-eclamptic toxaemia and antepartum haemorrhage.

NEPHROTOXIC INJURY

A wide range of therapeutic and toxic agents may cause acute tubular necrosis (see box).

Interstitial nephritis

This group of conditions affects the intertubular portion of the renal parenchyma. The aetiology is varied but most cases are non-infective. The pathogenesis is poorly understood. Histological changes are relatively uniform and consist of an inflammatory infiltrate, mainly of chronic type, in the interstitium during the acute phase of the disease, giving way to fibrosis and tubular atrophy later.

As with acute tubular necrosis, drugs and toxins are common causes of interstitial nephritis – particularly antibiotics, non-steroidal anti-inflammatory drugs, diuretics and heavy metals. Interstitial nephritis may be acute or chronic.

- **Acute interstitial nephritis** presents as acute renal failure.
- **Chronic interstitial nephritis** is more insidious and patients often present in established chronic renal failure.

An important variant of chronic interstitial nephritis is **analgesic nephropathy**. This was first recognized many years ago with analgesics such as phenacetin which are no longer used. The renal damage was shown to be potentiated by aspirin. Analgesic nephropathy still occurs in patients requiring long-term pain relief, for example for chronic arthritis. The pathogenesis is likely to be due to both nephrotoxic and ischaemic mechanisms. There is progessive diminution of renal function and renal papillary necrosis may ensue. Patients with chronic analgesic nephropathy have an increased frequency of transitional cell carcinoma of the renal pelvis.

Causes of acute tubular necrosis

- **Drugs**, including antibiotics, anti-inflammatory drugs, paracetamol overdosage
- **Chemical toxins**: mercuric derivatives, arsenic, carbon tetrachloride, paraquat, ethylene glycol (antifreeze)
- **Blood products**: myoglobin in severe crush injury leads to acute tubular necrosis, and haemoglobin in massive haemolysis

Renal transplantation

Renal transplantation is now a common alternative to haemodialysis and peritoneal dialysis in the management of chronic renal failure, particularly in younger patients. A successful transplantation offers a dramatic improvement in the quality of life in many chronic renal failure patients.

Most renal transplants are allografts and are thus susceptible to rejection by the host. Suppression of rejection is often successfully achieved by immunosuppressive drugs. Rejection when it occurs may be hyperacute, acute or chronic.

Hyperacute rejection

This is due to the action of preformed cytotoxic antibodies, principally against the endothelial cells of the graft organ. These antibodies may develop as a result of a previous blood transfusion or transplantation. Formerly, blood group incompatibility was a cause of hyperacute rejection. Renal damage occurs in the first day or so following transplantation, but occasionally signs of hyperacute rejection become evident to the surgeon almost immediately after blood flow to the graft commences. The grafted organ becomes dusky, soft and cyanosed. Progression to infarction is inevitable and requires removal of the graft. Histologically the changes are centred on vessels with widespread thrombosis in arterioles and glomerular capillaries. Appropriate matching of donor and recipient ensures that this serious complication is a rare occurrence.

Acute rejection

Acute rejection may occur a few days, weeks or months following a transplant, but rarely after more than one year. Acute rejection may be:

- **vascular**: due to cytotoxic antibodies, resulting in thrombosis and fibrinoid vascular necrosis with deposition of immunoglobulin and complement in the vessel wall
- **cellular**: by a cell-mediated immune response; histologically there is interstitial oedema, lymphocytic infiltration and tubular damage.

Chronic rejection

This is seen after many months or years. Chronic vascular damage (endarteritis obliterans) results in ischaemia, interstitial fibrosis and tubular atrophy (Fig 13.9).

Renal allografts are also susceptible to:

- **acute tubular necrosis** due to ischaemia after removal from the donor
- **ischaemic damage**, for example following anastomotic stricture of the renal artery
- **recurrence of the primary disease** in the transplant, for example some forms of glomerulonephritis, particularly IgA nephropathy and type II mesangiocapillary glomerulonephritis.

Renal transplant recipients require immunosuppressives, and complications of this therapy include:

- **opportunistic infections**

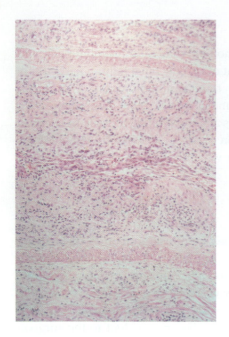

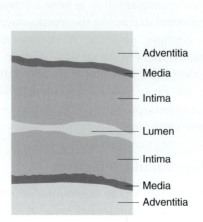

Adventitia
Media
Intima
Lumen
Intima
Media
Adventitia

Fig. 13.9   Severe vascular changes in chronic transplant rejection: note marked intimal fibrous thickening.

- **lymphoproliferative disorders**, including non-Hodgkin's lymphoma
- other **tumours**, such as skin tumours.

Obstructive uropathy

Obstruction of the ureters or bladder outflow causes variable effects on the kidney. Temporary acute obstruction of the ureter by a calculus causes renal colic, but long-term damage to the kidney may be minimal. More insidious renal damage ensues if the obstruction is partial or intermittent, particularly if it is unilateral. Chronic prostatic disease in men is a common cause of bilateral obstructive uropathy.

Obstruction of the urinary tract results in increased intraluminal pressure within the pelvicalyceal system of the kidney. This causes **hydronephrosis** – progressive dilatation of the pelvis and calyces with atrophy of the renal parenchyma (Fig. 13.10). Glomerular filtration is reduced and stasis predisposes to infection. Suppurative infection in a hydonephrotic kidney may occur.

Renal calculi

Stone formation in the urinary tract is relatively common. Calculi may form in any part of the urinary tract, but the most usual site is the renal pelvis

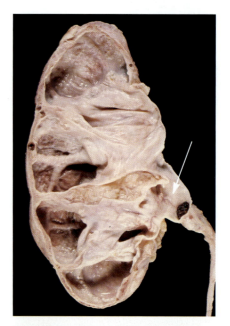

Fig. 13.10   Severe hydronephrosis: note calculus in pelviureteric junction (arrow).

Types of urinary calculi
- **Calcium oxalate calculi** are by far the commonest. They may also contain some calcium phosphate and uric acid.
- **Magnesium ammonium phosphate (triple) stones** are particularly associated with urinary tract infection due to urea-splitting bacteria, such as *Proteus* spp. Increased ammonia formation results in an alkaline urine and can result in the formation of a large calculus occupying most of the renal pelvicalyceal system. The shape of these stones resembles an antler – hence the name **staghorn calculus.**
- **Uric acid calculi** may occur in gout or sometimes as a result of chemotherapy for malignant disease which can cause massive tissue breakdown.
- **Rarer urinary calculi** may occur due to metabolic disorders such as oxalosis and cystinuria.

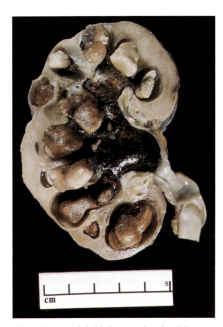

Fig. 13.11   Multiple renal calculi in a dilated pelvicalyceal system.

(Fig. 13.11). Passage down the ureter may result in renal colic. Most stones are eventually passed in the urine, but some remain in the bladder and can subsequently grow to a considerable size. About 90% of renal calculi are radio-opaque. The pathogenesis of renal calculi is poorly understood, but is related to:

- increased concentration of urinary solutes, resulting in precipitation
- alterations in urinary pH, for example during urinary tract infection and in disorders of metabolism.

Pyelonephritis

Bacterial infection is an important cause of renal disease. Rarely, other organisms such as fungi and viruses may be implicated, particularly in immunosuppressed patients. The kidneys may be involved by generalized septicaemia, but organisms also reach the kidney by vesicoureteric reflux or as a result of other risk factors (see box).

Acute pyelonephritis

There is acute inflammation of the renal pelvis and parenchyma, but the distribution may be patchy. Typically, streaks of pus extend throughout the parenchyma with destructive areas of suppuration (Fig 13.12). Scarring may ensue, but the other complications include:

- renal papillary necrosis
- pyonephrosis
- retroperitoneal abscess formation.

Chronic pyelonephritis

In the absence of urinary tract obstruction, chronic pyelonephritis is usually associated with congenital vesicoureteric reflux (see Chapter 16). Reflux of urine during micturition into the renal pelvis and calyces leads to increased intraluminal pressure in the proximal urinary tract. For pyelonephritis to develop, the infected urine must pass into the renal parenchyma (intrarenal or intraparenchymal reflux). The shape of the renal papillae is important in determining the degree of intraparenchymal reflux. Kidneys with blunt rather than conical papillae are more prone to intrarenal reflux and these papillae tend to be situated at the poles. This is

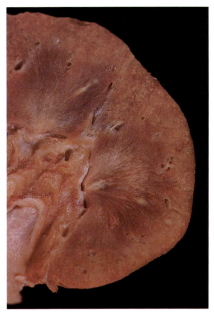

Fig. 13.12   Acute pyelonephritis: note multiple small yellowish abscesses.

Risk factors for pyelonephritis
- **Congenital abnormalities** of the urinary tract
- **Vesicoureteric reflux**
- **Urinary tract obstruction**: stasis of urine flow predisposes to infection
- **Diabetes mellitus**
- **Pregnancy**:
  - Obstruction due to the gravid uterus
  - Hormonal changes resulting in smooth muscle relaxation in the urinary tract
- **Operative procedures** and instrumentation of the urinary tract
- **Female sex**: urinary tract infection is more common in women

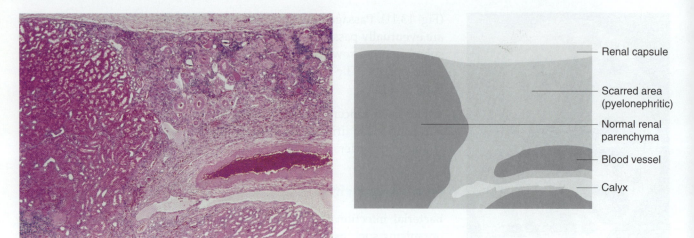

Fig. 13.13   Chronic pyelonephritis: note sharp demarcation between normal and diseased cortex.

reflected in the macroscopic appearance of chronic pyelonephritis. Indented coarse scars are seen at both poles of the kidney. Clinically significant disease is usually bilateral and extensive, and minor involvement is often not detected during life. The scarred areas are associated with underlying calyceal distortion.

It is likely that severe reflux of non-infected urine may cause renal damage, but superadded infection undoubtedly exacerbates renal damage.

Histologically, there is chronic inflammation, interstitial fibrosis, tubular atrophy and dilatation of remaining tubules which often contain eosinophilic casts resembling thyroid tissue (thyroidization) (Fig. 13.13). Later, glomerulosclerosis occurs to a variable degree. Many patients with chronic renal failure due to chronic pyelonephritis are also hypertensive and changes due to hypertension are often also seen.

Xanthogranulomatous pyelonephritis

This is an unusual variant of pyelonephritis seen in association with infection by *Proteus* sp. and *E. coli*, and with renal calculi. The condition is unilateral in most cases. The affected kidney is distorted by a pale tumour-like mass which may mimic renal cell carcinoma. Histologically there are abundant foamy macrophages and inflammatory cells.

Tuberculous pyelonephritis

Renal tuberculosis results from haematogenous spread of tubercle bacilli from another source, usually the lung. There may be miliary involvement with multiple small tubercles or larger, more localized, caseous lesions which may destroy a large area of renal parenchyma. Such foci may rupture into the calyces and renal pelvis with spread to the distal urinary tract. The renal lesions can also undergo suppuration, giving rise to the typical finding of **sterile pyuria**.

The kidney in systemic disease

Renal involvement in a variety of systemic disorders is common and often results in considerable morbidity and mortality.

Diabetes mellitus

Renal disease in diabetes mellitus may be due to:

- severe **atheroma** of the renal arteries leading to hypertension or ischaemia
- **pyelonephritis**: diabetic patients are more susceptible to infection
- **renal papillary necrosis**, often related to infection
- **diabetic glomerulopathy**.

DIABETIC GLOMERULOPATHY

Glomerular involvement leads to proteinuria or the nephrotic syndrome and eventually to chronic renal failure. In early onset diabetics, glomerular disease is often more severe. A variety of histological changes may be seen in affected glomeruli. The most important are:

- **hyaline thickening** of afferent and efferent arterioles
- increased mesangial matrix and capillary wall thickening, known collectively as **diffuse glomerulosclerosis**
- rounded hyaline nodules at the periphery of glomerular tufts, known as **Kimmelstiel–Wilson lesions** (Fig. 13.14).

Proteinuria in diabetic glomerulosclerosis is related to increased permeability of the glomerular basement membrane. The pathogenesis of this is poorly understood, but may be partly related to the altered anionic properties of basement membranes due to hyperglycaemia.

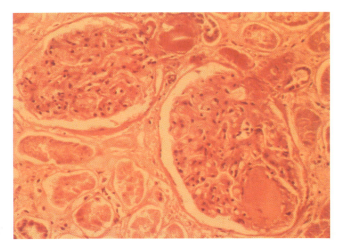
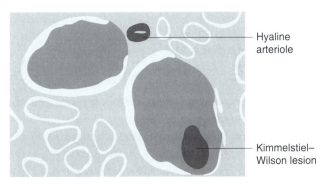

Hyaline arteriole

Kimmelstiel–Wilson lesion

Fig. 13.14 Diabetic glomerulosclerosis: note nodular (Kimmelstiel–Wilson) lesion and hyaline arteriolar change.

Amyloidosis

Amyloid is a proteinaceous material derived from plasma proteins (see Chapter 6). Deposition of amyloid in the kidney is associated with chronic inflammatory conditions (for example rheumatoid disease) and plasma cell dyscrasias, of which multiple myeloma is the most common. Amyloid is deposited in extracellular sites and in basement membranes (Fig. 13.15). In the kidney, proteinuria and the nephrotic syndrome are presenting features. Special histochemical stains such as Congo red highlight amyloid deposits in renal biopsies.

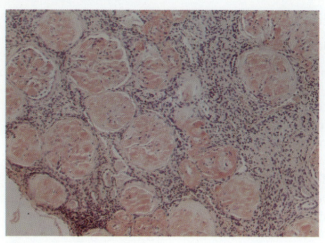
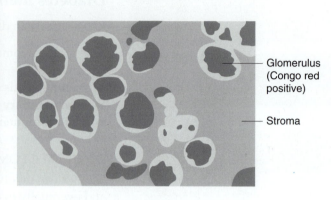

Glomerulus
(Congo red
positive)

Stroma

Fig. 13.15   Extensive glomerular amyloid deposition (Congo red stain).

Multiple myeloma

The degree of renal involvement in multiple myeloma is important in prognosis. There are several ways in which myeloma may involve the kidney.

Systemic lupus erythematosus

Renal disease is common, but of variable severity in this disease which is fully described in Chapter 7. Renal involvement may manifest as proliferative glomerulonephritis (diffuse and focal) or membranous glomerulonephritis. Different patterns of glomerular disease may be seen in any one case.

Infective endocarditis

Renal manifestations of infective endocarditis (see Chapter 8) include:

- wedge-shaped infarcts due to emboli from crumbling vegetations on cardiac valves
- immune complex-related glomerulonephritis (focal or diffuse).

Vascular disorders

Vascular disorders are discussed in detail in Chapter 8.

SYSTEMIC VASCULITIS

Polyarteritis nodosa

Polyarteritis nodosa (PAN) typically affects medium-sized or small arteries, but there is also a microscopic variant in the kidney involving arterioles and capillaries. Glomerular lesions include acute necrotizing or crescentic glomerulonephritis, and such severe glomerular disease often results in acute renal failure (Fig. 13.16).

Wegener's granulomatosis

Wegener's granulomatosis is a vasculitic disease typically affecting the upper respiratory tract and the kidney. Renal involvement is of variable

---

Renal invovment in multiple myeloma
- Deposition of amyloid
- Infection due to bone marrow suppression
- Myeloma kidney: casts of precipitated Bence Jones protein (immunoglobulin light chains overproduced by the myeloma cells) obstruct tubules and result in acute renal failure
- Hypercalcaemia leading to nephrocalcinosis and renal calculi
- Infiltration by neoplastic plasma cells

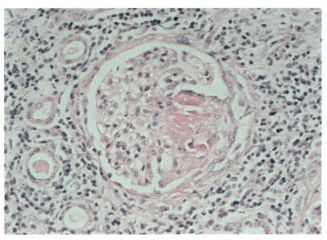 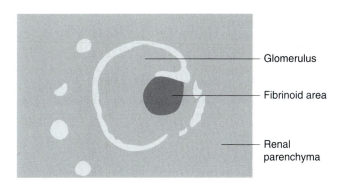

Fig. 13.16   Segmental necrotizing glomerulonephritis in systemic vasculitis.

severity, but histologically resembles PAN in more severe cases. Both PAN and Wegener's granulomatosis may respond well to immunosuppressive therapy.

THROMBOTIC DISORDERS

Thrombotic disorders include:

- haemolytic–uraemic syndrome (HUS)
- disseminated intravascular coagulation (DIC)
- idiopathic thrombocytopenic purpura (ITP).

Renal impairment due to these haematological conditions is often severe. The typical histological feature in these conditions is the presence of platelet and fibrin thrombi in arteriole and capillary lumina.

HYPERTENSION

The vascular changes in hypertension are discussed in Chapter 8. Systemic hypertension and renal failure are closely related. Primary renal failure often results in hypertension and, conversely, primary systemic hypertension has secondary renal manifestations.

- In **benign (essential) hypertension**, the renal damage is usually mild and renal function is at the most only slightly impaired. The most important histological change is **hyaline arteriolosclerosis** of afferent arterioles. Ischaemic damage of affected nephrons eventually results in glomerular sclerosis, but most glomeruli appear normal.
- In **accelerated (malignant) hypertension**, renal damage is more severe. Fibrinoid necrosis affects smaller arteries and afferent arterioles, often involving part of the glomerular tuft. Renal failure commonly follows.

INFARCTION

- **Emboli** may arise from atheromatous plaques, from thrombosis in cardiac chambers, or from crumbling valvular vegetations in infective endocarditis. Typical wedge-shaped infarcts are seen in the kidney.
- **Cortical necrosis**: patchy, but often extensive necrosis of the renal cortex is associated with complications of pregancy (such as pre-eclampsia) and with severe shock. It leads to acute renal failure and outcome depends on the extent of cortical involvement. The medulla is not involved.

Tumours of the kidney

Benign tumours

These are not uncommon but are rarely clinically significant.

FIBROMA

The commonest benign tumour is fibroma, which is often found incidentally at postmortem examination. They are usually located in the medulla and rarely exceed 10 mm in diameter.

CORTICAL ADENOMA

Cortical adenomas have similar macroscopic and histological appearances to renal cell carcinoma. Cortical tumours of this type less than 3 cm in size are generally regarded as benign, although this criterion must be arbitrary because early carcinomas may be of similar size.

ANGIOMYOLIPOMA

Angiomyolipoma is a distinctive lesion composed of mature fat, muscle and blood vessels. It may represent a hamartoma rather than a true neoplasm. It is often associated with tuberous sclerosis, one of the phakomatoses, but sporadic cases do occur.

OTHER BENIGN TUMOURS

Other benign renal tumours include angiomas and a renin-producing tumour of juxtaglomerular cells, which is a very rare cause of systemic hypertension.

Malignant tumours

RENAL CELL CARCINOMA

The case study on page 321 highlights several important features of renal cell carcinoma (also known as **hypernephroma** or **Grawitz's tumour**).

Wilms' tumour (nephroblastoma)

Nephroblastoma is one of the commoner solid paediatric malignant tumours. The majority occur in the first 10 years of life, although it is relatively rare in infancy. Occasional cases occur in adolescents and young adults. The tumour usually presents as a palpable abdominal mass. Hypertension and haematuria are also common features.

The histological appearance is extremely variable and several subtypes are recognized and can relate to prognosis. The classic appearance is that of a 'triphasic' tumour with admixture of primitive blastema, tubules and mesenchymal stroma. The tumour metastasizes predominantly to lungs and invasion of the renal vein is common. However, the prognosis of Wilms' tumour has considerably improved in recent years due to advances in therapeutic regimens including surgery, radiotherapy and chemotherapy.

Carcinoma of renal pelvis

TRANSITIONAL CELL CARCINOMAS

The pathological features of these tumours are identical to bladder

Features of renal cell carcinoma
- The most common presenting features are haematuria, loin pain and a palpable abdominal mass.
- Metastatic spread has often occurred at presentation, particularly to lung and bone.
- Cannonball lung metastases are a typical feature.
- Paraneoplastic phenomena may occur. In this case the high haemoglobin level is related to production of an erythropoietin-like substance by the tumour. Secretion of parathyroid hormone, renin and glucocorticoids has been described.
- Renal vein involvement is common.
- Prognosis is difficult to predict but if the tumour is confined to the kidney without renal vein involvement or metastatic spread up to 75% of patients survive 5 years.
- Increased incidence of renal cell carcinoma is found in tobacco smokers and in Von Hippel–Lindau disease.

CASE STUDY 13.2

A 55-year-old man presented to his general practitioner with a six-week history of right-sided loin pain, weight loss, lethargy and dyspnoea. He also said his urine had been 'discoloured' for some time. Physical examination revealed the suspicion of a right-sided abdominal mass and urinalysis confirmed the presence of blood in the urine. He was referred to hospital for further assessment. Haematological investigations showed a haemoglobin level of 19 g/dl and a chest radiograph revealed multiple cannonball-like lesions in both lungs. A mass was identified in the right kidney by ultrasound examination. At laparotomy, a tumour was confirmed in the right kidney. The tumour appeared well circumscribed but the renal vein was firm and dilated. Enlarged para-aortic lymph nodes were also noted.

A right nephrectomy and lymph node biopsy were performed. The cut surface of the kidney showed a 12 cm apparently well-circumscribed tumour with a yellowish, partly necrotic and haemorrhagic appearance (Fig. 13.17). A bulbous extension into the renal vein was seen. Histologically the tumour forms nests of cells with distinctive clear cytoplasm (clear cell carcinoma), separated by a fine connective tissue stroma (Fig. 13.18). The lymph node biopsy showed metastatic tumour of similar appearance.

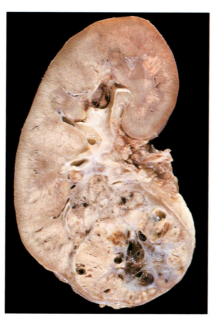

Fig. 13.17   Renal cell carcinoma: note typical yellow colour.

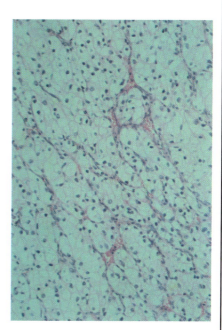

Fig. 13.18   Renal cell carcinoma with clear cell pattern.

---

transitional cell tumours discussed later in this chapter. They constitute up to 10% of malignant primary renal tumours. Haematuria is the commonest presenting symptom but the tumours are often infiltrative and advanced at this stage. Cytological examination of the urine may detect these tumours at an earlier stage.

SQUAMOUS CELL CARCINOMAS

Squamous cell carcinomas are rarer than transitional cell carcinomas and are often associated with calculi in the pelvicalyceal system.

Ureters and bladder

Congenital disorders

Ureters may be double (bifid), but this rarely leads to functional abnormalities.

VESICOURETERIC REFLUX

Abnormality of the course of the distal ureter through the bladder's muscular wall can give rise to vesicoureteric reflux. Micturition leads reflux of urine from the bladder into the proximal urinary tract, with the risk of renal infection and subsequent scarring.

EXSTROPHY

Exstrophy or extroversion of the bladder arises due to failure of development of the anterior bladder wall and the overlying abdominal wall. The ureters open onto the exposed posterior wall mucosa which is prone to infection, metaplastic change and increased risk of malignancy in the long term (adenocarcinoma).

URACHAL REMNANTS

Remnants of the urachal tract in the bladder dome may result in the development of adenocarcinoma. Complete persistence of the urachal tract may lead to the formation of a fistula opening at the umbilicus.

POSTERIOR URETHRAL VALVES

Congenital bladder outlet obstruction is usually caused by posterior urethral valves in male infants.

DIVERTICULA OF THE BLADDER

There may be congenital or aquired secondary to outflow obstruction (see Chapter 14).

Inflammation and infection: cystitis

COLIFORM BLADDER INFECTION

Bladder inflammation usually occurs in relation to urinary tract infection. This is commoner in women and presenting symptoms include urinary frequency, pain on micturition (dysuria) and haematuria. Coliform organisms, particularly *E. coli*, are the most frequent causes of bladder infection. Ascending infection may lead to ureteric inflammation and pyelonephritis.

OTHER BLADDER INFECTIONS

Other forms of infective cystitis include **tuberculosis**. The source of tubercle bacilli is most often rupture of caseous foci in the proximal urinary tract. Chronic bladder tuberculosis may lead to fibrosis and obstruction of ureteric orifices. Bladder involvement in **schistosomiasis** (*Schistosoma haematobium*) is important in endemic areas (Fig. 13.19). The parasitic infestation leads to a granulomatous inflammatory reaction with subsequent fibrosis and increased susceptibility to bladder tumours, particularly squamous cell carcinoma.

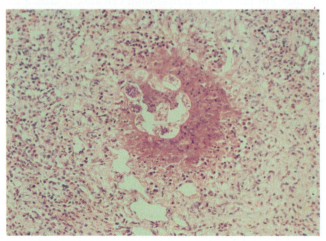
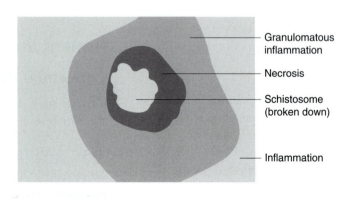

Granulomatous inflammation

Necrosis

Schistosome (broken down)

Inflammation

Fig. 13.19   Bladder schistosomiasis: note intense granulomatous inflammatory response to schistosome eggs.

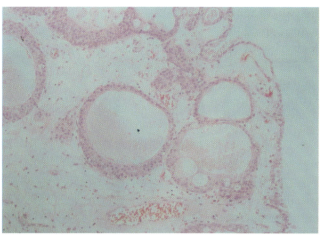

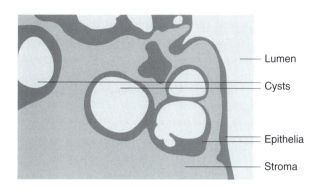

Fig. 13.20 Cystitis cystica.

CYSTITIS CYSTICA

Cystitis cystica results from chronic bladder inflammation. Small islands of transitional cells separate from the surface epithelium and give rise to cystic swellings which may be confused with tumours (Fig 13.20). Similar changes may occur in the ureter (**urethritis cystica**). In some cases there may be colonic-type glandular metaplasia in the cyst lining, known as **cystitis glandularis**.

MALAKOPLAKIA

Malakoplakia is a rare condition also associated with chronic cystitis. Cystoscopy reveals yellowish mucosal plaques which may clinically resemble bladder tumours. Histologically there is a mixed inflammatory infiltrate including macrophages which contain calcified inclusions called **Michaelis–Gutmann bodies**. A defective host response to chronic infective cystitis is the probable pathogenic mechanism.

INTERSTITAL CYSTITIS

Also known as **Hunner's ulcer**, interstitial cystitis is an inflammatory condition seen largely in middle-aged women. Its aetiology is uncertain.

Urinary tract obstruction

Obstruction of the ureters and bladder outlet are common clinical occurrences (Table 13.1). Acute ureteric obstruction is usually due to

Table 13.1   Causes of ureteric and bladder obstruction

Ureteric obstruction	
Luminal	Calculus, blood clot
Mural	Tumours (transitional cell carcinoma), strictures
Extrinsic	Advanced pelvic/abdominal tumours, pregnancy, congenital abnormalities, retroperitoneal fibrosis

Bladder obstruction	
Bladder	Tumours, neurogenic bladder, calculi
Prostate	Benign hyperplasia, cancer
Urethra	Strictures, posterior urethral valves, tumours

impaction of a calculus or blood clot, resulting in the severe pain of renal colic. The most common sites of impaction are the pelvic–ureteric junction, the pelvic brim and the distal ureter at the bladder wall. More chronic or intermittent obstruction may lead to hydronephrosis.

In men, bladder outlet obstruction is most commonly a result of prostatic disease. Chronic obstruction leads to smooth muscle hypertrophy with a typical pattern of trabeculation. This may result in the formation of diverticula (Fig. 13.21).

Bladder calculi

Calculi forming in the kidney may pass down the ureter into the bladder. Most disintegrate or are passed through the urethra, but some impact in the bladder and may grow to a considerable size within it (Fig. 13.22). Calculus formation in the bladder may occur in a diverticulum or in association with outlet obstruction and chronic inflammation. Many bladder calculi are asymptomatic, but they can cause chronic urinary frequency and dysuria with predisposition to infection. In the long term there is increased susceptibility to squamous carcinoma.

Bladder tumours

Tumours arising in the bladder epithelial lining are common. Most are transitional cell carcinomas, but squamous carcinomas and adeno-carcinomas occur.

TRANSITIONAL CELL CARCINOMA

Transitional cell carcinoma can arise from any part of the urinary tract lined by urothelium, from the renal pelvis to the bladder outlet. They are often multiple, reflecting widespread susceptibility to tumour formation (field change) within the urothelium. The commonest presenting symptom is painless haematuria. Most urothelial tumours have a papillary configuration (Fig. 13.23), but solid variants occur, particularly in higher-grade tumours (Fig. 13.24). Areas of squamous or glandular differentiation may be seen in otherwise recognizably transitional tumours.

The prognosis of bladder carcinoma is related to:

- **grade**: the degree of cytological differentiation, assessed histologically as grade I–III
- **stage**: the extent of invasion through the bladder wall.

In addition to papillary tumours, carcinoma in situ may be seen in adjacent flat mucosa or in some bladders with no identifiable tumour on cystoscopy. This change is often multifocal and carries a considerable risk of subseqent invasive malignancy.

SQUAMOUS CELL CARCINOMA

Pure squamous carcinomas are usually seen in association with bladder calculi or chronic schistosomiasis. Chronic mucosal inflammation and irritation lead to squamous metaplasia and dysplasia from which squamous carcinoma then arises. Histologically, these tumours are similar to those occurring elsewhere and carry a poor prognosis.

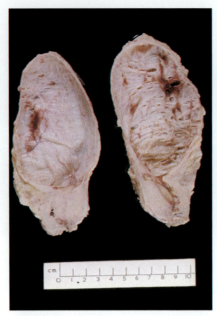

Fig. 13.21   Chronic bladder outlet obstruction resulting in hypertrophy of the bladder wall muscle seen as trabeculation in the mucosal surface.

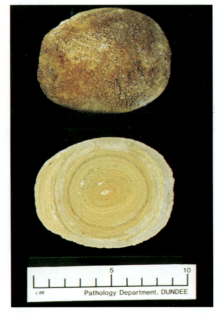

Fig. 13.22   Bladder calculi: these may be large.

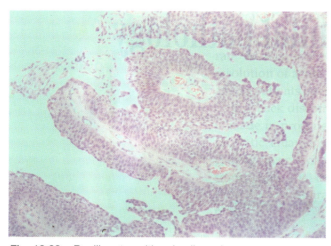

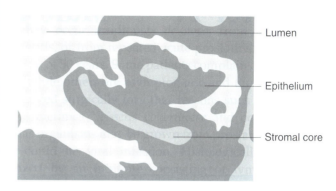

Lumen

Epithelium

Stromal core

Fig. 13.23   Papillary transitional cell carcinoma.

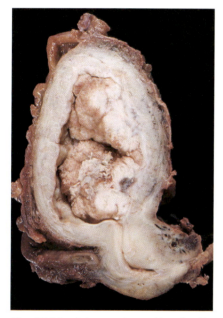

Fig. 13.24   Advanced transitional cell carcinoma of the bladder, filling almost the entire lumen.

> **Bladder carcinomas: aetiological agents**
> - **Industrial chemicals**: rubber, plastic and textile industries. Aniline dye derivatives such as β-naphthylamine are particularly implicated in the causation of transitional cell carcinomas.
> - **Cigarette smoking** (transitional cell carcinoma).
> - **Analgesic abuse** (transitional cell carcinoma of renal pelvis).
> - **Bladder calculi and schistosomiasis** (squamous carcinoma).

ADENOCARCINOMA

Adenocarcinoma of the bladder is relatively rare, but may arise from urachal remnants in the dome of the bladder, from bladders with cystitis cystica and cystitis glandularis, or in bladder exstrophy.

NON-EPITHELIAL TUMOURS

A variety of benign and malignant non-epithelial (mesenchymal) tumours may occur rarely in the bladder. The most important of these is **rhabdomyosarcoma**. While this can occur at any age, the childhood variant is the commonest paediatric bladder malignancy. This usually takes the form of oedematous polypoid mucosal lesions which have a grape-like appearance, hence the name **sarcoma botyroides**.

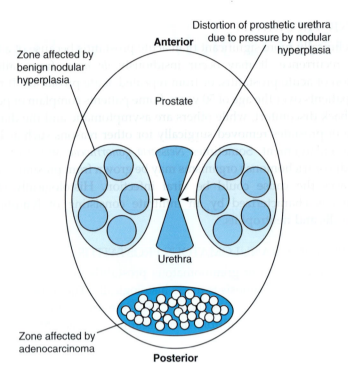

Fig. 14.1 Zones affected by benign nodular hyperplasia and adenocarcinoma of the prostate. In nodular hyperplasia, the nodules compress the urethra causing obstruction. The adenocarcinoma usually arises from the periphery of the gland posteriorly.

MORPHOLOGY

The middle lobe of the prostate in benign enlargement is most commonly affected, in contrast to carcinoma where the posterior lobe is affected (Fig. 14.1). The early changes occur in the areas surrounding the proximal part of the prostatic urethra. The enlarged prostate may medially compress the urethral lumen, causing obstruction. The lateral and posterior parts eventually compress the normal surrounding prostate. On cross-section, the gland appears to consist of multiple well-defined nodules, which are white–grey in colour. Cystic changes may be seen. Sometimes areas of haemorrhage and infarction may also be present (Fig. 14.2). In some cases the middle lobe assumes a polypoid slender structure which may bulge into the urethra and bladder neck region.

HISTOLOGY

The changes are mainly due to a combination of two processes, including hyperplasia of the epithelial elements in the glands and hypertrophy of stroma and smooth muscle. There is an increase in the number of glands which are lined by hyperplastic columnar or cuboidal epithelium thrown up into papillary structures (Fig. 14.3). A second layer of myoepithelial cells is seen lining the outer part of the glands. This layer is absent in adenocarcinoma. There is hypertrophy of smooth muscle fibres which usually surround the glands in a concentric manner.

COMPLICATIONS

The complications related to prostatic hyperplasia are mainly related to pressure on the prostatic urethra causing obstruction. This will increase pressure in the bladder during micturition, leading to hypertrophy of the detrusor muscles, with the end result of thickening the bladder wall. The lining of the bladder will first become trabecular, followed by herniation of the mucosa through the hypertrophied muscle fibres, forming diverticula

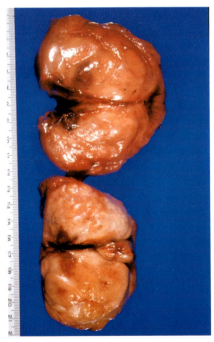

Fig. 14.2 Nodular hyperplasia of prostate. The cut surface shows well-defined nodules of various sizes.

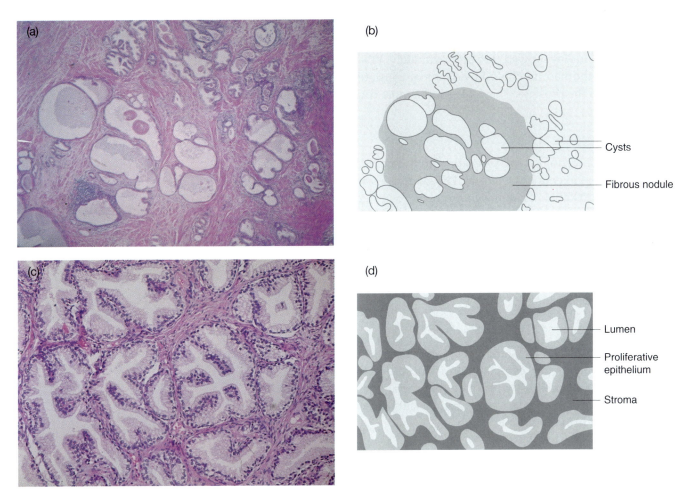

Fig. 14.3 Benign nodular hyperplasia of prostate: (a, b) cystic changes in glands; (c, d) proliferating glands lined by epithelial and myoepithelial cells.

(Fig. 14.4). Once these are formed, they are difficult to empty and accordingly stagnation of urine and infection may occur.

Increasing pressure in the bladder also causes increased pressure in the ureters and renal pelvis, resulting in hydroureters, hydronephrosis and ultimately impairment of renal function in severe cases.

CLINICAL FEATURES

The symptoms of prostatic hyperplasia are mainly related to urethral obstruction and increased pressure in the bladder. Patients present with frequency, dysuria, dribbling, and difficulty in starting and stopping micturition. Sometimes they may present with acute retention of urine. Treatment depends upon relief of the obstructing portion of the prostate by transurethral resection.

Prostatic adenocarcinoma

Prostatic carcinomas are among the commonest cancers of males in developed countries, usually only exceeded by carcinomas of the bronchus. The incidence is rare before the age of 50 years, and increases with age. Prostate cancer is responsible for approximately 3% of all deaths over the age of 55 years. Approximately 70% of clinically apparent prostatic carcinomas are in patients aged 60–79 years.

The term **latent carcinoma** is used for clinically undetectable carcinomas. This constitutes about 70% of all prostatic carcinomas. Postmortem studies showed that approximately 30% of men over the age of 50 years who had no clinical evidence of prostate cancer have foci of cancer within the prostate. This makes it the most common malignancy of human organs.

AETIOLOGY

Although the aetiology of prostatic carcinoma is unknown, there is special interest in endocrine effects. The evidence for that comes from the absence of prostatic carcinoma in eunuchs castrated before puberty, in contrast to postpubertal castration, and the responsiveness of metastatic disease to therapeutic castration or exogenous oestrogen. The incidence is also low in patients with hyperoestrogenism due to liver cirrhosis. Unfortunately, higher levels of serum androgens in patients with prostatic carcinoma have not been demonstrated and the pathogenesis remains unclear.

MORPHOLOGY

The commonest site of prostatic carcinoma is the periphery of the gland, in the subcapsular region, especially on its posterior aspect (see Fig. 14.1). This makes it possible to palpate by rectal examination. Prostatic carcinomas are usually multicentric and the cut surface of the gland shows yellow–white firm induration.

MICROSCOPY

Ninety-eight per cent of malignant prostatic tumours are adenocarcinomas (Fig. 14.5). Pathological diagnosis of prostatic carcinoma is based on nuclear anaplasia, architectural disturbance and invasion. The nuclei are usually larger than those of benign cells, but are generally uniform, with prominent nucleoli. Tumours may show a spectrum of differentiation varying from well-differentiated tumours to anaplastic poorly differentiated ones. Characteristically the best-differentiated tumours show well-formed glands of different sizes lined by single layer of neoplastic epithelial cells. Sometimes larger glands with a papillary or cribriform pattern may be seen. In less well-differentiated tumours the glands show increase variation in size and shape and epithelial proliferation. On the other side of the spectrum the tumour may be formed of single cells or sheets of cells without glandular differentiation. Different patterns are often present together in the same tumour. Invasion may be stromal, perineural, vascular or lymphatic.

CLINICAL FEATURES

Many patients present only with outflow obstruction. Rectal examination usually reveals an indurated area in the prostate. Sometimes the tumour is found accidentally when a prostatic specimen is removed and examined histologically. Other tumours may present with distant metastasis. These are usually bone metastases, giving rise to bone pain. The tumour may encircle the rectum by local spread and the patient may then present with intestinal obstruction. Patients may also present with uraemia or other symptoms due to infiltration and obstruction of the ureters.

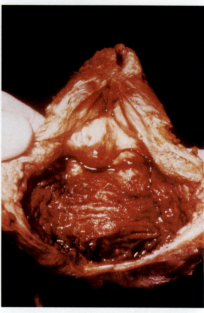

Fig. 14.4   Benign nodular hyperplasia of prostate. The enlarged prostate partially obstructing the urethra, causing muscular hypertrophy with increased mucosal trabeculation of the bladder wall.

Spread of prostate cancer
- **Local spread**: because of the common site of the tumour near the capsule, there is high frequency of capsular invasion. The tumour may also invade into the rectum posteriorly. Invasion into bladder neck and bladder may also take place
- **Perineural invasion**: this represents contiguous invasion of tumour along the nerve fibres
- **Haematogenous spread**: multiple metastasis to bone, lung and liver is common. Bony metastases are usually osteoblastic
- **Lymphatic spread**: usually to the pelvic lymph nodes

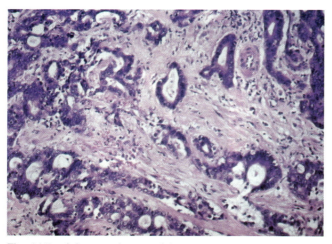 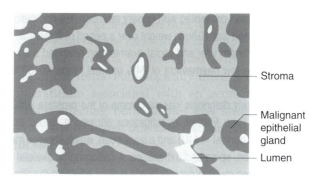

Stroma

Malignant
epithelial
gland

Lumen

Fig. 14.5 Adenocarcinoma of the prostate.

Staging of prostatic carcinoma
- **Stage A**: are incidental or clinically unsuspected cancers, detected in tissue removed for outflow obstruction (25% of patients)
- **Stage B**: tumours palpable by rectal digital examination but confined to prostate (30% of patients)
- **Stage C**: tumours have extended locally beyond the prostate, but have not produced clinically evident metastasis (15% of patients)
- **Stage D**: tumours with distant metastasis (30% of patients)

GRADING AND STAGING

Grading of prostatic carcinoma is based on degree of glandular differentiation, pattern of growth and nuclear anaplasia. There are four stages of prostatic carcinoma (see box). Prognosis is related to both stage and grade. The 5-year survival in stage A with a good grade of disease is about 85%, in comparison to stage C disease with poorly differentiated tumour, in whom the 5-year survival is about 15%.

MANAGEMENT

Management choice for prostatic carcinoma depends on grade and stage of tumour and age of patient. In general treatment may include prostatic surgical resection, radiotherapy or hormone treatment. Hormone therapy usually involves removal of androgen by either orchidectomy or oestrogen therapy.

OTHER TUMOURS OF THE PROSTATE

Other types of malignant tumours may arise in the prostate. **Transitional cell carcinoma** may either arise as a primary tumour in prostatic ducts, or spread from bladder. **Rhabdomyosarcoma** and **leiomyosarcoma** are uncommon soft tissue tumours of prostate which are highly malignant.

Diagnosis of prostatic adenocarcinoma
- Digital rectal examination
- Prostate-specific antigen (PSA) is a product of prostatic epithelium. Elevated levels of PSA occur in association with localized as well as advanced cancer. Serum levels of PSA are also raised in benign prostatic hyperplasia and some inflammatory conditions, although to a lesser extent.
- Prostatic acid phosphatase is produced by both normal and malignant epithelium. Increased serum levels of serum acid phosphatase are found only in cancers which have spread beyond the capsule or metastasized and is a useful marker of response to treatment
- Bone scan and radiography may show multiple osteoblastic lesions in the skeleton indicating metastatic disease
- Transrectal prostatic biopsy by aspiration or Tru-Cut needle biopsy (Fig. 14.6) to obtain cells/tissue for cytology/histology

Fig. 14.6 Tru-Cut needle.

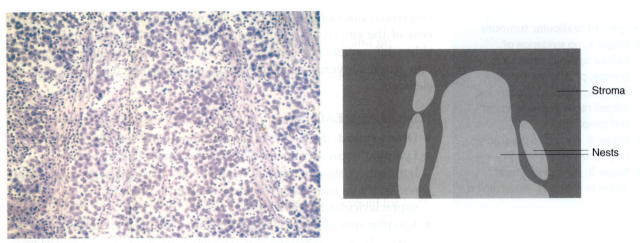

Fig. 14.9   Classic seminoma. The cells are present in nests, separated by fibrous septa with numerous lymphocytes.

Spermatocytic seminoma

This usually occurs in an older age group than seminoma – above the age of 50 years. Microscopically the cells are larger in size in comparison to those of typical seminoma, without a fibrovascular stroma and lymphocytic cell infiltrate. The prognosis is usually excellent.

Embryonal carcinoma

This tumour occurs in a younger age group than seminoma, usually within an age range of 20–35 years. It accounts for about 15% of all testicular germ cell tumours. The tumours are more likely to be clinically evident at an early stage, before becoming too large, due to testicular pain or early metastatic spread.

Macroscopically, cut section of the tumour shows a variegated surface, which is poorly demarcated from the testicular tissue, greyish in colour and containing areas of necrosis and haemorrhage.

Microscopically, the tumour consists of poorly differentiated pleomorphic epithelial cells with an ill-defined cell border, containing oval large nuclei with big nucleoli. They often show frequent mitoses (Fig. 14.10). The tumour cells can be arranged in solid sheets, glandular or tubular structures. Areas of haemorrhage and necrosis are common. Immunohistochemical stains show positivity for placental alkaline phosphatase and cytokeratins in both primary and metastatic tumours.

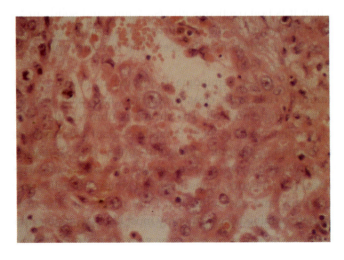

Fig. 14.10   Embryonal carcinoma. Sheets of poorly differentiated carcinoma. The cells show no distinct cell membranes.

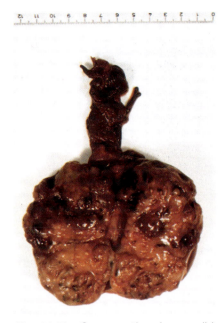

Fig. 14.11 Cross-section shows solid tumour containing multiple cysts associated with areas of necrosis and haemorrhage. Compare this with the much more uniform appearance of the seminoma in Fig. 14.8.

Metastasis is by both haematogenous and lymphatic spread to para-aortic lymph nodes, with lung and liver being the most common sites for haematogenous spread. The prognosis used to be bad for embryonal carcinoma, but with advances in combined chemotherapy, the prognosis has improved significantly. The 5-year survival rate is about 80%.

Teratoma

Teratoma accounts for about 30% of all testicular germ cell tumours. In general they occur in younger age groups with a few cases in early childhood. The peak incidence is in the 20s and there is a marked drop in the 40s. They are characterized by tissues with elements from the three germinal layers, including ectoderm, mesoderm and endoderm. These are present in different proportions.

Macroscopically, the tumour is formed of multicystic spaces alternating with solid areas, causing nodular enlargement of the testes. Areas of haemorrhage and necrosis may be present (Fig. 14.11).

Microscopically, teratomas are subdivided into mature teratoma, immature teratoma and teratoma with malignant transformation on the basis of their histology.

- **Mature teratomas** consist of well-differentiated tissue which may represent mature squamous, respiratory, gastrointestinal epithelium, cartilage, neural tissue, muscle and bone. All these elements are organized in organoid fashion simulating tissues such as gastric glands, respiratory epithelium, prostate, etc. (Fig. 14.12).
- **Immature teratomas** are teratomas where the elements of the three germ cell layers are incompletely developed and not arranged in organoid fashion. They are usually represented by a mixture of mature and immature elements.
- **Teratoma with malignant transformation** is characterized by the presence of one element of a mature teratoma which has undergone malignant change, such as the squamous epithelium showing changes of squamous cell carcinoma. Elements from other germ cell tumours could be present such as seminoma, embryonal carcinoma, yolk sac tumour or choriocarcinoma as part of the mixed germ cell tumours.

Metastases through lymphatics or blood vessels can take place to lymph nodes and different organs. The metastases can be formed of either

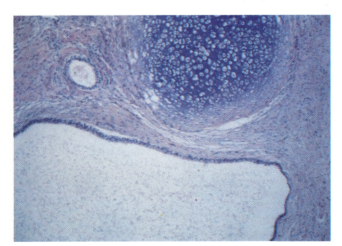

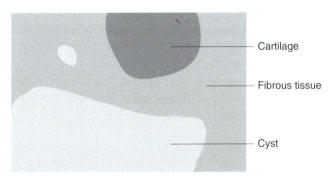

Cartilage

Fibrous tissue

Cyst

Fig. 14.12 Mature teratoma containing cartilage with cystic spaces lined by cuboidal epithelium.

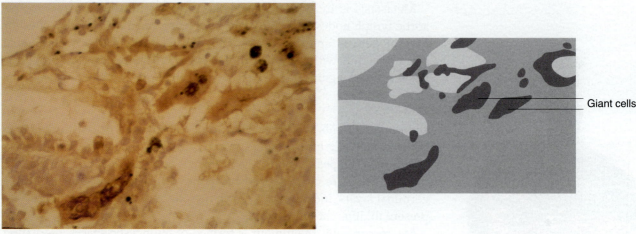

Giant cells

Fig. 14.13   Syncytiotrophoblastic giant cells from a choriocarcinoma stained positively (brown) for β-hCG by immunocytochemistry.

mature or immature elements, or both. Five-year survival after chemotherapy is about 92% in mature teratomas and 74% in immature teratoma.

Choriocarcinoma

Primary choriocarcinomas are extremely rare as primary tumours of the testis. It is more frequent to observe choriocarcinoma elements as a component in a mixed germ cell tumour. In addition, giant cells of syncytiotrophoblast type can be seen in seminoma or non-seminomatous germ cell tumours (Fig. 14.13).

Pure choriocarcinomas form only about 1% of all testicular germ cell tumours and occurs between the ages of 15 and 25 years. Most patients present with symptoms related to metastases, or with testicular enlargement. Some patients have gynaecomastia. Usually both serum and urine levels of β-hCG are high.

Pathologically the tumour consists of two types of cells: the syncytiotrophoblast and cytotrophoblast. Areas of haemorrhage and necrosis are present, and other elements of germ cell tumours may be seen. Usually immunohistochemical stains for β-hCG are positive (see Fig. 14.13). Usually these tumours invade early via blood vessels and spread to organs such as lung and brain. Prognosis is poor, with a 5-year survival of only about 18%.

Yolk sac tumour

Most of these primary tumours occur in infants and young children. In adults the pure form is rare and usually the tumour is part of a mixed germ cell tumour. Usually they are associated with raised serum α-fetoprotein (AFP). Pathologically, the tumour consists of multiple dilated tubular structures lined by flattened cells with intervening oedematous stroma. Immunohistochemical stains are positive for AFP.

Mixed germ cell tumour

Almost 60% of all testicular tumours are of more than one cell type. Mixtures of seminoma, embryonal carcinoma and teratomas can occur. All these tumours may also have either yolk sac elements or choriocarcinoma elements.

TUMOUR MARKERS

Tumour markers are hormones, proteins or enzymes formed by different types of germ cells. Using immunohistochemistry, it is relatively easy to document that there are cells expressing β-hCG, AFP and **placental alkaline phosphatase (PLAP)** on cell membranes in germ cell tumour tissue. They can also be measured in serum from patients with tumours, particularly if there are metastases.

Placental alkaline phosphatase can be demonstrated in seminomas and embryonal carcinomas, while β-hCG is usually demonstrated in tumours containing choriocarcinoma elements and in some seminomas with giant cells in the stroma. AFP is usually seen in tumours containing yolk sac elements. These markers could be used for diagnostic reasons and follow-up, especially to exclude recurrences.

CASE STUDY 14. 2

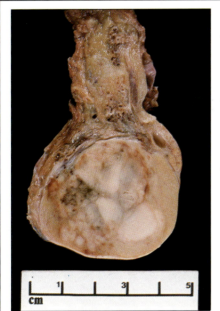

Fig. 14.14 Macroscopic view of the testicular tumour.

A 23-year-old man presented to his general practitioner with a swelling of his left testicle, associated with pain. There was no history of trauma. On examination he was found to have an enlarged left testicle, which was firm on palpation. There was no associated redness or oedema of the scrotum. In addition he was found to have gynaecomastia. The testicle was removed surgically. The specimen revealed replacement of the testis by a large tumour which weighed 100 g and measured 10 × 8 cm. The tumour was partly solid, partly cystic, with areas of haemorrhage and necrosis (Fig. 14.14).

Histology showed multiple cystic spaces, lined by respiratory, cuboidal and columnar type of epithelia. Areas of mature cartilage were seen. In areas the tumour was poorly differentiated with a high number of mitoses. Foci of necrosis and haemorrhage were noted with giant cells. The mature elements were in keeping with a mature teratoma while the poorly differentiated areas represented embryonal carcinoma. Special stains were performed for AFP, β-hCG and PLAP. The PLAP was positive in areas with embryonal cells, while β-hCG was positive in areas with the giant cells. The AFP was negative. This was therefore a mixed germ cell tumour, consisting of mature teratoma, embryonal carcinoma and areas of choriocarcinoma.

Further investigations including computed tomography, bone scan, chest radiograph and lymphogram were done to stage the tumour: all were negative in this case. Serum levels of β-hCG, AFP and PLAP were performed to confirm the diagnosis before surgery, and were repeated after surgery to ensure that there was no residual tumour. In this case the patient had raised levels of PLAP and β-hCG. The raised β-hCG level explains the presence of gynaecomastia. All of the investigations indicated that the tumour was limited to the testis. Accordingly this was stage 1 disease and the prognosis was very good with an expected 5-year survival of 85–90%.

MANAGEMENT

The therapy of testicular tumours depends largely on clinical stage and the histological type of tumour. The first step is to remove the tumour. Seminomas are radiosensitive and are usually treated by radiotherapy to para-aortic nodes if there is early stage disease. In stage 4 disease chemotherapy is also given.

Non-seminomas are treated as a group.

- In stage 1 disease orchidectomy with observation may be sufficient.
- In stage 2 disease, combination chemotherapy including bleomycin and vinblastine with radical removal of the retroperitoneal lymph nodes may give good results.
- In widespread disease chemotherapy and radiotherapy are recommended.

Non-germ cell tumours

SEX CORD TUMOURS

Sex cord tumours are rare tumours arising from the testicular stroma, and are usually not malignant. They account for approximately 2% of all testicular tumours. The two most important types are the Leydig cell and Sertoli cell tumours.

- **Leydig cell tumours** may produce testosterone resulting in precocious virilization.
- **Sertoli cell tumours** may secrete either oestrogen or androgens resulting in either precocious masculinization or feminization.

TESTICULAR LYMPHOMA

Lymphoma of the testis accounts for 5% of all testicular tumours and usually occurs in men above the age of 60 years. It generally involves the testis as part of generalized lymphoma, but in a few cases it may arise primarily in the testis.

ADENOMATOID TUMOURS OF THE EPIDIDYMIS

These benign tumours arise in the epididymis, and are of mesothelial origin. They present as a small well-demarcated mass in the epididymal region. They should be removed surgically to exclude malignancy.

OTHER TUMOURS

Tumours of the cord may cause scrotal swelling. These tumours are mainly of soft tissue origin, including lipomas, leiomyomas, liposarcomas, leiomyosarcomas and rhabdomyosarcomas.

Penis

Congenital abnormalities

Congenital abnormalities are uncommon in the penis. They include:

- **hypospadias**, in which the urethral opening is on the ventral surface of the glans penis
- **epispadias**, in which the urethral opening is on the dorsal surface of the glans penis
- **phimosis**, in which there is narrowing of the prepuce, which is difficult to retract over the glans penis. This is usually associated with chronic balanitis.

Other congenital abnormalities include agenesis, duplication, hypoplasia and congenital cysts.

Inflammation

PHIMOSIS

Inflammatory phimosis is more common than the congenital type. Histologically this is associated with oedema, and fibrosis and chronic inflammatory cell infiltrate affecting the upper dermis

BALANITIS

Balanitis is chronic inflammation of the glans, which is usually associated with inflammation of the prepuce, and is commonly associated with phimosis.

BALANITIS XEROTICA OBLITERANS

The unusual skin condition known as balanitis xerotica obliterans causes a whitish, irritating lesion around the prepuce and glans penis. The foreskin is thickened and shrunk, causing phimosis. The cause is unknown. It is associated with thinning of the epidermis, with basal layer degeneration, oedema and fibrosis of the upper dermis. It is similar to lichen sclerosus et atrophicus which affects mainly the vulva in females.

SEXUALLY TRANSMITTED DISEASES

Inflammation may also be caused by sexually transmitted conditions such as herpes, syphilis, granuloma inguinale and lymphogranuloma venereum.

Tumours

CONDYLOMA ACUMINATA

Condylomata acuminata are benign warts on the glans caused by transmissible infection by human papilloma virus. They are not premalignant and respond to treatment by podophyllin.

GIANT CONDYLOMA OR VERRUCOUS CARCINOMA

The giant condyloma or verrucous carcinoma is much larger than the condyloma acuminata. It is usually locally invasive and has tendency to recur. It is believed to be caused by a virus, such as human papilloma virus (hPV) 6 and 11 can be demonstrated. Macroscopically they are solitary fungating lesions which destroy the penis. Histology shows papillomatous thickening of the epidermis by cells with plenty of cytoplasm and small regular nuclei. No abnormal mitoses are seen. The tumour invades locally, but unlike squamous cell carcinoma it does not metastasize. Treatment is by wide local excision.

SQUAMOUS CELL CARCINOMA IN SITU (ERYTHROPLASIA OF QUEYRAT)

This in situ carcinoma mainly affects the glans penis and sometimes the prepuce. The patient presents with a well-demarcated, slightly raised, reddish shiny lesion. Histologically there is hyperkeratosis and thickening of the epidermis, with the presence of dysplastic cells and abnormal mitoses. The lesion is limited to the epidermis and there is often chronic inflammation in the upper dermis.

In about 5% of patients with carcinoma in situ, there is also an invasive squamous cell carcinoma. Treatment is by wide local excision.

SQUAMOUS CELL CARCINOMA OF THE PENIS

Carcinoma of the penis is a rare disease in Europe and the USA, accounting for about 0.5–1% of all malignancies in men. The incidence is much higher in African and south-east Asian countries, representing 12–20% of all male cancers. The disease is most prevalent in the age range of 40–70 years, and commoner in the lower socioeconomic groups.

Aetiology

Circumcision is an important factor in prevention of carcinoma of the penis, and the disease is very rare in cultures where ritual circumcision is

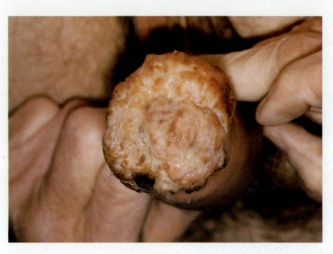

Fig. 14.15   A fungating squamous cell carcinoma of the shaft of the penis.

practised. However, there has been one case report of penile carcinoma in a young circumcised man in the recent literature. There is a definite association with poor personal hygiene, and the retention of smegma beneath the prepuce is thought to predispose to malignancy. There is also some evidence to suggest a possible association with hPV infection, types 16 and 18.

Macroscopically, the lesion may present as an ulcerated erythematous lesion, or as a fungating mass associated with phimosis and balanitis (Fig. 14.15). The urethra may be invaded, causing obstruction, and fistulae may develop.

Microscopically, the tumour is similar to squamous cell carcinoma that occurs in the skin. Usually they are well-differentiated keratinizing squamous cell carcinomas, but rarely they may be poorly differentiated.

Clinical course

Carcinoma of the penis is a slow-growing tumour, which usually spreads locally into the shaft of the glans penis and then via lymphatics to involve the inguinal and iliac lymph nodes. Vascular invasion is relatively late. Widespread metastasis is uncommon and usually seen in advanced cases. The prognosis depends mainly on the stage of the disease at diagnosis. In early stages, when the tumour is confined and not invading the shaft the 5-year survival is about 95%. If the stage of disease is advanced with lymph node involvement, then 5-survival is about 30% only. Treatment is usually amputation and radiotherapy.

Chapter 15   Female genital pathology

Learning objectives

To appeciate and understand:
- ❑ Diseases affecting the vulva and cervix, with emphasis on intraepithelial neoplasia
- ❑ Factors involved in endometrial disease, both benign and malignant
- ❑ Various types of ovarian disease, especially cysts and tumours
- ❑ Placental function, ectopic pregnancy, hydatidiform mole and choriocarcinoma

Developmental abnormalities

Congenital abnormalities of the female genital system can be classified by whether the patient has normal or abnormal chromosomes, gonads, genitalia and habitus. In patients with normal chromosomes, habitus and ovaries, congenital defects include failure of development or failure of fusion of the müllerian ducts. If partial, the latter results in a vagina and cervix with two uterine corpora forming two 'horns' (**uterus unicollis bicornis**) or, if more severe, a vagina with two cervices and corpora (**uterus bicollis bicornis**). Complete failure of fusion produces a uterus didelphys, the formation of two corpora and cervices and parts of two vaginas. Virilization of a female embryo can occur in congenital adrenal hyperplasia and other high androgen states, and result in ambiguous external and internal genitalia in the infant.

Women with Turner's syndrome have a deficiency of one X chromosome and have streak gonads. The genitalia are female but remain infantile. Some patients have an apparently normal female habitus but are chromosomally male: they have a defect in the metabolism or end-organ effect of testosterone called **androgen insensitivity syndrome**, which results in ambiguous external genitalia.

Vulva

The skin of the vulva is affected by the same diseases as the skin elsewhere in the body. Historically there has been some confusion in the terms used. For example, **lichenification** (in which the skin is thickened, roughened and hyperkeratotic) occurs commonly on the vulva. For a time, some of the types of lichenification were called **vulval dystrophies** as if they were specific to the vulva. This terminology is now obsolete, and the three main

---

Sex determination

There are six standpoints from which the sex of an individual can be defined:

- **Gonadal sex**: whether the gonads at birth are ovaries or testes
- **Chromosomal sex**: whether there is a Y chromosome or not
- **Genital sex**: whether the external and internal genitalia appear male or female
- **Phenotypic sex** other than that of genitalia: whether a person has the physique of a man or woman (may be important in patients with ambiguous genitalia)
- **Psychological sex**: whether the person behaves in a masculine or feminine way, and feels male or female
- **Assigned sex**: the sex that is decided upon by parents or carers, irrespective of the above

types of lichenification (lichen simplex, sclerosus and planus) are named as for the skin elsewhere.

Another obsolete term, leukoplakia, means a white patch and is a purely macroscopic description. The white appearance is produced largely by an increase in the thickness of keratin – the underlying condition can vary widely from lichen simplex to invasive carcinoma (Fig. 15.1).

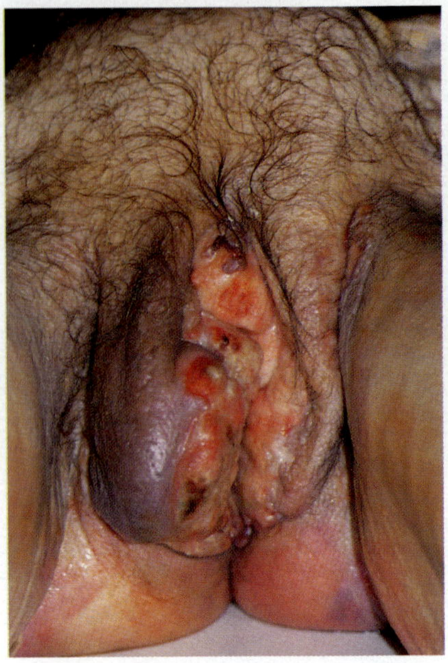

Lichen simplex, lichen sclerosus and lichen planus

All of these three conditions principally affect the labia majora. They all cause irregular white patches, which may spread on to the labia minora. The patient usually complains of pruritus, and ulceration with bleeding can develop.

Lichen simplex is also called squamous cell hyperplasia. There is epidermal thickening with a sparse chronic inflammatory cell infiltrate in the upper dermis. In **lichen planus** the infiltrate is denser and band-like. In **lichen sclerosus**, in contrast to the other two, the epidermis is thinner than normal but the overall thickness of the skin is increased because of accumulation of hyaline collagen in the dermis immediately below it. There is the typical band-like infiltrate of lymphocytes below this. When there is no evidence of cellular atypia, none of these conditions has significant premalignant potential.

Fig. 15.1 Squamous cell carcinoma of the vulva.

Benign neoplasms of the vulva

The commonest benign vulval tumour is **squamous cell papilloma**, which is usually related to human papilloma virus (hPV) infection. Other benign skin tumours such as neurofibroma, lipoma and haemangioma can also occur. A benign neoplasm of sweat glands, hidradenoma, is relatively common on the vulva and has the same features as this tumour elsewhere.

Vulval intraepithelial neoplasia

In most cases, vulval intraepithelial neoplasia (VIN) is graded in a similar fashion to cervical intraepithelial neoplasia (CIN), which is discussed later in this chapter.

In women between 40 and 60 years old, Bowen's disease may affect the vulva and may be termed **Bowenoid VIN**. This type of VIN is not graded. As in the cervix, papillomavirus infection in the epithelial cells is common and koilocytes may be found. Koilocytes (Greek *koilos*, a bubble) are large clear epithelial cells with crenated, hyperchromatic nuclei (see Fig. 15.7); they are not absolutely pathognomonic for hPV infection but are most commonly associated with this.

VIN may be associated with vaginal and cervical intraepithelial neoplasia, and when it is diagnosed it is important to examine the patient for these related conditions. Only a small percentage of women with VIN 3 progress to develop invasive carcinoma, but this is commoner in patients who are immunosuppressed and when the disease occurs on the perineum and clitoris.

Invasive carcinoma of the vulva

The commonest invasive neoplasm of the vulva is squamous cell carcinoma. Affected patients tend to be elderly, present late, and have large

> **Grading of vulval intraepithelial neoplasia**
> - **VIN 1**: only the lowest third of the epithelium is involved by the maturation abnormality, although its effects are evident throughout
> - **VIN 2**: the abnormality is confined to the lower two-thirds of the epithelium
> - **VIN 3**: more than two-thirds of the epithelium are involved

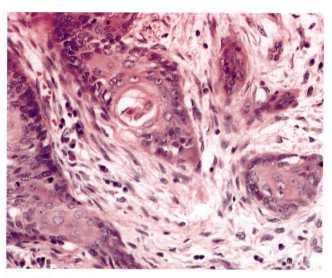

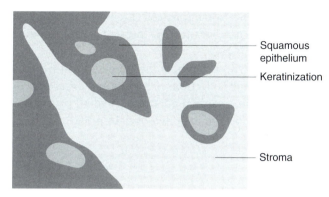

Squamous epithelium

Keratinization

Stroma

Fig. 15.2   Invasive islands of squamous cells in a moderately differentiated squamous cell carcinoma of vulva.

exophytic tumours that involve the labia, clitoris and perineum. Histologically the carcinoma is usually well or moderately differentiated (Fig. 15.2). Metastatic spread is to inguinal lymph nodes, and in advanced cases to iliac and lumbar nodes. When the tumour occurs in the region of the clitoris, spread to the pelvic nodes occurs earlier. The 5-year survival rate overall is good but falls steeply when the tumour is large or poorly differentiated, when the tumour arises on the clitoris or the perineum, and when the lymph nodes are involved.

Other malignant neoplasms of the vulva

Much rarer than squamous cell carcinoma are malignant melanoma and basal cell carcinoma. The features of these tumours on the vulva are similar to those occurring at other cutaneous sites. Adenocarcinoma may arise in Bartholin's gland and occasionally produces a clinical appearance on the vulva which is very similar to Paget's disease of the nipple, with an eczematoid, erythematous patch. Unlike in the breast, Paget's disease of the vulva is not always associated with a demonstrable underlying adenocarcinoma.

Vagina

Vaginal infections are common, especially in women in the reproductive years and women who have atrophic changes in the vagina after the menopause. Infecting organisms include *Chlamydia trachomatis*, *Candida albicans* and *Trichomonas vaginalis*. *Neisseria gonorrhoeae*, the gonococcus, does not involve the squamous epithelium of the vagina but infects the columnar epithelium of Bartholin's gland and the endocervix.

Neoplasms of the vagina

Vaginal intraepithelial neoplasia (graded as VAIN 1, 2 and 3) is diagnosed by the same criteria as basaloid VIN and CIN. Vaginal involvement by intraepithelial neoplasia is less common than cervical and vulval disease.

Squamous cell carcinoma rarely occurs in the vagina. When such a tumour is found, it is important to exclude spread to the vagina from the much commoner squamous cell carcinoma of the cervix or vulva. Patients with primary tumours tend to present late with widespread disease and the prognosis is poor.

In women whose mothers were treated with diethylstilboestrol during pregnancy, small collections of glands and cysts may develop in the wall of the vagina called **vaginal adenosis**. A small proportion of affected women develops adenocarcinoma in association with these.

Cervix

Normal anatomy and histology

The normal cervix is composed, in order from below, of:

- ectocervix
- external os
- endocervix
- internal os.

The ectocervical aspect is covered by stratified squamous non-keratinizing epithelium, and the canal by simple mucus-secreting columnar epithelium on the surface and in crypts.

The squamocolumnar junction does not have a constant position but moves under the influence of hormones, principally oestrogen. At puberty, the cervix enlarges. The glandular epithelium of the endocervix is everted and so exposed to the vaginal milieu. Squamous metaplasia occurs, and the squamocolumnar junction returns to around the site of the external os. This metaplastic squamous epithelium is called the **transition or transformation zone**. It is the site particularly affected by virus infection and neoplastic change. 'Erosion' of the cervix is almost always really eversion of the endocervical epithelium over the ectocervical face.

Cervical inflammation

Cervical inflammation may be acute or chronic, and may be non-specific or have a demonstrable cause. Acute cervicitis is uncommon. It may be caused by:

- *Neisseria gonorrhoeae*
- trauma
- parturition
- abortion
- pessaries.

Chronic cervicitis is much commoner than the acute form. It is usually non-specific but *Candida*, *Trichomonas* and *Chlamydia* spp. are relatively common causes. Tuberculosis of the cervix is common worldwide, and rarer causes include actinomycosis and cytomegalovirus infection.

Candida albicans is a very common pathogen in the lower female genital tract. The presence of fungi in the vagina or ectocervix is in itself not indicative of a pathological state. Candidiasis is seen often in the later stages of pregnancy, in diabetic patients and in patients treated with steroids or prolonged antibiotic therapy. *Trichomonas vaginalis* is a very common genital infection, affecting up to 20% of women in the sexually active period. Patients complain of a frothy yellow or green discharge with an unpleasant odour.

Chlamydia trachomatis is an obligate intracellular organism which is surrounded by a cell wall, contains both DNA and RNA, and divides by binary fission. In cervical infection lymphoid follicles form below the cervical mucosa, which are visible macroscopically as tiny white dots. A greater than expected incidence of CIN has been found in women with chlamydia.

Papillomavirus infection is common. Human papilloma viruses cause genital warts on the vulva, vagina and cervix, and have been linked to the development of cervical intraepithelial neoplasia and invasive carcinoma (see below). Over 65 different types of hPV have been identified, but hPV types 6, 11, 16 and 18 predominate in the female genital tract. Types 6 and 11 are found in warts and are uncommon in CIN and invasive carcinoma. Types 16 and 18, on the other hand, are demonstrable in cervical carcinoma cells, and the viral DNA can be shown to be integrated into the human DNA of the cell. There is no established proof that HPV causes carcinoma, but the evidence so far suggests that this is likely. The affected squamous cells become koilocytic (see Fig. 15.7).

Herpes simplex virus is one of the most prevalent viral infections of the cervix. Cervical infection can be completely asymptomatic: clinical illness develops in only 10% of carriers. Human immunodeficiency virus (HIV) may be present in cervical mucus and biopsy specimens from women carrying the virus. HIV-positive women have a higher prevalence of genital infection with HPV, and of cervical neoplasia, than women without HIV who are matched for HIV risk factors.

Hyperplasia of the cervix

Hyperplasia of the ectocervix occurs commonly in prolapse. The squamous epithelium becomes thicker and may keratinize. Glandular hyperplasia (the commonest type of which is **microglandular hyperplasia**, so called because the glands are small and crowded) occurs in women on oral contraceptives, on progesterone therapy alone, and in pregnancy. In many cases no aetiological agent is apparent. There is no definite relationship with age.

Endocervical polyps are common. They arise in the endocervical canal in most cases, and are considered to be a focal overgrowth of hyperplastic endocervical epithelium and its underlying stroma. Symptoms arise from excessive mucus secretion, surface ulceration with haemorrhage or infection.

Cervical cytology and screening

Cervical cytology specimens sample the superficial cells of the ectocervix and lower canal, and so are from a far wider field than cervical biopsy. Compared with biopsy, cytology is relatively inexpensive, is not invasive, and can be repeated an indefinite number of times given a suitable interval of sampling (Figs 15.3–15.5).

It is important to recognize the limitations of cervical cytology. Cells are wiped from the most superficial aspects of the cervical squamous mucosa,

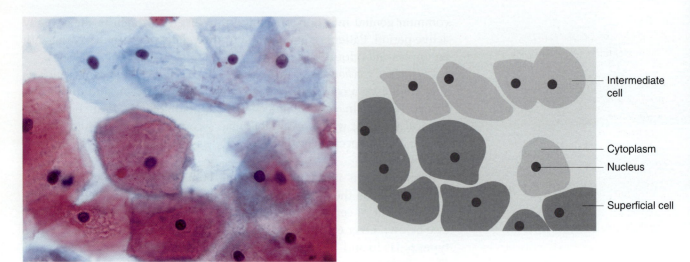

Fig. 15.3 Cytology from normal cervix. The superficial cells are large and flat, with acidophilic cytoplasm. Normal intermediate cells are also present (top) which have basophilic cytoplasm. The nuclei in both are small and pyknotic. The cells are equivalent to those removed from the surface of the cervix in Fig. 15.6.

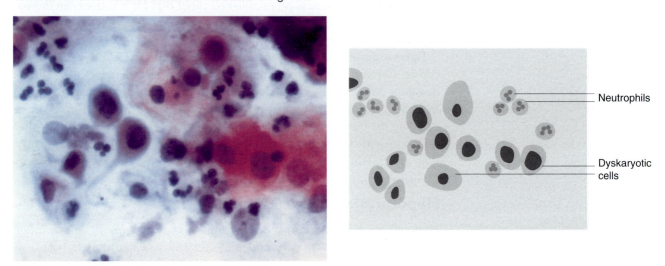

Fig. 15.4 Cytology from a patient with mild–moderate dyskaryosis, equivalent to cells obtained from the surface of the cervix in Fig. 15.9. The nuclear–cytoplasmic ratio is greater than normal, the nuclei are hyperchromatic and have clumping of chromatin, and pyknosis has not occurred.

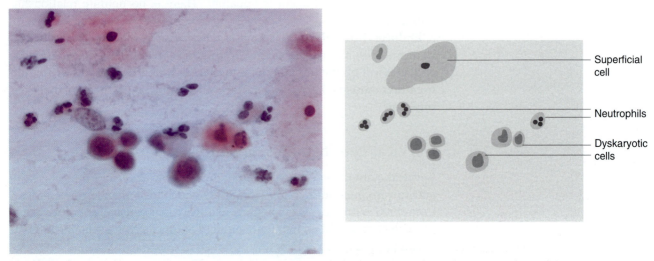

Fig.15.5 Cytology from a patient with severe dyskaryosis, equivalent to cells obtained from the surface of the cervix in Fig. 15.10. Large, darkly stained, irregular nuclei are present in cells with little cytoplasm.

Principles of screening
Screening for cervical neoplasia should be:
- **Easy to perform**
- **Cost effective**
- **Sensitive**: positive cases should not be missed
- **Specific**: cases should not be diagnosed as positive if they are not
- **Capable** of identifying a disease for which there is an effective management

and so only a presumptive diagnosis can be made of the changes that have occurred in the deeper cells. There is a correlation between the cytological and biopsy appearances, especially in the higher grades of intraepithelial neoplasia, but when an abnormal smear is found biopsy may be advised so that the abnormality can be confirmed and graded.

Most cervical smears from a screening clinic are from normal women and show normal cells or inflammatory changes only. In a small proportion, abnormal cells are present. These are usually smaller than normal and have larger, irregular nuclei. Depending on the degree of similarity to normal and the severity of the nuclear abnormalities, the smear is graded as having mild, moderate or severe dyskaryosis (equivalent, though not always exactly so, to CIN 1, 2 or 3). Using cytology it is possible to suggest that an invasive carcinoma is present, but biopsy is essential to confirm the diagnosis.

Cervical intraepithelial neoplasia

CIN is most commonly found in the transformation zone. The term refers to a range of changes in the stratified squamous mucosa in which there is failure of normal maturation, with mitoses and recognizably abnormal cells at different levels of the epithelium (Figs 15.6–15.10).

In all grades of CIN, nuclear abnormalities are present throughout the epithelium. These persist to the surface – if this were not so, of course, cervical cytology would be worthless.

CIN rarely regresses. It may stay the same, or progress to a worse grade. Progression is not automatic and may take years. Only about one-third of cases of CIN 3 go on to invasive carcinoma. Aneuploidy (abnormal amounts of DNA in the cells of the squamous mucosa affected by CIN) has been found to be associated with a tendency for the CIN to progress to a higher grade and to invasive carcinoma. It has been suggested that there may be two types of CIN, one that progresses quickly and one that is more indolent: the presence of HPV 16 has been linked with progressive disease, but this is not confirmed at present.

Staging of cervical intraepithelial neoplasia
- **CIN 1**: cytoplasmic and nuclear maturation is deficient but affects only the deepest one-third of the thickness of the epithelium, or less
- **CIN 2**: up to two-thirds of the thickness of the epithelium is abnormal
- **CIN 3**: more than two-thirds of the thickness of the epithelium is involved

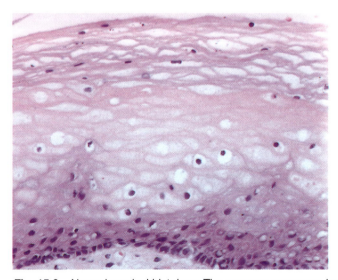 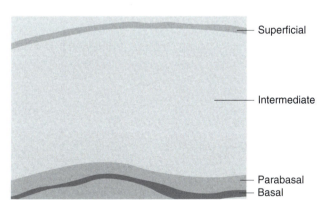

Superficial

Intermediate

Parabasal
Basal

Fig. 15.6 Normal cervical histology. The squamous mucosa has a single layer of basal cells covered by parabasal cells, intermediate cells and large, flat superficial cells. The surface cells removed for cervical cytology would correspond with those in Fig. 15.3.

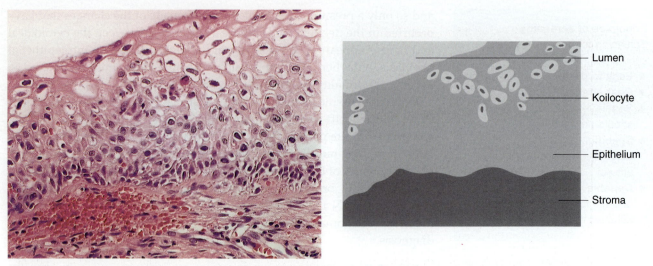

Fig. 15.7   Squamous mucosa of the cervix showing severe koilocytosis. The koilocytes have large amounts of clear cytoplasm, well-defined plasma membranes and irregular hyperchromatic nuclei.

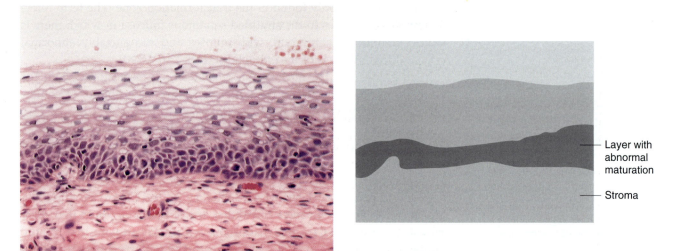

Fig. 15.8   Squamous mucosa of cervix with CIN 1. There is failure of proper maturation of the cells in the lowest third of the mucosa. Development remains abnormal to a mild extent throughout the thickness of the mucosa. The cells at the surface are mildly abnormal and so can be detected on cytology.

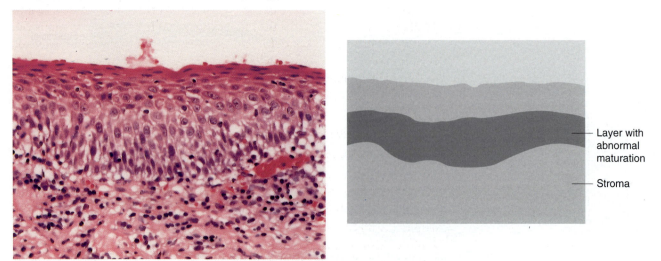

Fig. 15.9   Squamous mucosa of cervix with CIN 2. There is failure of maturation of the cells in the lower two-thirds of the mucosa. The cells that reach the surface reflect this, and on cytology would have the features seen in Fig. 15.4.

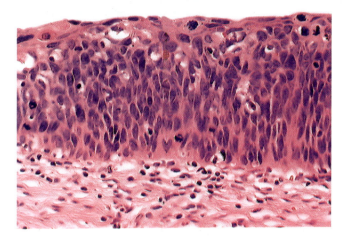 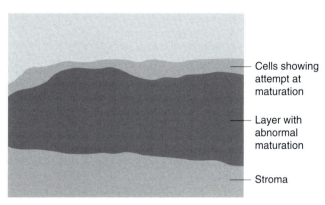

Cells showing attempt at maturation

Layer with abnormal maturation

Stroma

Fig. 15.10 Squamous mucosa of cervix with CIN 3. There is an abnormality of development affecting more than two-thirds of the epithelium. Mitoses are evident at all levels, and it is difficult to distinguish the cells near the surface from those in the basal layers. The cytology from this case would be equivalent to that in Fig. 15.5.

Carcinoma of the cervix

Most carcinomas of the cervix are squamous cell carcinomas. About 10% are pure adenocarcinomas, and up to 20% are mixed adenosquamous carcinomas. Squamous cell carcinoma of the cervix may be divided into superficially invasive carcinoma and invasive carcinoma. The term microinvasive carcinoma has been applied to small superficially invasive squamous cell carcinomas: there is no established microinvasive category for glandular tumours.

Aetiology and associations

Squamous cell carcinoma of the cervix is statistically commoner in women who are sexually active, women who have numerous male partners and women who smoke. It is also commoner in women who have a male partner who has many other partners. There is evidence that young age at first intercourse is a predisposing factor, and that barrier contraception is preventive. Some women have a family history of cervical cancer. In any one patient, however, none of these associations may apply. Types 16 and 18 of hPV are thought to be the main aetiological factors for squamous cell carcinoma but this is not definitely established, and herpes simplex virus type II may have an adjuvant role.

None of the above aetiological factors applies to adenocarcinoma of the endocervix. The only known cause is exposure to diethylstilboestrol *in utero*.

Squamous cell carcinoma of the cervix

Microinvasive carcinoma accounts for about 15% of all invasive squamous cell carcinomas of the cervix. It is defined as a carcinoma in which there is no or very little likelihood that metastasis has occurred at the time of diagnosis. Different classification schemes define it slightly differently, but essentially all of them require that there should be only a small tumour (of 7 mm or less in maximum width) with only a minimal depth of stromal invasion (of 3 mm or less) and no vascular invasion. The frequency of diagnosis of microinvasive carcinoma is increasing.

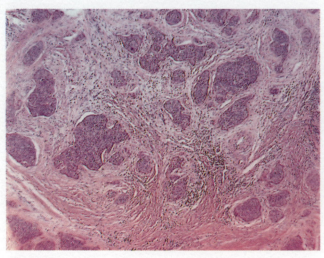
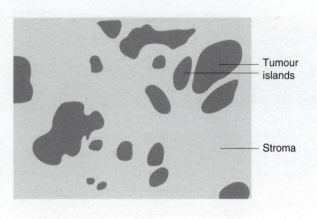

Fig. 15.11   Invasive squamous cell carcinoma of cervix of large cell non-keratinizing (moderately differentiated) type. Irregular tumour islands infiltrate the cervical stroma.

Invasive squamous cell carcinoma of the cervix may grow as a fungating, necrotic tumour on the surface of the cervix or occasionally invade deeply with little surface abnormality (Fig. 15.11). Local structures that are commonly invaded include the vagina, paracervical and parametrial tissues, and the uterine corpus. Lymph nodes in the lumbar, iliac and aortic groups are involved relatively early. Metastases to the liver, lungs and bone are uncommon and occur late in the disease. With current treatment the 5-year survival rate for patients who have tumour confined to the cervix is about 90%.

Staging of cervical carcinoma records the extent of spread. The 5-year survival for stages I–IV is approximately 90%, 70%, 30% and 10% respectively.

Mixed squamous and adenocarcinomas of the cervix occur, and are commoner than once thought, accounting for up to 20% of invasive carcinomas. Their behaviour is intermediate between that of pure squamous and glandular tumours.

Adenocarcinoma of the cervix

Adenocarcinoma in situ in the endocervix is becoming commoner. It may be associated with milder changes of epithelial atypia, and can also progress to invasive neoplasia so that a full range of epithelial abnormalities may be present. Invasive adenocarcinoma of the endocervix is a much more aggressive tumour than squamous cell carcinoma. Spread to iliac and para-aortic lymph nodes occurs relatively early, and the prognosis is poor.

Endometrium

Hormone control and the normal menstrual cycle

Oestrogen acts on endometrial cells in the first part of the cycle to cause them to make proteins that are used in the formation of cell structural components. Mitoses are induced, and this part of the endometrial cycle is therefore called the **proliferative phase** (Fig. 15.12). This corresponds to

---

Staging of cervical cancer
- **Stage I**: tumour is confined to the cervix
- **Stage II**: tumour extends beyond the cervix into the corpus or upper vagina, but not to the pelvic side wall
- **Stage III**: tumour has reached the pelvic side wall or the lower vagina, or both
- **Stage IV**: tumour involves tissues outside the female genital system such as the bladder or rectal mucosa

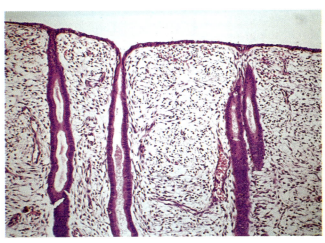

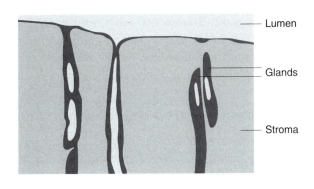

Lumen

Glands

Stroma

Fig. 15.12   Normal proliferative phase endometrium. The glands are straight and parallel-sided. Mitoses are numerous.

follicle development in the ovarian cycle, and so it is sometimes called the **follicular phase**. The length of the proliferative phase changes depends on the length of the cycle. In a cycle of 28 days the proliferative phase lasts for the first 14 days, and in a cycle of 35 days for the first 21.

In the second part of the cycle, progesterone is secreted by the corpus luteum of the ovary in addition to oestrogen. Progesterone switches the metabolism of the endometrial cells into making proteins for secretion into the endometrial glands, hence the name for this part of the cycle, the **secretory phase** (also called the **luteal phase**, by analogy with the ovarian cycle) (Fig 15.13). The effect of oestrogen is blocked, mitoses disappear and mucin accumulates in the glands. The arterioles in the endometrial stroma become prominent and tortuous. The secretory phase is constant at 14 days, irrespective of the length of the cycle.

Menstruation occurs with degeneration of the corpus luteum. The serum level of oestrogen falls sharply, the spiral arterioles contract, and there is necrosis and disaggregation of the upper levels of the endometrium. The stratum basale is not shed, and forms the site of regeneration for the next cycle. Menstruum is mostly fluid because of the plasmin that it contains.

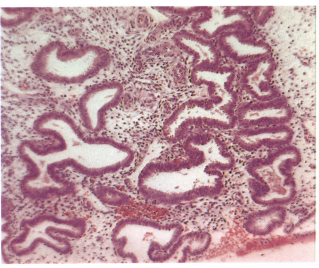

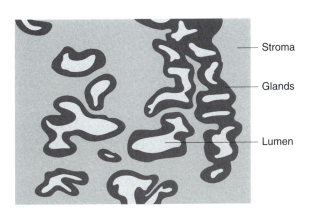

Stroma

Glands

Lumen

Fig. 15.13   Normal secretory phase endometrium. The glands have become tortuous and secretion is present in the lumina.

The changes in the proliferative phase are gradual and this phase is not subdivided. The secretory phase has clearly recognizable histological changes that permit division into early, middle and late secretory phase. This is important in the assessment of endometrium in women who are being investigated for infertility, as the response of the target organ to hormone stimulation can be assessed.

Other hormone-related changes in the endometrium

In pregnancy the corpus luteum persists and the effects of progesterone become more prominent. **Decidualization** occurs in the stromal cells, which become large and eosinophilic, and the glands develop an intensely secretory pattern called **Arias–Stella change**. The oral contraceptive pill alters the endometrium in relation to the balance of hormones contained: the most commonly used oral contraceptives produce inactive, small endometrial glands in a decidualized stroma. At the menopause, the endometrium becomes gradually more atrophic and thin (the climacteric, which is usually around the time of the menopause or slightly later, is when the hormonal function of the ovaries declines).

Endometritis

As in the cervix, inflammation in the endometrium may be non-specific or attributable to an identifiable organism. Acute endometritis of some degree almost always follows parturition: other causes include surgical instrumentation and radiotherapy. Neutrophil polymorphs are present in variable numbers in the stroma and glands.

Chronic endometritis, with a stromal infiltrate of plasma cells, is usually mild and without obvious cause. It may be associated with intrauterine contraceptive devices, retained products of conception and actinomycosis of the female genital tract. Tuberculosis of the endometrium is common in developing countries (Fig. 15.14). It may be diagnosable only as non-specific chronic endometritis, but if curettage of the endometrium is done late in the woman's menstrual cycle, such as in the late secretory phase, there may have been time for tuberculous granulomata to form.

Oestrogen and progesterone
■ **Oestrogen**
- attaches to oestrogen receptor
- moves to nucleus
- causes DNA to be transcribed to RNA specific for:
  ○ cell component proteins
  ○ oestrogen receptor protein
- makes endometrial cells grow and divide
- stimulates the formation of more oestrogen receptor to augment the loop

■ **Progesterone**
- attaches to progesterone receptor
- inhibits oestrogen receptor function by inhibition of oestrogen receptor formation
- moves to nucleus
- causes DNA to be transcribed to RNA specific for:
  ○ proteins for secretion into gland lumen
  ○ progesterone receptor protein

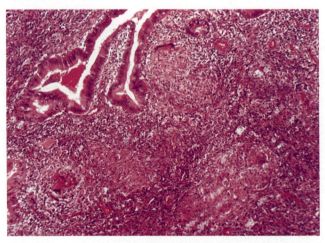
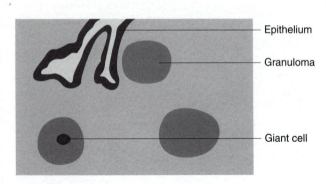

Epithelium

Granuloma

Giant cell

Fig. 15.14   Tuberculous endometritis. The stroma is severely inflamed with a dense infiltrate of lymphocytes and histiocytes. Langhans' giant cell formation is seen lower left.

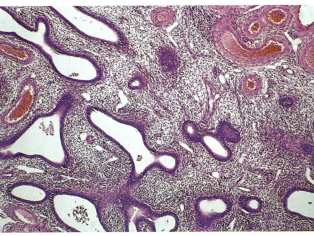
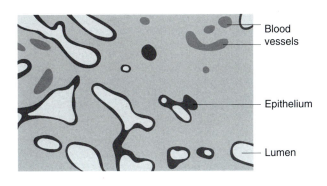

Fig. 15.15 Endometrial polyp. The glands are of widely differing sizes and shapes, and the stroma is inflamed and has prominent blood vessels (top right). A polyp represents focal endometrial hyperplasia.

Endometrial hyperplasia

This may be divided into focal endometrial hyperplasia (endometrial polyp formation) and diffuse hyperplasia.

ENDOMETRIAL POLYPS

Hyperplastic endometrial polyps are common. They are localized outgrowths of the endometrium with cystically dilated glands and thick-walled vessels (Fig. 15.15). Affected patients present with intermenstrual bleeding, menorrhagia and occasionally pelvic pain. An excessive local response to a normal level of oestrogen stimulation is thought to be the cause. Malignant change in endometrial polyps is rare. Polypoid hyperplasia can be caused by infective agents such as schistosomiasis, and submucosal leiomyomas can mimic endometrial polyps.

DIFFUSE ENDOMETRIAL HYPERPLASIA

In contrast to polyps, this type of hyperplasia is associated with an increased serum oestrogen concentration and affects the entire endometrium. The excess oestrogen may be exogenous (as oestrogen therapy) or endogenously produced. Ovarian tumours such as granulosa cell tumours and thecomas secrete oestrogens (Fig. 15.16), and in obese women (and men) there is peripheral metabolism of ovarian and adrenal androgens to oestrogen in adipose tissue.

Simple endometrial hyperplasia

This condition used to be called metropathia haemorrhagica. The endometrium develops cystically dilated glands lined by cuboidal cells in large amounts of stroma. The significant risk of malignant change in this type of hyperplasia is very small. Simple hyperplasia may be caused by unopposed oestrogen from anovulatory cycles (when progesterone is not secreted and so cannot switch off proliferation). This is commonest around the times of the menarche and menopause.

Complex endometrial hyperplasia

In this type there is proliferation of the endometrial glands out of proportion to the stroma. Complex architectural and nuclear changes occur

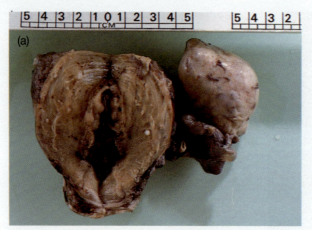

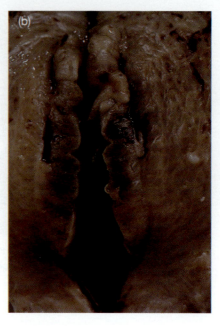

Fig. 15.16 (a) Diffuse endometrial hyperplasia: the endometrium is several times thicker than normal due to excessive proliferation. The reason for this, a thecoma that was secreting oestrogens, can be seen in the right ovary. (b) Detail of the hyperplastic endometrium.

(Fig. 15.17), with back-to-back formation of glands and cells with large, hyperchromatic nuclei. The risk of malignant change correlates with the degree of atypia, especially cytological atypia. In severe cases it may be impossible to distinguish atypical complex hyperplasia from intraendometrial neoplasia, and indeed some authorities consider atypical hyperplasia to be neoplastic. Evaluation of the likelihood of progression to adenocarcinoma is difficult as cases of atypical hyperplasia/intra-endometrial neoplasia are treated by hysterectomy, but the risk of a patient developing invasive malignancy eventually is considered to be over 50%.

Carcinoma of the endometrium

Carcinoma of the endometrium is usually well or moderately differentiated adenocarcinoma which characteristically occurs in postmenopausal women between the ages of 50 and 65 years. It is associated with a long cycling life (that is, early menarche and late menopause), nulliparity and anovulatory menstrual cycles. The frequency of endometrial

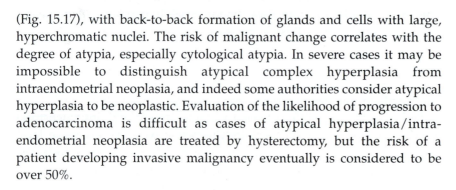

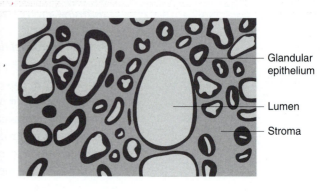

Glandular epithelium

Lumen

Stroma

Fig. 15.17 Atypical endometrial hyperplasia. When there is cytological and architectural atypia the chance of developing endometrial adenocarcinoma is increased.

adenocarcinoma is increasing, and now accounts for about 1% of deaths from malignant disease. Cervical carcinoma was more common than endometrial carcinoma 30 years ago, but the incidence is now about equal.

The association with hyperoestrogenic states such as oestrogen therapy, oestrogen-secreting ovarian tumours and obesity (see above) is convincing, but reports of an association with hypertension and diabetes have not been substantiated. Adenocarcinoma may develop in pre-existing atypical hyperplasia of the endometrium but most cases arise in previously atrophic endometrium.

Adenocarcinoma may be polypoid or diffuse, and is often both – there is extensive generalized thickening of the endometrium with outgrowths in some areas to form polyps. Necrosis is common, particularly in long-standing cases. Even in relatively late cases the myometrium may be invaded only in its innermost aspect, as the tumour is usually slow-growing and indolent. Surgery is the usual treatment but the tumours often respond well to progestogen therapy, which suppresses mitotic activity and slows growth.

Tumours that are poorly differentiated and have squamous areas are called **adenosquamous carcinomas**. They are usually aggressive. Spread into the myometrium and to iliac and lumbar lymph nodes is relatively early, and these patients have a poor prognosis.

Staging of endometrial carcinoma is on similar principles to that for cervical carcinoma.

Sarcomas of the endometrium

Sarcoma of the endometrium can form tissue that is normally present in those sites and also tissues that are not. An endometrial stromal sarcoma is an example of a pure homologous sarcoma. A pure heterologous sarcoma of endometrium might be a rhabdomyosarcoma, chondrosarcoma or osteosarcoma. Neoplasms also arise that are composed of both carcinomatous and sarcomatous elements, called carcinosarcoma or malignant mixed müllerian tumour. When malignant endometrial glands and endometrial stromal sarcoma or leiomyosarcoma are present, it is called a homologous malignant mixed müllerian tumour. When endometrial adenocarcinoma is associated with, for example, chondrosarcomatous elements, the tumour is a heterologous malignant mixed müllerian tumour. Low-grade endometrial stromal sarcoma has a relatively good prognosis but may recur locally. High-grade endometrial stromal sarcoma metastasizes early and has a poor prognosis. The presence of heterologous elements has no bearing on prognosis.

Endometriosis

Endometriosis is defined as the presence of endometrial glands and stroma at sites away from their normal position in the lining of the uterine corpus. It is divided into internal endometriosis (more commonly called **adenomyosis**) when endometrial tissue is found deep in the myometrium, and external endometriosis (usually simply called **endometriosis**) when it is outside the uterus altogether. Both are uncommon.

Affected women are typically aged 20–40 years and have deep pelvic pain and dyspareunia, especially before the menstrual period. Bowel

---

Staging of endometrial carcinoma
- **Stage I**: tumour is confined to the corpus
- **Stage II**: tumour extends to involve the cervix.
- **Stage III**: carcinoma has spread outside the uterus but is confined still within the true pelvis
- **Stage IV**: tumour has spread outside the true pelvis or involve rectal, bladder or other mucosa.

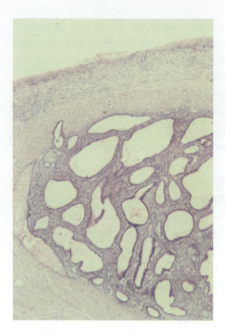

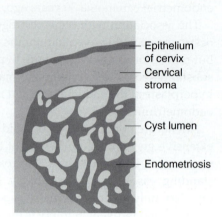

Epithelium of cervix
Cervical stroma
Cyst lumen
Endometriosis

Fig. 15.18   Endometriosis. There is a deposit of endometrial glands and stroma in the connective tissues of the ectocervix.

obstruction may occur. Endometriosis is commoner in the higher socioeconomic groups and is associated with infertility (even when there is no obstructive element contributed by the endometriosis itself).

Typical sites of involvement include the ovary, fallopian tubes, uterine pelvic ligaments, pouch of Douglas and peritoneum over the bladder and intestine. More rarely, the cervix (Fig. 15.18), vagina, omentum and inguinal canal are involved. Deposits may be found in surgical abdominal scars, especially after laparotomy in which the cavity of the uterus is breached. Very rarely endometriosis has been reported in the lung, pleura and diaphragm, the ureter, pelvic lymph nodes, and the breast, upper arm and nasal cavity.

Endometriosis in the ovary can be either diffuse as tiny pinpoint brown cysts scattered throughout, or form large endometriotic cysts many centimetres in diameter. These latter are referred to as 'chocolate' cysts of the ovary because of the appearance of the altered blood within them: externally they are in fact silver or bluish, because of the fibrous tissue surrounding the cyst. When endometriosis affects the serosa of an organ such as the bowel or bladder, it tends over time to penetrate deeper into the wall, and may in extreme cases reach the mucosa. The brisk fibrous reaction to endometriosis causes distortion, obstruction and dense adhesions with other adjacent organs.

The diagnosis of endometriosis rests on the demonstration of **endometrial glands and stroma** in sites outside the endometrium itself. Endometrial glands alone, without stroma, are very rarely seen. If glands alone are found in, say, the serosa of the appendix, they may represent spread from a very well-differentiated endometrial adenocarcinoma. The converse, of stroma without glands, is relatively common – the glandular element may be destroyed by the inflammatory reaction to the haemorrhage into the area. In these cases only a presumptive diagnosis of endometriosis can be made.

The aetiology of the condition is unknown but there are several theories, and more than one may apply. Endometriosis may very rarely undergo malignant change into endometrioid carcinoma. This is histologically

Aetiology of endometriosis
- **Metastatic theory**: the endometrium spreads to the site of endometriosis by reflux of endometrium through the fallopian tubes, or spread via lymphatics or the bloodstream. Implantation at the time of surgery, or in the cervix and vulva by menstruation, is also an example of metastatic spread.
- **Metaplastic theory**: the endometriosis arises at the site involved, by a process of metaplasia.
- **Direct local spread**: adenomyosis in the myometrium is an example of direct spread of endometrial tissue.

indistinguishable from endometrial adenocarcinoma but because it presents at a later stage than endometrial carcinoma, the prognosis is worse.

Myometrium

Tumours of the myometrium

LEIOMYOMA

Leiomyomas (or 'fibroids', a term used for historical reasons) are very common tumours of the myometrium. They affect about 20% of women over the age of 30 years and occur especially between the ages of 30 and 55 years. Leiomyomas give symptoms for the first time only rarely in women over 60 years, and pre-existing leiomyomas tend to regress at this time. The smooth muscle cells of some leiomyomas have oestrogen receptors, which may explain their tendency to regress after the menopause.

The size of leiomyomas varies widely, from only a few millimetres to many centimetres (Fig. 15.19). The largest recorded was over 50 kg. In most cases the diameter is 0.5–3.0 cm. Leiomyomas are usually intramural at their inception, but then may migrate to submucosal or subserosal sites. Submucosal leiomyomas distort the endometrial cavity and may descend through the cervix into the vagina. Intramural leiomyomas can grow large before symptoms develop. As a consequence, affected women complain of menorrhagia, abdominal pain and swelling, infertility and recurrent abortions, urinary symptoms and obstructed labour.

Macroscopically, leiomyomas are pale, round and rubbery. They compress the adjacent myometrium to form an apparent capsule and are easily shelled out from this: the danger at operation is that profuse haemorrhage may occur, especially when the uterus is distorted by numerous leiomyomas. Microscopically, there are smooth muscle bundles lying in different directions. Demarcation from the myometrium may be clear but usually the tumour merges imperceptibly with the non-neoplastic uterine wall. Only small amounts of fibrous tissue are present. Mitoses are rarely seen.

Changes (**degenerations**) that commonly occur in leiomyomas are hyaline change, in which the fibres are obscured by mucopolysaccharide material secreted by the smooth muscle cells; infarction (also called red degeneration) because of the dull red colour of leiomyomas that have this complication; and calcification, especially postmenopausally, when large amounts of calcium can be deposited in the leiomyoma. Infarction occurs especially in pregnancy. Less commonly, cystic change may be seen when mucopolysaccharide accumulates so much that central degeneration occurs, and fatty change results in the accumulation of adipocytes in the leiomyoma. Malignant change into leiomyosarcoma, which cannot be regarded as a degeneration, is also rare.

Leiomyosarcoma

The commonest site of leiomyosarcoma is in the uterus, though even here it is rare. It may arise from a recognizable previously benign leiomyoma, or *de novo*, and especially affects women between 50 and 65 years. Demarcation from the adjacent myometrium is less than for benign smooth muscle tumours. The prognosis of all except small, early tumours is poor. Metastasis to pelvic and lumbar lymph nodes occurs relatively early.

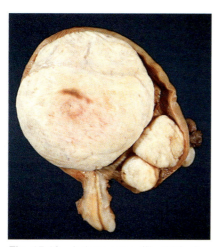

Fig. 15.19   Leiomyomas (fibroids) of the uterus. The myometrium has several pale whorled nodules which distort the endometrial cavity and the serosa of the uterus. (Reproduced, with permission, from Lowe DG, Jeffrey IM, *Macro Techniques in Diagnostic Histopathology*, 1989, London: Mosby Wolfe.)

Diagnosis of leiomyosarcoma rests on the demonstration of mitotic activity of over 10 mitoses per 10 high-power fields (HPFs). Such tumours have a definite tendency to metastasize and are considered to be malignant. Tumours with fewer than 3 mitoses/10 HPF are considered benign. Between these numbers, the behaviour is unpredictable and the tumour is diagnosed as a smooth muscle tumour of uncertain malignant potential.

Fallopian tubes

Salpingitis

Acute endosalpingitis may occur as an isolated event, or may be part of the loosely defined gynaecological condition known as pelvic inflammatory disease. In this, infection ascends through the fallopian tube to involve the ovary and surrounding peritoneum.

Salpingitis (principally endosalpingitis with infection spreading to involve all layers of the tube wall) is caused by *Neisseria gonorrhoeae*, mycoplasmas and chlamydiae, and in some parts of the world tuberculosis and schistosomiasis. Tuberculosis of the fallopian tubes is almost always secondary to pulmonary or intestinal disease. Tubal schistosomiasis is characteristically caused by *Schistosoma haematobium*, but *Schistosoma mansoni* is the prevalent type in some areas of Africa.

All of these infective agents result in fusion of the plicae, an infiltrate of inflammatory cells and varying degrees of fibrosis. In the early stages of infection there is pus formation and a pyosalpinx may form; if this partially resolves, a hydrosalpinx results. In chronic infections the residual scarring and distortion can lead to infertility, ectopic pregnancy and intraperitoneal adhesions.

Ectopic pregnancy

Most ectopic pregnancies occur in the fallopian tube, usually in the middle third. Other much rarer sites include the cervix, the ovary and the peritoneal cavity. Placentation proceeds normally at first, but the fallopian tube wall is inadequate to support the pregnancy: erosion of vessels and of the muscularis of the tube wall results in haemorrhage and rupture.

The incidence is increasing, and in most cases there is no apparent predisposing cause for it: the chromosomes of the fetus and the hormonal response of the ovary to the gestation may be normal. The rate of ectopic pregnancy is about 20 per 1000 live births, 15 per 1000 reported pregnancies and 10 per 100 000 women aged 14–44 years. When a cause can be established, it is usually tubal obstruction from previous inflammation and fibrosis. Some women with tubal pregnancy have no demonstrable obstruction. In them the cause may be inadequate ciliary function of the tube lining cells or ovulation from the ovary on the contralateral side to the ectopic gestation. Intrauterine contraceptive devices are associated with ectopic pregnancy, but the reason for this is unclear.

Tumours of the fallopian tube

All neoplasms of the fallopian tube are very rare. Adenocarcinoma presents as a watery, pink vaginal discharge and is often widespread at the time of diagnosis. Leiomyoma and haemangioma of the tube have been described.

Ovary

The normal ovary

The normal ovary is composed of **germ cells** or **oocytes** (not ova, which are formed when spermatozoa penetrate oocytes), Graafian follicles, fibrous stroma, surface epithelium and hilar cells. In the Graafian follicles the oocytes are surrounded by cells derived from the sex cords (**granulosa cells**) and cells from the stroma adjacent to them (**theca cells**) (Fig. 15.20). The granulosa cells, theca cells and other stroma-derived cells (the hilar cells) secrete steroid hormones. The **surface epithelium** (which used to be called 'germinal' epithelium) commonly invaginates to form tiny cysts below the surface. The lining epithelium of these is usually flat but may undergo metaplasia into tubal, endometrial or cervical type epithelium. The ovarian **stroma** is composed of dense fibrous tissue found only in the gonads.

All of the components of the ovary can become neoplastic. The name of the neoplastic component is the basis for the histological classification of ovarian tumours.

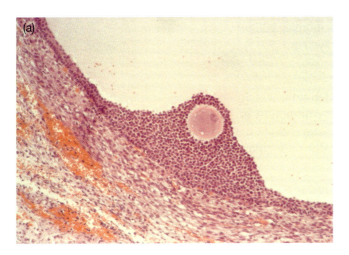

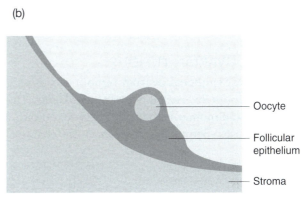

Oocyte

Follicular epithelium

Stroma

Fig. 15.20   (a, b) Part of a normal Graafian follicle showing the cumulus oophorus with oocyte, granulosa cell layer that contributes to the cumulus, and the surrounding theca cell layers. The granulosa cells have no blood supply until ovulation occurs, when blood vessels grow in from the theca. (c, d) Detail of (a) showing the oocyte.

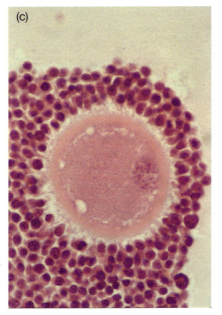

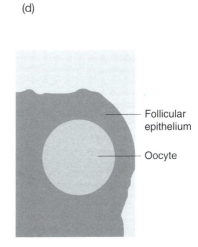

Follicular epithelium

Oocyte

Oophoritis

Acute inflammation of an ovary, especially the right ovary, may occur as part of pelvic inflammatory disease, acute salpingitis and acute appendicitis. Actinomycosis of the ovary can result in abscess formation that mimics an appendix abscess.

Non-neoplastic cysts of the ovary

There are four principal types of non-neoplastic cyst of the ovary. The clinical importance in the diagnosis of a non-neoplastic cyst of the ovary is that the patient can simply be followed up to make sure that the cyst is not increasing in size or persisting after a period of 3 months. If it is, laparoscopy or laparotomy with biopsy or excision is performed to confirm the nature of the cyst.

Neoplasms of the ovary

These are usually large and cystic but may be solid, especially when malignant. Neoplasms of the ovary may be composed of epithelium, germ cells, sex cord or stromal cells, or non-specialized ovarian tissues. Metastatic carcinoma to the ovary is common, particularly from carcinomas of the stomach, breast, colon and other parts of the female genital system.

EPITHELIAL OVARIAN TUMOURS

The commonest epithelial ovarian tumour is **serous cystadenoma**, which accounts for about 25% of all ovarian neoplasms. The next commonest is **mucinous cystadenoma**, at about 20%. These tumours are bilateral in about one-fifth of cases. Serous cystadenomas are characteristically unilocular,

---

Types of non-neoplastic ovarian cyst
- **Surface inclusion cyst** (by far the commonest type)
- **Follicular cyst**: from a Graafian follicle that has persisted after the normal physiological duration
- **Luteal cyst**: from a corpus luteum that has persisted after the normal physiological duration
- **Endometriotic cyst** (although there is some recent evidence that these are monoclonal and are therefore true neoplasms)

Tumours
- ■ **Epithelial tumours**
  - serous
    - ○ cystadenoma
    - ○ adenofibroma
    - ○ borderline tumour
    - ○ cystadenocarcinoma
  - mucinous
    - ○ cystadenoma
    - ○ adenofibroma
    - ○ borderline tumour
    - ○ cystadenocarcinoma
  - endometrioid
    - ○ cystadenoma
    - ○ adenofibroma
    - ○ borderline tumour
    - ○ cystadenocarcinoma
    - ○ clear cell variant
  - Brenner
    - ○ benign Brenner
    - ○ proliferative Brenner
    - ○ malignant Brenner tumour (very rare)
  - mixed epithelial tumours
  - undifferentiated epithelial tumours
- ■ **Germ cell tumours**
  - teratoma
    - ○ benign cystic teratoma
    - ○ mature solid teratoma (rare)
    - ○ predominant element in a benign cystic teratoma (such as thyroid, 'struma ovarii')
    - ○ malignant element in a teratoma
    - ○ immature teratoma
  - dysgerminoma
  - choriocarcinoma
  - yolk sac tumour
  - mixed germ cell tumours (dysgerminoma + choriocarcinoma, etc.)
  - mixed germ cell/sex cord/stromal tumours
    - ○ gonadoblastoma (germ cells + Sertoli cells)
- ■ **Sex cord/stromal tumours**
  - granulosa cell tumour
  - thecoma
  - fibroma
  - androblastoma (Sertoli cell tumour, Leydig cell tumour)
  - gynandroblastoma (androblastoma + granulosa cell tumour or thecoma)
  - other mixed sex cord/stromal tumours
- ■ **Ovarian tumours arising from non-specialized connective tissues**
  - haemangioma
  - lymphangioma
  - neurofibroma
- ■ **Metastatic tumours to the ovary**
  - from stomach, colon, breast, lung

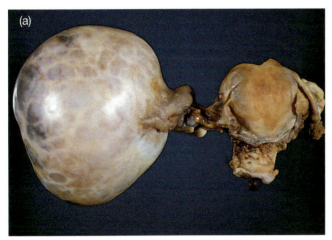
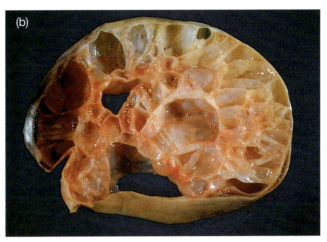

Fig. 15.21 (a) Mucinous tumour of ovary of borderline type: when these tumours (and their serous counterparts) are of medium size and smooth surfaced, they have a tendency to undergo torsion. No destructive stromal invasion was present in the tumour. (b) Cut surface of (a). (Reproduced, with permission, from Lowe DG, Jeffrey IM, *Macro Techniques in Diagnostic Histopathology*, 1989, London: Mosby Wolfe.)

contain thin straw-coloured fluid, and have thin walls. Mucinous tumours are usually multilocular, contain thick fluid and have thick walls, but it is not possible to differentiate reliably from macroscopic appearances alone. **Adenofibroma** (of both serous and mucinous types) has large amounts of fibrous tissues in addition to cystic spaces.

Small and medium-sized benign tumours may undergo torsion: larger benign tumours and malignant tumours seldom do so, as they are usually adherent to the pelvic wall. Haemorrhage into the cysts is quite common. Patients may therefore present in many ways – with an acute abdominal emergency, a mass, chronic weight gain or low-grade pelvic pain.

There is a category of ovarian tumour between benign and invasive malignant known as epithelial ovarian tumour (serous tumour, mucinous tumour, etc.) of borderline type. These are defined as having atypical proliferation of the epithelium lining the cystic spaces and on the surface, with multilayering of cells, atypical forms, mitotic figures, and shedding of cells into the lumina (Fig. 15.21). Borderline tumours are distinguished from invasive malignancy because they show no destructive stromal invasion. They are not considered carcinoma in situ as there may be extraovarian implants of the disease, but it is important for the category of borderline tumours to be separated as they have a significantly better prognosis than invasive carcinoma.

Malignant ovarian tumours, in which there is demonstrable destructive stromal invasion, are relatively common. They are bilateral in about half of cases.

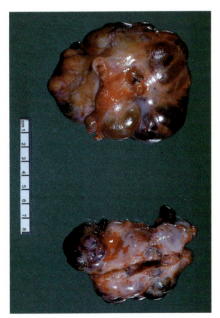

Fig. 15.22 Serous cystadenocarcinoma of ovary, in this case bilateral. The multiloculated cysts contain thin, clear, straw-coloured fluid with solid areas of invasive neoplasia.

- **Serous cystadenocarcinoma** is the commonest malignant tumour and accounts for about 40% of all invasive ovarian malignancy (Fig. 15.22). These tumours have solid areas and fine papillary processes that may be endophytic or exophytic. The 5-year survival is about 25%.
- **Mucinous** and **endometrioid carcinomas** are less common at about 10%, and have a better prognosis of about 60% at 5 years.
- **Clear cell carcinoma** was thought to be a distinct type but is now considered to be a subtype of endometrioid carcinoma. A clear cell component is quite common in endometrioid carcinoma; occasionally the tumour may be a pure clear cell carcinoma.

- **Brenner tumours** are almost always benign. They are composed of epithelium resembling urothelium, and are occasionally found in the walls of mucinous cystadenomas.

Staging of ovarian tumours is somewhat different from the staging of the other two main cancers of the female genital system.

GERM CELL TUMOURS

Teratomas account for about 20% of all ovarian neoplasms, and are almost always benign. The commonest age at presentation is 20–40 years. They contain all tissue types (skin, hair, gut epithelium, neural tissue) though oocytes are virtually never found (Fig. 15.23). Malignancy can rarely develop in one element (squamous cell carcinoma, adenocarcinoma, specific types of tumour such as thyroid carcinoma). More rarely, the entire teratoma can be immature and make fetal tissues; these are malignant and metastasize as immature teratomata.

Dysgerminoma is the female equivalent of seminoma, and has many features in common. The prognosis is worse than for testicular disease because the presentation is usually later. **Yolk sac tumour** (called endodermal sinus tumour in older literature) affects girls and young women. It has a poor prognosis but may respond to platinum-based chemotherapy. **Choriocarcinoma** of the ovary closely resembles gestational choriocarcinoma and has a relatively poor prognosis.

SEX CORD/STROMAL TUMOURS

These tumours are derived from cells that have an endocrine function, and secrete steroid hormones and inhibin. **Granulosa cell tumours** are malignant but often behave in an indolent fashion. They account for 5% of ovarian malignancies and may occur as a mixed form with theca cells in some areas (Fig. 15.24). They often secrete sex steroids such as oestrogen, and may therefore be associated with endometrial hyperplasia. It is not possible to predict the behaviour of these tumours on histological grounds, though there is some correlation between size and prognosis. The prognosis is 60–90% 5-year survival.

Thecomas (without any granulosa cell element) are benign. They may secrete hormones, and should be differentiated from the commoner **fibroma** of ovary which does not. Sertoli–Leydig cell tumours are sex cord

> **Staging of ovarian tumours**
> - **Stage I**: the cancer affects one or both ovaries and is limited to them
> - **Stage II**: there is involvement of one or both ovaries and pelvic tissues such as the fallopian tube or parametrium in addition
> - **Stage III**: tumours have metastases in the peritoneum outside the pelvis, and may have retroperitoneal lymph nodes
> - **Stage IV**: there are distant metastases

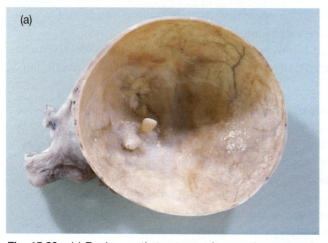
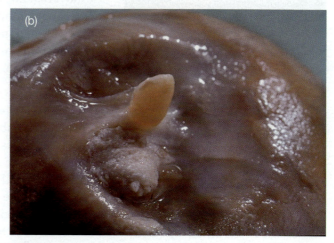

Fig. 15.23   (a) Benign cystic teratoma of ovary: the cyst cavity contained hairs and sebaceous material (now removed). In the wall is a lower incisor tooth adjacent to a mound of neural tissues. (b) Detail of (a).

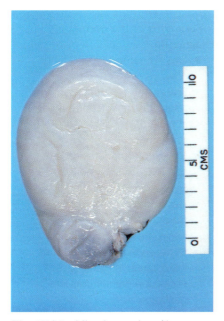

Fig. 15.24 Mixed granulosa/theca cell tumour of ovary. This tumour, like that in Fig. 15.16a, was oestrogen secreting and had induced endometrial hyperplasia.

stromal tumours that recapitulate the capacity of the primitive gonad to differentiate into male tissues as well as female. Rarely a mixed sex cord and germ cell tumour called **gonadoblastoma** may occur. This is commonest in dysgenetic gonads: about half of cases of gonadoblastoma will develop invasive germ cell neoplasia, particularly dysgerminoma, and the incidence is higher in gonads that have a Y chromosome.

METASTATIC TUMOURS

The commonest primary carcinomas which metastasize to the ovary include carcinomas of the breast, bronchus, large bowel, stomach and pancreas. Ovarian metastases, known historically as Krukenberg's tumours, tend to be bilateral. They can be difficult to distinguish from primary tumours macroscopically, though differentiation is usually possible microscopically in all but the most poorly differentiated tumours.

Placenta

Abnormalities of placental function may be because of the site of implantation or abnormal structure of the placenta. Most of the variants of gross placental structure (circummarginate placenta, circumvallate placenta, etc.) usually have no clinical significance. Twin placentas may be separate, fused or a single disc with two cords (Fig. 15.25). Inflammation of the placenta can be caused by non-specific ascending infection in cases of prolonged rupture of membranes before delivery, or by blood-borne organisms such as cytomegalovirus, *Listeria* and *Toxoplasma* spp.

The commonest abnormalities of the placenta include ectopic pregnancy (see section on Fallopian tubes on page 360), hydatidiform mole and choriocarcinoma.

Hydatidiform mole

The prevalence of hydatidiform mole varies widely in the world. Common places for it to occur include Nigeria and parts of Japan and China: in industrialized countries the incidence is less common, at about 1 in 1000 gestations.

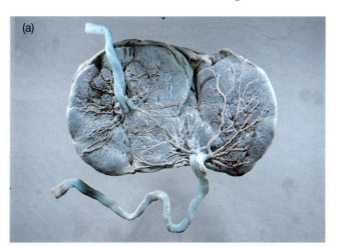
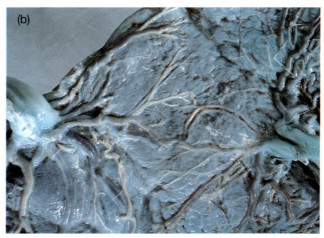

Fig. 15.25   (a) Twin placentas: any of the four types of placenta (monoamnionic monochorionic, diamnionic monochorionic, and diamnionic fused and separate) can occur in association with monovular twins. (b) Detail of (a) showing a common vessel running across the fetal aspect of the joint placental disc. These can result in fetofetal transfusions when one umbilical cord becomes compressed at the time of delivery.

In hydatidiform mole, the development of the embryo and placenta is abnormal. The placental villi become distended and vesicular, hence the name of the condition as a grape-like mass. In a **complete** mole, the embryo is absent and the mole is usually paternally derived – the molar tissue has an XX karyotype with both X chromosomes contributed by the male partner. The origin of these moles is probably the development of diploid cells from a degenerating oocyte that is fertilized by a paternal X spermatocyte which then undergoes duplication. The small proportion of complete moles that are XY are also paternally derived, probably from diploid cells developing from two spermatozoa (one X bearing, one Y) entering a degenerating oocyte.

Partial moles, in which only some of the villi have hydatidiform changes, may be associated with a recognizable fetus. These are usually triploid, with a chromosomal complement of 69.

CHORIOCARCINOMA

Choriocarcinoma is a soft, haemorrhagic mass in the uterus that invades the wall and metastasizes early. Common sites of involvement include the lungs, brain, liver, skin and other places in the female genital system such as the vagina or cervix. Choriocarcinoma follows hydatidiform mole in about half of cases: a quarter are associated with an apparently uncomplicated abortion: and the remaining quarter follow a normal gestation.

The prognosis nowadays is much better than previously with the use of potent cytotoxic drugs. Persistence and recurrence of disease can be monitored by hCG measurements, though the precise tumour load is not directly proportional to the degree of elevation of the hCG.

Functions of the normal placenta
- **Gas transfer**: the fetal lungs have no respiratory function
- **Water and pH balance**: the fetal kidneys function properly in acid–base balance only late in gestation
- **Excretion**: the fetal kidneys can excrete to some extent, but this is suboptimal
- **Catabolic and resorptive functions**: in place of the immature fetal bowel
- **Synthesis and secretion of hormones**: in place of most endocrine glands until late in gestation
- **Metabolic and secretory functions of the liver**: the fetal liver takes over functions gradually from about week 28
- **Haemopoiesis in the early stages**: before the fetal liver and spleen take over
- **Heat transfer**: the fetal skin is maintained at 37°C and the fetus has no other efficient means of heat exchange
- **Immunological functions**: to an unknown degree

Chapter 16 Paediatric pathology

Learning objectives

To understand and appreciate:
- ❑ How genetic disorders lead to childhood disease
- ❑ Importance of developmental biology in the causation of systemic malformation
- ❑ Pathology associated with birth trauma and prematurity
- ❑ Dangers of infection to the infant
- ❑ Factors which may be involved in sudden infant death
- ❑ Commoner types of childhood malignancy
- ❑ Pathological conditions associated with handicap

Although the basic pathological processes (abnormalities of cellular growth and differentiation, inflammation, degenerative conditions, thrombosis, etc.) are essentially similar in children and adults, the importance of developmental abnormalities, the rarity of degenerative disorders and the differing susceptibility of the organs in the young mean that the pattern of disease is very different from that in adults. This chapter addresses the important problems of infancy and young life which are not covered elsewhere, including some which are unique to childhood.

Genetic disorders

An individual's overall genetic make-up determines his or her response to numerous environmental stimuli. It is one factor which underlies the chances of cellular damage resulting from exposure to infectious agents, chemicals (including drugs and food substances) and other physical agents. Polygenic inheritance is therefore important in determining underlying susceptibility to a wide range of diseases, especially those which tend to run in families. However, in addition to the contributions of multiple genes to the risk of many common disorders, specific defects of the cellular DNA may occur. These often cause problems evident before or immediately after birth or may present in childhood. They fall into two major groups: **chromosomal abnormalities** and **single gene defects**.

The basic biology associated with such abnormalities is covered in Chapter 2; the present section is concerned with the way in which these genetic defects lead to disease in childhood.

Chromosomal abnormalities

Chromosomal abnormalities are characterized by aberrations in the number or structure of the chromosomes. The consequences of an abnormal chromosomal constitution depend on the nature and extent of the defect and whether the autosomes or sex chromosomes are affected.

ABNORMAL NUMBERS OF CHROMOSOMES

Most embryos with an abnormal number of **autosomes** do not survive, and abort spontaneously in the first or second trimester of pregnancy. Only around 1% of the total number of polyploid or autosomal aneuploid zygotes conceived survive into infant life. The same is true when there is loss of a sex chromosome, but an increased number of sex chromosomes is not a lethal condition.

Autosomal aneuploidies are usually due to the presence of a single extra autosome resulting in a **trisomy**. Trisomies of most of the autosomes have been recorded, with varying incidence. All result in abnormal development of many organs and tissues – hence the reason why most are lethal *in utero* (Fig. 16.1). The small number of affected fetuses who survive have a high perinatal and infant mortality rate, mental handicap, growth retardation and a variety of major congenital malformations. The commonest autosomal aneuploidies found in liveborn children, and their range of characteristic effects, are shown in Table 16.1. The precise abnormalities present, and their severity, vary in different individuals with an apparently identical chromosomal abnormality.

Polyploidy is the presence of a complete extra set of chromosomes which is an exact multiple of the haploid number ($1N$). With tetraploidy ($4N$) and triploidy ($3N$) placental tissue is usually present, so the mother develops symptoms and signs of early pregnancy, but no proper embryo forms. Triploid conceptuses may result in formation of a partial hydatidiform mole (see Chapter 15).

Absence of a sex chromosome is also usually lethal during embryogenesis. Complete absence of an X chromosome is incompatible with life, so the genotype 45 Y0 is unknown in formed fetuses. A 45 X0

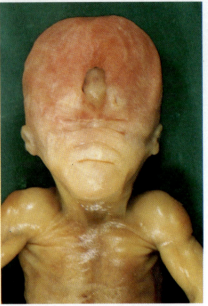

Fig. 16.1 Fetus with trisomy 13 (Patau's syndrome). Note very abnormal face with proboscis above rudimentary orbits, and absent nose. The brain has not developed into two cerebral hemispheres.

Table 16.1   Major effects of trisomy 21, 18 and 13

	Down's syndrome (trisomy 21)	Patau's syndrome (trisomy 13)	Edward's syndrome (trisomy 18)
Incidence per number of live births	1:700	1:7000	1:5000
Brain and CNS	Mental handicap	Mental handicap CNS malformations	Mental handicap
Craniofacial	Slanted eyes Large tongue	Facial clefts Cyclops	Globular head Small chin
Musculoskeletal	Hypotonia Single creases in palms	Polydactyly	Overlapping fingers Rockerbottom feet
Cardiovascular	Cardiac septal defects	Variable defects	Ventricular septal defects
Other	Duodenal atresia	Exomphalos Genitourinary anomalies	Exomphalos Genitourinary anomalies

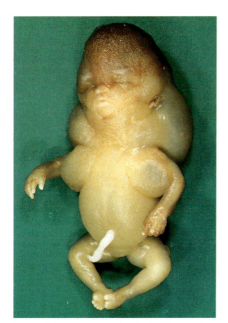

Fig. 16.2 Fetus with a lethal form of monosomy X (Turner's syndrome). Note generalized oedema with large lymphangioma at the back of the neck.

Major features of monosomy X (Turner's syndrome) in liveborn individuals
- Short stature
- Broad chest, wide spaced nipples
- Webbing of the neck
- Aortic coarctation
- Horseshoe kidney
- Lack of oocytes in ovaries

Classes of proteins which may be affected by single gene defects
- **Cell membrane proteins**: receptors, transport molecules
- **Extracellular proteins**: haemoglobin, collagen
- **Cellular growth regulators**: proto-oncogenes
- **Enzymes**

---

karyotype produces **Turner's syndrome**; most affected zygotes are lost early in pregnancy, but some survive into the second trimester and are recognized because they are growth retarded and oedematous (Fig. 16.2).

Less than 10% of X0 fetuses survive to the stage of viability (24 weeks' gestation and over). Those which do have a range of physical defects, but usually no mental handicap (see box).

Increased numbers of sex chromosomes, such as 47 XXY (Klinefelter's syndrome), 47 XYY, 47 XXX or 48 XXXY for example, can also occur and are fairly common (present in approximately 3 in 1000 people). Such karyotypes do not result in abnormal development of the major organ systems. Thus, unlike the trisomies, individuals with increased numbers of sex chromosomes survive. They may initially appear normal, but many develop behavioural problems and are infertile.

ABNORMAL CHROMOSOME STRUCTURE

Balanced translocations, in which there is interchange of parts of two different chromosomes with no loss of genetic material, may have no adverse effects except for problems with formation of normal germ cells, and thus with reproduction.

Duplication or **deletion** of parts of chromosomes and **unbalanced translocations** produces variable effects. Appreciable loss of genetic material is generally lethal, whereas abnormalities resulting in the presence of extra genetic material may have effects similar to the trisomies. Small deletions can present in a similar manner to single gene defects (see below).

Fragile sites are areas where the structure of the DNA is abnormal, resulting in chromosomal breakage when affected cells are grown in certain culture conditions in the laboratory, such as in a low folate medium. The best-known fragile site is on the X chromosome and is linked with mental handicap.

Single gene defects

In this group of disorders, there is absence of a gene or an abnormality in its DNA sequence. The problem cannot be seen by looking at metaphase chromosomal preparations, although in some cases presence of the error can be demonstrated using molecular biology techniques. With some defects, the presence of one normal gene is sufficient to supply the needs of the cell. There is no clinical effect unless the copies of the gene on both the maternally and paternally derived chromosomes are abnormal (recessive). With other defects, abnormalities arise even if only one copy of a gene is abnormal (dominant). Most single gene defects are inherited, although some autosomal dominant disorders are new mutations.

Consequences of a defective gene

A change in the DNA sequence which alters the genetic code may result in absence or abnormality of the gene product or it may alter expression of the gene if the abnormality is in the regulatory sequence. The net result is excessive, reduced or defective production of the protein coded for or regulated by the abnormal or absent gene. The pathological consequences are extremely variable. They depend upon the nature of the protein produced by the affected gene (see box), and whether it is possible to compensate for the abnormality.

A large number of different single gene defects have been described. Thus diseases as variable as those listed in Table 16.2 and illustrated in Figs 16.3–16.5 are all the result of single gene disorders. Although all of these are congenital in that the underlying genetic abnormality is present from birth, many do not present clinically for some months or years, and a few are not manifest until adulthood.

Some single gene defects are reasonably common, although many are extremely rare and have only been described in a small number of families. The incidence of the more frequent defects varies in different ethnic groups: cystic fibrosis is common in people of northern European descent, but is almost unknown in Africans, whilst the converse is true of sickle-cell disease.

Some diseases caused by single gene defects

CYSTIC FIBROSIS

This disease occurs when the cystic fibrosis transmembrane conductance regular (*CFTR*) gene on both the maternally and paternally derived chromosome 7 is defective. The transmembrane protein coded for by the normal *CFTR* gene is involved in the transport of chloride ions. In patients with the disease, there is disruption of normal electrolyte and water secretion by cells. This results in increased loss of chloride and sodium in the sweat and reduced hydration of the secretions from all the exocrine glands. The secretions become viscid and plug acinar and ductal lumina which may lead to cellular damage and death, chronic inflammation with fibrosis, and reduced function of the gland. The major clinical effects are seen in the pancreas, gastrointestinal tract and respiratory system in both sexes, and in the male reproductive system.

Infants may present with bowel obstruction due to intestinal blockage with viscid meconium (Fig. 16. 4). In older children, reduced clearance of secretions in the lungs predisposes to infection and bronchiectasis. Ductal obstruction in the pancreas ultimately results in acinar loss and pancreatic fibrosis, with secondary malabsorption. Blockage of the ejaculatory and

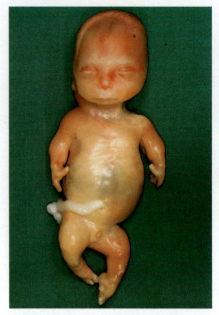

Fig. 16.3 Fetus with diastrophic dysplasia. Note the very short limbs, small mandible and 'hitch-hiker' thumbs. This is an autosomal recessive condition.

Table 16.2   Examples of diseases due to single gene defects

Disease	Inheritance	Defect	Major consequences
Cystic fibrosis	AR	Abnormal membrane protein	Abnormal cellular electrolyte transport
Sickle-cell disease	AR	Abnormal haemoglobin	Haemolysis, anaemia
Haemophilia	X-linked	Low/absent factor XIII	Bleeding
Achondroplasia	AD	Abnormal human fibroblast growth factor 2	Short stature
Duchenne muscular dystrophy	X-linked	Abnormal dystrophin	Progressive muscle weakness
Familial retinoblastoma	AD	Absent *RB1* tumour suppressor gene	Retinal malignancy
Meckel's syndrome	AR	Unknown	Multiple malformations
Inborn metabolic errors	Variable, mostly AR	Absent/abnormal enzyme	Abnormal metabolism
Immune deficiency disorders	Variable, X-linked, AR	Variable T-cell or antibody deficiency, or neutrophil or macrophage dysfunction	Recurrent infections

Fig. 16.4 Meconium ileus: intestinal obstruction due to blockage of the lumen of a loop of small bowel with abnormal sticky meconium in an infant with cystic fibrosis.

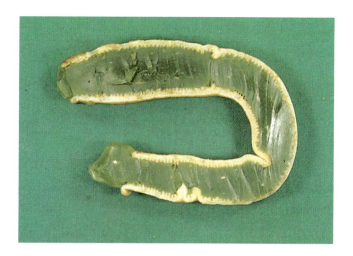

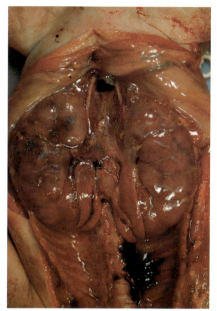

Fig. 16.5 Kidneys of a full-term infant which are grossly enlarged owing to autosomal recessive (infantile) polycystic kidney disease.

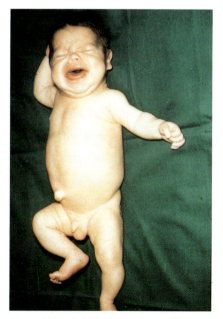

Fig. 16.6 Infant with untreated congenital hypothyroidism. Note coarse facial features with large tongue and umbilical hernia.

other ducts in the wolffian system by viscid secretions leads to male infertility.

RETINOBLASTOMA

Retinoblastoma is a malignant tumour of the retina which develops in infancy or early childhood. It arises when both copies of the retinoblastoma (*Rb1*) gene, a tumour suppressor gene located on chromosome 13, are absent. In familial forms of the disease, the child inherits one deletion. During development there is a high probability that the second *Rb1* gene will be lost from occasional retinal cells, usually as the result of a mitotic error. This loss, the so-called 'second hit', results in malignant transformation of the affected cell and retinoblastoma results. Inheritance of the abnormality is associated with a greater than 90% incidence of the tumour and, because there is a high chance of this second hit occurring in more than one retinal cell, familial retinoblastoma tends to be bilateral and multiple. The same tumour can arise in an individual with no family history who therefore inherits two normal *Rb1* genes. In this case two separate events are required to delete or damage both *Rb1* genes in a single cell. Non-familial retinoblastoma is therefore rare, and the tumours are typically single and unilateral.

POLYCYSTIC KIDNEY DISEASE

Some types of cystic kidney disease are due to single gene defects. Autosomal dominant (or adult) polycystic kidney disease usually presents with renal failure between the ages of 30 and 40 years, by which time the development of multiple tubular cysts has resulted in destruction of the functioning renal tissue. In contrast, autosomal recessive (or infantile) polycystic kidney disease is much less common, and results in renal failure and death in early infancy (Fig. 16.5).

Inborn errors of metabolism

Inborn errors result from abnormalities in the enzymes or cofactors controlling metabolic pathways. Most result from autosomal recessive or sex-linked inherited genetic defects. A huge number of different conditions have been described affecting most known metabolic pathways, for example carbohydrate, lipid, protein and organic acid metabolism, the urea cycle, the function of lysosomes and the turnover of mucopolysaccharides

Table 16.3   Neonatal screening in the UK

Disease	Abnormality	Effect
Phenylketonuria	Defective breakdown of phenylalanine	Progressive brain damage
Hypothyroidism	Abnormal thyroxine synthesis enzymes (dyshormonogenesis) or absent thyroid	Cretinism

and sphingolipids. An enzyme abnormality may result in the slowing down or complete blockage of a metabolic pathway, with failure to manufacture vital substances. This lack may be the major reason for clinical disease. However, in some conditions the main problem results from the accumulation of the substrates for the defective enzyme (examples are fatty acid oxidation defects and congenital adrenal hyperplasia). These may be small molecules which have a directly toxic effect, or macromolecules which cannot be excreted and have to be stored indefinitely within cells. Individually most inborn errors of metabolism are rare, but their effects can be devastating (see box). In the UK at present, all neonates are screened for phenylketonuria and hypothyroidism (Fig. 16.6) by means of the Guthrie test (Table 16.3).

Congenital malformations

Congenital malformations are structural abnormalities present at birth which result from anomalies of intrauterine growth and/or developmental processes. They range from minor single defects such as a bifid uvula to multiple major lethal anomalies affecting several different organs. Approximately 3% of babies are born with a single major congenital malformation, and 0.7% have multiple defects. See the box at the bottom of the page for some of the major terms relevant to the discussion of developmental abnormalities.

Aetiology and pathogenic mechanisms

In most cases no specific agent can be identified, although there are some recognized causes of congenital malformations (see box on p. 373). In these, the aetiology is probably multifactorial and due to the action of various adverse environmental factors in a genetically susceptible fetus (see second box on p. 373). The major **pathogenic mechanisms** involved in the production of congenital structural anomalies are primary malformation, disruption and deformation.

Some manifestations of inborn errors of metabolism
- **Fetal**: abortion, intrauterine death, generalized fetal oedema
- **Neonatal**: coma, convulsions, hypoglycaemia, acidosis
- **Older infants and children**: failure to thrive, sudden unexpected death, progressive mental and motor dysfunction, hepatosplenomegaly, coarse facies, liver failure

---

Effects of hypothyroidism in infants and children
- Mental handicap
- Protuberant abdomen and tongue
- Umbilical hernia
- Dwarfism
- Constipation

Congenital malformations: terminology
- **Hypoplasia**: underdevelopment of part of the body due to a decreased number of cells
- **Hyperplasia**: overdevelopment of part of the body due to an increased number of cells
- **Hypertrophy**: increase in size of part of the body due to increase in number or size of cells
- **Atrophy**: reduction in size of a previously normally developed part of the body due to reduced cell size or number
- **Agenesis**: absence of part of the body due to failure of the primordium to form
- **Aplasia**: formation of only a rudimentary structure due to failure of primordium to develop properly – an extreme form of hypoplasia
- **Dysplasia**: abnormal organization of cells into tissues (note that the term 'dysplasia' used in the context of abnormal development carries no implication of a preneoplastic condition)

Recognized causes of congenital malformations
- Chromosomal abnormalities
- Mutant genes
- Environmental factors

Environmental factors leading to congenital malformation
- **Maternal disorders**: diabetes mellitus, maternal phenylketonuria
- **Drugs**: including alcohol and cocaine
- **Intrauterine infection**: rubella, toxoplasmosis
- **Physical agents**: irradiation, chemicals
- **Dietary deficiencies**: folic acid

In **primary malformation**, the developmental process is intrinsically abnormal. There is a failure in the formation, migration or rearrangement of cells. This is generally the result of a chromosomal abnormality or a defective gene. It may also occur after exposure to a teratogen at a critical stage of development.

Disruption to a tissue or organ which is developing normally is a second major mechanism leading to a congenital abnormality. It may result from an intrauterine infection which destroys normally grown and positioned cells, from an intrauterine vascular catastrophe or from a teratogen. Anomalies caused in this way are not inherited. However, if disruption occurs very early in development it may be difficult to distinguish from a primary malformation with a genetic aetiology.

Deformation results from unusual mechanical forces, most commonly resulting from reduced amniotic fluid or a malformed uterus. Although affected tissues are initially normally formed, abnormal forces subsequently cause derangement of further intrauterine growth and development, manifest at birth as a congenital anomaly.

Multiple malformations

The pattern of multiple malformations in an individual may be random, or form a recognizable pattern. It is important to identify the latter, because based on previous observations it is usually possible to assess the risk of recurrence of the abnormalities in a future pregnancy.

Table 16.4 Common clinically significant congenital malformations

		Approximate incidence per 5000 births
Central nervous system	Neural tube defects	10
	Hydrocephalus	2
Congenital heart disease	Ventricular and atrial septal defects	14
	Aortic stenosis	4
	Coarctation of the aorta	2
	Tetralogy of Fallot	2
	Transposition of the great vessels	1
Soft tissue and musculoskeletal defects	Inguinal hernia	55
	Congenital dislocation of the hip	50
	Varus, valgus and other foot deformities	10
	Cleft lip and/or palate	7
	Diaphragmatic hernia	2
Genitourinary anomalies	Undescended testis	20[a]
	Hypospadias	7[a]
	Renal agenesis	2
	Urinary tract obstruction	2
Gastrointestinal problems	Congenital hypertrophic pyloric stenosis	10
	Gut atresias	2
	Meckel's diverticulum	75[b]
	Hirschsprung's disease	1

[a] Incidence in male babies.
[b] Many will never become symptomatic.

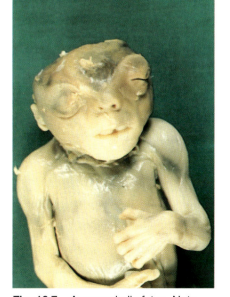

Fig. 16.7 Anencephalic fetus. Note absence of cranium and underlying brain, associated with grotesque facies with bulging eyes.

Common malformations

Some of the commonest clinically significant malformations are listed in Table 16.4. The incidence is given per 5000 births, which is roughly the number of babies a large obstetrics unit would deliver each year. Certain types of anomalies may not be evident at birth, and present later in infancy or in childhood and, in some cases, a clinically significant malformation only comes to light in adult life.

Central nervous system

NEURAL TUBE DEFECTS

Neural tube defects (NTDs) are the commonest type of major congenital malformation. They result from failure of closure of the neural tube 21–28 days after conception, with secondary failure of formation of the overlying bone. If the cranial end of the neural tube is affected, the result is anencephaly (Fig. 16.7). This is incompatible with postnatal life. Failure of closure of the caudal end of the neural tube results in lumbosacral spina bifida and myelomeningocele (Fig. 16.8). The latter is usually accompanied by a brain-stem abnormality (**Arnold–Chiari malformation**) which obstructs the flow of cerebrospinal fluid and produces hydrocephalus (see below). Many infants with spina bifida die in early infancy. Those which survive usually have varying degrees of paralysis and sphincter disturbance and may be mentally handicapped secondary to hydrocephalus. Neural tube defects may occur as part of a genetic multiple malformation syndrome. However, in most cases, no specific chromosomal or single gene defect can be demonstrated. The increased incidence of NTDs in malnourished mothers and in some racial groups suggests a multifactorial aetiology. Reduced folate levels in the mother are thought to be a major environmental factor. Recent research has revealed that, if women who have had one affected baby take folic acid for a few months before they conceive again, the risk of recurrence is greatly reduced.

Spina bifida occulta, due to the non-fusion of a single neural arch with no other abnormality, is present in approximately 5% of the population. It is not classified as a neural tube defect.

HYDROCEPHALUS

Hydrocephalus is defined as excess **cerebrospinal fluid** (CSF) in the cranial cavity, and is manifest as ventricular dilatation (Fig. 16.9).

In children, hydrocephalus is usually the result of a lesion which obstructs the flow of CSF. It may also occur as a secondary phenomenon after destruction of cerebral tissue by infection or infarction. The commonest cause of congenital hydrocephalus is an Arnold–Chiari malformation associated with lumbosacral spina bifida. In this, the brain stem is displaced downwards. The medulla extends through the foramen magnum into the upper cervical canal, blocking the free flow of CSF from the third and fourth ventricles (where it is produced by the choroid plexus), into the subarachnoid space. The result is accumulation of fluid and dilatation of the ventricular system. The reason why spina bifida is almost always accompanied by an Arnold–Chiari malformation is unclear; it may be due to tethering of the spinal cord in the region of the spina bifida with the result that the brain is pulled downwards through the foramen magnum as the body elongates.

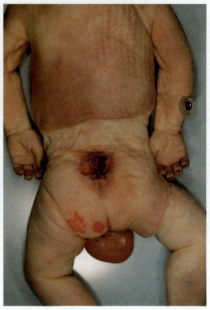

Fig. 16.8   Infant with spina bifida and associated myelomeningocele.

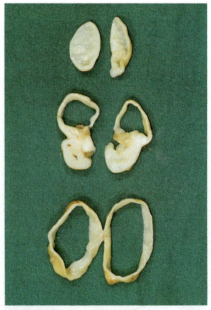

Fig. 16.9   Hydrocephalus: note massive dilatation of the lateral ventricles in the occipital, parietal and frontal regions with a relative sparing of the temporal region in this case.

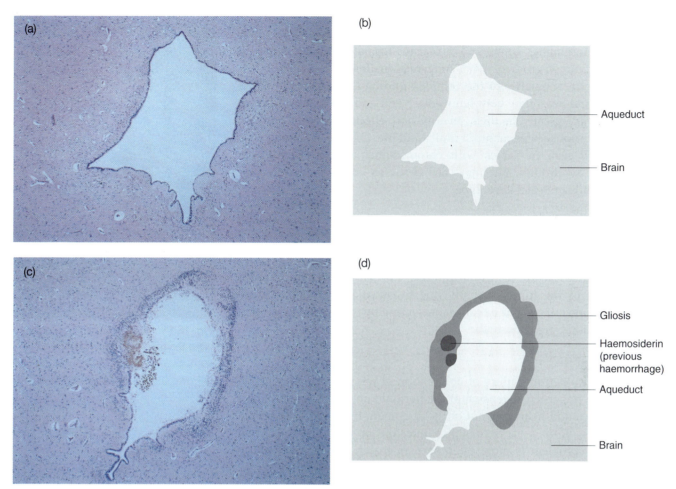

Fig. 16.10   (a, b) Normal mid-brain acqueduct. (c, d) Acquired aqueduct stenosis owing to intraventricular haemorrhage in the perinatal period.

Congenital hydrocephalus may also be due to failure of the foramina of the fourth ventricle to develop (**Dandy–Walker syndrome**). This prevents passage of CSF from the ventricular system into the subarachnoid space. Narrowing of the aqueduct of Sylvius (the channel which runs between the third and fourth ventricles) or other complex CNS anomalies may also be accompanied by hydrocephalus. The aetiology of this group of malformations is generally unknown. However, in male infants, congenital hydrocephalus may be an X-linked inherited genetic abnormality. On occasions, CNS abnormalities producing hydrocephalus are part of a multiple malformation syndrome.

Some cases of hydrocephalus in children are not congenital, but are acquired after birth. Intraventricular haemorrhage in pre-term infants (see below) is a well-recognized risk factor for the development of hydrocephalus. Cellular reaction to the blood as it passes down the aqueduct and out of the exit foramina of the fourth ventricle (foramina of Luschka and Magendie) results in reduced flow of CSF to the subarachnoid space (Fig. 16.10).

Ventricular dilatation secondary to loss of brain tissue from infarction, infection or other causes may be congenital or acquired. A hind brain tumour such as a medulloblastoma (see below) is a rare cause of acquired hydrocephalus.

Cardiovascular system

After CNS abnormalities, congenital cardiac malformations (see Chapter 8) are the most common group of major congenital malformations (Fig. 16.11). They result from anomalies in the complex folding and septation of the primitive ventral heart tube between weeks 3 and and 8 after fertilization. The lesions vary greatly in their severity and effects, and some minor anomalies may not become manifest until adult life. Cardiac malformations are commonly seen in babies with chromosomal and other multiple malformation syndromes, but may also occur as an isolated defect in individuals with a normal karyotype.

Soft tissue and musculoskeletal defects

CONGENITAL DISLOCATION OF THE HIP

Congenital dislocation of the hip (also known as **developmental displacement of the hip**) is usually due to capsular laxity. It is more common in male infants and in babies presenting by the breech, and there is some hereditary predisposition.

INGUINAL HERNIA

This hernia results from failure of obliteration of the processus vaginalis. The latter is a finger-like extension of the peritoneum which accompanies the testes or around ligaments out of the abdomen. If the inguinal hernia persists it may form a sac into which intestine or uterine adnexa can herniate. This problem is more often seen in males, and is particularly common in small pre-term infants.

DEFORMITIES OF THE FEET

Foot deformities may occur in association with a variety of other conditions (see box), but in many infants no obvious cause is found. The commonest problem is **talipes equinovarus** in which the foot is plantar flexed (equinus), the heel is inverted and the mid and forefoot are adducted (varus). Splinting from birth or operative correction is usually required to enable the child to walk properly.

CLEFTS OF THE LIP AND PALATE

Cleft lip and palate result from failure of fusion of the facial swellings around 6 weeks' gestation. They may be unilateral or bilateral, isolated or associated with other defects. They are commonly seen in trisomy 13 and are associated with numerous other syndromes. Some isolated cases are the result of maternal phenytoin ingestion. Multifactorial hereditary factors are important in other infants in whom this is the only defect. Palatal clefts interfere with feeding and speech development, and affected babies need specialist care.

DIAPHRAGMATIC HERNIA

This hernia results from failure of proper formation of the diaphragm, so the pleural and peritoneal cavities remain in communication. It is generally unilateral and affects the left hemidiaphragm. The result is the displacement of abdominal viscera into the chest (Fig. 16.12). The lung on the affected side fails to develop properly and is small. If the hernia is very

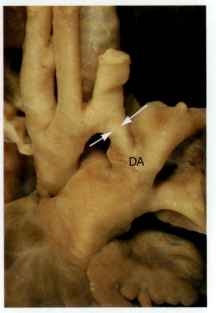

Fig. 16.11   Coarctation of the aorta. Note the marked narrowing of the aorta distal to the left subclavian artery (arrows) and immediately proximal to the ductus arteriosus (DA).

Conditions associated with foot deformities
- Oligohydramnios
- Abnormal intrauterine position
- Sacral agenesis
- CNS abnormalities
- Congenital short talus

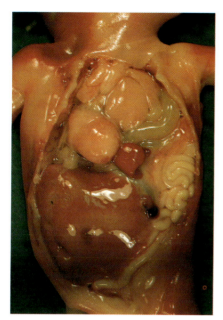

Fig. 16.12 Large left-sided congenital diaphragmatic hernia: note loops of bowel in the left chest.

large, with displacement of the heart and mediastinum, the contralateral lung may also be hypoplastic. Although reduction of the hernia and repair of the defective diaphragm are possible postnatally, many affected babies die of respiratory failure because there is insufficient pulmonary parenchyma to support independent life. Diaphragmatic hernias may be associated with an abnormal karyotype or other malformations, or may occur in the absence of any other major anomalies.

Genitourinary system

UNDESCENDED TESTES

Testes descend through the inguinal canal at months 7–8 of intrauterine life. Thus in many premature infants, but also in some babies born at term, the testes are not in the scrotum. Most descend after birth, but at 3 months of age in 1.6% of males, the testes still cannot be manipulated into the scrotum. This may be due to arrest of descent in the normal pathway (cryptorchidism) or the result of ectopic placement of the testis, usually in the superficial inguinal region. Undescended testes may occasionally be associated with other abnormalities, including intersex states. Untreated, maldescended testes undergo tubular and interstitial cell atrophy, and there is a significantly increased risk of germ cell neoplasia, especially seminoma (see Chapter 15).

HYPOSPADIAS

Reduced testosterone or diminished testosterone responsiveness during early intrauterine development can result in incomplete formation of the urethra in the male. The commonest problem is hypospadias in which the urethra opens on the ventral aspect of the penis at the base of the glans, more proximally along the penile shaft or occasionally in the perineal region. As well as aberrant siting of the external urethral meatus, there is deformity of the foreskin and angulation of the penile shaft (see Chapter 15).

RENAL AGENESIS

The ureteric bud, formed from the metanephros, induces differentiation of the mesoblast into renal parenchyma during embryonic life. If the ureteric bud fails or degenerates, there is absence of the kidney and ureter. The cause of renal agenesis is generally unknown, but some cases are familial. Unilateral renal agenesis is relatively common, and in the absence of disease in the second kidney or other genitourinary defects produces no clinical effects and may go unnoticed during life. Bilateral renal agenesis (**Potter's syndrome**) is fatal, and affected infants die shortly after birth (see Chapter 13). The immediate cause of perinatal death is respiratory failure due to pulmonary hypoplasia. In order to develop normally, fetal lungs *in utero* must be distended with fluid. The marked reduction in the volume of amniotic fluid, caused by lack of fetal urine production, results in a net loss of liquid from the lungs and failure to form and mature adequate numbers of terminal air sacs in the pulmonary parenchyma. Severe oligohydramnios also results in an abnormal face (**Potter's facies**) and positional deformities of the limbs.

CONGENITAL URINARY TRACT OBSTRUCTION

Abnormalities which prevent free flow of urine through the ureters or urethra cause urinary tract obstruction. Lower urinary tract obstruction usually results from accentuation of a pair of mucosal folds in the posterior urethra in infant boys, so-called **urethral valves**. Higher up in the urinary tract, obstruction at the junction of the renal pelvis and upper ureter is the most frequent lesion. In these cases no luminal blockage can be demonstrated and the cause is thought to be a narrow segment where there is no peristalsis, possibly due to abnormal arrangement of the muscle bundles at this point or to some defect in innervation. Both these anomalies may have severe complications (see box). The prognosis depends upon the site and degree of obstruction, the stage of development at which the problem developed and, in the case of upper urinary tract obstruction, whether the disorder is unilateral or bilateral. Severe early obstruction is associated with failure of proper development of the renal parenchyma (renal dysplasia – see below). If both kidneys are affected, the condition is lethal early in the perinatal period due to the combination of pulmonary hypoplasia resulting from oligohydramnios and little or no renal function. The cause of urinary tract obstruction is generally unknown although a few cases are associated with multiple malformation syndromes and chromosomal abnormalities.

Complications of congenital urinary tract obstruction
● Hydronephrosis, hydroureter
● Renal dysplasia
● Oligohydramnios

RENAL DYSPLASIA

Abnormal development and organization of the renal parenchyma is known as renal dysplasia. The renal parenchyma forms from the metanephros, and requires induction by a normal ureteric bud. Ureteric atresia and severe intrauterine urinary tract obstruction in the first and second trimesters of pregnancy both result in abortive nephrogenesis. The renal parenchyma is disorganized and may be solid or contain multiple large cysts. Small areas of dysplasia may sometimes be seen in otherwise normal kidneys, reflecting local abnormalities in induction of nephrogenesis. However, if the dysplasia is severe, widespread and bilateral, there will be little or no urine production *in utero*. The results will thus be similar to bilateral renal agenesis (see above).

VESICOURETERIC REFLUX

Vesicoureteric reflux results from a defect in the normal mechanisms at the lower end of the ureter which prevent back flow of urine into the ureters. There is reflux of urine from the bladder back up the ureters and secondary renal damage (**reflux nephropathy**). Although reflux is congenital, the problem usually presents in infants or older children and is more common in girls. Small degrees of reflux may not be diagnosed unless they are associated with urinary tract infection. Severe degrees of reflux produce dilatation of the renal collecting system on the affected side and reflux nephropathy (Fig. 16.13). Reflux is often complicated by infection, and there is controversy whether this, or the reflux per se, is more important in causing renal damage. Chronic infection is probably a prerequisite of renal scarring with lesser degrees of reflux, but it is possible that renal damage may result from back flow of sterile urine if the grade of reflux is sufficiently severe.

Errors of sexual differentiation

When normal gonads are present but there is abnormal differentiation of the internal or external genitalia, errors of sexual differentiation result. The

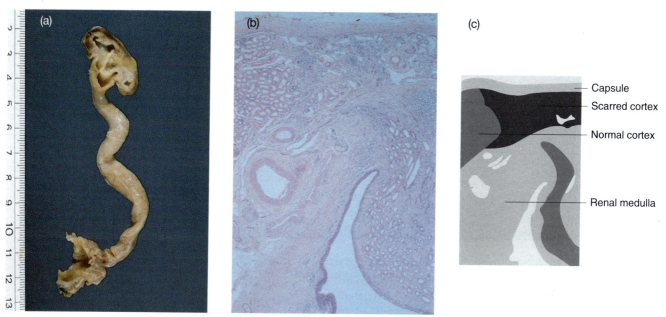

Fig. 16.13   (a) Reflux nephropathy: note the dilatation of the pelvis (hydronephrosis) and a characteristic pattern of renal scarring with marked thinning of the cortex and atrophy of the papillae overlying distended, deformed calyces. (b, c) Histology showing marked thinning of the cortex and atrophy of the papillae overlying distended deformed calyces. Away from the calyces, some normal renal tissue remains.

anomalies are usually the result of an intrauterine endocrine disorder. The most common is virilization of a genetic female: the external genitalia are like those of a male except that no testes are present in the scrotum. The problem is usually due to excessive production of androgens as a result of congenital adrenal hyperplasia. Defective virilization of a genetic male is the result of absent androgen receptors, a congenital abnormality known as **testicular feminization syndrome**.

Gastrointestinal system

CONGENITAL HYPERTROPHIC PYLORIC STENOSIS

Pyloric stenosis produces marked narrowing of the pylorus with gastric outlet obstruction. It is much more common in males than females, first-born sons being particularly affected. Pathologically, the pylorus is increased in length and diameter with a marked increase in the thickness of the circular muscle and attenuation of the longitudinal muscle. Clinical presentation is usually after the age of 1 week, characteristically around 6 weeks after birth. The cause is unknown; abnormal pyloric innervation inducing circular muscle hypertrophy and obstruction is one hypothesis.

INTESTINAL ATRESIA

Intestinal atresia is an abnormality resulting in loss of continuity of the bowel lumen producing intestinal obstruction. The most common sites are the ileum, jejunum and duodenum, and the atretic segments of bowel can be multiple. On gross examination, there may be complete interruption to the intestine and a gap in the adjacent mesentery.

More commonly, the atretic bowel is represented by a fibrous cord with an intact mesentery or by a continuous bowel wall with a lumen occluded by fibrous tissue. Jejunal and ileal atresia is thought to represent a

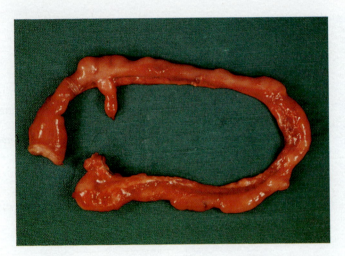

Fig. 16.14 Meckel's diverticulum. A narrow out-pouching of the small intestine wall is present a short distance from the ileocaecal valve. These may give rise to ulceration and bleeding, intussusception or acute inflammation mimicking acute appendicitis.

disruption due to intrauterine intestinal ischaemia with mucosal and submucosal necrosis and subsequent granulation formation and fibrosis. In contrast, duodenal atresia (which is often associated with trisomy 21, Down's syndrome) is probably a primary malformation resulting from initial failure of canalization of the gut.

MECKEL'S DIVERTICULUM

This diverticulum is an out-pouching of the bowel wall along the antimesenteric border of the ileum, a few centimetres proximal to the ileocaecal valve (Fig. 16.14). It is due to failure of complete obliteration of the **omphalomesenteric duct**, the structure which runs from the primitive gut through the umbilicus to the yolk sac in embryonic life. The reason why part of the duct sometimes persists is unknown. Meckel's diverticula are lined by small intestinal mucosa although heterotopic epithelium, particularly gastric mucosa, is present in many cases. They may give rise to a number of complications (see Chapter 11).

HIRSCHSPRUNG'S DISEASE

Hirschsprung's disease (or **intestinal aganglionosis**) is due to abnormal innervation of the bowel. During the first trimester neuroblasts migrate down the gut in a craniocaudal direction, and mature to ganglion cells in the submucosa and muscle (Fig. 16.15). If migration ceases early, varying

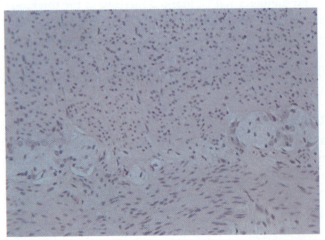

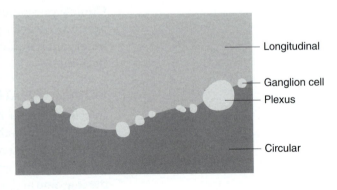

Longitudinal

Ganglion cell

Plexus

Circular

Fig. 16.15 Normal myenteric plexus between the circular and longitudinal muscle layers of the bowel wall. Note delicate fibrillary plexus with ganglion and Schwann cells.

Complications of Hirschsprung's disease
- **Newborn infants**: intestinal obstruction, intestinal perforation
- **Older children**: constipation

lengths of the distal intestine are aganglionic (see Chapter 11). The rectum, being the most distal part of the bowel, is always affected. The earlier migration ceases, the further up the bowel the abnormal segment extends. Rarely the whole gut is aganglionic. The disease is diagnosed histologically; biopsies of rectal submucosa or of full thickness rectal wall show a complete absence of ganglion cells but enlarged nerve trunks. The complications of Hirschsprung's disease (see box) usually result in diagnosis in the neonatal period. Occasionally, however, this is delayed into childhood, or exceptionally into adult life.

The aetiology of Hirschsprung's disease is unknown, although there is some familial tendency, this being more evident the longer the affected segment. Recently, mutation of the *ret* oncogene has been implicated in this disorder.

The infant of the diabetic mother

Congenital malformations are appreciably more common in babies born to mothers who have diabetes prior to pregnancy. The commonest malformations are in the central nervous system but failure of adequate development of the sacral spine and heart defects are also seen. Other complications may occur in the infants of mothers with either established or gestational diabetes. Sudden unexpected intrauterine asphyxial death of the infant in the third trimester is also more common than normal. The infants of diabetic mothers tend to be large and cherubic and there is an increased risk of trauma during delivery. In spite of their large size, the organs of the infants of diabetic mothers are often immature and respiratory distress in the newborn as a result of hyaline membrane disease (see below) is also a problem. Hypoglycaemia secondary to hypertrophic islets of Langerhans is a further potential complication in this group of infants.

Fetal alcohol syndrome

Abnormalities in the fetal alcohol syndrome
- Abnormal face
- Small head
- Cleft palate
- Heart malformations
- Growth retardation
- Mental handicap

Excessive heavy maternal drinking during pregnancy is associated with a variety of characteristic abnormalities in the baby, collectively known as the fetal alcohol syndrome (see box).

Birth

The process of birth requires rapid, major adaptation on the part of the infant to the extrauterine environment. The chief problems encountered in full-term births are:

- interference with the supply of nutrients during delivery resulting in hypoxia and acidosis, known as **birth asphyxia**
- **trauma** to the infant due to excessive forces applied in order to effect delivery; birth trauma is often associated with coexisting hypoxia
- infection if membranes are ruptured for a long time during labour (see below).

Birth asphyxia

Interference with the supply of nutrients (including oxygen) to the fetus during labour and delivery causes hypoxia and acidosis. Mild degrees of

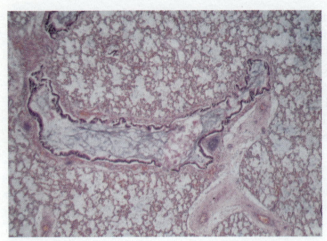
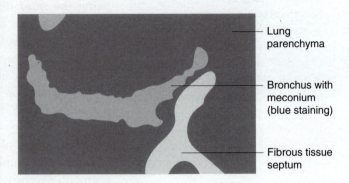

Lung parenchyma

Bronchus with meconium (blue staining)

Fibrous tissue septum

Fig. 16.16   Massive inhalation of meconium in an asphyxiated term infant. Note the presence of mucoid material in the airways, derived from the bowel.

asphyxia are relatively common. The fetus is better adapted to withstand the effects of a low Po_2 and low pH than children and adults, and minor abnormalities are soon corrected after birth with no apparent short- or long-term ill effects. More severe degrees of intrapartum hypoxia are less common. If the fetus is recognized to be hypoxic *in utero*, a decision is usually taken to expedite delivery, either by performing an emergency caesarean section or, if labour has advanced to the second stage, by the use of forceps or vacuum extraction.

Hypoxia during delivery can result from cord abnormalities, premature separation of the placenta from the uterus before the infant has been delivered, and a few other recognized problems. However, in most cases the reason for the intrauterine asphyxia remains unknown. Intrauterine hypoxia and acidosis at term may cause the baby to pass meconium *in utero*, and this can then be inhaled into the lungs which compromises oxygenation after birth if the infant is born alive (**meconium aspiration syndrome**) (Fig. 16.16).

Other major features of birth asphyxia are damage to the endothelium of capillaries, causing small haemorrhages especially in the thoracic organs, damage to the myocardium resulting in marked congestion of the organs, and damage to neurons in the brain. The last, if severe, produces the clinical syndrome of hypoxic–ischaemic encephalopathy with fitting in the neonatal period and a high incidence of neurodevelopmental handicap. If the baby dies during delivery or soon after birth, no macroscopic or microscopic abnormalities, except for congestion, may be seen in the heart or brain. Morphological changes take a few hours to develop, and it is only if the baby survives for a few days that neuronal necrosis and other forms of brain damage are visible histologically.

Birth trauma

Minor bleeding into the scalp is almost universal after a normal cephalic delivery, and is of no significance. Modern obstetric practice has meant that serious trauma is much less of a problem than in previous times. It usually results from the application of excessive force in attempts to deliver an infant who is only advancing down the birth canal very slowly, or indeed has got 'stuck'. Serious birth trauma is more common with large infants

Serious birth injuries
- **Bony fractures**: skull, limbs, clavicle
- **Subdural haemorrhage**: tearing of the bridging veins due to marked and uneven deformation of the head
- **Tears** of the falx cerebri and tentorium cerebelli
- **Spinal cord, nerve root or brachial plexus injury** secondary to excessive traction
- **Hepatic injury**: subcapsular haematoma which may rupture and give haemoperitoneum

born at full term; pre-term infants are smaller and more malleable and less subject to serious damage. See box on p. 382 for a summary of the major traumatic lesions.

Premature birth

Premature birth is defined as birth occurring before 37 completed weeks of gestation. It is an important public health problem. In terms of parental anxiety, the chance of handicap and the cost of neonatal intensive care, it has major socioeconomic implications. In a proportion of cases, pre-term birth results from spontaneous premature onset of labour for which no reason can be discovered. For some of the recognized causes see box.

Although the excellence of modern intensive care means many very premature babies now survive, there are major problems resulting from immaturity of the organ systems and the risks are increased the earlier the gestation at delivery. The immediate, major, pathological problems are in the lungs, brain and intestines (see box), but acidosis, hypoglycaemia, electrolyte disturbance, abnormal cardiac and hepatic function also result in major clinical problems. In very premature babies who require long-term ventilation, chronic changes may develop in the lungs (**bronchopulmonary dysplasia**) and abnormalities of the retina, resulting from toxic effects of long-term ventilation with oxygen, are an important consideration. In addition, immaturity of the immune system with lack of protective maternal antibodies means premature babies have an increased risk of developing an infection. The difficulty of introducing sufficient nutrients in babies with small bowel problems may lead to impaired mineralization of the skeleton and rickets.

Hyaline membrane disease (infant respiratory distress syndrome)

Hyaline membrane disease is a pathological term used to describe amorphous eosinophilic material lining the terminal airways of a neonate. It is usually due to lack of **surfactant**, a deficiency which results in high surface tension in small air sacs. Thus large pressures and increased inspired oxygen concentrations need to be used to inflate the lungs and oxygenate a pre-term baby. Unfortunately these interventions result in damage to lung epithelium and endothelium by sheer stress and oxygen-related free radicals. Necrotic epithelial cells and plasma proteins which leak from damaged capillaries form the hyaline membranes. Good care of pre-term babies requires balancing the need for adequate blood gases against the damage caused by excessive ventilatory pressures and high inspired oxygen concentrations. At postmortem examination, lungs affected by hyaline membrane disease are solid and deep red in colour with typical microscopic changes (Fig. 16.17). Hyaline membrane disease gives rise to neonatal respiratory distress and may be complicated by interstitial emphysema or pneumothorax.

LEAKAGE OF AIR

The high pressures required to expand stiff lungs affected by hyaline membrane disease often cause tearing of delicate respiratory tissue. Leakage of air into the lung connective tissues produces interstitial

Some causes of premature birth
- Chorioamnionitis
- Multiple pregnancy
- Retroplacental haemorrhage/placental abruption
- Placenta praevia
- Pre-eclampsia
- Fetal growth retardation
- Rhesus disease
- Maternal disease
- Hypertension
  - Renal disease
  - Cardiac disease

Potential problems in the premature infant
- **Lungs**: hyaline membrane disease, interstitial emphysema, bronchopulmonary dysplasia
- **Brain**: intraventricular haemorrhage, white matter infarction
- **Intestines**: necrotizing enterocolitis
- **Liver**: jaundice, coagulation defects
- **Blood**: hypoglycaemia, electrolyte imbalance
- **Heart**: hypotension, cardiac failure with haemorrhagic pulmonary oedema
- **Lymphoreticular**: immune deficiency, infection
- **Eyes**: retinal fibrosis
- **Skeleton**: neonatal rickets

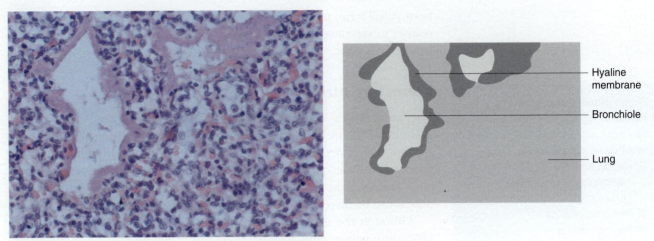

Fig. 16.17   Hyaline membrane disease. Note dilatation of terminal and respiratory bronchioles which are lined by eosinophilic hyaline membranes, and collapse of more distal airspaces.

emphysema (Fig. 16.18). If there is rupture of the visceral pleura, the result is a **pneumothorax**. These complications further compromise satisfactory ventilation, and thus oxygenation of pre-term neonates.

BRONCHOPULMONARY DYSPLASIA

Bronchopulmonary dysplasia is defined clinically as the continuing requirement for oxygen after 28 days of life, with persisting clinical, radiological and blood gas abnormalities, in an infant who had an acute lung injury (such as hyaline membrane disease) in the first 2 weeks of life. At postmortem examination, affected lungs are voluminous with random areas of collapse and overdistension. Microscopically there are emphysematous areas and poorly expanded areas, the latter showing septal oedema and fibroblast proliferation with macrophages in air spaces (Fig. 16.19). This intractable problem only develops in a small number of pre-term neonates. However, it may lead to pulmonary hypertension and right heart failure (**cor pulmonale**), and death at several months of age.

Intraventricular haemorrhage

In the developing brain during the first two trimesters, there is a dense layer of immature, proliferating cells around the cerebral ventricles which

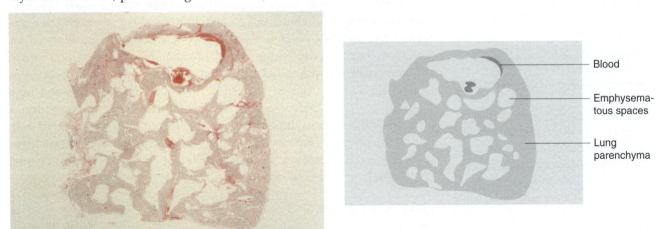

Fig. 16.18   Pulmonary interstitial emphysema. Note large spaces within the pulmonary parenchyma due to massive leakage of air into the interstitial connective tissues. Some of the spaces contain small amounts of blood.

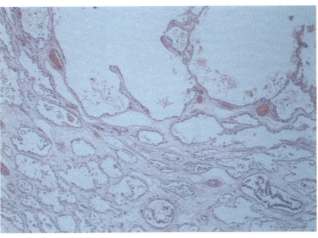

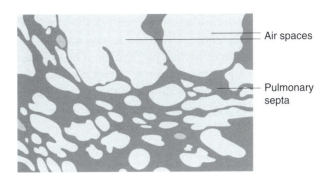

Air spaces

Pulmonary septa

Fig. 16.19 Bronchopulmonary dysplasia. Note the large variation in the size of the air spaces with septal fibroblast proliferation in poorly expanded areas.

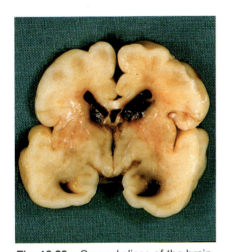

Fig. 16.20 Coronal slices of the brain of a premature infant showing subarachnoid haemorrhage with blood in both lateral ventricles.

give rise to cerebral neurons and glial cells. This is the **germinal matrix** from which cells migrate out into the cortex. It contains numerous endothelium-lined capillaries, which are easily damaged by hypoxia. Disruption of the endothelium results in germinal matrix haemorrhage. This often ruptures through the ependyma producing intraventricular haemorrhage (Fig. 16.20). The blood tracks down the route taken by the CSF, through the aqueduct and out through the exit foramina of the fourth ventricle into the subarachnoid space (Fig. 16.20). Intraventricular haemorrhage is very common in pre-term neonates. If the amount of bleeding is small there may be no adverse effects. Larger bleeds may cause haemorrhagic infarction of the adjacent brain, or block the flow of CSF producing hydrocephalus.

White matter infarction

Infarction of the white mattter results from ischaemic damage to the cerebrum, and is a typical lesion of the immature brain. Classically, the white matter around the angles of the lateral ventricles is involved. This is in the watershed area of vessels coming from the surface of the brain and those derived from the periventricular zone. It is thus relatively poorly perfused and vulnerable to damage whenever blood flow is reduced. Early on, the infarcts appear as small white spots (hence the technical term of **periventricular leukomalacia**), but with time there is removal of the necrotic material and gliosis. If the infarcted area was large, small cysts may be left at the site (Fig. 16.21). Such lesions disrupt the internal capsule, and can result in severe motor disability.

Necrotizing enterocolitis

Necrotizing enterocolitis (NEC) is a form of ischaemic necrosis of the intestines which is largely confined to very pre-term neonates. It is an important problem estimated to occur in 8–12% of babies born before 28 weeks' gestation or with a birth weight of less than 1500 g. The mortality rate in infants with established NEC is of the order of 30%. The aetiology and pathogenesis of the condition are not well understood. It is associated with oral feeding (especially with formula milk), and the presence of bacteria in the gut; medical management of the problem involves treatment with antibiotics, and withdrawal of enteral feeds and substitution with total parenteral nutrition. Abnormal activity of the physiological mechanisms designed to redistribute blood away from the gut, and thus excessive shut-down of the splanchnic circulation in response to hypotension, has been postulated to be an important mechanism. The presence of luminal bacteria and milk may injure the ischaemic bowel, leading to damage and necrosis of the mucosa and bowel wall. The major complications are perforation and peritonitis in the acute phase, and stricture formation later on if the baby lives and an affected area heals by fibrosis.

Infection

Infections are an important cause of morbidity and mortality in mid-pregnancy, in the perinatal period, in infancy and later in childhood.

Intrauterine infection

Infections acquired *in utero* may lead to miscarriage, stillbirth and/or fetal damage. Two major groups are recognized: **ascending infections** and **haematogenous infections**.

ASCENDING INFECTIONS

The vagina in many pregnant women contains bacteria and organisms such as chlamydia which do not cause local cell damage or symptoms, but can prove to be harmful pathogens if they gain access to the uterus. Bacteria may ascend through the cervix when the membranes rupture, but it is now increasingly realized that they can also infect the intact gestational sac. Either way, the result is acute inflammation of the chorion and amnion with outpouring of a polymorph-rich exudate into the amniotic fluid. For major causes of chorioamnionitis, see the box.

Inflammation weakens the membranes and may cause them to rupture. The mediators of the inflammatory reaction, such as prostaglandins, cause uterine contractions and onset of labour. Before 24 weeks' gestation there is little in the way of bacteriostatic and bactericidal substances in the amniotic fluid. Inhalation of infected liquor by the fetus leads to an intrauterine pneumonia.

Ascending infection of the gestational sac is one of the major causes of miscarriage in the second trimester before 24 weeks' gestation. It is now

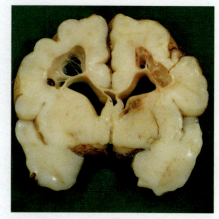

Fig. 16.21   Infarction of the periventricular white matter (periventricular leukomalacia). The baby has lived for some weeks after the acute insult and the dead white matter has been gradually removed leaving large cystic spaces around the ventricles. Such lesions disrupt the internal capsule and can result in severe motor disabilities.

Major causes of acute chorioamnionitis
- Group B streptococci
- Coliforms, e.g. *E. coli*
- *Listeria monocytogenes*
- *Gardnerella vaginalis*
- Gram-negative anaerobes, e.g. *Bacteroides* spp.
- Gram-negative cocci, e.g. *Peptostreptococcus*
- *Chlamydia* spp.
- *Candida* spp.

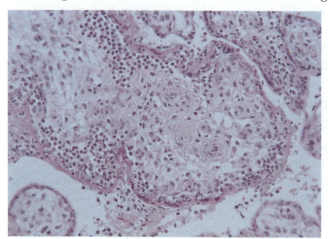

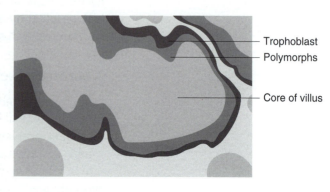

Trophoblast
Polymorphs

Core of villus

Fig. 16.22   Acute villitis due to listeria infection. Note large collections of polymorphs below the surface trophoblast of the villi.

thought to be the underlying problem in many cases of premature onset of labour in the third trimester.

HAEMATOGENOUS INFECTIONS

Haematogenous infections are spread to the fetus and placenta from the maternal blood stream. Organisms in the maternal blood space in the placenta damage the villi leading to an inflammatory response.

The infecting organism then gets access to the fetal circulation, with variable results including:

- miscarriage
- intrauterine death
- malformations and other forms of fetal damage
- growth retardation
- acute neonatal illness and/or inflammatory sequelae in childhood.

The precise effects depend upon the host susceptibility, nature of the organism, the infective dose and the stage of gestation. The potential consequences of intrauterine infection with the major pathogens are shown in Table 16.5.

It is important to realize that:

- not every fetus whose mother develops a haematogenous infection during pregnancy is infected
- not every infected fetus is damaged
- in some cases the consequences of an intrauterine infection may not be apparent at birth.

Thus deafness due to intrauterine infection of a fetus with rubella virus may only be recognized after infancy, and the effects of intrauterine infection with toxoplasmosis may only present as a visual disturbance due to retinitis in late childhood.

Infection in infancy and childhood

Infections remain an important cause of morbidity and mortality throughout childhood, especially in the early months and years. They are

Table 16.5 Haematogenous intrauterine infection

Infection	Possible effects
Rubella	Miscarriage, congenital abnormalities (mental handicap, cataract, cardiac malformations, deafness)
CMV	Miscarriage, intrauterine death, acute neonatal illness, later encephalitis, chorioretinitis, mental handicap
Toxoplasmosis	Low birth weight, neonatal illness, hydrocephalus, chorioretinitis
Herpes simplex	Skin scarring, eye and cerebral abnormalities
Listeria	Stillbirth, neonatal meningitis; no malformations reported
HIV	Infant or childhood AIDS; no malformations reported
Influenza	Miscarriage or stillbirth; no malformations reported
Syphilis	Rhinitis, skin lesions, osteochondritis, neurosyphilis
Varicella	Skin lesions, limb hypoplasia, small eyes, cerebral atrophy, neonatal illness
Parvovirus	Intrauterine death, fetal anaemia and oedema

an important cause of childhood death in the UK after perinatal problems, congenital malformations, trauma/accidents/poisonings, sudden unexpected infant deaths and malignant tumours. Respiratory infections are numerically the most important, but gastrointestinal infections (including food poisoning) and meningitis are also of concern, especially with the recent decrease in the number of cases of measles.

Neonatal pneumonia

Neonatal lung infection may result from intrauterine chorioamnionitis, or be acquired during delivery or in the first few days of life. Intrapartum and postnatal bacterial infections usually produce non-specific acute bronchopneumonia. However, group B haemolytic streptococci are very virulent in the neonate, and if death is rapid the lungs may show congestion and oedema with minimal inflammation.

Bronchiolitis and bronchitis

Most lower respiratory tract infections in children are caused by viruses (see first box) although secondary bacterial invasion may occur. In fatal cases of bronchiolitis, which are most common under the age of two years, there is necrosis of bronchial and bronchiolar epithelium and infiltration of the wall by mononuclear cells. This results in obstruction of the lumina of affected bronchioles, and severe respiratory difficulties. In some cases, the mononuclear infiltrate may extend into the surrounding lung parenchyma resulting in focal areas of pneumonia.

Meningitis

Inflammation of the meninges is a potentially serious condition. In children this is usually caused by a bacteria, although viral cases also occur. Among the most common bacterial pathogens, different organisms are important at different ages (see second box). With the exception of tuberculosis, all cause a brisk acute inflammatory reaction in the meninges with collection of pus

> **Viral causes of bronchiolitis and bronchitis in children**
> - Respiratory syncytial virus (commonest in first 2 years)
> - Adenovirus
> - Parainfluenza viruses
> - Influenza A and B virus
> - Measles virus

> **Bacterial meningitis in children**
> - Neonatal meningitis
>   - Group B haemolytic streptococci
>   - Gram-negative organisms (*E. coli*, *Pseudomonas*)
>   - *Listeria* spp.
> - Pre-school age group
>   - *Haemophilis influenzae*
> - Older children
>   - *Streptococcus pneumoniae*
>   - *Neisseria meningitidis*
> - Other
>   - *Mycobacterium tuberculosis*

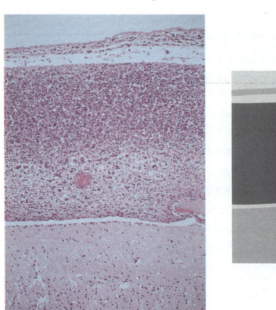

Inflamed meninges

Cortex

Fig. 16.23 Acute bacterial meningitis in a 4-month-old infant. Note the gross thickening of the meninges which are infiltrated with acute inflammatory cells. The underlying cerebral cortex is not inflamed.

Fig. 16.24 Haemorrhagic necrosis of the adrenal glands.

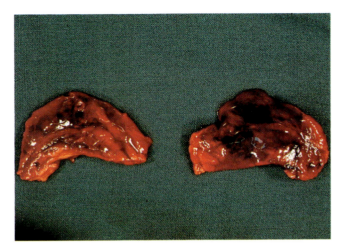

in the subarachnoid space (Fig. 16.23). Neonatal meningitis has a high mortality rate. Later in childhood the outcome is more favourable provided there has been early diagnosis and treatment. However, the septicaemia which accompanies meningitis may result in death from haemorrhagic necrosis of the adrenal glands (Fig. 16.24), especially with severe *N. meningitidis* infection (Waterhouse–Friderichsen syndrome). Another serious complication is local infarction of the brain due to cerebral swelling and inflammation and thrombosis of blood vessels. In survivors, organization of the exudate around the outlet foramina of the fourth ventricle may lead to obstruction to the flow of cerebrospinal fluid and hydrocephalus.

Recurrent infections

A variety of different mechanisms protects the body against invading micro-organisms. These include:

- Non-specific barrier and clearance mechanisms, for example intact skin, stomach acid and the normal production and movement of mucus in the respiratory tract.
- A good inflammatory response which may be sufficient to contain an infection before it becomes generalized.
- The immune response, including both specific reactions and non-specific components.

Defects in any of these protective mechanisms (see box) may lead to recurrent infection.

Primary immunodeficiency disorders

A wide variety of primary immunodeficiency disorders have been recognized in both the specific and the non-specific components of the immune system. Many are complex, in terms of both their causation and their effects. Some are familial, with classic autosomal recessive or X-linked patterns of inheritance. In others the exact aetiology is unknown, although small abnormalities in chromosome structure are increasingly being recognized in this group. Many patients with severe immunodeficiency syndromes have associated congenital malformations of organs and tissues outwith the immune system.

Conditions leading to an increased susceptibility to infection

- Primary immunodeficiency
  - B-cell disorders
  - T-cell deficiency states
  - Combined immunodeficiency diseases
  - Phagocytic cell deficiencies
  - Complement deficiency
- Malnutrition
- Prematurity
- Acquired immunodeficiency syndrome (HIV infection and AIDS)
- Other chronic diseases
  - Chronic diarrhoea
  - Metabolic disease, etc.
  - Cystic fibrosis

Primary immunodeficiency disorders are generally classified according to the component of the immune system which is defective. With the exception of selective immunoglobulin deficiencies, most are rare. Antibody and complement deficiencies predispose to recurrent infection with organisms such as pneumococci, staphylococci and *Haemophilus influenzae*. T-cell dysfunction results in severe infection with non-pathogenic bacteria and fungi or with agents that usually do not give serious illness such as *Toxoplasma* spp., atypical mycobacteria, *Cryptococcus* spp., fungi and viruses.

B-CELL DISORDERS

B-cell disorders range from complete **agammaglobulinaemia** to selective deficiency of some immunoglobulin classes or subclasses. In the rare X-linked agammaglobulinaemia (**Bruton's disease**), there is arrested development of B cells and antibodies are not formed in response to bacterial infections or immunization. **Selective IgA deficiency** is, in contrast, relatively common with a prevalence in the population of 1 in 5000. Not all affected individuals are symptomatic; those who are tend to have increased numbers of respiratory and intestinal infections.

T-CELL DEFICIENCIES

Primary T-cell deficiencies are rare and tend to result in clinically severe disease. A variety of different syndromes have been reported, most of which have associated abnormalities in other systems. One example is the **DiGeorge syndrome** in which the third and fourth branchial arches fail to develop properly. The result is absence or hypoplasia of the thymus and parathyroid glands and abnormal T-cell function, frequently associated with abnormalities of the heart and aorta such as an interrupted aortic arch. Some cases are familial, and in others a small chromosomal defect can be demonstrated.

SEVERE COMBINED IMMUNODEFICIENCY

Severe combined immunodeficiency is characterized by almost total absence of immune function. There is an abnormality of thymic development with absent Hassall's corpuscles and marked lymphocyte depletion. Lymph nodes are small and lack germinal centres. No natural killer cells are present in the peripheral blood. The disease is inherited, in either an X-linked or an autosomal recessive manner. In some families it is associated with an abnormality of an enzyme (adenosine deaminase) which results in multisystem defects as well as immune deficiency.

PHAGOCYTIC CELL DEFICIENCIES

Primary phagocytic cell deficiencies are rare and are characterized by abnormal uptake or intracellular killing of micro-organisms by monocytes/macrophages or neutrophils. In **chronic granulomatous disease of childhood** the production of superoxide by neutrophils is defective. The result is a failure of intracellular lysis of engulfed catalase-positive bacteria such as *Staphylococcus aureus*, and chronic infection with such organisms. Most cases are X-linked, but autosomal recessive inheritance has also been reported.

COMPLEMENT DEFICIENCIES

Deficiencies of all the components of the complement cascade have been described, and abnormalities of complement inhibitors have also been recognized. Deficiency of some components is associated with recurrent infections.

SECONDARY IMMUNE DEFICIENCY

Malnutrition or any chronic disease in childhood may result in defective production of antibodies and other immune system proteins. In pre-term infants, the immune system is immature and there are low circulating levels of maternal antibody which predispose them to infection. Acquired immune deficiency syndrome results from destruction of T-helper lymphocytes secondary to infection with the human immunodeficiency virus (see Chapter 6).

DEFECTIVE NON-SPECIFIC PROTECTIVE MECHANISMS

In cystic fibrosis, the excessively viscous respiratory tract secretions impede the normal mucus clearance mechanisms. The result is a predisposition to retain secretions and inhaled bacteria, resulting in recurrent bronchial and pulmonary infections.

Sudden unexpected death in infancy

Many problems and diseases in infancy can present with sudden unexpected death. Such a tragedy is likely to be followed by a postmortem examination performed at the request of the local coroner. The pathologist responsible for such an examination should be given full information about the circumstances surrounding the death. If death is sudden and witnessed, the cause is usually obvious (accident or trauma), or due to sudden airway obstruction, or a cardiac problem (see first box).

More commonly, unexpected death in infancy is unobserved, and the infant is found lifeless in his or her cot. In approximately 20% of these, a definite cause will be found provided a full postmortem examination is performed, including histological and microbiological examination of the internal organs (see second box). However, in the majority of cases of unobserved death, neither the history nor a thorough postmortem examination will reveal a satisfactory explanation. These are designated **sudden infant death syndrome** (SIDS) or **cot death**.

Sudden infant death syndrome

SIDS is defined as 'the sudden death of any infant which is unexpected by history and in which a thorough postmortem examination fails to reveal an adequate cause of death'.

Recently this definition has been expanded to include the requirement for an examination of the scene of death before a baby's death is classified as SIDS. In the UK, this inspection is generally carried out by police officers, and any suspicious features conveyed to the pathologist performing the postmortem examination.

SIDS is probably the result of a common mode of death that has many precipitating causes. Epidemiologically, there is no difference between unobserved sudden infant death for which a cause is found *post mortem*

Causes of witnessed sudden infant death
- ■ Accident, trauma
- ■ Airway foreign body
- ■ Laryngeal cyst
- ■ Cardiac problems
  - ● Myocarditis
  - ● Malformations
  - ● Cardiomyopathies
  - ● Coronary arteritis

Causes of unobserved sudden infant death
- ● Infection
- ● Heart disease
- ● Seizure disorders
- ● Non-accidental injury
- ● Poisoning
- ● Inborn errors of metabolism
- ● SIDS

Characteristic epidemiological associations in explained sudden infant death and SIDS
- ● Age peak 3–4 months
- ● Male predominance
- ● Commoner in autumn and winter
- ● High incidence with young mothers
- ● Higher risk with increasing birth order
- ● Higher incidence in social classes IV and V
- ● Higher incidence with maternal smoking

Postulated causes of SIDS

■ Infection, including anaphylaxis secondary to infection, and toxin production by common bacteria in respiratory tract
■ Overheating, including malignant hyperthermia trait
■ Hypothermia
■ Respiratory anomalies including prolonged sleep apnoea, surfactant deficiency, upper respiratory tract obstruction during sleep
■ Cardiac problems, including abnormal conduction pathways
■ Immunological defects, including anaphylaxis to cows' milk, house-dust mites, etc.
■ Metabolic problems, including hypoglycaemia, hypernatraemia, inborn errors of metabolism
■ Nutritional abnormalities, including deficiency of trace metals, vitamin deficiency
■ Endocrine disorders, including
  ● elevated triiodothyronine
  ● absent parathyroid glands
■ Toxins, including:
  ● common drugs and poisons
  ● carbon monoxide
  ● lead
■ Vaccination/immunization

and cases which are diagnosed as SIDS. Numerous different causes for SIDS have been postulated (see box above).

Recent work on the development of thermoregulation and breathing control in normal infants has shed light on possible underlying pathogenic mechanisms in SIDS. In young infants, control of breathing and temperature is unstable. Immediately after birth, a newborn baby is very susceptible to hypothermia. However, after the first month of life the increase in subcutaneous adipose tissue and development of the hypothalamus mean that the balance changes in favour of heat retention. There is evidence from animal studies that small changes in hypothalamic temperature affect control of respiration, and anecdotal evidence that heat stress may be associated with sudden death of human infants. It is therefore possible that the sudden apnoea leading to SIDS is triggered by a rise in body temperature. Hence minor infections, allergic reactions and many other conditions, not in themselves life-threatening, may be associated with SIDS if they result in a critical increase in core body temperature. The latter is likely if heat loss is compromised by too high an environmental temperature or excessive clothing. In an infant in a cot, most loss of body heat occurs through the head especially the face. If heat loss from these sites is reduced because the head is covered or the infant is face down, this could be associated with a rise in brain temperature and subsequent apnoea. The mechanism by which a thermal stress might trigger apnoea in an infant remains unknown. The recent UK guidelines aimed at reducing the numbers of cases of SIDS are based on this hypothesis.

Over the last 2–3 years there has been a reduction in the numbers of sudden unexpected deaths in infancy attributed to SIDS in the UK. Whether this is due to the change in infant sleeping position consequent upon these guidelines remains to be established.

Diagnosis of SIDS requires that a thorough postmortem examination has been performed, but no adequate cause of death has been discovered. However, this does not mean that there are no findings *post mortem*. In many cases the clinical details and macroscopic and microscopic changes

Department of Health guidelines to help prevent SIDS (summary of recommendations)
● Babies should be laid down to sleep on their backs
● Do not let babies get too warm
● Create a smoke-free zone for your baby

found in the body organs *post mortem* are so characteristic that a positive diagnosis of SIDS can be made (see box).

Some characteristic postmortem findings in SIDS
- Well-nourished baby
- Froth around nose
- Cyanosis of lips and nailbeds
- Prominent thymus
- Pleural, thymic, heart petechiae
- Pulmonary congestion and oedema

Childhood tumours

Neoplastic disease in children differs quantitatively and qualitatively from that in adults. Many tumour-like masses in children are not true neoplasms and are more properly regarded as hamartomas. A hamartoma is a tumour-like mass composed of an overgrowth of mature cells and tissues that normally occur in the affected part.

Many of the common haemangiomas, lymphangiomas and naevi which are present at birth in a large percentage of the population come into this category. Benign tumours are also found in the young and many of these involve mesenchymal tissues. The mucosal and glandular adenomas common in adults are infrequent in children except in some inherited disorders like familial polyposis coli. The incidence of malignant disease is much lower than in adults, but it is an important cause of death in the 0–15 year age group.

Malignant disease in childhood

In the UK, approximately 1 child in every 600 develops cancer between birth and the age of 15 years, that is, an annual incidence of roughly 1 in 10 000.

Adenocarcinomas and squamous carcinomas, which are the commonest malignancies in adults, are rare in childhood. Instead **leukaemia** and **lymphoma**, the so-called 'embryonic tumours', **tumours of bone** and some types of **germ cell neoplasms** are the predominant malignancies in the paediatric age group. **Brain tumours**, although rarely spreading outwith the CNS, are also an important cause of morbidity and mortality in childhood.

Pathogenesis of childhood cancer

As with adult tumours, genetic mechanisms are thought to be crucial in the pathogenesis of childhood malignancies. Development of a tumour requires aberrations in cellular proto-oncogenes and/or antioncogenes (tumour suppressor genes). Such abnormalities may result from point mutations, amplification or translocation either of the growth controlling gene itself, or of its regulatory sequences. Development of most tumours requires more than one genetic event. In some childhood tumours the first event has already taken place because an abnormal gene has been inherited. Familial retinoblastoma (see above) is a good example of this situation.

Round blue cell (embryonic) tumours

The common **solid**, malignant childhood tumours (excluding lymphomas, germ cell, bone and brain tumours which also occur in adults) are composed of cells which resemble those of embryonic tissues. The neoplastic cells are generally round or oval and have a high nuclear to cytoplasmic ratio, thus appearing dark blue in routinely stained histological sections. The commonest types of embryonic tumours, and their usual sites, are listed in

Table 16.6   Common embryonic tumours of childhood

Tumour	Percentage of childhood malignancies	Major site(s)
Neuroblastoma	6.8	Adrenal medulla, sympathetic ganglia
Rhabdomyosarcoma	6.5	Numerous, including orbit, nasopharynx, nose, ear, bladder, vagina, paratesticular region Rarely in the limbs
Nephroblastoma (Wilms' tumour)	5.2	Kidney
Medulloblastoma	5.0	Cerebellum
Retinoblastoma	2.7	Eye
Hepatoblastoma	0.9	Liver

Table 16.6. Of these, neuroblastoma, rhabdomyosarcoma and Wilms' tumour (Fig. 16.25) are the most common. Most embryonic tumours present as an abnormal mass, but medulloblastomas commonly cause hydrocephalus and attention is usually brought to a retinoblastoma because of the development of a white pupil or a squint. All these tumours are highly malignant, but the prognosis has been transformed by modern surgery, chemotherapy and radiotherapy.

Childhood handicap

Disease in a child, as in an adult, affects the general wellbeing of that individual. However, chronic disorders in childhood also interfere with growth and development. This has serious implications for individual families, local health and community services and the education system. The major causes of severe childhood handicap are shown in Table 16.7.

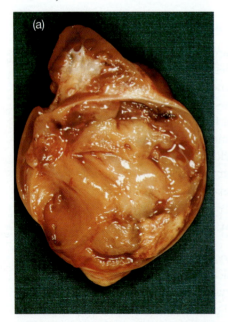
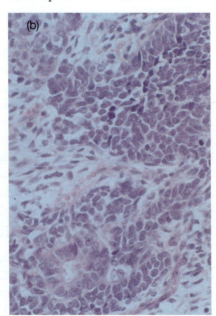
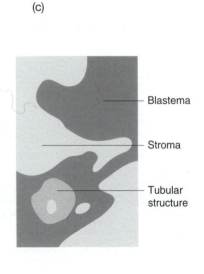

Fig. 16.25   (a) Nephroblastoma (Wilms' tumour). (b, c) Histological appearance showing undifferentiated small blue cells (blastema), occasional tubular structures and some tumour stroma – the typical components of a triphasic nephroblastoma.

Table 16.7 Causes of severe handicapping disorders in a series of 10 000 affected children

Mental handicap	38%
Neurological disorders	37%
Psychiatric disorders	6%
Bone, joint and muscle disorders	6%
Alimentary disorders	4%
Heart and great vessel abnormalities	3%
Metabolic and endocrine disorders	2%
Tumours	2%
Asthma	1%
Genitourinary disorders	1%
Others	<1%

Brain and central nervous system abnormalities are of major importance. Mental handicap often has a genetic basis, **trisomy 21** and the **fragile X syndrome** being the most common causes. Brain damage leading to neurological impairment is often also accompanied by mental handicap. The low percentage of children who are severely handicapped by common conditions like asthma reflects the fact that effective treatment is available for most sufferers.

Brain development and injury

At birth, the brain stem and other areas responsible for control of reflex actions like breathing are relatively more developed than the cerebral hemispheres. However, the higher centres develop rapidly during the tremendous growth spurt which occurs in the early years. The latter results in an increase in the weight of the brain from around 350 g at term to about 1000 g at 4 years of age. It is mainly the result of production of large amounts of myelin and development of increased numbers of dendrites which interconnect nerve cells. Growth is slower after this, but continues until adulthood under genetic control. Development of movement, manipulation, visuospatial abilities, speech and ability to learn occurs during this period. As well as normal brain growth, development requires normal environmental stimuli. Brain damage during childhood has numerous causes (see box).

If an insult is not followed by rapid recovery, the result is interference with growth, development and rate of learning, and lifelong neurological impairment. The degree of handicap resulting from an injury to the brain depends on the nature and severity of the injury, and on the maturation of the brain at the time of injury. Early in life, injury often has a generalized profound effect, but in some cases part of the function of the destroyed brain will be taken over by other areas. Later there is more specific damage to particular structures and the ability to compensate for lost tissue is more limited.

Some causes of childhood brain damage
- Genetic, familial, chromosomal disorders
- Non-genetic brain malformations
- Fetal alcohol syndrome
- Perinatal asphyxia and haemorrhage
- Birth trauma
- Neonatal jaundice
- Hypoglycaemia
- CNS infections
- Survival after 'near miss cot death'
- Head injury
- Non-accidental injury
- Status epilepticus
- Near drowning
- Poisoning
- Metabolic disorders

Cerebral palsy

Cerebral palsy is defined as a disorder of movement resulting from non-progressive brain damage sustained during a period of rapid brain growth in children. Thus:

- all affected children have motor dysfunction
- children with spinal cord disease are not classed as having cerebral palsy.

Although by definition the abnormality in the brain does not spread or get worse, the symptoms and clinical signs may change. Many children with the motor problems of cerebral palsy have associated abnormalities such as epilepsy, learning problems, behavioural disturbance and/or mental handicap.

The prevalence of cerebral palsy in the UK is approximately 2.5 in 1000 children. It may result from any of the causes of brain damage in which the damage is static. In many cases the aetiology is unknown. Recent careful epidemiological and other studies have revealed no evidence for the widespread belief that intrapartum care commonly influences the risk of cerebral palsy.

Chapter 17   Neurological and eye disease

Learning objectives

To appreciate and understand:
- ❏ The cell types and their interactions within the central nervous system (CNS)
- ❏ The causes and consequences of intracranial space-occupying lesions
- ❏ The congenital, traumatic, metabolic, inflammatory, infective, degenerative and neoplastic conditions affecting the central and peripheral nervous systems
- ❏ The main types of muscle disease

Central nervous system

The cells in the central nervous system (CNS) can be considered in five main groups (Fig. 17.1):

- **Neurons** are the most metabolically active cells and responsible for functional diversity in the CNS.
- **Glial cells: astrocytes, oligodendrocytes, ependymal cells** and **choroid plexus cells** (see box).
- **Microglial cells** belong to the monocyte/macrophage family and react to CNS injury by hyperplasia and hypertrophy.
- **Blood vessels**: CNS capillaries possess a unique non-fenestrated arrangement with tight junctions between adjacent cells which form

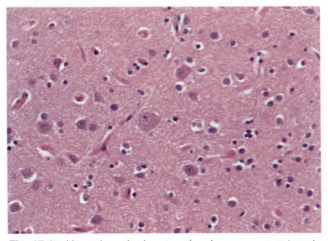
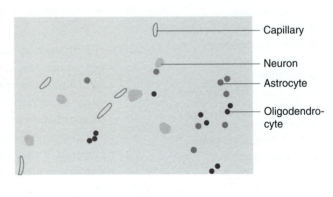

Fig. 17.1   Normal cerebral cortex showing neurons, astrocytes, oligodendrocytes and capillaries.

Types of glial cells

- **Astrocytes** provide a supportive framework for the CNS and regulate the blood–brain barrier; they respond to many types of CNS injury by hypertrophy and hyperplasia
- **Oligodendrocytes** are responsible for the synthesis and maintenance of myelin
- **Ependymal cells** line the CSF pathway within the brain and spinal cord
- **Choroid plexus cells** are resonsible for the secretion of CSF

the so-called **blood–brain barrier** to restrict the movement of amino acids, glucose, lipids, ions and drugs into and out of the CNS.
- **Connective tissue cells** in the meninges and around blood vessels.

Developmental disorders

Malformations of the CNS occur in 3–4 of every 100 000 live births. Most are multifactorial in origin, with genetic, dietary and social factors implicated in their aetiology.

NEURAL TUBE DEFECTS

Neural tube defects are the most common developmental abnormalities (see Chapter 16). Failure of the neural tube to close can be detected *in utero* by ultrasonography. The maternal serum and amniotic fluid usually contain high levels of α-fetoprotein (AFP); this is used in antenatal screening. These defects usually occur as spina bifida in the lumbosacral region (Fig. 17.2); cranial involvement may occur as anencephaly or cranial meningocele.

OTHER CONGENITAL MALFORMATIONS

Agenesis and dysgenesis

These usually involve the corpus callosum and olfactory bulbs. Failure of neuronal migration may result in agyria, polymicrogyria and neuronal heterotopias.

Destructive lesions

Lesions such as **ulegyria** occur as a consequence of infection, for example rubella, or hypoxia *in utero*.

Posterior fossa malformations

These malformations are of two types:

- **Arnold–Chiari malformation**, involving the cerebellum, brain stem and spinal cord, which may be associated with spina bifida
- **Dandy–Walker malformation**, where the cerebellar vermis is hypoplastic and the fourth ventricle distended to form a cystic structure.

Phakomatomoses

The phakomatomoses are a group of autosomally dominant inherited neurocutaneous disorders, including:

- neurofibromatosis
- von Hippel–Lindau syndrome
- tuberous sclerosis.

Fig. 17.2 Spina bifida: in meningocele (a), the vertebral arch (1) is incomplete, exposing a large sac of meninges (2) within which lies the spinal cord (3). In meningomyelocele (b), the spinal cord is located high within the meningeal sac, and in spina bifida aperta (c) the meningeal sac and overlying skin are absent, exposing the spinal cord.

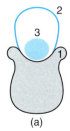
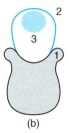
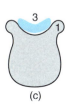

(a)   (b)   (c)

Chromosomal abnormalities

Chromosomal abnormalities may be associated with CNS malformations, for example in trisomy 21 (Down's syndrome), where the brain exhibits irregular contours with neuronal heterotopias and abnormal myelination.

Hydrocephalus

This term is used to describe disorders where an excess quantity of CSF is present in the cranial cavity. Two main types are recognized:

- **primary hydrocephalus**, usually accompanied by raised intracranial pressure
- **secondary hydrocephalus**, compensatory to tissue destruction or cerebral atrophy.

Primary hydrocephalus commonly results from:

- obstruction of the CSF pathway by congenital malformations (such as the Arnold–Chiari malformation)
- tumours growing in the CSF pathway, such as medulloblastoma, ependymoma (Fig. 17.3)
- organization of inflammatory exudate or haemorrhage.

Obstructive hydrocephalus results in progressive ventricular enlargement which can be relieved by surgical drainage.

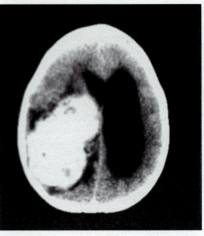

Fig. 17.3 This computed tomography scan shows a large ependymoma growing in the right lateral ventricle which has obstructed the foramen of Monro, resulting in hydrocephalus affecting both lateral ventricles.

SYRINGOMYELIA

In this uncommon condition, a cavity develops within the spinal cord, sometimes following spinal cord injury. The clinical features are loss of pain and temperature sensation, and progressive neurogenic muscle atrophy, which is described on p. 418.

Intracranial space-occupying lesions

Expansion of the intracranial contents usually results from an enlarging extracerebral mass, or brain swelling.

DIFFUSE BRAIN SWELLING

Diffuse brain swelling results from cerebral vasodilatation and oedema due to:

- cytotoxic oedema in hypoxic states
- vasogenic oedema caused by disruption of the blood–brain barrier
- interstitial oedema in hydrocephalus.

These may occur together – in head injury, both vasogenic and cytotoxic oedema are common complications.

FOCAL BRAIN SWELLING

A neoplasm or abscess is often accompanied by cerebral oedema which contributes to the overall mass effect. The clinical consequences of intracranial mass lesions all result from the effects of raised intracranial pressure.

Intracranial herniation is the most serious consequence of raised intracranial pressure. The features observed depend upon the site of herniation, as shown in Table 17.1 and Fig. 17.4.

Clinical consequences of raised intracranial pressure
- Blurred vision with **papilloedema**, due to an accumulation of axoplasm in the optic nerves
- **Headache**, due to distortion of pain fibre-carrying structures
- **Nausea** and **vomiting**, due to pressure on the brain stem
- **Neck stiffness**, due to compression of the dura matter in the posterior fossa
- **Deterioration in consciousness**, due to pressure on brain-stem vital centres

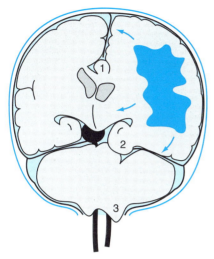

Fig. 17.4 A representation of the three main sites of intracranial herniation resulting from an expanding intracerebral mass. The cingulate gyrus (1) may herniate below the falx cerebri, the parahippocampal gyrus (2) may herniate across the edge of the tentorium cerebelli, and the cerebellar tonsils (3) may herniate down into the foramen magnum. The clinical consequences of these herniations are listed in Table 17.1.

Table 17.1   Consequences of intracranial herniation

Hernia site	Consequences
Subfalcine	Anterior cerebral artery compression
Transtentorial	IIIrd nerve compression
	Cerebral peduncle compression
	Posterior cerebral artery compression
	Brain-stem compression and fatal haemorrhage
Foramen magnum	CSF obstruction
	Brain-stem compression and fatal haemorrhage

Trauma

HEAD INJURY

Head injuries are classified in two main groups, according to the traumatic agent:

- **Missile injury** is typically caused by bullets or other objects propelled through the air. These impacts may result in skull fractures and perforating or penetrating brain injuries, and are associated with severe cerebral destruction, infection and epilepsy.
- **Non-missile injury** to the brain ranges from severe injuries which are rapidly fatal to relatively minor concussion injuries.

Non-missile injury occurs most commonly in falls and road traffic accidents, and may be considered in two stages: **primary** and **secondary brain damage**.

Primary brain damage

Primary brain damage may be focal, for example:

- Cerebral contusions at impact and contrecoup sites.
- Brain-stem disruption with a basal skull fracture.
- Vascular rupture, resulting in intracranial haemorrhage (see Table 17.2): this may be amenable to neurosurgical drainage, if diagnosed early.
- Diffuse brain damage results from shearing and tensile strains damaging axons within the white matter. It may occur in the absence of a skull fracture and accounts for around one-third of all deaths from head injury.

Table 17.2   Pathology of traumatic intracranial haemorrhage

Site	Vessel damaged	Clinical consequence
Cerebrum	Intracerebral artery or arteriole	Intracerebral haematoma: often fatal
Subdural space	Bridging veins	Subdural haematoma: Acute: often fatal Chronic: slowly enlarging intracranial mass
Extradural space	Middle meningeal artery	Acute haematoma: surgical drainage can be curative

Secondary brain damage

Secondary brain damage occurs as a result of cerebral oedema and brain swelling with intracranial herniation, hypoxia (which may result from other injuries) and meningitis, particularly with an open skull fracture. Following a severe head injury, 20% of survivors make a good recovery, while 19% remain severely disabled due to post-traumatic epilepsy and the persistent vegetative state, which occurs as a consequence of severe diffuse brain damage; the remainder have a residual neurological deficit.

CASE STUDY 17.1

A 23-year-old man was knocked from a motorbicycle in a road traffic accident. He was said to have lost consciousness immediately and had bleeding from the left ear. On arrival at hospital, he sustained a grand mal seizure and became comatose with a fixed dilated left pupil. Skull radiography showed a basal fracture, and computed tomography demonstrated an acute left **subdural haematoma**, which was evacuated. Postoperatively, he remained comatose with persistently raised intracranial pressure and developed pulmonary oedema and bronchopneumonia, which failed to respond to antibiotic therapy. At postmortem examination, widespread **cerebral contusions** and **diffuse axonal injury** with small **intracerebral haemorrhages** were demonstrated (Fig. 17.5).

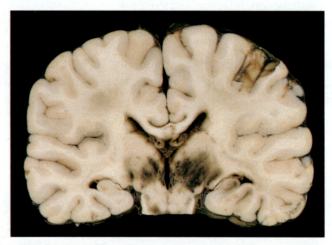

Fig. 17.5   The fixed brain from this head injury case shows numerous haemorrhages within the thalamus, basal ganglia and brain stem. Small cortical contusions were also present, and histology revealed diffuse axonal injury.

SPINAL INJURIES

Two main groups of spinal injuries are recognized clinically:

- **open injuries** caused by direct trauma to the cord, such as bullet wounds
- **closed injuries**, which are are often accompanied by a fracture or dislocation of the vertebral column. Cord damage results from physical disruption, oedema and ischaemia.

SPINAL CORD AND NERVE ROOT COMPRESSION

Compression often occurs due to subacute disease processes, such as intervertebral disc prolapse and cervical spondylosis. Disc prolapse occurs most frequently at the L5–S1 and C5–C6 levels, when tears in the annulus fibrosus allow the nucleus of the disc to herniate backwards, causing nerve

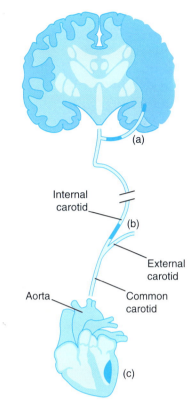

Fig. 17.6 Cerebral infarction may result from thrombosis or embolism from various sites in the arterial tree. Common lesions include: (a) thrombosis or embolic occlusion of the middle cerebral artery or one of its branches; (b) thrombosis of the internal carotid artery at its bifurcation, which may also cause emboli; (c) cardiac mural thrombus, a source of emboli.

Fig. 17.7 This old cerebral infarct in the territory of the right middle cerebral artery involved the internal capsule, resulting in contralateral hemiparesis. The lesion is now represented by a gliotic cystic cavity.

root compression. Other causes of non-traumatic spinal cord compression include:

- **neoplasms** involving the vertebral column or the extradural space
- **bony disorders**, such as rheumatoid arthritis
- **infection**, such as tuberculosis.

Vascular disorders

CEREBROVASCULAR DISEASE

Cerebrovascular disease is the third most common cause of death and a major cause of morbidity in the UK. CNS damage occurs as a consequence of hypoxia: neurons can only survive hypoxia for a few minutes, following a cardiac arrest for example.

PATHOLOGY OF STROKE

Stroke is a clinical term used to describe a sudden event which produces persisting CNS damage due to vascular disease. The annual incidence of stroke in the UK is around 2 per 1000, and several major risk factors have been identified, including ischaemic heart disease, systemic hypertension and diabetes mellitus. The major causes of stroke are **cerebral infarction** (accounting for around 80% of cases) and **intracerebral haemorrhage**.

Cerebral infarction

Cerebral infarction occurs after a critical reduction in blood flow or arterial oxygenation (Fig. 17.6). The major causes are:

- **myocardial infarction** with cardiac arrest
- **embolic occlusion** from thrombus in the heart or carotid arteries
- **localized thrombosis** within the arterial supply to the CNS or intracranial arteries.

The site and size of the infarct is influenced by the vascular lesion and the anastomotic blood supply from the circle of Willis. Most infarcts occur in the distribution of the middle cerebral artery territory, where damage to the corticospinal pathway results in contralateral hemiparesis (Fig. 17.7). Following infarction, the brain undergoes colliquative necrosis and a cystic cavity lined by glial fibres is formed. Some infarcts are haemorrhagic, probably as a result of vascular reperfusion. Venous infarction occasionally causes stroke, usually as a consequence of cerebral sinus thrombosis in debilitated patients or those with intracranial sepsis.

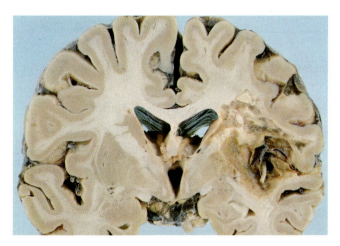

Intracerebral haemorrhage

Most spontaneous intracerebral haemorrhages occur within the basal ganglia region in hypertensive adults over 50 years of age. The morbidity and mortality from a haemorrhagic stroke are higher than those for an ischaemic stroke, since the accumulating haematoma acts as a rapidly expanding lesion (Fig. 17.8). It was previously thought that these haematomas occurred following rupture of microaneurysms on intracerebral arterioles in hypertensive patients, but recent studies indicate that vascular rupture close to arteriolar bifurcations may also be important.

Subarachnoid haemorrhage

Spontaneous subarachnoid haemorrhage usually occurs following rupture of a saccular ('berry') aneurysm on the anterior portion of the circle of Willis, in middle-aged adults. These are sited at branching points on the anterior circle of Willis, particularly on the internal carotid, middle cerebral and anterior communicating arteries. Their pathogenesis relates to defects in the smooth muscle of the arterial media at a site of bifurcation (Fig. 17.9). Hypertensive patients are more likely to have multiple aneurysms, and other vascular abnormalities, for instance atheroma may influence aneurysm formation. Aneurysm rupture is usually accompanied by sudden onset of severe headache followed by vasospasm, which can cause cerebral infarction. One-third of survivors suffer hypoxic brain damage following subarachnoid haemorrhage.

Other forms of intracranial haemorrhage are summarized in Table 17.3.

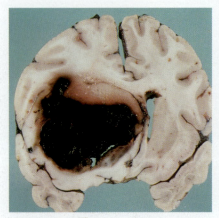

Fig. 17.8   Rupture of a small intracerebral arteriole in this hypertensive patient resulted in a rapidly accumulating left-sided haematoma, producing a marked rise in intracranial pressure and shift of the intracranial contents to the right.

Table 17.3   Other types of intracranial haemorrhage

Site	Pathology	Associated conditions
Ventricular system	Rupture of vessels in periventricular germinal layer in neonates	Hyaline membrane disease; hypoxia
Subdural space	Rupture of venous sinus in neonate	Birth trauma
Cerebrum	Vasculitis	Meningitis Connective tissue diseases
	Vascular malformations	Sturge–Weber syndrome
	Blood dyscrasia	Haemophilia Anticoagulant therapy

Infections of the CNS

BACTERIAL INFECTIONS

Bacterial infection of the CNS occurs by two routes:

- **haematogenous spread** as a consequence of septicaemia or as septic emboli, for example in bacterial endocarditis
- **direct spread** from an adjacent focus of infection – in the middle ear, for example.

Meningitis

The term meningitis usually refers to inflammation in the subarachnoid

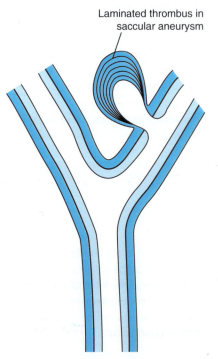

Fig. 17.9   Saccular aneurysms on the circle of Willis lack the elastic and muscle tissues present in the wall of the adjacent normal artery. As they progressively enlarge, the aneurysm lumen often becomes filled with laminated thrombus.

Laminated thrombus in saccular aneurysm

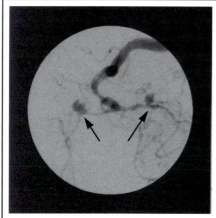

CASE STUDY 17.2

A hypertensive 56-year-old man collapsed at work after complaining of a sudden severe headache 'like being hit on the back of the head'. On arrival in the hospital accident and emergency department he was comatose but responding to painful stimuli. Computed tomography of the head demonstrated **subarachnoid haemorrhage**, and angiography found a **ruptured aneurysm** on the right middle cerebral artery (Fig. 17.10). This was clipped surgically and the patient improved. On follow-up review 2 months later he complained of a dull headache and occasional blurring of vision. Further computed tomography demonstrated **obstructive hydrocephalus**, which was relieved by a ventriculoperitoneal shunt. The patient remains well 2 years later.

Fig. 17.10   This digital subtraction angiogram demonstrates two saccular aneurysms (arrows) on the right middle cerebral artery and the anterior communicating artery. The proximal middle cerebral artery also exhibits vasospasm. (Courtesy of Dr R Sellar.)

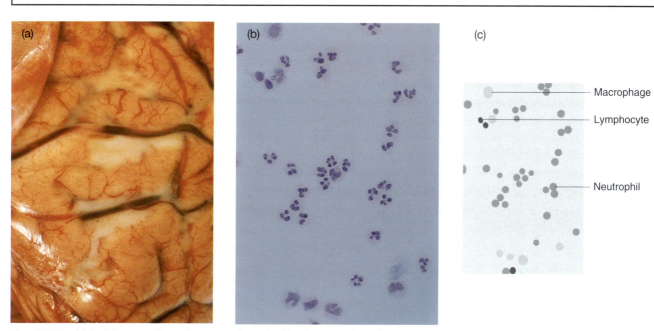

Fig. 17.11   (a) In this case of meningococcal meningitis, the vessels in the subarachnoid space are markedly congested and surrounded by pus. (b, c) A centrifuged preparation of the CSF in a case of meningococcal meningitis shows numerous neutrophil polymorphs with occasional lymphocytes and macrophages.

space (**leptomeningitis** – Fig. 17.11a). The main pathogens involved in acute bacterial meningitis are listed in Table 17.4. Meningococcal meningitis may be complicated by disseminated intravascular coagulation (**Waterhouse–Friderichsen syndrome**) which is often fatal. Other complications of acute meningitis include vasculitis with cerebral infarction, abscess formation, epilepsy and hydrocephalus. Chronic meningitis may develop in inadequately treated patients. Patients with meningitis usually suffer from headache, photophobia and neck stiffness with pyrexia. Examination of the CSF is essential for diagnosis (Fig. 17.11b) and to investigate antibiotic sensitivity of the responsible organisms (Table 17.5).

Cerebral abscess

Cerebral abscess causes similar clinical features to bacterial meningitis, although epilepsy and focal neurological signs are more common.

Table 17.4   Common organisms in bacterial meningitis

Age group	Organism
Neonates	*E. coli, Listeria monocytogenes, Salmonella* spp.
Infants and young children	*Haemophilus influenzae* type b
Children and young adults	*Neisseria meningitidis*
Adults	*Streptococcus pneumoniae* type 3

Table 17.5   CSF changes in meningitis

	Appearance	Mononuclear cells (/ml)	Polymorphs (cells/ml)	Protein (g/l)	Glucose (relative to blood glucose)
Normal	Clear	<5	Nil	0.2–0.4	>0.5
Bacterial	Purulent, turbid	>10	>50	0.5–2.0	<0.3
TB	Viscous, turbid	>25	>15	0.5–2.5	<0.3
Viral	Clear	10–100	Nil	0.4–1.0	<0.5

Antibiotic therapy is effective in the early stages of abscess formation, but surgical excision or drainage may be required once a capsule has formed.

Extradural abscess and subdural empyema

Both extradural abscess and subdural empyema are extracerebral suppurative lesions which usually occur as a complication of open skull fractures. They may act as space-occupying lesions, requiring surgical drainage and antibiotic therapy.

Tuberculosis

Tuberculosis in the CNS usually results from haematogenous spread of infection from the lung. Two main forms occur in the CNS:

- **tuberculous meningitis** (see Table 17.5) with caseating granulomata around vessels in the subarachnoid space; focal neurological signs with isolated cranial nerve palsies are well-recognized complications
- **tuberculomas**, foci of granulomatous caseation and fibrosis in the cerebellum.

VIRAL INFECTIONS

CNS infection by viruses may occur by **haematogenous spread** as part of a systemic infection, or by **neural spread** – retrograde axonal transport along peripheral nerves to the CNS, for example by rabies virus.

Viral meningitis

Viral meningitis is a common, self-limiting illness in which the CSF exhibits characteristic features (see Table 17.5). Common pathogens include mumps virus, Coxsackie A and B viruses and echo virus.

Viral encephalitis

Viral encephalitis may occur in a mild form during common illness, such as mumps, measles or chickenpox. Herpes simplex I virus is the most common cause of acute viral encephalitis in the UK, producing a lytic infection of neurons and chronic inflammation with reactive gliosis and cerebral oedema. This infection can now be successfully treated with acyclovir.

Latent viral infections

Herpes zoster is caused by the varicella-zoster virus, and results from reactivation of latent virus within sensory ganglia. Spread along peripheral sensory nerves is accompanied by a painful cutaneous rash, usually in the midthoracic region or trigeminal nerve distribution.

Other viral infections

Some rare infections are summarized in Table 17.6.

Table 17.6   Rare viral infections of the CNS

Virus	Disease
Measles	Acute measles encephalitis
	Subacute sclerosing panencephalitis
Cytomegalovirus	Necrotizing encephalitis *in utero*
Rubella	
JC papovavirus	Progressive multifocal leukoencephalopathy

AIDS and associated infections

Early CNS involvement in HIV infection occurs as a lymphocytic meningitis, but the virus is thought later to enter the brain by crossing the blood–brain barrier in monocytes. Patients dying with AIDS show a wide range of CNS abnormalities which are listed in Table 17.7.

Table 17.7   CNS abnormalities in AIDS

Abnormality	Associated lesion	Clinical features
Giant cell encephalitis	HIV infection	Dementia
Spinal cord demyelination	Vacuolar myelopathy	Ataxia
		Sensory loss
		Weakness
Cerebral abscess	Toxoplasma	Pyrexia
	Fungi	Seizures
Progressive multifocal leukoencephalopathy	JC papovavirus	Multiple neurological abnormalities
Cerebral lymphoma	Epstein–Barr virus infection	Raised intracranial pressure
		Focal neurological signs
Meningitis	Cryptococci	Pyrexia
	Amoebae	Neck stiffness
	Atypical mycobacteria	Headache

FUNGAL INFECTIONS

Fungal infections of the CNS are uncommon and usually arise as a consequence of haematogenous spread from the lungs, for example *Candida albicans* and *Aspergillus fumigatus*. Fungal meningitis with abscess formation may be accompanied by vasculitis and haemorrhage.

CASE STUDY 17.3

A 28-year-old heterosexual man presented with a short history of pyrexia and right-sided seizures. Computed tomography of the brain showed a well-defined focal lesion in the left cerebral hemisphere which was biopsied, showing **toxoplasmosis**. HIV serology was positive. The patient was treated with azathioprine, and remained reasonably well for the next 2 years until the onset of severe seizures, visual disturbances and left hemiparesis. He died suddenly, and on postmortem examination was found to have a **primary cerebral lymphoma** (Fig. 17.12a), along with **HIV encephalitis** (Fig. 17.12b) and **cytomegalovirus retinitis**, but no recurrent toxoplasmosis: *Pneumocystis carinii* was cultured *post mortem* from the lung.

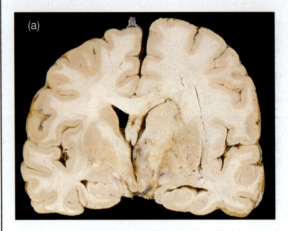

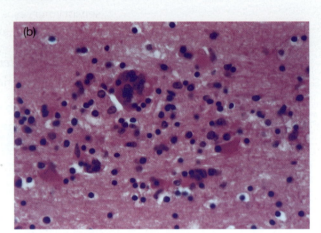

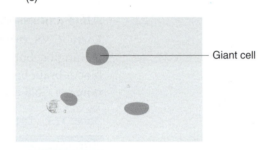

Giant cell

Fig. 17.12   (a) Examination of the fixed brain from this case of AIDS found a large necrotic tumour in the right basal ganglia, which on histology was a high-grade B-cell non-Hodgkin's lymphoma. (b, c) Elsewhere in the brain there was evidence of HIV encephalitis, with characteristic multinucleate giant cells.

Degenerative disorders

In normal ageing, the brain weight decreases slowly after the third decade of life and more rapidly from the seventh decade onwards, accompanied by cortical atrophy and a variable loss of neurons. Surviving neurons may exhibit a range of structural abnormalities with changes in neurotransmitter activity.

DEMENTIA

Dementia can be defined clinically as an acquired global impairment of intellect, personality and reason, without impairment of consciousness, which affects 15% of adults over the age of 80 years in the UK. Many disorders affecting the CNS can result in dementia (Table 17.8). In some cases, such as **Wernicke's encephalopathy**, an effective treatment is available; in others, such as **Huntington's disease**, genetic counselling may be required

ALZHEIMER'S DISEASE

Alzheimer's disease is the most common cause of dementia in the UK, affecting 5% of people over the age of 65 years. Most cases occur sporadically, and females are affected almost twice as frequently as

Table 17.8   Categories of dementing illnesses

Disease type	Examples
Primary (organic) dementia	Alzheimer's disease Huntington's disease Pick's disease
Cerebrovascular disease	Multi-infarct dementia
Transmissible diseases	Creutzfeldt–Jakob disease HIV encephalitis Syphilis
Metabolic disorders	Wernicke's encephalopathy Myxoedema Uraemia
Drugs	Barbiturates Anticholinergic agents
Intracranial space-occupying lesions	Chronic subdural haematoma

males. The aetiology is unknown: no consistent genetic component exists, and the possibility of an underlying toxin, such as aluminium, has been suggested. The illness usually lasts 2–10 years, terminating in cachexia and bronchopneumonia.

In Alzheimer's disease the brain is atrophied, particularly the frontal, temporal and parietal cortex. The characteristic histological lesions are the senile plaque and neurofibrillary tangle, the severity of which correlates with the severity of the dementia (Fig. 17.13a). Senile plaques consist of an extracellular amyloid core with surrounding neuritic processes and reactive glial cells. This amyloid is formed from a precursor encoded on a gene on chromosome 21, which is abnormal in some familial cases, whilst in Down's syndrome (trisomy 21) Alzheimer-like changes develop at an early age. Neurofibrillary tangles are intraneuronal structures composed of paired helical cytoskeletal filaments. A reduction in cortical cholinergic activity also occurs in Alzheimer's disease.

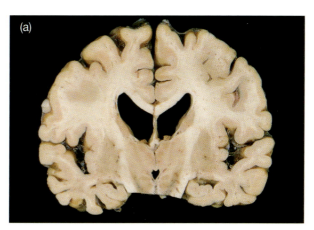
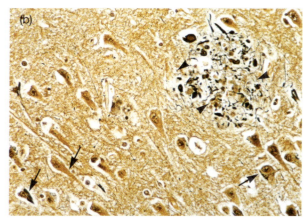

Fig. 17.13   (a) Examination of the fixed brain in this case of Alzheimer's disease shows marked cortical atrophy with compensatory hydrocephalus. (b) This silver-stained section from the hippocampus in Alzheimer's disease shows numerous neuritic processes at the periphery of a plaque (arrowheads) and several neurons containing dark-staining neurofibrillary tangles (arrows).

CASE STUDY 17.4

A 72-year-old woman developed progressive memory impairment with personality disintegration over a 12-month period. Psychometric testing showed evidence of a global dementia, and the patient was placed in a psychogeriatric unit. Computed tomography of the brain showed cerebral cortical atrophy, but no evidence of infarction. The patient deteriorated over the next 30 months, and became profoundly demented and incontinent until she died from bronchopneumonia. At postmortem examination, the brain weighed only 995 g (Fig. 17.13a) and showed the characteristic features of Alzheimer's disease on histology (Fig. 17.13b).

VASCULAR DEMENTIA

Patients who sustain multiple cerebral infarcts involving the cerebral cortex may develop progressive dementia. Other forms of cerebrovascular disease, such as widespread arteriosclerosis, may also be associated with dementia, sometimes with coexisting Alzheimer's disease.

SYSTEMS DEGENERATIONS

The group of neurodegenerative diseases known as systems degenerations is characterized by loss of functionally related nerve cells and their associated pathways. Some are inherited diseases, but their pathogenesis is poorly understood. Considerable overlap of the clinical and pathological features occurs, but several well-defined examples exist (Table 17.9 and Fig. 17.14). These disorders may occur in combination as **multiple systems degeneration**.

Table 17.9   Systems degenerations

Example	Pathway involved	Clinical features
Motor neuron disease	Corticospinal pathway	Muscle wasting and fasciculation Progressive weakness
Parkinson's disease	Striatonigral pathway	Rigidity, tremor, bradykinesia
Holmes' cerebellar atrophy	Pontocerebellar pathway	Ataxia, nystagmus
Friedreich's ataxia	Spinocerebellar and sensory pathways	Ataxia, deafness, sensory loss Autosomal recessive disorder

Demyelinating diseases

Primary demyelination in the CNS occurs when the myelin sheath is destroyed but the underlying axons remain intact. Oligodendrocytes cannot effectively remyelinate in the adult CNS, hence the progressive clinical dysfunction seen in many demyelinating conditions.

MULTIPLE SCLEROSIS

Multiple sclerosis is the most common demyelinating disease in the UK. Patients usually present in early adult life with limb weakness, paraesthesiae and visual disturbances. Females are affected more often than males, and the disease follows a characteristic relapsing and remitting course. Multiple sclerosis is most prevalent in populations living at

Fig. 17.14 In the normal brain (a), the cells in the substantia nigra release dopamine as a transmitter in the basal ganglia. In Parkinson's disease (b), death of the nigral neurons results in a deficiency of dopamine in the projection sites. This deficiency can often be replaced therapeutically with L-dopa, resulting in a clinical improvement.

(a) (b)

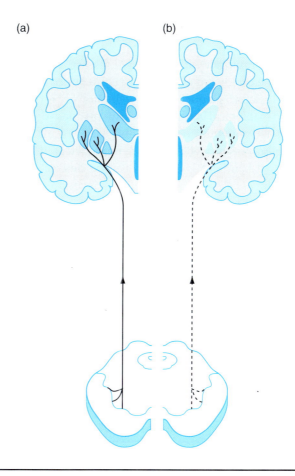

CASE STUDY 17.5

A 54-year-old man developed progressive weakness and muscle wasting in the hands and legs. On examination, the lower limb reflexes were brisk, with increased tone and reduced power in all limbs. Electromyography suggested an acute denervating process, which was confirmed on muscle biopsy (see Fig. 17.24). The patient deteriorated over the next 12 months, with widespread muscle wasting and fasciculation of the tongue. Death occurred following aspiration pneumonitis. Postmortem examination showed widespread loss of motor neurons in the cerebral cortex, brain stem and spinal cord, with degeneration of the corticospinal pathways, confirming the clinical diagnosis of motor neuron disease (Fig. 17.15).

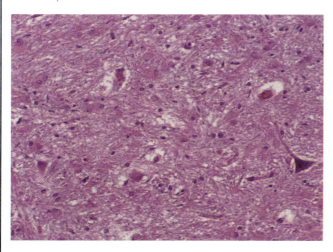

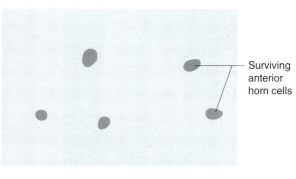

Surviving anterior horn cells

Fig. 17.15 The spinal cord in this case of motor neuron disease showed a marked loss of anterior horn cells, with only a few degenerate surviving cells.

latitudes remote from the equator, and is associated with HLA antigens DR2 and DQ1 in the UK.

Some patients die rapidly with progressive disease, while many develop complications of the prolonged immobility, such as urinary tract infections. With each clinical relapse, plaques of demyelination are formed in the brain or spinal cord. Histological studies of early plaques show widespread myelin breakdown, cerebral oedema and perivascular cuffing with inflammatory cells (plasma cells and T lymphocytes). The plasma cells produce oligoclonal bands of IgG which can be detected in the CSF. As myelin breakdown subsides, reactive gliosis is established and is the dominant feature in chronic plaques.

OTHER DEMYELINATING CONDITIONS

Other conditions are summarized in Table 17.10.

> **Multiple sclerosis: suggested aetiologies**
> - A **circulating toxin** in the CSF
> - A **viral infection** of the CNS
> - An abnormality of the lipid component of **myelin**
> - An **autoimmune disorder** (possibly virus-induced): this is currently the most favoured hypothesis, but conclusive evidence is still awaited

Table 17.10   Miscellaneous demyelinating disorders of the CNS

Disease type	Examples
Viral infections	Progressive multifocal leukoencephalopathy (JC papovavirus)
Toxins	Hexachlorophene
Metabolic disorders	Central pontine myelinolysis
Leukodystrophies	Metachromatic leukodystrophy Krabbe's leukodystrophy

---

CASE STUDY 17.6

A 34-year-old woman developed weakness of the lower limbs, with two episodes of blurred vision. On examination, the lower limbs were weak and flaccid. CSF studies found oligoclonal IgG bands, with increased numbers of lymphocytes and macrophages. Visual evoked responses showed marked slowing of impulse conduction, and magnetic resonance imaging of the brain showed multiple lesions in the periventricular white matter (Fig. 17.16a). Over the next 10 years the patient sustained several episodes of remission and relapse, with progressive deterioration. She became immobile, and developed chronic pyelonephritis, complicated by a fatal septicaemia. Postmortem examination found multiple chronic multiple sclerosis plaques in the cerebrum, spinal cord and optic nerves (Fig. 17.16b), along with chronic pyelonephritis and cystitis.

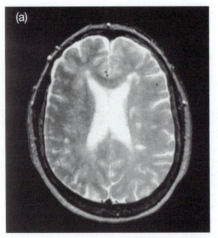
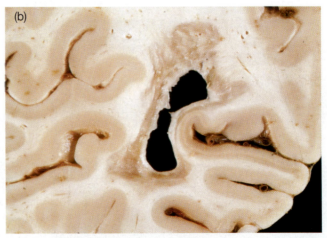

Fig. 17.16   (a) A T2-weighted magnetic resonance imaging scan in a case of multiple sclerosis shows multiple areas of high signal intensity in a typical periventricular distribution. Some of the lesions are longitudinal in the direction of the draining veins. (Courtesy of Dr R. Sellar.) (b) Examination of the fixed brain from this case confirmed the clinical diagnosis of multiple sclerosis, with chronic demyelinated plaques present in the white matter around the lateral ventricles.

Toxic and metabolic disorders

CNS damage may result from the effects of toxins, deficiency of vitamins and other compounds, or the effects of specific metabolic diseases. Many inherited metabolic diseases have a well-defined biochemical basis, which allows antenatal diagnosis. Examples of the more important disorders are listed in Table 17.11; alcohol is a common CNS toxin whose main effects are summarized in Table 17.12.

Table 17.11   Toxic and metabolic disorders affecting the CNS

Agents	Examples	CNS disorder
Drugs	Phenytoin	Microcephaly (exposure *in utero*)
	Vincristine	Axonal degeneration
Metals	Inorganic lead	Encephalopathy
	Organic mercury	Cerebellar degeneration and peripheral neuropathy
Industrial chemicals	Hexacarbons	Axonal degeneration Anticholinesterase action
Vitamin deficiency	Vitamin B_{12}	Subacute combined degeneration of spinal cord
	Vitamin E	Spinocerebellar degeneration
Lysosomal storage diseases	Tay–Sachs disease	Neuronal degeneration
	Batten's disease	Neuronal degeneration

Table 17.12   Effects of excess alcohol on the nervous system

Disorder	Mechanism	Clinical features
Sudden death	Acute toxicity	Collapse and coma
Wernicke's encephalopathy	Vitamin B_1 deficiency	Memory and personality changes
Hepatocerebral syndrome	Liver damage	Acute confusional state, coma
Central pontine myelinosis	Hyponatraemia	Brain-stem dysfunction, death
Peripheral neuropathy	Axonal degeneration	Sensory loss and weakness in hands and feet
Fetal alcohol syndrome	Direct toxicity	Microcephaly, mental handicap

CNS tumours

Primary CNS tumours occur in around 6 per 100 000 of the population. They are the second most common group of neoplasms in children, but the sixth most common group in adults. In children the most common site for tumours is the cerebellum and brain stem, but in adults most brain tumours are supratentorial. Brain tumours usually present with the effects of raised intracranial pressure and/or localizing signs due to tissue destruction, for example visual loss with an optic nerve tumour. The pathogenesis of most brain tumours is unknown, but experimental tumours can be produced following exposure to chemical and viral carcinogens. Phakomatoses are associated with both intrinsic and extrinsic CNS tumours and immunosuppression is implicated in the pathogenesis of primary CNS lymphoma.

Treatment with radiotherapy has improved the prognosis for this tumour in recent years.

Lymphoma

The incidence of primary CNS lymphoma has increased greatly in association with immunosuppressed states, particularly AIDS (see Fig. 17.12a). Most are high-grade B-cell non-Hodgkin's lymphomas and carry a poor prognosis. Recent investigations have implicated the Epstein–Barr virus in the pathogenesis of some neoplasms.

EXTRINSIC TUMOURS

Tumours arising from the coverings of the brain, spinal cord and nerve roots are less common than intrinsic CNS tumours, and occur most frequently in adult women. Most are benign and produce symptoms by compression rather than invasion (Fig. 17.19), so complete removal is often possible and curative. The major types are listed in Table 17.14.

Table 17.14 Extrinsic CNS tumours

Tumour	Site	Clinical features
Angioma	Cerebral convexity, base of skull, spinal cord	Raised intracranial pressure, seizures, focal neurological signs
Schwannoma	Vestibular branch of nerve VIII	Deafness, tinnitus, vertigo
Neurofibroma	Spinal sensory nerve	Sensory loss with an anatomical level
Haemangioblastoma	Cerebellum	Ataxia, nystagmus, hydrocephalus

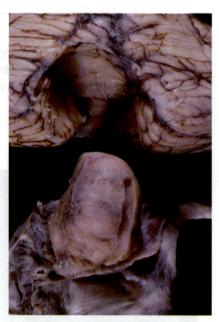

Fig. 17.19 A posterior fossa meningioma shows a typical dural attachment, with a rounded margin which has compressed (but not invaded) the adjacent cerebellum.

METASTATIC TUMOURS

The most common metastatic tumours are carcinomas of the bronchus, breast and kidney, and malignant melanoma, which reach the CNS by haematogenous spread. Metastases usually occur as multiple lesions within the brain, and in carcinomatous meningitis the CSF space may become infiltrated by malignant cells. The prognosis in most cases of metastatic CNS tumours is very poor. Metastases to the skull or extradural spinal space may cause bony collapse and compression of neural tissue. Tumours arising in adjacent organs may also compress or invade the CNS, for example pituitary adenomas, which compress the optic chiasma causing visual impairment.

Skeletal muscle

The diagnosis of skeletal muscle disorders requires multiple investigations, including muscle biopsy, electrophysiological techniques and biochemical studies, for example creatine phosphokinase (CPK) measurement in the serum. Muscle disorders can be classified into three main groups: **myopathies**, **neurogenic disorders** and **disorders of neuromuscular transmission**.

Myopathies

MUSCULAR DYSTROPHIES

These are inherited disorders which result in progressive muscle fibre destruction.

CASE STUDY 17.8

A 70-year-old man – a smoker – presented with multiple cranial nerve palsies and headache. Computed tomography showed mild hydrocephalus with obstruction of the basal cisterns. Chest radiography showed an irregular opaque lesion in the upper lobe of the left lung and **CSF cytology** showed irregular clusters of malignant cells (Fig. 17.20a, b). The patient deteriorated and died 3 months later. Autopsy confirmed an **adenocarcinoma** of the left upper lobe of lung, with metastases in hilar lymph nodes, the adrenal glands, liver and brain (Fig. 17.20c).

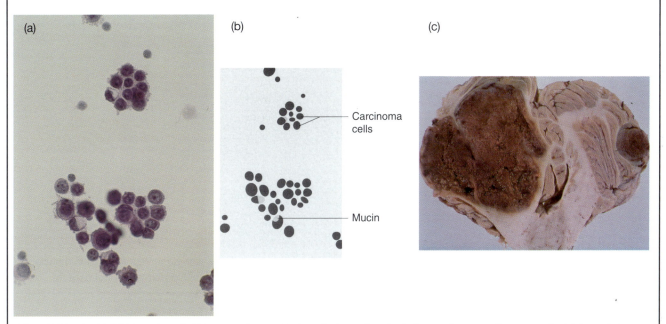

(a)

(b)

Carcinoma cells

Mucin

(c)

Fig. 17.20 (a, b) CSF cytology in this case demonstrated clusters of metastatic carcinoma cells, some of which contain droplets of mucin in the cytoplasm, suggestive of an adenocarcinoma. (c) Examination of the fixed brain showed multiple deposits of metastatic carcinoma, which in the cerebellum appeared necrotic and haemorrhagic.

Duchenne muscular dystrophy

The most common of the muscular dystrophies is Duchenne muscular dystrophy, an X-linked disorder affecting around 1 in 3000–5000 live male births. It presents at 2–4 years of age with progressive muscle weakness, motor delay and elevation of serum CPK. Muscle histology shows large hyaline necrotic fibres, progressive fibre destruction and replacement of the muscle by fibrous tissue and fat. Most patients die before the age of 20 years, often as a consequence of cardiac muscle involvement.

The gene for this disorder has been mapped to the p21 band of the X chromosome. Genetic deletions in Duchenne dystrophy result in abnormalities of the protein **dystrophin**, which helps maintain structural integrity during fibre contraction.

Becker muscular dystrophy

Becker muscular dystrophy has a milder clinical course than Duchenne dystrophy, with a later age of onset. Genetic studies of Becker patients have found deletions of the p21 band on chromosome X, suggesting that Becker and Duchenne dystrophies are allelic variants.

Other muscular dystrophies

Some other types of muscular dystrophy are summarized in Table 17.15.

CASE STUDY 17.9

A 4-year-old boy presented with progressive weakness and motor regression. On examination, he had marked weakness in the proximal limb muscles with pseudohypertrophy of the calves, and demonstrated Gower's manoeuvre on attempting to stand. The serum CPK was greatly elevated, and electromyography showed myopathic changes. Muscle biopsy confirmed the clinical diagnosis of **Duchenne dystrophy** (Fig. 17.21), with widespread fibre destruction and absence of dystrophin on immunocytochemistry. Genetic analysis found a deletion on the p21 band of the X chromosome, and the family received genetic counselling. The patient became progressively weak, and died 12 years later of an associated **cardiomyopathy**.

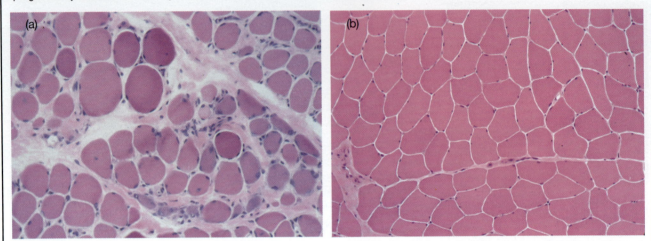

Fig. 17.21   Muscle biopsy in this case (a) showed the features of Duchenne dystrophy, with a marked variation in muscle fibre size, large hyaline fibres and an excess quantity of connective tissue in comparison with a normal control case (b).

Table 17.15   Other inherited muscular dystrophies

Type	Inheritance	Clinical features
Limb girdle dystrophy	Autosomal recessive	Progressive proximal weakness of limbs
Facioscapulohumeral dystrophy	Autosomal dominant	Slowly progressive weakness of the face and proximal muscles
Myotonic dystrophy	Autosomal dominant	Weakness and wasting of face, limb girdle and proximal muscles with myotonia Systemic effects include cataract, gonadal atrophy and diabetes mellitus

INFLAMMATORY MYOPATHIES

Skeletal muscle can be involved in a variety of infections. The pathogens may be:

- **bacteria**, such as clostridia and group A streptococci
- **viruses**, such as influenza and Coxsackie B
- **parasites**, such as *Trichinella* and *Toxoplasma* spp.

Polymyositis

Polymyositis is the most common inflammatory myopathy, occurring most frequently in adult females. Muscle fibre damage results from immunological injury by cytotoxic T lymphocytes (Fig. 17.22); treatment with immunosuppressive drugs such as corticosteroids is often beneficial. Polymyositis may be associated with collagen diseases, such as SLE, or

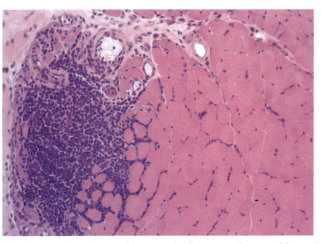
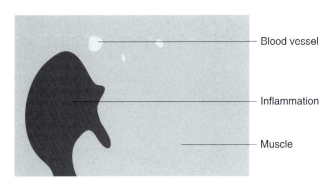

Blood vessel

Inflammation

Muscle

Fig. 17.22 In polymyositis, muscle fibres are damaged by an inflammatory reaction in which cytotoxic T lymphocytes and macrophages predominate. Although extensive fibre damage may occur, as in this case, immunosuppressive drugs can help restore the muscle structure.

bronchial carcinoma. A variant of this disorder, **dermatomyositis**, is accompanied by a characteristic facial rash, particularly in children.

METABOLIC AND TOXIC MYOPATHIES

A summary of metabolic and toxic myopathies is given in Table 17.16.

Table 17.16   Metabolic and toxic myopathies

Disease group	Example
Glycogen storage disease	McArdle's disease (glycogenosis V)
Mitochondrial cytopathy	Cytochrome oxidase deficiency
Endocrine disease	Myxoedema, Cushing's disease
Drugs	Corticosteroids, penicillamine
Toxins	Ethanol

CONGENITAL MYOPATHIES

The congenital myopathies are rare diseases presenting in infancy with floppiness and hypotonia, which are occasionally progressive and fatal. Many are inherited diseases affecting muscle fibre maturation.

Neurogenic disorders

Most denervating diseases are accompanied by progressive weakness and atrophy of skeletal muscles, although re-innervation may sometimes occur (Fig. 17.23). Neurogenic muscle disease can be classified into four main groups: **motor neuron disease**, **spinal muscular atrophy**, **peripheral neuropathies** and **spinal cord disorders**.

MOTOR NEURON DISEASE

Motor neuron disease is a progressive system atrophy in the CNS which results in muscle denervation and neurogenic atrophy (Fig. 17.24).

SPINAL MUSCULAR ATROPHY

Spinal muscular atrophy is a group of rare inherited conditions affecting motor neurons in the CNS. The most severe form is **Werdnig–Hoffman**

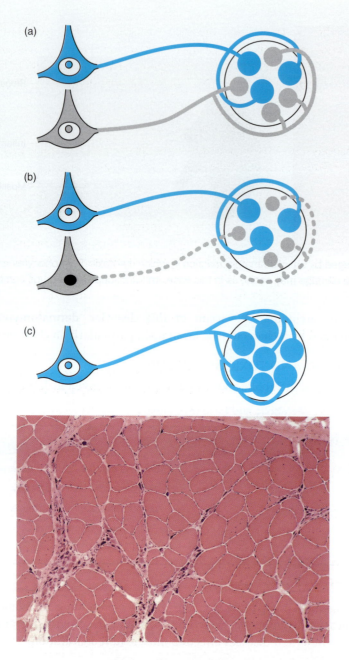

Fig. 17.23 (a) Normal muscle consists of a mosaic pattern of type 1 and 2 fibres; muscle fibre type is determined by the innervating anterior horn cell. (b) In neurogenic disorders, such as motor neuron disease, damage to a motor nerve cell or its axon results in denervation of the supplied muscle fibres, which undergo atrophy. (c) Adjacent surviving axons can sprout to re-innervate these atrophied fibres. The re-innervated fibres assume the fibre type of the new axonal unit, resulting in a large population of uniform fibres.

Fig. 17.24 In this case of motor neuron disease, muscle biopsy shows numerous groups of small angulated fibres, characteristic of denervation atrophy. Many of these atrophied fibres contain scanty cytoplasm, with a prominent hyperchromatic nucleus.

disease, a cause of congenital muscle weakness which is progressive and fatal before the age of 18 months.

PERIPHERAL NEUROPATHIES

Pure motor neuropathies are uncommon, and many peripheral nerve disorders present with muscle wasting and weakness accompanied by sensory loss.

SPINAL CORD DISORDERS

Any disease involving the corticospinal fibres, anterior horn cells or ventral nerve roots may result in neurogenic muscle disease: examples are **poliomyelitis** and **syringomyelia**.

Disorders of neuromuscular transmission

This group of uncommon conditions includes **myasthenia gravis**, an autoimmune disorder in which most patients have circulating antibodies against the acetylcholine receptor in the muscle endplate, and **Lambert–Eaton myasthenic syndrome**, a rare non-metastatic complication of malignancy, in which affected patients have a circulating IgG antibody to channels controlling neurotransmitter release at motor nerve terminals.

Peripheral nervous system

The reactions of peripheral nerve to injury are limited and consequently the clinical manifestations of peripheral nerve disorders can be classified clinically into three main groups:

- **mononeuropathy**, where a single nerve is involved, for example the median nerve in the **carpal tunnel syndrome**
- **mononeuritis multiplex**, where several isolated nerves are involved, for example in polyarteritis nodosa and sarcoidosis
- **polyneuropathy**, the most common group, where numerous sensory and/or motor nerves are involved.

Pathological reaction to disease

Three main groups of pathological reactions to disease can be seen in peripheral nerve biopsy (Fig. 17.25); they are **axonal degeneration**, **demyelinating neuropathies** and **other inflammatory neuropathies**.

AXONAL DEGENERATION

Axonal degradation is accompanied by secondary myelin breakdown and is of two types:

- **Wällerian degeneration**, where damage to the axon results in degeneration distal to the site of injury. Axonal regeneration can begin around 3–4 days following injury, but re-innervation may be hindered by factors which inhibit nerve growth, such as ischaemia or scar tissue.
- **Distal degeneration**, where neuronal metabolism is impaired, for example deficiency of vitamins B_1 and E.

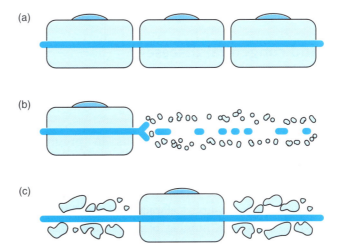

Fig. 17.25 (a) In normal peripheral nerve, the larger axons are surrounded by a myelin sheath arranged in uniform internodal segments derived from the cell membrane of a Schwann cell and its nucleus. (b) Damage or transection of the axon results in distal axonal degeneration, with fragmentation of the axon and secondary myelin sheath breakdown. (c) In primary demyelinating neuropathies the axon is intact, but the myelin sheath is damaged and disintegrates, often in internodal segments. Remyelination may occur following Schwann cell proliferation, with recovery of function.

DEMYELINATING NEUROPATHIES

Demyelinating neuropathies, where primary damage occurs to the myelin sheath and the underlying axon is preserved intact, can be classified into two groups:

- **Primary segmental demyelination**, which results from damage to Schwann cells in a variety of conditions, e.g. inherited metabolic disorders (including leukodystrophies). Demyelination may be accompanied by Schwann cell proliferation in attempts to restore myelin structure.
- **Inflammatory demyelinating neuropathies**, where myelin sheaths are damaged by macrophages in the presence of T lymphocytes. This mechanism operates in the Guillain–Barré syndrome, in which a complete clinical recovery can occur once Schwann cell proliferation and remyelination are established. It is also apparent in leprosy.

OTHER INFLAMMATORY NEUROPATHIES

Other inflammatory neuropathies are summarized in Table 17.17.

Table 17.17   Other inflammatory neuropathies

Disorder	Mechanism of nerve damage
Vasculitis	Ischaemia, haemorrhage
Sarcoidosis	Multiple granulomata in nerve fibre bundles
Leprosy	Granulomatous inflammation, necrosis

Interstitial neuropathies

The structure and function of nerve fibres can be impaired by conditions primarily involving the connective tissue and blood vessels within the nerve, for example vasculitis, diabetes mellitus and amyloid deposition.

Pathology of the eye

The normal structure of the eye is shown in Fig. 17.26. It is a complex organ with an equally complicated embryological origin from neuroectodermal, mesodermal and ectodermal tissues. The following section gives a brief description of some of the more common problems affecting the eye.

Genetic and congenital disease

Many of those who develop eye disease have a genetic predisposition to do so, but certain diseases of childhood are particularly important.

RETINITIS PIGMENTOSA

This group of inherited diseases results in progressive loss of photoreceptors leading to progressive reduction in the visual field until vision is restricted to the macula (**tunnel vision**). The name comes from secondary proliferation of the retinal pigment epithelium which causes patchy retinal hyperpigmentation. Cataracts occur, and their removal helps preserve vision. There are a number of genetic defects. The autosomal dominant form of the disease appears to be due to mutation of a gene for **rhodopsin**, the rod photoreceptor pigment.

ANATOMICAL ABNORMALITIES

Embryological malformations may occur at any stage of the development of the eye. Partial defects of the iris, cililary body and retinal defects are

Fig. 17.26 Structure of the normal eye.

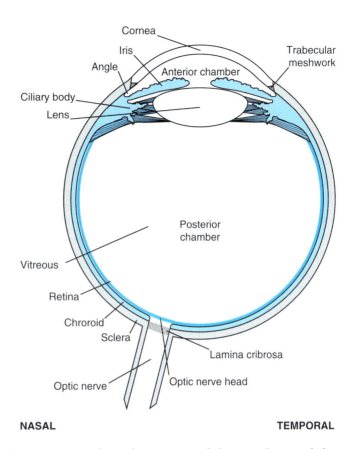

Cornea

Iris

Angle

Ciliary body

Lens

Anterior chamber

Trabecular meshwork

Posterior chamber

Vitreous

Retina

Chroroid

Sclera

Lamina cribrosa

Optic nerve

Optic nerve head

NASAL   **TEMPORAL**

relatively common and are known as **colobomas**. Larger failures of iris formation cause **aniridia**. This is associated with Wilms' tumour and other congenital syndromes. Hamartomatous conditions affecting the eye (phakomatoses) include neurofibromatosis, tuberous sclerosis, von Hippel–Lindau and Sturge–Weber syndromes.

Trauma

Corneal injuries, usually mechanical tears, are common and extremely painful. Penetrating injuries are much more serious and require early diagnosis to allow surgery which can prevent complications leading to loss of the eye (Fig. 17.27). Damage to the anterior segment can lead to secondary angle-closure or open-angle glaucoma (see below). Corneal epithelium can grow down defects in the cornea to form cysts within the anterior chamber. Dislocation of the lens leads to its degeneration, but rupture of the capsule leads to a giant cell granulomatous reaction against lens antigens known as **lens-induced uveitis**. Retinal detachment follows a tear and is almost always present after severe blunt injury (from a squash ball, for example) or a penetrating injury.

SYMPATHETIC OPHTHALMIA

Perhaps the most serious condition resulting from trauma to one eye is sympathetic ophthalmia, since it can lead to loss of the other eye if it is not recognized and treated. The normal eye 'sympathizes' with the injured eye by mounting a cell-mediated non-caseous granulomatous response in the choroid, and it is important to realize that this is a bilateral disease. This immune reaction can occur when retinal antigens come into contact with the immune recognition system of the uveal tract.

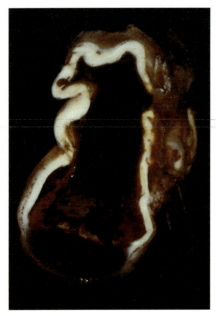

Fig. 17.27 The end result of trauma to the eye, showing loss of scleral shape and internal disruption.

Glaucoma

Pressure within the eye is maintained at 13–21 mmHg by a balance between aqueous inflow from the ciliary epithelium and outflow via the trabecular meshwork and canal of Schlemm. Glaucoma occurs when the intraocular pressure rises to an extent which causes damage to tissues within the eye, particularly the optic disc and retina. The problem appears to be the outflow tract, which can become dysfunctional or blocked by a variety of mechanisms. Glaucoma may be primary or secondary to other disease in the eye and generally causes severe headache. It is further classified morphologically by whether or not the angle is open or closed (Fig. 17.28).

- **Primary open-angle glaucoma (POAG)** is an acquired disease of the trabecular meshwork which has an increased resistance and shows hyalinization histologically. It is most common in elderly people.
- **Primary acute angle-closure glaucoma** is unilateral or bilateral. It is occurs in middle–old age. The iris becomes directly apposed to the inner surface of the trabecular meshwork and cornea, thus closing the angle. Treatment involves perforation of the iris (by surgery or laser) allowing the pressures in the anterior and posterior chamber to equilibrate. The iris then resumes its normal position, the angle is open again and the patient is cured. However, if the condition is not treated quickly, the iris may stick to the trabecular meshwork leading to persistent glaucoma.
- In **secondary open-angle glaucoma** the trabecular network can be blocked by particulate or cellular elements which accumulate in the anterior chamber, for instance after injury, release of melanin from the iris or surgery (especially if silicon oil is used to treat retinal detachment). Interference with trabecular endothelial cell function by steroids is an important iatrogenic cause.
- Many conditions, but especially diabetes, lead to formation of fibrovascular membranes on the iris. This causes adhesion between the iris and the cornea in the limbus shutting off the trabecular meshwork from the anterior chamber. **Secondary closed-angle glaucoma** results, and is often termed neovascular glaucoma to emphasize the importance of vascularization in its pathogenesis.

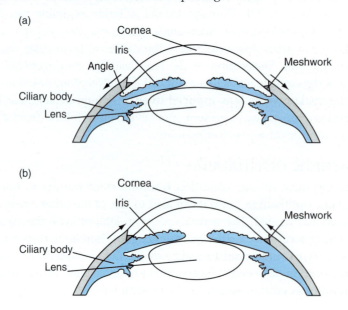

(a)
Cornea
Iris
Angle
Meshwork
Ciliary body
Lens

(b)
Cornea
Iris
Meshwork
Ciliary body
Lens

Fig. 17.28   In (a) open-angle glaucoma, the trabecular meshwork is abnormal but the angle is not physically occluded by anterior synechiae (adhesion between the iris and the cornea). A diagram of the anterior chamber of the eye showing the way in which blockage of the trabecular meshwork by anterior synechiae leads to (b) closed-angle glaucoma.

Vascular disease of the eye

Retinal ischaemic disease may be so severe that infarction results. Total retinal infarction may occur as the result of blockage of the central retinal artery, and occlusive disease of small vessels produces small infarcts. Examination of the fundus allows the macroscopic pathology to be seen in the patient; pathologists usually only see end-stage disease in eyes removed because of intractable glaucoma.

Features of focal ischaemia

- **Microinfarcts** (cotton-wool spots): these are seen on ophthalmoscopy as small white swellings where the retina has infarcted due to sudden occlusion of a small artery. The swollen ends of axons at the edge of the infarction form cytoid bodies.
- **Plasma (hard) exudates**: plasma-rich exudates form yellow clusters on the retina which persist until they are removed by macrophages after several months
- **Haemorrhages**: these may be intra- or subretinal and follow endothelial breakdown in the wall of capillaries or small venules. Circular haemorrhages with white centres (**Roth's spots**) are classically seen in subacute bacterial endocarditis. Haemorrhage into the vitreous may occur and can be treated by vitrectomy.
- **Microaneurysms**: focal swellings in capillaries due to degeneration in the supporting pericytes, particularly in diabetes
- **Neovascularization**: as in other organs, ischaemia leads to the formation of new vessels. In the retina and vitreous these tend to bleed. A vicious circle of organization and further bleeding leads to retinal detachment.
- **Retinal detachment**: in vascular disease this is usually due to contraction of fibrovascular tissue on the inner surface of the retina.

DIABETES

All of the features of focal ischaemia may be seen in diabetic retinopathy, with vascular proliferation being the major problem. This is often controlled by laser coagulation.

CENTRAL RETINAL VEIN OCCLUSION

Occlusion of the central retinal vein is a relatively common problem of elderly, often hypertensive, people causing sudden loss of vision in one eye. There is extensive haemorrhage in the fundus and neovascular glaucoma is a common complication. Occasionally younger patients may be seen with this condition due to vasculitis or thrombosis, which may be associated with oral contraceptive use.

HYPERTENSION

In malignant hypertension, there is papilloedema, haemorrhage and plasma exudation with fibrinoid necrosis of vessels in the retina. Thickening of arterioles (arteriolosclerosis) is a more common finding, although similar changes are seen in old age.

OTHER CONDITIONS

- Vascular changes are thought to underlie **macular degeneration** which is a common cause of visual loss in elderly people (Fig. 17.29).
- **Temporal (giant cell) arteritis** can affect the eye.
- **Embolization** of the central retinal artery may occur.
- **Telangiectasia** and **haemangiomas** are relatively common in the eye.

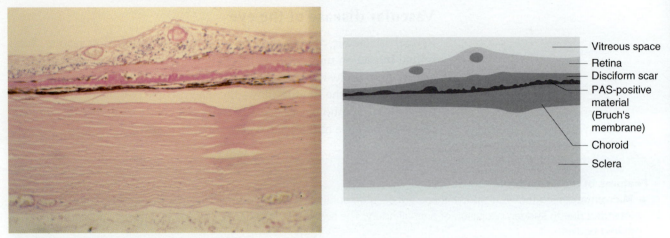

Fig. 17.29   Macular degeneration due to deposition of PAS-positive material on Bruch's membrane with consequent 'disciform scar' formation and retinal degeneration.

Inflammation and infection

The eye is often thought of as an immunologically privileged site partly because of its shape and physical separation from the environment. Nevertheless, it can be infected by a vast number of different pathogens and can be the site of inflammatory disease.

CONJUNCTIVITIS

Conjunctivitis is commonly associated with type I hypersensitivity as part of hay fever. However, other causes such as Sjögren's syndrome, chlamydial infection (trachoma), sarcoidosis and dermatological disorders may also affect the conjunctiva.

CORNEAL ULCERATION

Ulceration of the cornea is common and is usually viral or bacterial. Rarer causes include fungi and protozoa, both of which are more likely in immunosuppressed patients. *Acanthamoeba* sp. (Fig. 17.30) infects the

Fig. 17.30   A corneal ulcer with acanthamoeba cysts in the corneal stroma demonstrated by immunostaining.

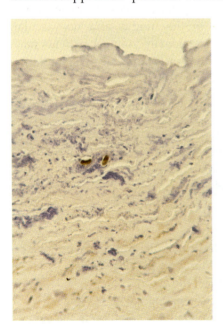

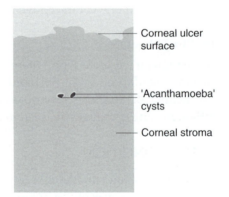

cornea in contact lens wearers. Viral pathogens include herpes simplex, cytomegalovirus and zoster, while bacteria are usually of pyogenic type (staphylococci, streptococci and Gram-negative bacilli).

INTRAOCULAR INFECTION

Infection within the eye is caused by a similar array of pathogens to those causing corneal ulceration. Accidental or surgical perforation of the cornea or sclera carries a risk of infection. Abscesses may form in any of the chambers of the eye. Other organisms may reach the eye via the bloodstream. Acid-fast bacilli are particularly prone to do this, forming granulomata within the uveal tract. Non-infectious causes such as sarcoidosis form part of the differential diagnosis. Larger blood-borne organisms including protozoa (such as *Toxoplasma* spp.) and helminths such as *Toxocara canis* may invade the eye. The vast load of toxocara eggs shed by dogs and cats in public parks is a source of considerable danger, and much of the population is exposed in childhood.

ONCHOCERCIASIS

River blindness remains common in certain parts of Africa. It is caused by a helminth, *Onchocerca volvulus*, which is spread by the blood-sucking *Simulium* sp. blackfly. Migrating larvae spread to the eye via the bloodstream where they cause a granulomatous reaction in the choroid.

Cataract

Cataract refers to opacity of the lens from any cause. The normal lens is formed of soluble transparent crystallin proteins enclosed in long spindle cells which are attached to one another by peg and socket joints. There is a thin rim of lens epithelium behind the elastic anterior lens capsule. Metabolism of the lens is maintained by diffusion of nutrients from the aqueous. Biochemical disturbances (such as diabetes or hypercalcaemia) can therefore cause lens opacification (cataract).

Congenital cataracts form if there is malformation or toxic damage to the lens fibres, for instance as a result of rubella infection. Degenerative changes in the lens with age (**senile cataract**) may be accelerated by exposure to ultraviolet light, irradiation, inflammation within the eye or blunt trauma to the eye. The changes are usually non-specific with nuclear sclerosis, cortical clefting and liquefaction histologically.

Tumours

Tumours in the eye are subdivided into **melanoma** and metastases (adults), and **retinoblastoma** (children). Retinoblastomas are dealt with in Chapter 16.

Melanoma (Fig. 17.31) may occur in any part of the eye, but is most common in the choroid. If less than 7 mm in maximum diameter, the prognosis is excellent with less than 2% metastasizing to the liver following enucleation. Histological type is a further guide, with 80% of pure spindle cell (low-grade) melanomas surviving more than 5 years. However, larger tumours and those of epithelioid cell type do poorly with a 50% 5-year survival rate. Overall, ocular melanoma accounts for 13% of melanoma deaths.

(a)

(b)

(c)

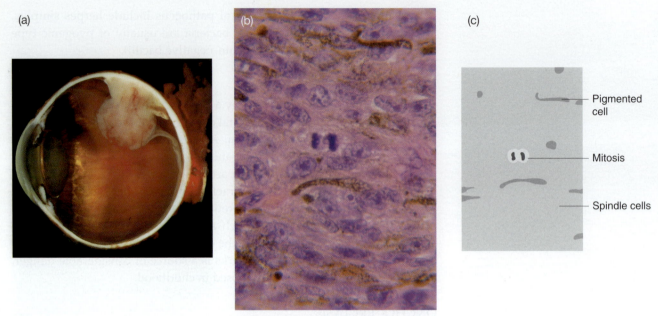

Pigmented cell

Mitosis

Spindle cells

Fig. 17.31   Melanoma of the choroid showing (a) the classic mushroom shape caused by penetration through Bruch's membrane into the subretinal space and (b, c) the typical spindle cell histology.

Chapter 18   Endocrine disease

Learning objectives

To appreciate and understand:
- Different types of endocrine disease which may occur, and their features
- Effects of excess or lack of different hormones as they relate to endocrine disease
- Role of the pathologist in diagnosis and treatment of endocrine disease

The endocrine system

The classical endocrine system comprises the pituitary, thyroid, parathyroid and adrenal glands, the islets of Langerhans in the pancreas, the testis and the ovary. All secrete hormones into the blood which interact with target cells at distant sites, as discussed in Chapter 3. Sometimes these glands secrete too much or too little hormone, which results in specific clinical syndromes. Alternatively, the gland may increase in size owing to hyperplasia or tumour development, and this may be apparent to the patient, or cause local symptoms due to pressure on adjacent tissues which lead to clinical presentation.

Diseases/disorders by organ

■ **Pituitary gland: anterior lobe**
- Hyperfunction
  - Acromegaly
  - Hyperprolactinaemia
  - Cushing's disease
- Hypopituitarism
- Pituitary adenomas
- Inflammatory conditions
- Circulatory disturbances

■ **Pituitary gland: posterior lobe**
- Diabetes insipidus
- Inappropriate secretion of vasopressin

■ **Thyroid gland**
- Hyperthyroidism
- Hypothyroidism
- Non-toxic nodular goitre

- Autoimmune thyroid disease
  - Graves' disease
  - Hashimoto's thyroiditis
  - Primary myxoedema
- Thyroid tumours
  - Follicular adenoma
  - Papillary carcinoma
  - Follicular carcinoma
  - Medullary carcinoma

■ **Adrenal cortex**
- Adrenocortical hyperfunction
- Cushing's disease
- Hyperaldosteronism
  - Primary Conn's syndrome
  - Secondary Conn's syndrome
- Adrenogenital syndrome
- Adrenocortical tumours

- Adrenocortical hypofunction
  - Acute
  - Chronic – Addison's disease

■ **Adrenal medulla**
- Phaeochromocytoma

■ **Parathyroid glands**
- Hyperparathyroidism
- Hypoparathyroidism

■ **Endocrine pancreas**
- Diabetes mellitus
  - Insulin dependent (type I)
  - Insulin independent (type 2)
- Multiple endocrine neoplasia
  - Type 1
  - Types 2a and 2b

It is now realized that endocrine cells are also scattered singly or in small groups throughout other organs such as the gastrointestinal and respiratory tracts – the **diffuse endocrine system**. These are thought to act in a paracrine fashion in the regulation of local function. Their pathology is as yet not understood.

Therefore, the diseases considered in this chapter are those well-recognized syndromes associated with the classical endocrine glands. None is common, but they are important to recognize because, apart from some of the malignant tumours, most are treatable, and patients thereafter have a significantly better quality of life.

Pituitary gland

The pituitary gland comprises the anterior lobe (adenohypophysis) arising from the oral cavity which accounts for about 75% of the weight, and the posterior lobe (neurohypophysis) which grows down from the brain and remains connected to the hypothalamus by the pituitary stalk. It sits in the sella turcica, a bony cavity in the base of the skull, covered by a layer of dura, the diaphragma sellae, through which the pituitary stalk passes. It lies below the optic chiasma and is bounded laterally by the cavernous sinuses. If the pituitary enlarges significantly it can cause pressure on these structures.

The anterior lobe produces:

- **growth hormone (GH)**
- **prolactin (PRL)**
- **adrenocorticotrophin (ACTH)**
- **thyroid-stimulating hormone (TSH)**

and the gonadotrophins:

- **follicle-stimulating hormone (FSH)**
- **luteinizing hormone (LH)**

as discussed in Chapter 3 (Fig. 18.1). The cells of this lobe and the tumours arising from them have traditionally been classified on the basis of histochemical stains as eosinophil, basophil and chromophobe, but this is now outdated. Immunohistochemistry now identifies specific hormones (Fig. 18.2).

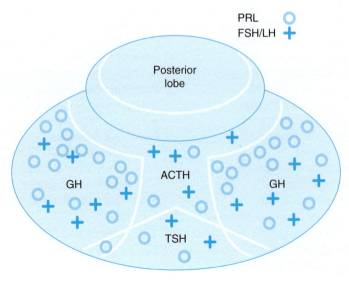

Fig. 18.1 Diagrammatic representation of the distribution of the various cell types in a transverse section of the pituitary. ACTH cells are sited chiefly in the median wedge and around the junction with the posterior lobe; GH cells in the lateral wings; TSH cells in a wedge-shaped area on the anterior rim. Gonadotrophs (FSH/LH) are randomly distributed. PRL cells are also distributed throughout the gland, but in higher numbers posteriorly.

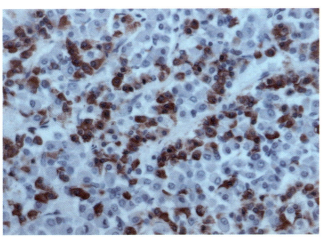
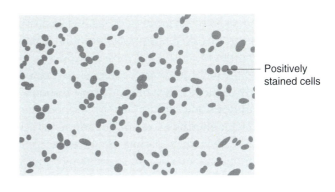

Positively
stained cells

Fig. 18.2   Immunocytochemical localization of growth hormone in cells in the lateral wings, interspersed with other cell types.

Cell types identified by immunohistochemistry
- GH cells (**somatotrophs**)
- PRL cells (**lactotrophs**)
- ACTH cells (**corticotrophs**)
- TSH cells (**thyrotrophs**)
- FSH and/or LH cells (**gonadotrophs**)

The blood supply of the anterior lobe is mainly via the hypothalamic–pituitary portal system. The primary capillary plexus is in the median eminence of the hypothalamus, draining blood into venous channels which run down the pituitary stalk to the secondary capillary plexus in the anterior lobe. This permits direct access of high concentrations of hypothalamic regulatory factors to their target cells in the anterior pituitary.

The posterior pituitary secretes **oxytocin**, which is involved in lactation and in uterine contraction in labour. No diseases have been identified in association with excess or lack of secretion of this hormone. It also produces **vasopressin (antidiuretic hormone, ADH)** which has actions on water balance and blood pressure. Both of these hormones are synthesized in neuronal cell bodies of the supraoptic and paraventricular nuclei of the hypothalamus and pass down axons in the pituitary stalk to be secreted into the systemic circulation.

Anterior pituitary hyperfunction

Hyperfunction of the anterior pituitary is almost invariably due to hypersecretion of a hormone by a pituitary adenoma. Prolactin is the only hormone commonly secreted in excess for other reasons, as discussed below.

ACROMEGALY

Acromegaly is caused by excessive GH secretion in adult life. There is overgrowth of bone and soft tissues; hands and feet enlarge and a characteristic facial appearance develops with prognathism and widening of the nose (Fig. 18.3). Osteoarthritis often ensues. Growth of internal organs leads to cardiomegaly and hypertension and patients have a greatly increased risk of dying from cardiovascular disease. Effects on general metabolism give rise to abnormal glucose tolerance and sometimes frank diabetes mellitus. **Gigantism** occurs when GH excess occurs before epiphyses close. Some patients show features of both conditions. Almost all patients have a pituitary adenoma.

HYPERPROLACTINAEMIA

If a PRL-secreting tumour occurs in a premenopausal woman, the menstrual cycle is abnormal and the patient presents with amenorrhoea and

Fig. 18.3   Patient showing typical features of acromegaly with general coarsening of features, prominent supraorbital ridges and a degree of prognathism.

infertility, and occasionally galactorrhea, whether the tumour is small or large. In men hyperprolactinaemia occasionally results in loss of libido or infertility, but is usually asymptomatic, as it is in postmenopausal women. Thus, in these groups, PRL-secreting tumours usually present clinically only if large enough to cause local pressure effects.

In contrast to the other pituitary hormones, hypersecretion of PRL occurs not infrequently in the absence of a pituitary tumour. This is because PRL secretion is under tonic inhibition by hypothalamic dopamine and therefore any factor altering access of dopamine to the anterior pituitary or dopamine metabolism may permit enhanced secretion of PRL. Physiological hyperprolactinaemia occurs in pregnancy and lactation.

CUSHING'S DISEASE

Cushing's syndrome (see below) is caused by excessive glucocorticoid secretion from the adrenal glands. In about 70% of patients this is due to hypersecretion of ACTH from the pituitary resulting in hyperstimulation. This condition is known as Cushing's disease. Almost all are due to an ACTH cell adenoma. A few have ACTH cell hyperplasia, possibly caused by excessive hypothalamic secretion of **corticotrophin-releasing factor (CRF)**.

OTHER SYNDROMES

Occasionally, TSH-secreting tumours cause secondary hyperthyroidism. Gonadotrophin excess rarely gives rise to clinical symptoms.

Hypopituitarism

Multiple hormone deficiencies are usually caused by destruction of the pituitary gland, preventing synthesis of the hormone, or destruction of the pituitary stalk or hypothalamus leading to deficiency of hypothalamus-stimulating factors. In industrialized countries, the most common cause is now pressure from an expanding pituitary adenoma, or damage following pituitary surgery. In developing countries, **Sheehan's syndrome (postpartum necrosis)** is still the major cause. Pituitary irradiation may result in hypopituitarism after several years' delay. Trauma, inflammation (including autoimmune hypophysitis) or other intrasellar tumours are rare causes. Infiltration of the hypothalamus by histiocytosis X or granulomatous diseases, or destruction by suprasellar tumours including craniopharyngioma, may interfere with the production of releasing factors by the hypothalamus.

The clinical presentation depends on the degree of loss of each hormone. Gonadotrophin deficiency usually becomes apparent first, with loss of secondary sex characteristics and libido, and amenorrhea in women and impotence in men. Deficiency of GH does not usually give rise to symptoms. If not recognized, hypothyroidism and hypoadrenalism may eventually present acutely with nausea, vomiting, hypotension and, rarely, fatal collapse. Isolated hormone deficiencies are usually due to congenital abnormalities in the production of specific hormones or of their releasing factors. GH deficiency is one cause of short stature; occasional deficiencies of gonadotrophins or ACTH have been reported.

Pituitary adenomas

These are the most common pathological lesion in the pituitary. In clinical neurosurgical practice, they account for 10% of intracranial neoplasms.

Causes of hyperprolactinaemia
- Prolactin-secreting **adenoma**
- **Pituitary stalk pressure**, for example by other type of adenoma
- **Hypothalamic destruction**, by tumour or inflammatory process
- Drug therapy:
  - **dopamine receptor antagonists** (phenothiazines, metoclopramide)
  - drugs affecting **dopamine turnover** (methyldopa, reserpine)
- Primary **hypothyroidism**
- **Idiopathic**
- **Physiological** (pregnancy)

They may be found more frequently than this in the pituitaries of patients who undergo postmortem examinations, indicating that most do not give rise to any clinical signs or symptoms. They are classified as **microadenomas** (less than 10 mm diameter) and **macroadenomas** (more than 10 mm). Small tumours usually present only if they secrete excess hormone. Larger tumours may also cause hormonal symptoms, but may present even when not secreting because of local pressure symptoms. They may compress surrounding structures causing visual disturbances (classically homonymous hemianopia) when the optic chiasma or nerves are involved, or headache. Pressure on the normal para-adenomatous gland may induce atrophy and hypopituitarism. Complex hormonal profiles may be seen when a hormone-secreting tumour causes destruction of the normal gland and lack of other hormones.

A small minority of tumours show aggressive local spread into the hypothalamus and brain, causing increased intracranial pressure. These are still regarded as benign, however, and the diagnosis of carcinoma is made only in those extremely rare cases where metastasis is identified, usually to extracranial sites. Lateral spread into the cavernous sinus may make it impossible to remove the tumour fully and such patients may have continuing hypersecretion of hormone after surgery, or may have an initial period of remission followed by recurrence of their clinical syndrome as such a remnant grows and produces significant hormone output.

Occasionally, major haemorrhage may occur into a tumour (**pituitary apoplexy**) causing a sudden increase in intracranial pressure which precipitates a medical emergency. If the patient survives, the tumour necrosis usually causes regression of the symptoms of hormonal excess.

As with the cells of the normal gland, classification of tumours should now be based on the immunohistochemical identification of hormone production (Fig. 18.4), with ultrastructural analysis as a second level, without which some diagnoses cannot be made. Cases should be referred to centres with specialist expertise for such investigations. These approaches are now beginning to provide data on more aggressive subgroups, thus permitting the implementation of adjunctive therapy (such as irradiation) following initial surgery. It is important to realize, however, that patterns of drug therapy may alter the types of tumours coming to surgery. For example, many microadenomas secreting PRL are

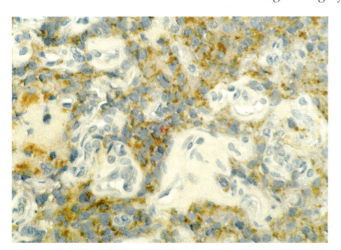
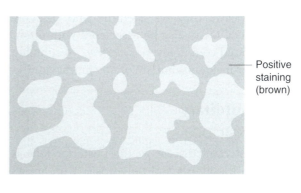

Positive staining (brown)

Fig. 18.4   PRL cell adenoma showing a dot pattern of positive staining for the hormone.

now treated pharmacologically with the dopamine agonist bromocriptine, which inhibits their secretion of PRL; these patients do not come to surgery.

The pathogenesis of pituitary adenomas is unclear. Most are sporadic, but some are part of the multiple endocrine neoplasia syndrome type 1 (MEN1, Wermer's syndrome, see below). Few molecular genetic abnormalities have as yet been identified, apart from a mutation in the subunit of a stimulatory G protein (G_s) in a subgroup of GH cell adenomas (the *gsp* oncogene). Mutations of the *ras* oncogene family appear rare.

The role of hypothalamic hormones is unclear, but they may act as tumour promoters. For example, there is a higher incidence of TSH cell adenomas in patients with primary hypothyroidism who have increased levels of thyrotrophin-releasing hormone (TRH), than in the general population.

OTHER TUMOURS

Craniopharyngiomas may occur in an intrasellar location, although more usually suprasellar. Rarely, a tumour may arise from the other elements of the gland, for example angioma or fibroma. Occasional cysts arising in remnants of Rathke's cleft may mimic a tumour, causing pressure effects by local expansion.

INFLAMMATORY CONDITIONS

Inflammatory processes are rare in the pituitary. Acute inflammation usually reflects direct extension of infection from neighbouring structures. Granulomatous inflammation such as tuberculosis and sarcoidosis may involve the gland. Autoimmune hyophysitis is rare compared with autoimmune diseases of the other endocrine glands. It usually follows pregnancy and often undergoes spontaneous remission. In AIDS, cytomegalovirus appears to be the only common opportunistic infection.

CIRCULATORY DISTURBANCES

Infarction has to be extensive (greater than 70%) before clinical evidence of hormone deficiency is seen. This most often occurs in Sheehan's syndrome – postpartum pituitary necrosis following post- or intrapartum haemorrhage. The pituitary is rendered vulnerable to the effects of the hypotension because of the low pressure in the portal vascular system and the increase in size which occurs in pregnancy. Long-term ventilation, sickle-cell disease, diabetes mellitus and disseminated intravascular coagulation (DIC) may also be associated with infarction. Small pituitary infarcts are found commonly *post mortem*, presumably the results of minor cardiovascular incidents, but are of no clinical significance.

Posterior pituitary

DIABETES INSIPIDUS

The most important disease of the posterior lobe is diabetes insipidus, presenting with polyuria and polydipsia, with an inability to concentrate the urine even when fluid intake is restricted. It is due to lack of vasopressin. It may be idiopathic, and some of these cases are familial. Destruction of the hypothalamic nuclei synthesizing vasopressin by granulomatous disease, histiocytosis X or tumour may also be a cause. It may also follow pituitary surgery or head injury (usually transient).

INAPPROPRIATE SECRETION OF VASOPRESSIN

This is usually due to ectopic secretion by an oat cell carcinoma of bronchus, but may also occur in some cases of meningitis, subarachnoid haemorrhage, head injury, on ventilation or in pneumonia. The mechanisms in the last cases are unclear, but patients have hyponatraemia and hypo-osmolality due to water retention. Muscle cramps, vomiting and weakness develop; coma and death may follow.

TUMOURS

Primary tumours of the posterior lobe are rare. Metastases, particularly from breast and lung, may be found in 1–3% of cancer patients but are rarely of clinical significance.

Thyroid gland

The thyroid gland consists of two lateral lobes joined by an isthmus, and lies just below the cricoid cartilage. In the normal adult, it weighs 15–25 g. Follicles of varying size, lined by cuboidal epithelium, store colloid containing thyroglobulin on which **thyroid hormones** are synthesized (Fig. 18.5). These are derived from a downgrowth of the primitive pharynx. In the middle and upper portions of the lateral lobes, C cells which produce **calcitonin** are scattered among the follicles. These derive from the ultimobranchial bodies and are thought to be neuroectodermal in origin.

Secretion of thyroid hormones is stimulated by TSH and they in turn exert negative feedback at both hypothalamic and pituitary levels to control TSH release. Calcitonin release is regulated by serum calcium levels, although there is a suggestion that TSH may also be involved.

Most clinical thyroid disease relates to the thyroid follicles. Patients may present clinically with a thyroid swelling – **goitre** – which may be diffuse or nodular. Alternatively, patients may have symptoms related to excess or

Fig. 18.5 Normal thyroid gland consists of follicles of varying sizes storing colloid, which contains thyroglobulin on which thyroid hormones are synthesized.

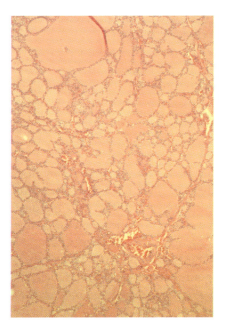
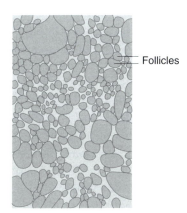

Follicles

deficiency of thyroid hormones. The wide-ranging physiological roles of thyroxine (T_4) and tri-iodothyronine (T_3) mean that such abnormalities have significant general metabolic effects. These syndromes are outlined below.

Hyperthyroidism

This is also known as **thyrotoxicosis**. There is a general increase in metabolic activity. Patients are hyperkinetic, irritable and emotionally labile. Despite an increase in appetite, they lose weight. There is heat intolerance, excessive sweating and a fine tremor. Palpitation, tachycardia and increased cardiac output are present. Atrial fibrillation and cardiac failure are not uncommon in older patients. There is eyelid retraction (Fig. 18.6) and infrequent blinking due to increased sympathetic tone, causing contraction of levator palpebrae superioris. In some patients there is true **proptosis** – protuberance of the eyeball due to inflammatory infiltration of the extraocular tissues of the orbit.

The most common cause (more than 80% of cases) is **Graves' disease** (see below). Toxic nodular goitre accounts for about 10% and a toxic nodule (adenoma) for a further 5–10%. It may occur in early **Hashimoto's thyroiditis**, sometimes referred to as hashitoxicosis. Rarely, a TSH-secreting pituitary adenoma may be implicated. Occasional patients ingest large doses of thyroid hormones. In some patients with multinodular goitre the administration of iodine leads to a sudden marked increase in synthesis of thyroid hormones (**Jod–Basedow phenomenon**).

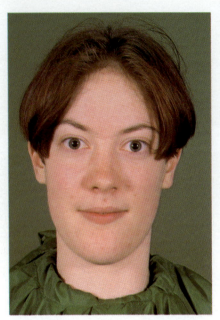

Fig. 18.6 Thyrotoxic patient showing a degree of eyelid retraction, owing to increased sympathetic tone.

Hypothyroidism

This is known as **myxoedema**, and the symptoms depend on the degree of hormone deficiency. There is general lethargy and weight gain. The patient feels cold and may indeed develop hypothermia if the diagnosis is missed, resulting in emergency medical admission. The skin and hair are dry and excess deposition of mucopolysaccharides in connective tissue causes thickening of the skin, pain and paraesthesiae, and hoarseness. There is intellectual impairment and change of mood which may proceed to frank psychosis (myxoedema madness). Blood cholesterol is raised.

Autoimmune thyroiditis is the most common cause, either primary myxoedema or Hashimoto's thyroiditis. Less commonly, severe iodine deficiency or dyshormonogenesis may be implicated. It may also follow thyroid surgery or radioiodine therapy or as the result of ingestion of goitrogens or antithyroid drugs. Hypopituitarism may result in secondary hypothyroidism, usually in association with deficiencies of other target gland hormones.

In infancy, severe hypothyroidism is known as **cretinism**. The baby may appear normal at birth because of the effects of maternal hormones. Signs of mental handicap, neuromuscular abnormality, retarded growth and deaf mutism develop. The child has a characteristic appearance with coarse features and an enlarged tongue, again due to deposition of mucopolysaccharides. Where thyroid agenesis or hypoplasia is the cause, there is no goitre. In areas of endemic goitre, maternal iodine deficiency may be the cause, the baby having a goitre. Deficiencies of enzymes involved in the pathways of thyroxine biosynthesis, or of peripheral

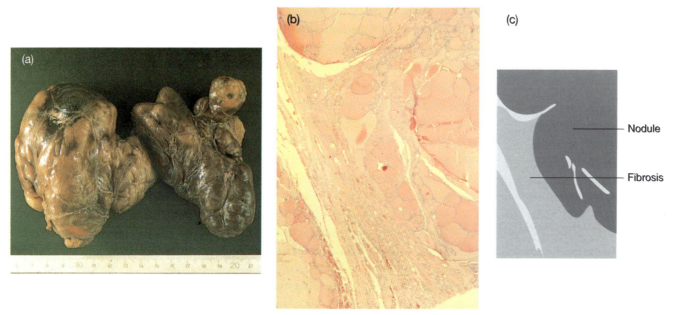

Fig. 18.7 Non-toxic goitre: (a) the thyroid is generally enlarged and nodular, fibrous tissue extending between the nodules. (b, c) The microscopic appearance confirms the initial impression of nodularity.

response to the hormone result in sporadic goitrous cretinism. To prevent the dangerous sequelae of this condition, early diagnosis is important for the implementation of replacement therapy.

NON-TOXIC NODULAR GOITRE

The most common pathological lesion of the gland is non-toxic nodular goitre (Fig. 18.7). In the face of absolute or relative iodine deficiency, reduced thyroid hormone levels increase TSH secretion, and this induces compensatory hyperplasia in an attempt to re-establish euthyroidism. Initially, there is diffuse hyperplasia with colloid depletion (parenchymatous goitre). Involution leads to accumulation of colloid (colloid goitre). Succeeding cycles of iodine deficiency and involution eventually result in the well-recognized picture of multinodular goitre, with nodules consisting of follicles of varying size, with fibrosis, evidence of haemorrhage and focal inflammatory infiltrate. The gland may weigh up to several hundred grams and is usually asymmetrical. Sometimes one nodule may be much larger than the others (dominant nodule) suggesting a possible tumour. Fine-needle aspiration cytology or even partial thyroidectomy may be required to make the final diagnosis. Rarely, in older patients, the individual may develop hyperthyroidism – **toxic nodular goitre**. Occasionally, a goitre may cause tracheal or oesophageal compression or involve the recurrent laryngeal nerve.

On epidemiological grounds, in areas where more than 10% of the population is affected, it is defined as **endemic goitre**. Endemic goitre occurs in areas of **absolute dietary iodine deficiency**. Because seafood is the major natural source of dietary iodine, these areas are usually far from the sea and/or mountainous, like the Himalayas, the Andes and the Alps. The incidence has decreased in developed countries since the introduction of iodized salt. Goitre usually develops in childhood and males and females are equally affected.

Sporadic goitre is defined as goitre occurring in less than 10% of the community and is caused by **relative deficiency of iodine** in an individual patient. It is ten times more common in women and often presents around puberty or in pregnancy or lactation because of the increased requirement for iodine. Most patients are clinically euthyroid, but TSH levels may be slightly raised. The iodine deficiency may be the result of poor dietary intake, deficiencies of enzymes involved in thyroxine synthesis or the ingestion of goitrogens. These include vegetables of the Brassica family (cabbage, Brussels sprouts) and excessive fluoride in water; drugs such as p-aminosalicylic acid and sulphonylureas; and, in some individuals, iodides in cough expectorants. Finally, it has been suggested, but not proved, that some cases may represent a variant of autoimmune thyroid disease with the production of growth-stimulating immunoglobulins.

Autoimmune thyroid disease

The autoimmune thyroid diseases are **Graves' disease**, **Hashimoto's thyroiditis** and **primary myxoedema**. They are characterized by the presence of lymphoid infiltration in the gland and circulating autoantibodies to components of thyroid follicular cells including antithyroglobulin, antimicrosomal (now known to react with peroxidase enzyme) and anti-C2 (second colloid antigen). These are found in 80% of patients with autoimmune thyroid disease and in 10% of the general population. **Thyroid-stimulating immunoglobulins** (TSI) are TSH-receptor antibodies which activate the receptor once bound, causing hyperthyroidism. **Thyroid growth-stimulating immunoglobulins** (TGI) are thought to stimulate growth, and may have a role in goitrogenesis in Hashimoto's thyroiditis. Receptor blocking antibodies may help contribute to the hypothyroidism by preventing TSH gaining access to the receptor, thus reducing thyroid activity.

These diseases have a familial association with specific autoimmune diseases including Addison's disease, type 1 diabetes mellitus and pernicious anaemia.

GRAVES' DISEASE

This disease is characterized by hyperthyroidism. Women are affected five times more than men, mainly between 20 and 40 years of age. There is a reported increased prevalence of HLA-DR3. The gland is diffusely hyperplastic, up to three times normal size. When untreated, the follicular epithelium is columnar, and there is little colloid storage. The lymphocytic infiltrate is usually less marked in Graves' disease than in the other variants of autoimmune thyroiditis. Surgical specimens do not usually show these classic changes because the hyperthyroidism must be controlled by antithyroid drugs before operation. These increase the extent of hyperplasia, while iodine pre-treatment reduces vascularity and increases colloid accumulation.

HASHIMOTO'S THYROIDITIS

This disease occurs mainly in middle-aged women, occurring 20 times more commonly than in men. An increased prevalence of HLA-DR5 has been reported. There is a diffuse, firm, painless goitre. The patient is usually euthyroid at presentation, but 80% will become hypothyroid. Occasional patients present with hyperthyroidism, presumably due to production of TSI. There is widespread infiltration with lymphocytes,

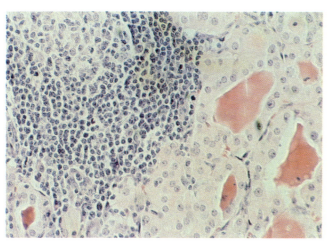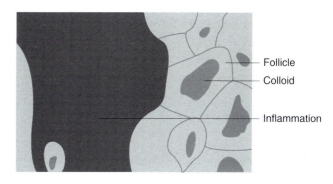

Fig. 18.8 Hashimoto's thyroiditis showing marked chronic inflammatory infiltrate and follicular cells with typical Askanazy cell changes.

plasma cells and macrophages, and germinal centre formation is common. The thyroid follicular cells become enlarged and granular, due to accumulation of mitochondria (Fig. 18.8). This is known as **Askanazy** or **Hürthle cell change**.

PRIMARY MYXOEDEMA

This occurs mainly in elderly women. There is no goitre, the thyroid being atrophic and largely replaced by fibrous tissue with a lymphoid infiltrate. These patients are severely hypothyroid.

FOCAL CHRONIC THYROIDITIS

Focal lymphoid infiltrates may be found in about 15–20% of thyroids from patients with no clinical evidence of thyroid disease. These may represent subclinical autoimmune disease, since the incidence correlates with that of thyroid autoantibodies in the general population, but this is not proven.

LYMPHOCYTIC THYROIDITIS

Lymphocytic thyroiditis occurs in children and young adults, presenting usually with a goitre, sometimes with hyperthyroidism. A diffuse lymphoplasmacytic infiltrate is seen with germinal centre formation, but no Askanazy cell change. If present, thyroid autoantibodies are in low titre. It has been suggested that it is an early form of Hashimoto's disease.

OTHER TYPES OF THYROIDITIS

- **Acute thyroiditis** is uncommon, but may develop in bacteraemia, with focal abscess formation, or as a result of local extension of infection.
- **Giant-cell (de Quervain's) thyroiditis** is also known as **subacute thyroiditis** and presents with painful goitre. It is thought to have a viral origin and there is often a preceding upper respiratory infection or general malaise and fever. Women are affected three times more commonly than men. Hyperthyroidism may be present initially, but resolves. Thyroid autoantibodies are present transiently in some cases. There is initial infiltration with neutrophil polymorphs, followed by a granulomatous response with giant cell formation and varying degrees of fibrosis. Complete resolution may occur, but a degree of fibrosis remains in some glands.

- **Reidel's thyroiditis** is a rare condition, in which the thyroid is replaced by dense fibrous tissue, often extending into perithyroidal tissues, mimicking a malignant tumour. The patient may present with goitre or there may be tracheal involvement or entrapment of the recurrent laryngeal nerve. The aetiology is unknown, but some patients also have mediastinal or retroperitoneal fibrosis.

Thyroid tumours

Thyroid tumours usually present as clinical solitary nodules; most are 'cold' on scan – they are less active in concentrating iodine than the normal gland. However, only about 30% of clinical solitary nodules are tumours, the remainder representing dominant nodules in a multinodular goitre (see above). Thus, in men and young women, a solitary thyroid nodule is more likely to be a tumour than in a middle-aged woman, where non-toxic goitre is common. Most thyroid tumours are benign: malignant tumours account for less than 1% of all cancers, and less than 0.5% of all cancer deaths.

Most tumours arise from follicular cells, the most common being the **follicular adenoma**. Two forms of carcinoma arise from follicular cells, **papillary** and **follicular**, with different morphology and behavioural patterns. The C cells give rise to **medullary carcinoma** of the thyroid.

FOLLICULAR ADENOMA

This adenoma is the most common thyroid neoplasm and it occurs most frequently in women over 30 years of age. Most are non-functional and appear 'cold' on scan but rare tumours cause hyperthyroidism (toxic adenoma) and appear 'hot'. They are usually encapsulated and compress the surrounding gland. They range in histological appearance from those resembling normal thyroid through microfollicular to patterns resembling the fetal gland, but none of these differences has any influence on tumour behaviour. It may be difficult to distinguish an adenoma from a circumscribed hyperplastic, cellular nodule in a nodular goitre. However, in practical terms, there is no difference in the clinical management of the two. Removal results in complete cure.

PAPILLARY CARCINOMA

All true papillary lesions of the thyroid are regarded as carcinoma. They account for 60–70% of all thyroid cancer, are three times more common in women and the peak incidence is between 30 and 40 years. They are not usually encapsulated and may appear multifocal, possibly due to intraglandular lymphatic spread. Lymph node metastases may be found in the neck at presentation in about 40% of cases. However, this does not worsen the prognosis, the 5-year survival approaching 90%. The primary tumour may be extremely small and the lymph node metastasis may be the presenting symptom. Distant metastases are uncommon, but when present at time of diagnosis reduce the 5-year survival to about 75%.

These tumours have a characteristic cytology, with optically clear nuclei, and many show sclerosis and calcispherites (**psammoma bodies**). Most are papillary in appearance (Fig. 18.9b), but mixed papillary and follicular variants occur and some tumours are purely follicular but have the typical cytological features. All of these behave in the same non-aggressive fashion as the classic papillary lesion.

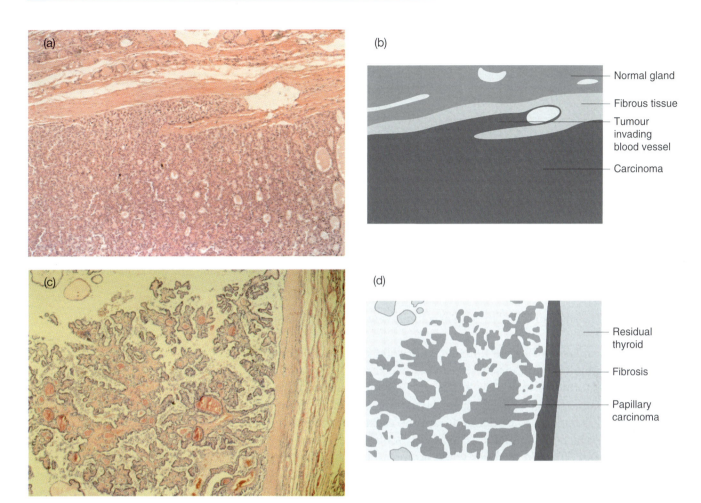

Fig. 18.9 (a, b) Follicular carcinoma. This tumour shows some evidence of follicle formation and vascular invasion. (c, d) Papillary carcinoma. In contrast, this tumour consists of fibrovascular papillae, with no evidence of follicular formation.

FOLLICULAR CARCINOMA

Where iodine intake is adequate, follicular carcinomas account for 15–20% of all thyroid cancers, but in areas of endemic goitre constitute a higher proportion of cases. They are more common in women, with a peak incidence between 40 and 50 years of age. They metastasize via the bloodstream chiefly to bone and lung. The overall survival rate is 50%. They may be divided into two groups – widely invasive tumours, which obviously infiltrate the gland, surrounding tissues and vessels, and encapsulated tumours where capsular and/or vascular invasion is detected only by microscopic examination (Fig. 18.9a). This latter group have a much better prognosis than the former.

MEDULLARY CARCINOMA

These carcinomas arise from the C cells and account for 5–10% of thyroid cancers. Most are sporadic, but 10–20% are familial, mostly forming part of the MEN2 syndromes (see below). Women are slightly more commonly affected than men. Sporadic cases usually present between 40 and 60 years of age. The familial variant arises on a background of C-cell hyperplasia and is thus usually bilateral and multifocal and may present before the age of 25 years. Where this diagnosis is made, family members should be screened for evidence of MEN2. Prophylactic thyroidectomy should be

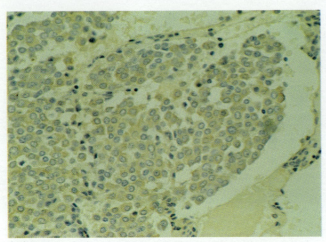
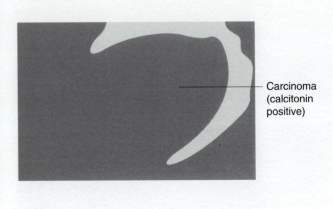

Carcinoma
(calcitonin
positive)

Fig. 18.10 Medullary carcinoma showing immunopositivity for calcitonin. The tumour cells are arranged in sheets and alveolar structures.

performed at the stage of C-cell hyperplasia to prevent the development of tumour.

Medullary carcinoma (Fig. 18.10) consists of solid groups and cords of cells and calcitonin immunoreactivity can be detected. The tumours may produce other hormones including ACTH, and serotonin and occasionally give rise to ectopic hormone syndromes. Amyloid is present in about half the cases, and is thought to be derived from the calcitonin precursor. The tumour spreads by both lymphatic and vascular routes. The overall 10-year survival is about 50%, but is better when no metastases are identified at time of initial presentation. Tumours in MEN2b syndrome (see below) are, however, extremely aggressive and invariably fatal.

ANAPLASTIC TUMOURS

About 5–10% of thyroid carcinomas are anaplastic. They are found mainly in women aged 60–70 years, and grow rapidly. They are highly malignant and have often both local invasion and distant metastases at presentation. There is often a history of a long-standing thyroid mass, and it is thought that most arise in pre-existing papillary or follicular carcinomas. Histology shows an undifferentiated tumour often with giant cell formation; small foci of papillary or follicular carcinoma may be found.

AETIOLOGY OF THYROID CARCINOMA

It is unclear whether iodine deficiency alters the overall incidence of thyroid cancer, but it does change the proportions, increasing follicular tumours. The addition of iodine to the diet in areas of endemic goitre has reversed this change. External irradiation may have a role in the pathogenesis of some papillary cancers – an increased incidence has been reported after the atomic bombs in Hiroshima and the nuclear accident at Chernobyl, and following therapeutic exposure of the head and neck in childhood.

The molecular genetic analysis of thyroid cancers indicates that different events are involved in the pathogenesis of follicular and papillary tumours. Although activating mutations of *ras* oncogenes occur as early events in follicular neoplasia, being present in adenomas, they are rare in papillary tumours, where alterations in the *ret* oncogene occur in some cases. In contrast to other tumours, alterations in expression of the *p53* tumour suppressor gene appear uncommon, and are important only in the progression from differentiated to anaplastic tumours. Mutations of the *ret* proto-oncogene are now known to be involved in MEN2 and in some cases of sporadic medullary carcinomas.

LYMPHOMAS

B-cell lymphomas of follicle centre cell type can arise in the thyroid. Over 75% are in women with long-standing Hashimoto's thyroiditis, the patient usually complaining of a sudden increase in size of a pre-existing goitre. Some 1–2% of patients with Hashimoto's disease develop lymphoma. Some of the tumours show features in common with MALT (mucosa-associated lymphoid tissue) lymphomas, the thyroid having originated in the primitive gut. They are originally confined to the thyroid, and thyroidectomy may at this point result in cure; however, they may then disseminate and prognosis worsens. Plasmacytoma may also rarely arise in Hashimoto's disease.

OTHER TUMOURS

Occasional tumours arise in the connective tissue elements of the gland (haemangioma, for example). Metastases are also seen rarely, mainly from lung, breast and gastrointestinal tract.

Miscellaneous conditions

Congenital absence (**agenesis**) or hypoplasia of the gland may cause cretinism. Occasionally the thyroid may not descend properly, the most common variant being **lingual thyroid**. Persistence of the lower part of embryonic tubal downgrowth gives rise to **thyroglossal duct cyst**. These lie in the midline, and usually become inflamed and may rupture. They are lined by respiratory or squamous epithelium and lymphoid tissue and thyroid follicles are found focally in the wall.

Amyloid may be found in systemic amyloidosis or as an isolated finding and may result in goitre.

Adrenal glands

The adrenal glands lie above the kidneys and comprise the outer cortex of mesodermal origin which surrounds the medulla derived from neuroectoderm. In the adult the normal gland weighs 4–4.5 g at surgery or in cases of sudden death. Stress causes stimulation by ACTH and an increase in weight and so the average weight at hospital autopsy is about 6 g because of the stress of the terminal illness. The cortex and medulla are discussed separately, as their functions and pathology differ.

Adrenal cortex

As outlined in Chapter 3, the cortex consists of the **zona glomerulosa**, active in mineralocorticoid secretion, and the **zona fasciculata** and **zona reticularis** which produce glucocorticoids and sex steroids. Patients with cortical disease usually present with symptoms of excessive or deficient secretion of one or more of the cortical steroids. Those with malignant tumours may have evidence of metastases or other general symptoms of malignant disease.

ADRENOCORTICAL HYPERFUNCTION

Cushing's syndrome is the result of excess cortisol, **Conn's syndrome**, of primary hyperaldosteronism, and adrenogenital syndrome of hypersecretion of sex steroids, more usually androgens.

Cushing's syndrome

This disease occurs most commonly in women, but occasionally in men and even more rarely in children. There is a characteristic appearance. Centripetal deposition of fat causes a moon face, buffalo hump and truncal obesity. Protein catabolism results in reduced muscle bulk, most noticeable in the limbs. Abdominal striae are the result of abnormal collagen maturation. Patients are hypertensive. Osteoporosis may cause vertebral collapse. Hyperglycaemia and glycosuria are found in about 20% of cases. Psychological symptoms are common with depression and, in some cases, frank psychosis. Androgens may also be secreted in excess, producing hirsutism, amenorrhea and virilization.

CASE STUDY 18.1

A 35-year-old woman presented to her primary care physician with mild headaches and vague symptoms of depression. On examination, her blood pressure was 130/95 on three occasions. There were no obvious indications of secondary hypertension and she was started on mild antihypertensive therapy. Over the next year, her depressive symptoms worsened, she complained of feeling weak and tired, and she had now back pain. Her physician noted that she was gaining weight, particularly in the trunk and face, was becoming plethoric and was bruising easily. She was referred to the endocrine clinic with a putative diagnosis of Cushing's syndrome. On biochemical testing, cortisol levels were raised and there was a loss of the normal circadian rhythm of cortisol. Plasma ACTH levels were detectable despite high cortisol. These cortisol levels were not suppressed after the administration of 0.5 mg dexamethasone four times a day for 48 hours, but were suppressed on 2 mg four times a day. These findings suggested pituitary-dependent Cushing's syndrome, usually caused by an ACTH-secreting adenoma of the pituitary gland. Magnetic resonance imaging suggested a 3 mm left-sided pituitary adenoma. At trans-sphenoidal surgery abnormal tissue was identified in this area and removed. Histology and immunocytochemistry confirmed an ACTH cell adenoma. The patient received cortisol replacement therapy for eight months because of the inhibition of the normal hypothalamic–pituitary–adrenal axis resulting from the increased negative feedback of the excessive glucocorticoids, which may take some time to recover. She remains well 5 years after the gradual withdrawal of steroid therapy, with no evidence of recurrence of her disease.

About 70% of cases are due to **excessive secretion of ACTH by the pituitary gland**, usually by a pituitary adenoma. This is known as **Cushing's disease**. It results in bilateral hyperplasia of the adrenals. The plasma cortisol levels are high, but can be suppressed by high doses of the synthetic glucocorticoid dexamethasone, and this forms the basis for a diagnostic test. ACTH levels are slightly high and the normal circadian rhythm is lost.

A further 20% of patients have an **adrenal tumour**, secreting cortisol in an autonomous fashion. Half are adenomas, the other half carcinomas. In children, in contrast to adults, adrenal tumours are the cause of about half of the cases of Cushing's syndrome and a higher proportion are malignant. When there is also evidence of androgen secretion (**'mixed' Cushing's syndrome**), malignant tumours are more common. Glucocorticoid levels cannot be suppressed by dexamethasone, and ACTH levels are low or undetectable owing to increased negative feedback. Because of this the normal adrenal tissue atrophies and patients must therefore receive steroids following tumour removal until the normal function of the pituitary–adrenal axis is re-established.

In some patients, ACTH is secreted by a non-pituitary tumour – **ectopic ACTH syndrome**. Most commonly these are small cell carcinomas of lung, thymic carcinoids and islet cell tumours of the pancreas. In patients with lung tumours, the classic syndrome may not be apparent because of the superimposed effects of the cancer. Very high levels of ACTH are usually found, and high levels of glucocorticoids which do not suppress with dexamethasone. The adrenal glands are hyperplastic and are usually bigger than in Cushing's disease.

It should be noted that excessive administration of exogenous glucocorticoids for therapeutic reasons may produce a Cushing-like syndrome.

HYPERALDOSTERONISM

Primary hyperaldosteronism, or **Conn's syndrome**, causes hypertension, periodic weakness or paralysis, muscle cramps, tetany, and nocturia and polyuria. Many of these changes are related to the hypokalaemia and metabolic alkalosis (high serum bicarbonate). Aldosterone levels are high and renin low, indicating autonomous secretion of aldosterone. An adrenal adenoma is found in about 80% of cases. The remainder have bilateral hyperplasia of the zona glomerulosa, although its cause is unknown. Carcinomas are extremely rare.

Secondary hyperaldosteronism occurs when the renin–angiotensin system is stimulated and plasma renin and aldosterone are both high. This will occur in renal disease associated with ischaemia, in oedema, as a result of oestrogen administration and, rarely, in the presence of a renin-secreting tumour.

ADRENOGENITAL SYNDROME

A group of diseases exists due to the congenital deficiency of one of the enzymes involved in the biosynthesis of **cortisol**. Most present in infants and young children. In the full-blown form, these are rare conditions, although some occur more frequently in specific ethnic groups. They are important to recognize because early administration of replacement steroids is necessary for normal life. Reduction in cortisol secretion causes decreased negative feedback at pituitary level and, therefore, ACTH secretion is increased in an attempt to produce normal levels of cortisol. This usually also results in an increase in androgen secretion. Excessive levels of intermediate steroids with mineralocorticoid effects may also result. The clinical picture depends on the combination of steroids secreted.

The most common form is the **21-hydroxylase deficiency**, occurring with a mean frequency of 1 in 14 000. Female infants have an enlarged clitoris and variable degrees of labial fusion. Internal genitalia are normal. Male children undergo precocious puberty. In two-thirds of cases, aldosterone synthesis is also affected and neonates show evidence of salt wasting, with dehydration, vomiting and hypotensive collapse. Deficiency of **11β-hydroxylase** is five times less common. Hypertension accompanies virilism, due to accumulation of deoxycorticosterone.

The adrenals show massive hyperplasia, about five times the normal weight. In most, the cortex is composed of reticularis-like cells with no lipid storage. Only in the rare **20,22-desmolase deficiency**, in which cholesterol cannot be metabolized, is there significant lipid accumulation.

In adults, adrenocortical tumours may secrete sex steroids, more usually androgens. In women, this will result in loss of secondary sex characteristics with virilization (development of clitoromegaly and hirsutism). While this may be seen in association with both benign and malignant tumours, it is more common in the latter. It may occur as an isolated finding or in association with hypersecretion of cortisol as a 'mixed' Cushing's syndrome. Rarely, an adrenal carcinoma may secrete oestrogens, causing gynaecomastia and penile and testicular atrophy in males.

ADRENOCORTICAL TUMOURS

It is not clear how common **adrenal adenomas** are, since the diagnosis is usually made clinically only when excess hormone secretion occurs (Fig. 18.11). At postmortem examination, nodules can be found in about 5% of glands; however, it is not known whether these are neoplastic or represent hyperplastic nodules. More of these are being identified in life during abdominal scanning for the investigation of other intra-abdominal disease. The problem is what to do with them. At present, if the lesion is less than 3 cm in diameter with no evidence of growth on sequential scanning and there is no evidence of excess hormone secretion, most surgeons would not remove it. This approach is based on the low probability that any such lesion has malignant potential and the fact that carcinomas tend to be larger tumours.

Adrenocortical carcinoma has an incidence of only 1–2 per million of the population. Most are obviously malignant at presentation with local spread and/or metastases. The prognosis is poor. The histological distinction between benign and potentially malignant intra-adrenal tumour is difficult and is based on analysis of many factors. Clinical and biochemical features such as virilism or lack of hormone secretion and a tumour weight of over 100 g are also suggestive of malignancy.

ADRENOCORTICAL HYPOFUNCTION

Clinical signs of cortical failure do not become apparent until about 90% of the cortex is destroyed. This may happen as an acute event, or as the result of chronic disease.

Acute adrenocortical insufficiency

Acute insufficiency has been associated with septicaemic states, particularly meningococcal infection and is known as the **Waterhouse-Friderichsen syndrome**. It has also been reported with pneumococci, staphylococci and *Haemophilus influenzae*. There is vomiting, salt loss, hyponatraemia, hyperkalaemia, hypoglycaemia and dehydration. Hypotensive collapse may be fatal. Fever is often present and a purpuric rash. Intra-adrenal haemorrhage occurs with cortical necrosis. It was

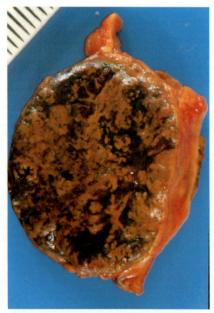

Fig. 18.11 A small, circumscribed, pale yellow and brown adenoma of the adrenal cortex in a patient with Cushing's syndrome. The adjacent cortex is atrophic because the cortisol released by the tumour has suppressed the secretion of ACTH from the pituitary gland.

previously thought that adrenocortical failure was primarily responsible for the vascular collapse. It is now appreciated that bacteraemia and endotoxaemia are the main pathogenic factors.

Acute failure may be superimposed on chronic failure when, for example, infection or trauma place increased demands on a cortical reserve which is working at maximum output (**addisonian crisis** – see below). Lack of glucocorticoid replacement in adrenalectomized patients or withdrawal of glucocorticoids from patients on long-term treatment may also precipitate failure. Neonates with severe congenital adrenal hyperplasia may also present in acute failure.

Chronic adrenocortical insufficiency: Addison's disease

In developed countries, the most common cause of chronic adrenal failure is autoimmune adrenalitis, accounting for 75% of cases. There is cortical atrophy with an infiltrate of lymphocytes and plasma cells (Fig.18.12). The medulla is not affected. There is an association with other organ-specific autoimmune diseases including autoimmune thyroid disease, pernicious anaemia, vitiligo and insulin-dependent diabetes mellitus.

Patients have general lethargy, weight loss, hypotension, muscle weakness, anorexia and pigmentation of the skin and mucous membranes.

Tuberculosis is the second most common cause in industrialized countries and is the most common cause in developing countries. Both medulla and cortex are destroyed. The adrenals are enlarged and replaced by caseous material with calcification, often obvious on abdominal radiography. Amyloidosis, fungal infection or tumour metastases are very rare causes.

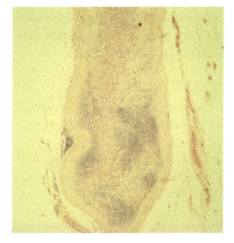
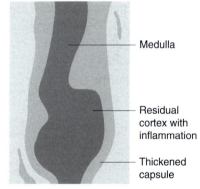

Fig. 18.12 Autoimmune Addison's disease. The adrenal cortex is infiltrated by chronic inflammatory cells and few cortical cells remain.

Adrenal medulla

The medulla synthesizes and secretes catecholamines from the phaeochromocytes or chromaffin cells – the main component. Ganglion cells and nerves are also identified. Tumours are the only important pathology.

PHAEOCHROMOCYTOMA

Phaeochromocytoma arises from the chromaffin cells (Fig. 18.13). Symptoms and signs relate to the excessive secretion of catecholamines, which at first may be episodic, and include hypertension, headache, palpitation, sweating and occasionally collapse. Hyperglycaemia and

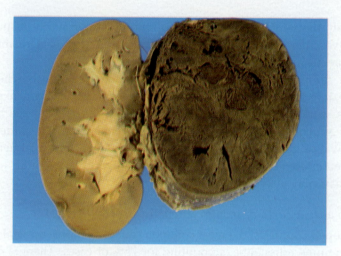

Fig. 18.13   Phaeochromocytoma. This large benign tumour is dark in colour after being exposed to chrome salts.

glycosuria are present. These tumours occur in both sexes at all ages, although they are rare in children:

- 10% are bilateral
- 10% are familial, most often as part of the MEN2 syndrome, where they are preceded by medullary hyperplasia
- 10% are malignant.

As in cortical tumours, it is difficult to predict malignant potential, the presence of metastases being the only absolute indicator of malignancy. They may occasionally produce ectopic hormones, secreting **vasoactive intestinal polypeptide (VIP)**, which causes the **watery diarrhoea, hypokalaemia and achlorhydria (WDHA)** syndrome, ACTH or occasionally other hormones.

Similar tumours may be found in extra-adrenal paraganglia, where they are known as **paragangliomas**. These are more likely to be malignant than adrenal tumours. The most common site is the organs of Zuckerkandl.

OTHER TUMOURS

In children, **neuroblastoma** arises from the primitive cells of the medulla. Neurofibroma, ganglioneuroma, fibroma or angioma may arise from other components.

Haemopoietic tissue is commonly seen as an incidental finding and when associated with fat is known as **myelolipoma**. Metastases are not uncommon, particularly from bronchial carcinoma.

Parathyroid glands

The parathyroid glands develop from the third and fourth branchial pouches. There are usually four, lying behind the thyroid, two at the lower and two at the upper poles. One or more may, however, be intrathyroidal or lie in the lower neck or upper mediastinum in close relationship to the thymus, also of third branchial pouch origin. They weigh in total up to 120 mg in males, and 140 mg in females, with 50 mg the upper limit of normal for an individual gland. They consist of chief cells, the main hormone-secreting cells and oxyphil cells, larger and granular due to large numbers of mitochondria. Stromal fat is seen after puberty and comprises up to 30% of the normal adult gland. They secrete **parathyroid hormone** which regulates serum calcium levels by effects on bone, kidneys and gut.

Hyperparathyroidism

- In **primary hyperparathyroidism**, hypersecretion of parathyroid hormone appears to be autonomous.
- In **secondary hyperparathyroidism**, the glands secrete excess hormone in response to increased physiological stimulation, most commonly in chronic renal failure.

PRIMARY HYPERPARATHYROIDISM

This disease occurs mainly in middle age, and is slightly more common in women. Patients may present with general tiredness and muscular weakness and, with heightened awareness, an increasing number of patients are diagnosed at the stage of such general symptoms before significant pathology develops. In the past, the majority of patients presented with renal calculi and some developed severe bone disease with osteitis fibrosa cystica. Duodenal ulceration and acute pancreatitis can also occur. Metastatic calcification may cause nephrocalcinosis and renal failure may affect the heart, other organs and soft tissues.

In 80% of patients a single adenoma is identified and surgical removal can result in cure. In 15–20% of cases, more than one gland is enlarged. This is regarded as primary hyperplasia. Surgeons should always look for and examine all parathyroids to exclude this diagnosis. Parathyroid carcinoma is rare, accounting for 2–3% of cases. Such cases are often obviously infiltrative at the time of surgery. If not, again it can be difficult for the pathologist to predict malignant potential.

Primary hyperparathyroidism may occur as part of the MEN1 and MEN2 syndromes. Hyperplasia is the more common finding in these patients.

SECONDARY HYPERPARATHYROIDISM

When there are consistently low serum levels of ionized calcium, parathyroid stimulation will result in increased parathyroid hormone release. Hyperplasia of the glands ensues, indistinguishable on morphological grounds from primary hyperplasia. This is most commonly the result of chronic renal failure but may also occur with malabsorption and vitamin D deficiency.

Occasionally, hypercalcaemia develops in patients with secondary hyperparathyroidism. This is thought to represent the development of autonomy in a group or clone of cells within the hyperplastic glands. Sometimes an adenomatous nodule may be identified. This syndrome is referred to as **tertiary hyperparathyroidism**.

Hypoparathyroidism

Lack of parathyroid hormone causes hypocalcaemia and hyper-phosphataemia. The low calcium results in increased muscle tone and tetany. Cataracts commonly occur, and patients may show psychological changes and convulsions. The most common cause is surgical removal of the glands. In **DiGeorge syndrome**, which presents more commonly in children and infants (see Chapter 16), it is coupled with immunological deficiencies, due to hypoplasia or aplasia of both parathyroids and thymus, as a result of maldevelopment of the third and fourth branchial arches. Occasionally, autoimmune parathyroiditis may be the cause, sometimes in association with other organ-specific autoimmune diseases.

Endocrine pancreas

The islets of Langerhans are scattered through the exocrine gland (Fig. 18.14). They consist of aggregates of cells producing insulin, glucagon, somatostatin and pancreatic polypeptide. The main function of these hormones is in the control of blood glucose levels.

The two main groups of disease to be considered are **diabetes mellitus** and **islet cell tumours**.

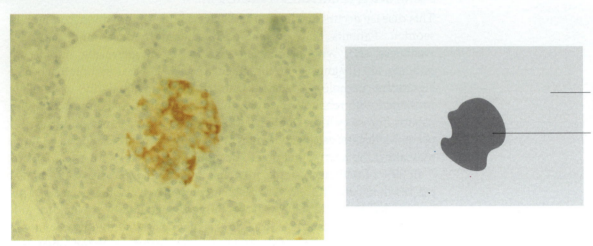

Fig. 18.14   Normal pancreas immunostained for insulin. An islet of Langerhans lies surrounded by exocrine tissue.

DIABETES MELLITUS

This is a group of diseases resulting from an absolute or relative lack of insulin coupled with a relative or absolute excess of glucagon. The symptoms are related to the insulin excess and comprise thirst, polyuria, polyphagia. A raised plasma glucose level is associated with glycosuria and weight loss, reduced protein synthesis and lipolysis. Fatty acids are metabolized to ketone bodies and the patient may develop ketoacidosis, with eventual coma. In contrast, where very high glucose levels are present without ketoacidosis, the patient may develop significant dehydration and hyperosmolar non-ketotic coma. There are two major categories – **type 1** and **type 2** diabetes mellitus. The disease may occasionally occur as a complication of haemochromatosis, chronic pancreatitis, Cushing's syndrome or acromegaly.

Type 1 diabetes (insulin dependent)

Insulin-dependent diabetes occurs in a younger age group (less than 40 years of age) and is characterized by selective destruction of the insulin-producing cells (β cells) within the islets. There is infiltration of islets by chronic inflammatory cells with eventual absence of β cells. Clinical symptoms do not appear until about 80% of the β-cell mass is lost. It is likely that the disease results from an interaction of genetic predisposition and environmental factors. There is an increased association with HLA-DR3 and HLA-DR4, but the concordance rate in monozygotic twins is less than 50%. Putative environmental factors include viruses and evidence of Coxsackie B infection has been found in up to 65% of new cases. Rubella, and possibly mumps viruses, have also been implicated. The case for all is unproven. If involved, it is likely that the infection triggers an autoimmune response, and both islet cell antibodies and cell-mediated immunity to β cells may be identified in patients. There are also associations with other organ-specific autoimmune diseases including autoimmune thyroiditis, adrenalitis and pernicious anaemia. Treatment involves the administration of insulin.

Type 2 diabetes (insulin independent)

Type 2 disease is significantly more common than type 1 disease but varies with the population. It is more common in obese people and is characterized by relative resistance to the action of insulin. Development of the disease is thought to be multifactorial, although a concordance rate of 100% in monozygotic terms indicates a strong genetic influence. The insulin resistance causes hypersecretion of insulin but this may not be sufficient to lower glucose levels. Peripheral resistance to insulin actions may also be present. The islets contain amyloid in about 70% of cases, derived from a peptide amylin, now thought to be a normal constituent of β-cell granules, which may be secreted in excess in type 2 diabetes.

Islet cell tumours

Islet cell tumours are uncommon. Most are benign and present only if they secrete excess hormone. They are usually circumscribed masses within the gland, and consist of cords or groups of small regular cells, often in a fibrous stroma. Amyloid may be present, especially in insulinomas. Most are sporadic, but they may occur as part of the MEN1 syndrome.

Patients with **insulinoma** present with episodes of fainting or dizziness, which are relieved by food. Hypoglycaemic coma may occur. Almost all are benign and surgery is curative.

Gastrinomas are associated with the **Zollinger–Ellison syndrome**. Hypersecretion of gastrin stimulates excessive acid secretion from the stomach. This leads to ulcers, often multiple, in the duodenum and sometimes the jejunum. The majority of these tumours are malignant (Fig. 18.15).

Occasional tumours secrete glucagon, somatostatin, VIP or ectopic hormones. The details of the clinical syndromes associated with these may be found in textbooks of endocrinology.

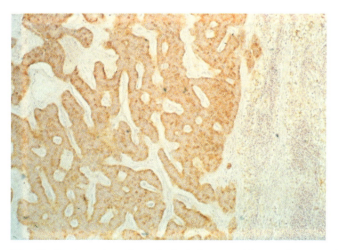
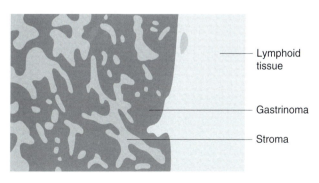

Lymphoid tissue

Gastrinoma

Stroma

Fig. 18.15   Lymph node metastasis from gastrinoma, immunostained to confirm gastrin content.

Multiple endocrine neoplasia (MEN) syndromes

The MEN syndromes are uncommon familial syndromes in which tumours or hyperplasia occurs in more than one endocrine gland, either in the same individual or in different members of the family. They are inherited in an autosomal dominant manner and are of two main distinct groupings. Despite their rarity, they are important to recognize because, once an index case is diagnosed, biochemical and molecular genetic techniques are now available for family screening to detect affected individuals or those at risk. Hyperplasia usually precedes tumour development and preventive surgery may be undertaken at this stage.

MEN type 1 (Wermer's syndrome)

Parathyroid adenomas are present in 95% of MEN1 patients. Pancreatic islet cell tumours producing insulin, gastrin and, more rarely, pancreatic polypeptide or glucagon occur. Pituitary tumours, mainly PRL cell or GH cell type are also found. This is now thought to be linked to mutations in a gene on the long arm of chromosome 11.

MEN type 2

There are two variants of MEN2. These are associated with activating germline mutations in the different codons of the *ret* proto-oncogene on chromosome 10, which encodes a tyrosine kinase receptor.

MEN2A (SIPPLE'S SYNDROME)

Medullary carcinoma of thyroid is present in most cases of MEN2a, with phaeochromocytoma in about 50% and parathyroid adenoma or hyperplasia in about 40%.

MEN2B

In MEN2b, medullary carcinoma of thyroid and phaeochromocytoma are associated with neuromas in the mucosa of the lips and tongue and on the eyelids and cornea. Ganglioneuromas develop in the gut. Medullary carcinoma is more aggressive in this variant and is invariably fatal. Thus, diagnosis of C-cell hyperplasia and thyroidectomy is important in preventive therapy.

Chapter 19   Skin disease

Learning objectives

To understand and appreciate:
- ❏ Principles underlying diagnosis of skin disease and knowledge of the descriptive terms used
- ❏ Role of infection and inflammation in causing skin disease
- ❏ Distinction between basal cell carcinoma and squamous cell carcinoma
- ❏ Role of ultraviolet light in the aetiology of skin cancer, with emphasis on melanoma

Functional morphology of the skin

The skin consists of three layers: an outermost epithelial layer (**epidermis**), a connective tissue layer (**dermis**) (Fig. 19.1), and a layer of fat tissue (**subcutis**). Downgrowths of the epidermis are embedded in the dermis and the subcutis (**skin appendages: hair follicles, sebaceous glands, eccrine** and **apocrine sweat glands, nails**).

Epidermis

The main cellular constituent of the epidermis is the **keratinocyte**, which forms multiple cell layers (Fig. 19.2). Cell division takes place in the basal cell layer and in the suprabasal cells. The spinous cell layer shows prominent bundles of **cytokeratin filaments** inserting into **desmosomes**, which link neighbouring keratinocytes to each other. In the granular layer, the cytokeratin filaments are rearranged by forming transient basophilic granules, and the nucleus is degraded and the keratinocyte transforms into the non-living **corneocyte**. The latter constitute the corneal layer, by being arranged like bricks in a wall, glued by a lipid interphase.

Dermis

The dermis consists of two parts: the **papillary dermis**, immediately beneath the epidermis, consists of loose connective tissue, forming papillary projections towards the epidermis, and contains numerous small blood vessels, nerves, sensory structures, lymphocytes, cells of the monocyte–macrophage lineage and mast cells. It can readily react to a variety of stimuli; most inflammatory skin disorders take place in the papillary dermis, with some involvement of the epidermis. The **reticular**

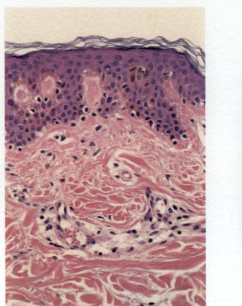

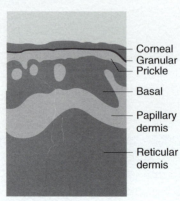

- Corneal
- Granular
- Prickle
- Basal
- Papillary dermis
- Reticular dermis

Fig. 19.1   Histology of normal human skin.

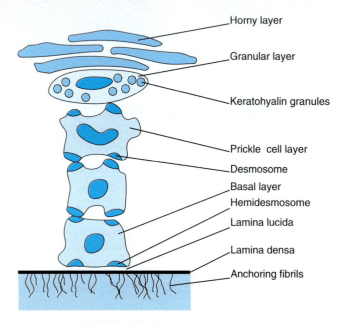

- Horny layer
- Granular layer
- Keratohyalin granules
- Prickle cell layer
- Desmosome
- Basal layer
- Hemidesmosome
- Lamina lucida
- Lamina densa
- Anchoring fibrils

Fig. 19.2   The epidermal layers.

dermis, in contrast, contains mainly coarse connective collagen fibres with only a few cells. It is much less liable to inflammatory reactions.

Subcutis

Lobules of unilocular fat cells are located between connective tissue septa. The subcutis provides thermal insulation, mechanical resistance to pressure and storage of lipids.

Pigment cell system

During embryological development, **melanoblasts** migrate from the neural crest through the dermis into the basal layer of the epidermis, where they remain throughout life. They produce **melanin**, which protects the body from the DNA-damaging effect of ultraviolet light. Melanin synthesis

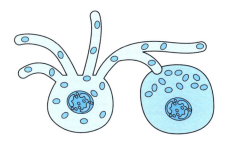

Fig. 19.3 Melanocyte in the skin. The melanocyte synthesizes melanin within specific organelles (melanosomes). These melanosomes are transferred to neighbouring keratinocytes via melanosomal dendrites. In the keratinocytes, the melanosomes form a cap over the nucleus, shielding DNA from being damaged by ultraviolet light.

takes place in melanosomes, which are finally transferred into keratinocytes by long, branching dendrites of the **melanocyte** (Fig. 19.3).

Skin immune system

As a barrier to the surrounding, the skin contains a highly developed immune system for the induction of early reactions to various environmental hazards. As a peripheral outpost, dendritic **Langerhans' cells**, a subtype of the monocyte–macrophage lineage, are located in the mid-epidermis (Fig. 19.4). These cells have characteristic **Birbeck's granules** resembling tennis rackets in their cytoplasm and express MHC class II antigens on their surface. They can internalize antigen, move downward to the dermis and present the antigen to T-helper lymphocytes either in the dermis or in the regional lymph node. A certain number of recirculating **T lymphocytes** is always present in the skin, particularly around small blood vessels of the papillary dermis. Various toxic, allergic or infectious stimuli can trigger cytokine signalling, which in turn leads to the recruitment of other inflammatory cells, which stick to the endothelium of postcapillary venules, leave the bloodstream and move into the connective tissue of the dermis or even into the epidermis. The recruited cells are mostly T lymphocytes, providing a non-specific superficial T-cell reaction in the papillary dermis and the epidermis. In some cases, however, granulocytes, eosinophils or monocytes and their derivatives may predominate.

Besides these largely T-cell-mediated responses, circulating immunoglobulins may cause immune complexes in vessel walls, thus inducing vasculitis. **Type E immunoglobulins** adhere to the cell membrane of mast cells and may cause mast cell degranulation after allergenic provocation.

Principles of diagnosis

Macroscopic aspects

In contrast to most other medical disciplines, inspection of skin disease with the naked eye allows direct examination of the macroscopic

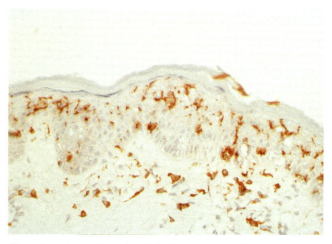

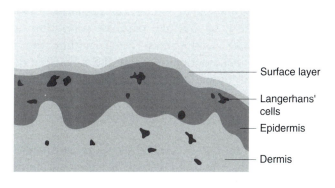

Surface layer

Langerhans' cells

Epidermis

Dermis

Fig. 19.4 Langerhans' cells in the epidermis (immunoperoxidase staining). Note dendritic cells situated within the malpighian layer.

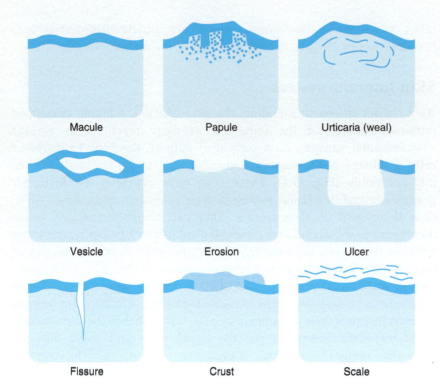

Macule	Papule	Urticaria (weal)
Vesicle	Erosion	Ulcer
Fissure	Crust	Scale

Fig. 19.5 Basic skin lesions.

Skin lesions
- **Macules** or **patches** are just changes of skin colour
- **Papules** or **nodules** are raised over the surface of the skin, consist of solid tissue and are <1 cm in diameter
- **Nodes** or **tumours** are similar, but >1 cm
- **Urticariae** or **weals** are also raised, but consist of dermal oedema instead of solid tissue
- **Vesicles** are elevated lesions due to fluid in a superficial cleft; if they contain pus, they are called **pustules**
- **Erosion** is a superficial defect of the epidermis only
- **Excoriation** also includes the papillary dermis and is usually due to scratching
- **Ulcers** involve the reticular dermis or even the subcutis
- **Fissures** are small clefts penetrating into the dermis
- **Crusts** are the air-dried remnants of oozing tissue fluid, pus or blood
- **Scales** consist of horny material

pathological features. One has first to take into account the distribution of the skin lesions, since particular diseases prefer particular body sites (for example, sun-exposed skin in photodermatoses, seborrheic areas in acne, segmental distribution in herpes zoster). Subsequently, the individual skin lesions may be classified according to their size, shape and colour: most skin disorders are described by a specific and limited set of these well-defined skin lesions (Fig. 19.5).

Histological aspects

A skin biopsy is usually scanned for pathological changes starting from the horny layer down to the subcutaneous fat. The horny layer may be thickened (**hyperkeratosis**) and/or contain nuclear remnants (**parakeratosis**) (Fig. 19.6). The granular layer may be missing, which is often found underneath a parakeratotic horny layer, or may be thickened (**hypergranulosis**). The spinous layer may be thickened (**acanthosis**), which is often associated with an accentuated wavy dermal–epidermal interface with long dermal papillae projecting into the epidermis (**papillomatosis**). Clefts may occur within the epidermis, at the dermal–epidermal junction or within the superficial dermis, giving rise to intraepidermal, junctional or subepidermal (dermolytic) blisters. Intraepidermal blisters may be due to loss of keratinocyte cohesion (**acantholysis**). Intercellular oedema within the epidermis is called **spongiosis**.

In the dermis, the accumulation of inflammatory cells is the most common feature. The infiltrate may be superficial (limited to the papillary dermis) or deep. It may be nodular or diffuse, and it may also involve the epidermis as cells move into it from the dermis (**epidermotropism**). Regarding the cells involved, lymphocytes with some histiocytes, neutrophils with or without eosinophils, and histiocytes–epithelioid

Fig. 19.6 Basic patterns of histological skin changes: (a) normal, (b) inflamed.

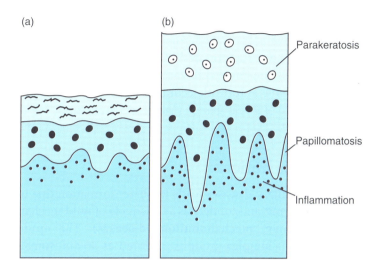

(a)   (b)

Parakeratosis

Papillomatosis

Inflammation

> **Histological skin changes**
> - **Hyperkeratosis** is an increase in thickness of the stratum corneum
> - **Parakeratosis** is retention of keratinocyte nuclei in the stratum corneum
> - **Spongiosis** is intercellular oedema in the malpighian layer
> - **Papillomatosis** is an increase in dermal papillae length
> - A **dermal infiltrate** is an accumulation of inflammatory cells, mostly lymphocytes and histiocytes, in the dermis

cells–giant cells may predominate. The most common finding in many inflammatory dermatoses is that of a superficial lymphohistiocytic infiltrate consisting of T-helper cells, T-suppressor cells and some Langerhans' cells (**superficial T-cell reaction**). Besides the cellular infiltrate, the dermis may show accumulation of fluid (oedema) or proteoglycans (**mucinosis**), vasculitis, increase of collagen (**sclerosis**) and changes of the skin appendages.

Congenital abnormalities

Ectodermal disorders

A normal corneal layer depends on a complex interaction of proliferative activity, the molecular composition of the cytokeratin filaments, of the cytokeratin-associated filaggrins in the granular layer, and on the lipid metabolism within the horny layer. Hereditary defects in any of these mechanisms may lead to hyperkeratosis and/or scaling.

ICHTHYOSIS

In the various forms of ichthyosis, large body areas or the entire skin are affected. The most common form is the autosomal dominant **ichthyosis vulgaris** (Fig. 19.7), with polygonal scales on the trunk and on the extensor surfaces of the extremities. There is a molecular defect of the filaggrins, resulting in absence of the granular layer and in delayed desquamation of corneocytes, called **retention hyperkeratosis**. **X-linked ichthyosis**, which affects exclusively male patients, shows fine white scales on the entire body surface. In this disease, a defect of steroid sulphatase leads to a disturbance of the lipid composition of the horny layer and subsequently to the clinically visible scales. In contrast to these two relatively benign conditions, the heterogeneous group of **congenital ichthyoses** may represent a life-threatening disease in the newborn with thick hyperkeratoses and deep fissures in the flexures (**harlequin fetus**).

In palmoplantar **keratoderma**, hyperkeratosis is limited to the palms and soles. A diffuse, a striated and a papular variant can be discerned. Additionally, there are transgradient forms, which extend gradually beyond the lateral margins of the palms and soles and may be associated with other defects (abnormalities of the teeth).

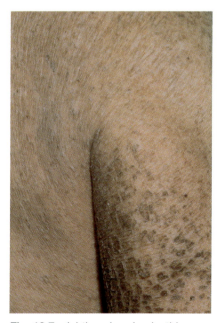

Fig. 19.7 Ichthyosis vulgaris: this autosomal dominantly inherited disorder shows brown, polygonal scales on trunk and extremities preferring the extensor surfaces. Life expectancy is normal, but the continuous application of emollients is necessary.

ECTODERMAL DYSPLASIA

There are several variants of ectodermal dysplasia, which are characterized by variable defects of structures derived from the ectoderm: sweat glands, nails, hair and teeth are affected to variable degrees. The most severe form is that of **X-recessive anhidrotic ectodermal dysplasia**. In these patients, the virtual absence of sweat glands results in a sometimes life-threatening intolerance to heat.

Epidermolysis bullosa

A variety of hereditary diseases leads to blister formation due to impaired cohesion of epidermis and/or dermis as a sequela of mild mechanical injury (hence the synonym **mechanobullous diseases**). The **epiderm-olysis bullosa hereditaria simplex** group is inherited as an autosomal dominant trait and runs a benign course. Blisters occur after mild trauma particularly on the hands and feet. Ultrastructurally, there is an intraepidermal cleft, in some cases due to an abnormal structure of certain cytokeratins. **Epidermolysis bullosa hereditaria junctionalis** displays clefts within the basement membrane zone; there is a benign variant and a lethal variant, with the latter involving the oesophagus and leading to death usually during the first year of life. Intradermal blisters occur in the **epidermolysis bullosa hereditaria dystrophica** cases. In this disease group, the blisters leave scars, and in the severe variants mutilation of the extremities, nail dystrophy and mucous membrane involvement may occur (Fig. 19.8).

CASE STUDY 19.1

A 15-year-old male patient presented with severe mutilations of fingers and toes. There were large areas of erosion on the hands and feet, but also on the knees and buttocks. Some erosions were covered with dry yellow crusts, others showed oozing and bleeding. On the elbow an apple-sized bulla was evident. The patient had had this condition since early childhood. Various treatment modalities had been of virtually no effect, except for some control of intermittent bacterial infection. The diagnosis was epidermolysis bullosa hereditaria dystrophicans.

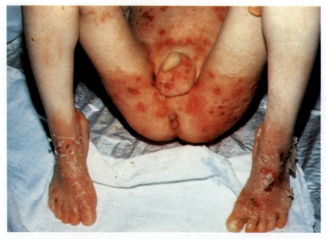

Fig. 19.8   Epidermolysis bullosa hereditaria dystrophica: this autosomal recessive disorder shows a structural defect in the basement membrane zone of the epidermis. There are blisters, erosions, scars and mutilations.

Fig. 19.9 Ehlers–Danlos syndrome (cutis hyperelastica): in this heterogeneous group of hereditary disorders defects of collagen cross-linking have been described. There is hyperelasticity of the skin, hyperextensibility of the joints and occasionally aortal aneurysms and eye changes.

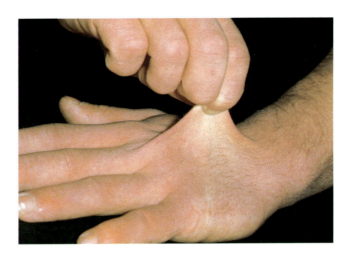

Connective tissue abnormalities

Other hereditary defects may affect the connective tissue of the dermis and other organs. In the various forms of **Ehlers–Danlos syndrome** (cutis hyperelastica, Fig. 19.9), there is a defect in collagen synthesis, processing or crosslinking. Since the elastic fibres are unimpaired, the skin is thin, fragile, but highly elastic. Additionally, the joints may be hyperextensible, and blood vessels and the eyes may be involved. The mild forms carry a normal life expectancy, but in the severe forms death may occur due to rupture of the large arteries. Other syndromes with collagen defects are **Marfan's syndrome** (tall, slender people with 'spider' fingers and loose joints), and **osteogenesis imperfecta** with a pronounced fragility of the long bones and multiple fractures from an early age. In **pseudoxanthoma elasticum**, the synthesis of elastic fibres is impaired. Functionally, insufficient clumps of elastic material are stored in the dermis and appear clinically as yellow ('pseudoxanthomatous') papules, particularly in the large body folds. In **dermatochalasis**, absence of elastic fibres leads to large, hanging skin folds without elasticity.

Other congenital disorders

Various congenital defects may involve the skin:

- **Neurofibromatosis (von Recklinghausen's disease)** may show light brown macules (*café-au-lait* macules) in addition to cutaneous neurofibromas.
- A **port wine stain** (**naevus flammeus** or **naevus telangiectaticus**, Fig. 19.10) may be found in the skin area innervated by the trigeminal nerve, or may occur on one extremity and can be associated with arteriovenous malformations and hypertrophy of the limb.
- Some congenital defects show themselves in a segmental fashion, but do not strictly follow the spinal nerve segments. Instead, they show a wavy pattern following the so-called **Blaschko's lines**, which are determined by the movement of epidermal cells during early embryological development. The most typical example is **linear epidermal naevus** (Fig. 19.11), which shows warty lesions distributed throughout a segment along Blaschko's lines. Histologically, there is hypertrophy of the epidermis and occasionally also of the sebaceous glands. It is considered to be due to a somatic mutation in the particular dermatome.

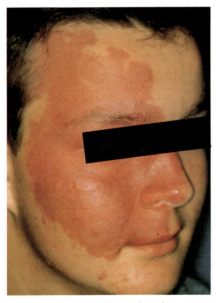

Fig. 19.10 Port wine stain: when port wine stains are distributed within the skin area innervated by the trigeminal nerve, choroidal and meningeal angiomas may be additionally present.

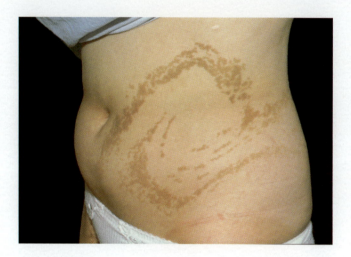

Fig. 19.11   Linear epidermal naevus: brown, warty, keratotic papules are linearly arranged along embryonic developmental lines.

Infectious skin diseases

Common viral exanthemas

Many viral infections present with a more or less specific skin rash. Pathogenically, the rash may be due to the initial viraemia. In this case, the rash consists of transient light red macules, and is associated with prodromal symptoms. Most viral exanthemas, however, are due to the immune reaction of the host against virus-infected cells. These exanthemas are more pronounced and consist of red macules or flat papules, densely distributed throughout the skin, which may show confluence. Typical examples are measles and rubella.

Herpes simplex, herpes zoster and varicella

Herpes simplex and varicella-zoster virus have in common that both affect keratinocytes and lead to intraepithelial clefts with multinucleated giant cells histologically and umbilicated vesicles clinically. The initial infection with herpes simplex virus is most often without clinical manifestation. In some cases, however, there may be an extensive vesicular eruption in the face (**primary herpes simplex**), sometimes involving the oral cavity (**gingivostomatitis herpetica**), or of the genital region (**vulvovaginitis** or **balanoposthitis herpetica**). Particularly in the newborn and immunocompromised, herpes encephalitis may evolve. Both clinically apparent and inapparent infections leave humoral immunity. Some virus particles, however, may survive in the sensory ganglia of the cerebral or spinal nerves. Due to trigger factors (sun exposure of the skin, irritation of

---

CASE STUDY 19.2

An adult male patient presents with grouped pinhead-sized, umbilicated vesicles situated on an inflammatory erythema on the upper lip. History reveals that in childhood there was a severe vesicular eruption of the perioral region and aphthous (ulcerative) lesions of the oral cavity. Since then, vesicular eruptions of the lip have occurred every few months, often following sun exposure or fever. A diagnosis of recurrent herpes simplex is made. The eruption in childhood is interpreted as primary herpes simplex infection with the clinical presentation of gingivostomatitis herpetica.

Fig. 19.12 Herpes simplex: there are grouped, tiny vesicles giving rise to small crusts distributed around the mouth.

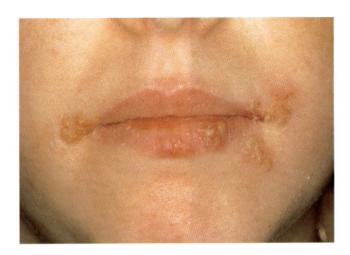

the ganglia, fever), recurrent eruptions in a localized skin area innervated by the particular neurons may occur (Fig. 19.12). These recurrent eruptions are usually milder and more circumscribed then the primary infections.

The varicella-zoster virus shows a similar pathogenesis. The primary infection may be inapparent or – more likely – present as varicella, with disseminated vesicles preferring the scalp and the trunk, which occur over a period of a few days. The single lesion becomes crusty or even necrotic, and bacterial superinfection is not uncommon. In later life, the virus may cause a vesicular eruption in one or two skin segments of a spinal or cerebral nerve. There is no tendency to recurrence, but due to involvement of the nerve ganglia, severe pain may persist for months and even years (**postzoster neuralgia**). In immunocompromised patients, particularly in those with leukaemia or other malignancy, herpes zoster may become necrotic or disseminated.

Human papilloma virus infections

Human papilloma viruses (HPV) are DNA viruses infecting primarily the keratinocytes. So far, more than 60 subtypes have been detected. Though certain subtypes have a tendency to cause particular clinical manifestations, there is no strict association between virus subtype and the morphology of the lesion. The most common manifestation is **warts**. With a preference for the dorsa of the hands and the periungual area, sharply circumscribed, dome-shaped, skin-coloured papules with a papillomatous, hyperkeratotic (verrucous) surface occur (Fig. 19.13a). Due to scratching, new skin areas may become infected. Histologically, elongated dermal papillae, acanthosis, hypergranulosis and columnar parakeratosis is evident (Fig. 19.13b). Additionally, densely packed virus particles form inclusion bodies at the light microscopic level. The warts persist for months or years. Spontaneous regression, accompanied by an inflammatory T-cell infiltrate, is not uncommon. Particularly in the face of children, numerous small **juvenile plane warts** may be found, which regularly show spontaneous resolution. On the soles, deeply penetrating, painful **plantar warts** (verrucas) may occur, particularly in pressure-bearing areas. In the moist skin areas of the anogenital region, HPV infection presents as aggregated, papillomatous, macerated **condylomata acuminata**. Additionally, flat, pigmented HPV-induced lesions can be sometimes found on the genitalia, which look histologically like carcinoma in situ (see

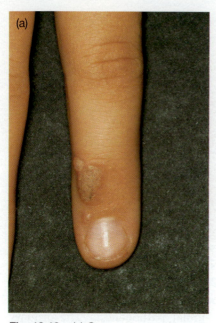
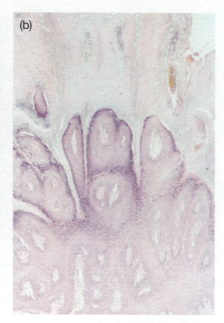
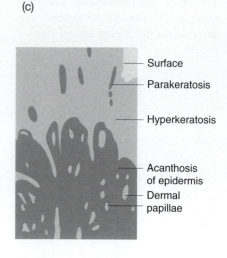

Surface
Parakeratosis

Hyperkeratosis

Acanthosis
of epidermis
Dermal
papillae

Fig. 19.13   (a) Common wart: these dome-shaped papules with a hyperkeratotic, verrucous surface are due to papilloma virus infection. (b, c) Histology of a common wart. There is marked hyperkeratosis, acanthosis and papillomatosis with elongated dermal papillae.

Chapter 15). These are often caused by particular HPV subtypes, which are associated with an increased risk of cervical cancer. A particular congenital immune defect (**epidermodysplasia verruciformis**) is characterized by widespread HPV infection, which eventually gives rise to squamous cell carcinoma.

Pox virus group infections

The pox virus group consists of DNA viruses with a peculiar ultrastructure. **Variola vera (smallpox)**, a severe, often lethal disease with involvement of the skin, the lymph nodes and inner organs is now extinct due to a successful worldwide vaccination campaign. However, infections by **cowpox** virus are quite frequently found. Inoculation with this virus takes place on the hand; the infective source is usually cattle. A solitary papule appears, which subsequently becomes vesicular and pustular. Regional lymphadenitis and fever may be present. The disease is usually self-limiting. Similarly, but milder, are **milker's nodule** and **ecthyma contagiosum** (derived from sheep).

The most common infection of the pox virus group is **molluscum contagiosum**, caused by **poxvirus mollusci** (Fig. 19.14). Particularly in children, numerous skin-coloured, umbilicated, pinhead-sized papules appear at any body site. Histologically, there are lobes of acanthosis with large inclusion bodies full of mature viruses. Autoinoculation and contact infection of other children are common. The disease is self-limited. Extensive involvement with large papules is sometimes observed in AIDS patients (see Chapter 7 for further information about HIV infection).

Streptococcal and staphylococcal infections

Streptococci and staphylococci may cause a variety of infectious skin diseases. **Impetigo contagiosa** is a superficial (subcorneal) infection. A

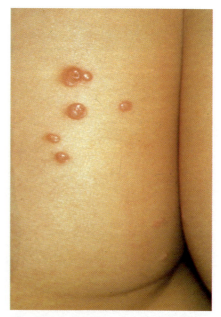

Fig. 19.14   Molluscum contagiosum: mollusca are characterized by dome-shaped, skin-coloured papules with a central depression. The causative agent belongs to the pox virus group.

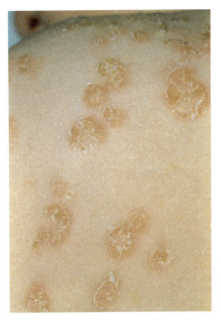

Fig. 19.15 Impetigo contagiosa: there are extensive yellow crusts. The disease is due to streptococcal or staphylococal infection and prefers children.

purulent rhinitis or tonsillitis may precede the eruption, which often starts in the perinasal or perioral area. Sometimes there are large bullae filled with pus, but sometimes there are only tiny, transient pustules, which rapidly give way to pustular crusts; these are the predominant clinical feature in most cases (Fig. 19.15). Due to scratching, new lesions develop and other children may become infected. The condition clears rapidly with proper treatment. In the newborn and in early infancy, staphylococci may produce life-threatening large bullous and erosive lesions, not only by direct skin infection, but also due to the secretion of an epidermolytic exotoxin from internal foci.

CASE STUDY 19.3

A 5-year-old boy shows numerous coin-sized erythematous macules covered by thick yellow crusts in the perinasal region and scattered over the trunk. In very recent lesions, tiny superficial pustules are evident. History reveals that a couple of other children attending the same kindergarten have the same problem. The clinical appearance is that of impetigo contagiosa. It clears rapidly on topical and oral antibiotic therapy (see Fig. 19.15).

Infection of the dermal lymphatic vessels and the interstitium by streptococci causes **erysipelas** (Fig. 19.16). Streptococci enter the dermis via fissures of the epidermis, and give rise to a localized, red, tender, oedematous, sharply demarcated patch associated with regional lymphadenitis and fever. The lower leg and the face are most commonly affected. The lesion may become vesicular, haemorrhagic or necrotic. Recurrent attacks can lead to chronic lymphoedema, which in turn is a precipitating factor of further recurrences.

The most common skin site of bacterial infection is the hair follicle. In simple **folliculitis** a follicular papule with a central pustule occurs. In a **furuncle**, the perifollicular tissue becomes necrotic and the surrounding skin shows intensive inflammation. In some patients, there may be recurrent furuncles over years (**furunculosis**). A **carbuncle** is mainly located at the nape of the neck and consists of a group of confluent furuncles, often associated with fever and deterioration of the general condition (Fig. 19.17).

Besides these specified diseases, staphylococci may secondarily affect pre-existing skin lesions, particularly various types of eczema, leg ulcers or sebaceous cysts.

Mycobacterial infections

Tuberculosis is discussed in detail in Chapter 7. In the skin, **lupus vulgaris** with yellow–brown, scarring plaques, **tuberculosis verrucosa cutis** with a solitary, elevated, warty lesion, and **tuberculosis cutis colliquativa** with draining fistulas and ulcers overlying the cervical lymph nodes are the most frequent clinical presentations. All skin manifestations are characterized histologically by epithelioid cell (tuberculoid) granulomata, but the extent of caseation necrosis varies according to the clinical picture. Rarely, **miliary tuberculosis** may affect the skin with multiple small nodules and the mucous membranes with miliary ulcers.

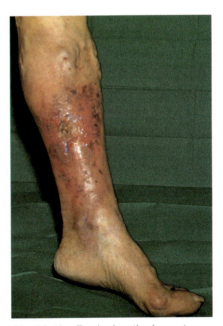

Fig. 19.16 Erysipelas: the lower two-thirds of the lower leg show an intense, sharply circumscribed erythema. Varicose veins and brown hyperpigmentation are signs of chronic venous insufficiency, which is a promoting factor for erysipelas.

Skin tuberculosis may occur as the result of implantation of *Mycobacterium tuberculosis* via skin abrasions. *Mycobacterium marinum*, an atypical mycobacterium, may be acquired from aquariums in this manner and leads to tuberculoid granulomata on the arms, mostly aligned along the lymph vessels (Fig. 19.18). **Buruli ulcer**, caused by *Mycobacterium ulcerans*, is also thought to be caused by implantation due to infection of cuts acquired from elephant grass. It has a restricted distribution within Africa, where it causes very large undermined ulcers. These ulcers initially contain large numbers of bacilli, but these disappear as granulomata develop later on in the course of the disease. **Leprosy** is a disease of skin and nerve, caused by *Mycobacterium leprae*. It has a worldwide distribution and demonstrates a spectrum of disease with granuloma formation in tuberculoid cases and macrophage infiltration in lepromatous cases.

Gonorrhoea

Gonorrhoea is a very common sexually transmitted disease caused by Gram-negative diplococci. In male patients, acute urethritis with an extensive leukocytic exudate is the usual presentation. Subsequently, the prostate and the epididymis may be involved and infertility may result. In females, onset is often less severe and only discrete cervicitis is evident. However, involvement of the corpus uteri, the salpinx and even the peritoneal cavity with fibrinous exudate, adhesion and scarring with subsequent infertility can occur. Rarely, mild septicaemia with mono- or oligoarthritis and haemorrhagic pustules on the extremities can evolve. In the neonate, infection can cause conjunctivitis and blindness.

Treponematoses

Treponemas are slowly growing, filiform, spiral bacteria. *Treponema pallidum*, which is best recognized by dark-field microscopy, causes **syphilis** (Fig. 19.19). The primary infection is usually acquired by sexual intercourse.

In tropical regions, **framboesia (yaws)** and **pinta** occur, both of which represent treponematoses that are similar to, but milder than syphilis.

Borreliosis is also a treponematous disease transmitted by certain ticks (ixodes). It may cause a ring-like erythema surrounding the tick bite (**erythema chronicum migrans**, Fig. 19.20) and may in rare cases lead to cutaneous atrophy (**acrodermatitis chronica atrophicans**), neural involvement, myocarditis and arthritis.

Fungal infections

Fungal skin diseases include dermatophytoses, candidiasis, *Pityrosporum ovale* and deep systemic fungal infections.

CASE STUDY 19.4
A 60-year-old woman has noted scaling on the soles and interdigital maceration and fissuring between the toes for a couple of years, worsening in hot weather and after wearing occlusive shoes. Gradually, the nails have become thickened and acquired yellowish-brown discoloration. Microscopic examination of horny material revealed hyphae and spores, confirming the diagnosis of a dermatophytic fungal infection (**tinea pedum**).

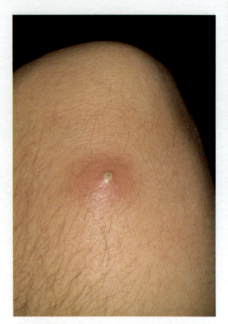

Fig. 19.17 Furuncle: there is an erythematous, inflammatory papule associated with a hair follicle, showing a central pustule.

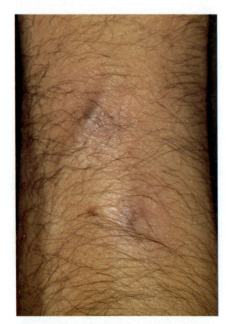

Fig. 19.18 *Mycobacterium marinum* infection: on the forearm there is a granulomatous nodule extending along perivenous lymphatic channels.

Fig. 19.19 Syphilis (primary lesion): at the site of inoculation syphilis starts with a primary lesion, which is usually a flat nodule with central ulceration located in the genital area. Subsequently regional lymphadenitis occurs.

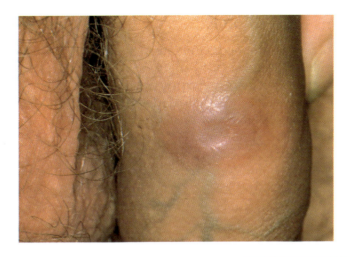

Syphilis
- **Stage I**: on the genitalia or elsewhere a hard papule with a central indolent ulceration appears 2–3 weeks after infection, followed by non-suppurating regional lymphadenitis.
- **Stage II**: generalized lymphadenitis and recurrent exanthemas, initially consisting of inconspicuous red macules (**roseola syphilitica**), later of brown–red papules, become evident. Highly infective eroded papules occur in the perigenital region (**condylomata lata**).
- **Stage III**: several years after infection, syphilitic **gummata** with central necrosis may evolve in various organs, with reniform ulcers in the skin. Additionally, **serpiginous tuberous syphilids** may develop.
- **Stage IV**: in rare cases disease with specific syphilitic involvement of the frontal lobe of the brain (**progressive paralysis**) or of the spinal cord (**tabes dorsalis**) develops after years or decades.

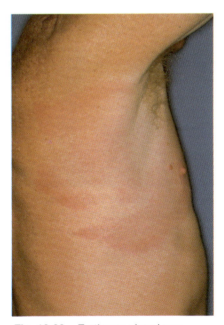

Fig. 19.20 Erythema chronicum migrans: the lesion is characterized by a ring-like erythema, which enlarges at the periphery and clears in the centre. Erythema chronicum migrans is caused by *Borrelia* spp. which are transmitted by tick bites.

Dermatophytes exclusively affect horny material: the horny layer of the epidermis in various body regions (tinea pedum, tinea inguinalis, tinea corporis), the nails (tinea ungium) or the hair apparatus. Involvement of the superficial portion of the hair follicles may occur on any body site and presents as a round erythema with papules and scaling at the periphery (**ringworm**, Fig. 19.21). Involvement of the deep portion of the hair follicles occurs particularly on the scalp of children (kerion celsi) and in the beard area of adult males (**trichophytia barbae**).

Candidiasis affects intertriginous areas, particularly the groin and the perianal and perigenital regions, and the mucous membranes. In the intertrigines, moist erythemas with individual pustules at the periphery occur. In mucous membranes, whitish adherent plaques are found on an erythematous base. The vulva, vagina and oral cavity are most commonly involved. Oesophageal candidiasis is often found in advanced HIV infection (see Chapter 7). In severe immunodeficiency, candida septicaemia and involvement of inner organs may occur.

Pityrosporum ovale is a saprophyte on normal skin. In predisposed individuals, it may cause discrete, scaly brown or hypopigmented macules on the trunk. Hypopigmentation is due to a dicarboxylic acid released by the fungus, which impairs the function of melanocytes.

Systemic fungal infection is uncommon in middle and northern Europe, but is often found in South and North America, Asia and Africa. In the skin, nodules, ulcers and cold abscesses are the most common presentations. With respect to inner organs, the lung is most commonly affected. Typical examples are **histoplasmosis**, **lobomycosis**, **cryptococcosis** and **blastomycosis**.

Reactions to arthropods

The sting of various arthropods can cause toxic or allergic reactions in the skin, presenting as a weal, an itchy papule which becomes excoriated in the centre, a haemorrhagic lesion or even a necrotic lesion. Histologically, dermal oedema, vasodilatation and a mixed cellular infiltrate of lymphocytes, histiocytes and eosinophils are usually found. In bee and wasp **stings**, generalized allergic reactions with extensive urticaria, bronchoconstriction and even anaphylactic shock may occur. The venom of certain arthropods (such as the **black widow spider**) may cause severe systemic toxic reactions.

Scabies mites (*Sarcoptes scabiei*) are ectoparasites, living in the stratum corneum. The individual mite is 0.5 mm in diameter. The dorsum of the finger webs, the axilla, the buttocks and the genital region are particularly affected: there are linear scales, itchy papules, excoriations and eczematous lesions (Fig. 19.22). Other mites do not live in the skin, but may cause similar clinical changes by contact (for example trombidiosis).

Non-specific reactions to infectious agents

Besides the skin changes caused directly by infectious agents, there are others where the infectious agents cannot be found in the skin, but in which the skin shows an allergic reaction to an infection elsewhere (see Fig. 19.23 and the box on p. 465). These **'-id'** reactions may be due to viruses (**virusid**), bacteria (**bacterid**), tuberculosis (**tuberculid**) or fungus (**mycid**).

Non-infectious inflammatory skin diseases

Reactions to physical and chemical hazards

Skin diseases may be due to excessive exposure to physical hazards (heat, cold, ionizing radiation and ultraviolet light) or chemicals. Changes similar to these caused by heat (see box) can also be due to cold exposure and to chemicals. Ionizing radiation may cause an acute erythema, or – often years after irradiation – telangiectasia, fibroplasia, pigmentary disturbances and ulceration. Ultraviolet light may also cause acute erythema (sunburn), characterized by vasodilatation and by individual necrotic keratinocytes (sunburn cells). Prolonged exposure to ultraviolet light leads to persistent connective tissue changes with coarse wrinkles and a yellowish discoloration, histologically characterized by accumulation of elastotic material in the dermis (**solar elastosis**). Finally, recurrent attacks of **sunburn** in childhood may cause the development of malignant melanoma, and prolonged ultraviolet exposure may give rise to epithelial skin tumours. These neoplastic changes are accelerated, when the defence of the skin against ultraviolet light is disturbed: in albinism, where melanin synthesis is impaired, and in **xeroderma pigmentosum**, where the repair of ultraviolet-induced DNA changes is defective.

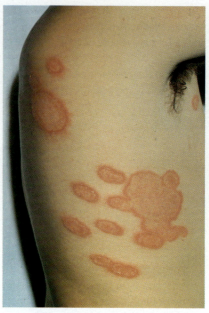

Fig. 19.21   Ringworm (tinea corporis): there are numerous, confluent, erythematous and scaly lesions with a raised, infiltrated border. Mycotic lesions of this type are often acquired from cattle.

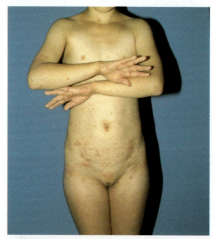

Fig. 19.22   Scabies: the child shows highly pruritic papules and excoriations particularly on the hands and on the lower abdomen.

CASE STUDY 19.5

A 20-year-old female hairdresser presents with itchy skin changes on the dorsa of fingers and hands. There is indistinct erythema, tiny vesicles, scaling, erosions and crusts. The diagnosis is acute allergic contact dermatitis, later proved to be due to nickel allergy.

Effects of heat on the skin
- **Grade I**: erythema
- **Grade II**: blister formation
- **Grade III**: necrosis of the skin

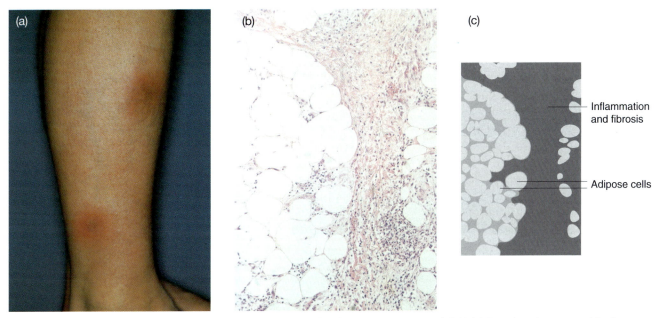

Fig. 19.23 (a) Erythema nodosum: there are deeply situated, subcutaneous, very painful bluish-red nodes symmetrically distributed on the lower legs. The lesions are larger on palpation than they appear on inspection. Erythema nodosum is a variant of panniculitis, usually caused as an -id reaction to a streptococcal infection of the upper airways. (b, c) Erythema nodosum. Fibrosis and inflammatory infiltration of septa in the subcutis (septal panniculitis).

Non-specific reactions
- **Erythema nodosum** (Fig. 19.23): a septal panniculitis (inflammation of the subcutis) showing painful bluish-red nodes on the lower leg, often following upper respiratory tract infection
- **Erythema multiforme**: showing annular lesions with a central vesicle on the extremities, often following a herpes simplex eruption; the condition is also commonly associated with drug reactions

Contact dermatitis

Contact dermatitis (contact eczema) is a reaction of the skin to topically applied stimuli. The classic example is acute allergic contact dermatitis. There is erythema, followed by papules and tiny vesicles. Histologically, there is pronounced exudation of tissue fluid and lymphocytes from the dermis into the epidermis, which shows widened intercellular spaces (spongiosis) accentuated focally to form spongiotic vesicles, along with intraepithelial lymphocytes (Fig. 19.24). Pathogenically, the allergen is processed by Langerhans' cells and presented to specifically sensitized T lymphocytes, which in turn release inflammatory mediators aggravating the inflammatory reaction non-specifically. In chronic forms of contact eczema, there is less spongiosis, but pronounced acanthosis and hyperkeratosis associated with a dermal lymphohistiocytic infiltrate, clinically characterized by plaque-like infiltration, scaling and fissures. Contact allergy may evolve to various allergens after long exposure, including metal ions, external medications and industrial products. A similar picture can be elicited by a non-allergic, cumulative toxic mechanism (**toxic contact dermatitis**), due to substances such as detergents or technical oils.

Atopic dermatitis

A skin disorder morphologically similar to chronic contact dermatitis may occur in atopic individuals, prone to develop allergic conjunctivitis, allergic asthma, urticaria and **atopic dermatitis (neurodermatitis)**. All these manifestations seem to be linked to grossly elevated serum IgE levels, since IgE is not only found on mast cells (responsible for conjunctivitis, asthma and urticaria), but also on Langerhans' cells (responsible for eczematous

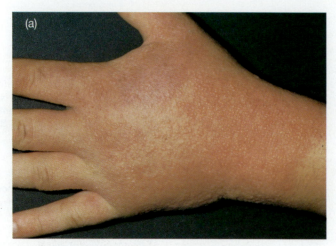

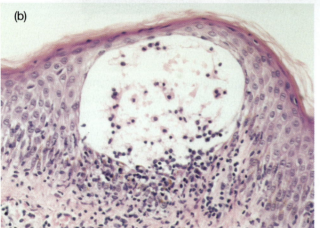

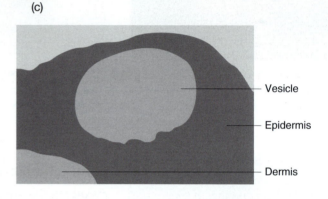

Vesicle

Epidermis

Dermis

Fig. 19.24   (a) Acute allergic contact dermatitis: the back of the hands shows densely aggregated, tiny papules and vesicles. The whole affected area is irregularly outlined. (b, c) Acute allergic contact dermatitis: histology shows an intraepidermal vesicle with spongiosis in the adjacent dermis and numerous lymphocytes in the dermis and epidermis.

reactions) in patients with atopy. Children are particularly affected, with itchy lesions on the flexure surfaces of elbows and knees.

Systemic allergic reactions

Allergic reactions of the skin due to systemically applied allergens often manifest themselves as acute **urticaria**. Allergens (certain food, spices, preservatives, medications) bind specifically to mast-cell bound IgE in sensitized patients. Mast cell degranulation leads to the wealing of the skin (Fig. 19.25), but may also cause systemic symptoms including anaphylactic shock. A similar reaction can be due to substances which induce mast cell degranulation without binding to IgE (such as aspirin). Besides, urticaria, particularly chronic urticaria, is often triggered by non-allergic mechanisms.

Lichen planus

Lichen planus is a highly characteristic, benign chronic skin disease without known aetiology, producing flat papules on the flexure surface of

---

CASE STUDY 19.6
A couple of minutes after a bee sting, a patient developed a general urticarial eruption of the entire integument, leading to grossly disfiguring oedema of the lips and eyelids. Concomitantly, dyspnoea and nausea occurred. With appropriate parenteral treatment, the symptoms resolved within 2 hours.

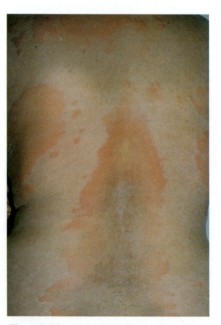

Fig. 19.25   Urticaria with numerous confluent weals on the back due to degranulation of mast cells. Mast cell degranulation can be due to specific IgE antibodies or can be triggered non-specifically by various chemical stimuli including some drugs.

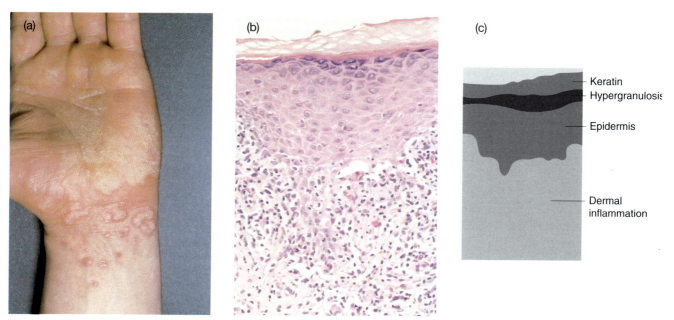

Fig. 19.26 Lichen planus: (a) lichen planus prefers the flexor surface of the wrist and shows pink, flat-topped, coalescing papules with a smooth surface. (b, c) Histology shows acanthosis, hypergranulosis, basal cell liquefaction and a dense dermal infiltrate pressed against the epidermis.

the wrist and on other body sites (Fig. 19.26). Histologically, there is a band-like (lichenoid) infiltrate in the papillary dermis immediately adjacent to the acanthotic epidermis, with liquefaction of the basal cell layer. Additionally, there is pronounced hypergranulosis. Since similar changes have been observed in graft-versus-host disease, lichen planus is considered as a local manifestation of self-reactive T lymphocytes.

Acne and related disorders

Sebum produced by the sebaceous glands is secreted through the upper portion of the hair follicle (follicular infundibulum). In **acne vulgaris**, increased sebum excretion and/or hyperkeratosis of the follicular infundibulum leads to sebum retention, clinically visible as a **comedo**. An increase in androgen levels and increased sensitivity of peripheral tissues to androgens are considered to be operative in some cases. Release of free fatty acids into the adjacent tissue and overgrowth of saprophytic or pathogenic bacteria may subsequently cause inflammation, clinically represented as folliculitis. Finally abscesses, scars and cysts may develop. Acne vulgaris is very common in adolescents and affects the body areas with particularly large and numerous sebaceous glands: the face, and the medial regions of the anterior and posterior upper trunk. There is usually remission after a few years, but severe variants of acne may persist for decades and may leave disfiguring scars.

Rosacea, a disease which also affects the sebum-rich areas, occurs in middle-aged people and shows erythema, telangiectasia and papulopustules, but no comedos.

Psoriasis

Psoriasis is characterized by hyperproliferation of the epidermis, triggered in genetically predisposed individuals by various exogenous and

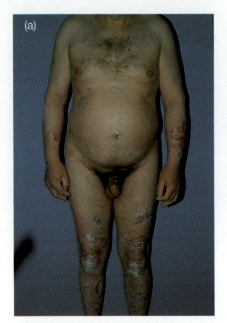
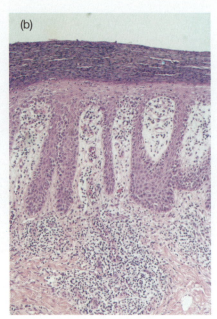
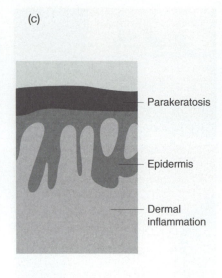

Parakeratosis

Epidermis

Dermal
inflammation

Fig. 19.27   Psoriasis vulgaris: (a) psoriasis vulgaris prefers the extensor surfaces of the extremities and shows coalescing, red plaques covered by an abundance of white scales. (b, c) Histology shows a band-like parakeratosis, acanthosis, papillomatosis and a mixed dermal infiltrate consisting of lymphocytes, histiocytes and neutrophils.

endogenous factors. Histologically, there is acanthosis, papillomatosis with tortuous capillaries in the papillae, absence of a granular layer and hyper-parakeratosis. There is a dermal infiltrate with histiocytes, lymphocytes and neutrophils, with the last migrating into the epidermis at the tip of the papillae. Clinically, there are erythematous plaques with extensive scaling (Fig. 19.27). In the pustular variant, which may either be localized to the acral skin or which may involve the entire integument, neutrophils dominate the histological picture, resulting in spongiform pustules.

CASE STUDY 19.7
A middle-aged man shows numerous erythematous scaly plaques on the elbows, knees, extensor surfaces of the lower legs and in the presacral region. Additionally there is erythema and scaling on the scalp and a noticeable dystrophy of several fingernails. The general condition is unimpaired. The initial manifestation of the disease was in early adult life; since then, relapses have occurred every one or two years. The diagnosis is psoriasis vulgaris, plaque type (see Fig. 19.27).

Autoimmune bullous diseases

There is a group of diseases characterized by autoantibodies to the epidermis or dermoepidermal junction, which lead to blister formation either by complement activation or by inducing the release of proteolytic enzymes from keratinocytes or granulocytes. In **pemphigus**, autoantibodies to desmosomes induce acantholysis with intraepithelial cleft formation. Clinically, fragile blisters and large erosions occur (Fig. 19.28). In **bullous pemphigoid**, autoantibodies impair the function of the hemidesmosomes at the dermal–epidermal interface, resulting in tense bullae. **Dermatitis herpetiformis** is mediated by IgA immune complexes deposited at the tip of the dermal papillae. Clinically, tiny, itchy vesicles

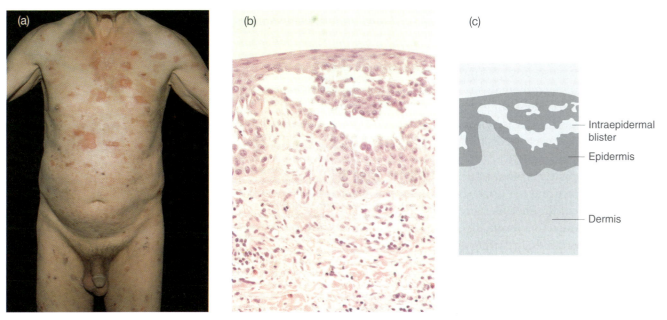

Fig. 19.28 Pemphigus vulgaris: (a) there are large erosions scattered over the trunk and the proximal extremities. (b, c) Histologically, pemphigus shows an intraepidermal vesicle with acantholytic cells due to disintegration of desmosomal contacts. Release of desmosomal contacts is caused by circulating autoantiabodies to desmosomal components.

occur. There is a strong clinical association with coeliac disease. The definitive diagnosis of autoimmune bullous skin diseases is established by immunohistological demonstration of the autoantibodies in skin biopsies and serum (Fig. 19.29).

Fig. 19.29 Level of blistering in autoimmune bullous diseases.

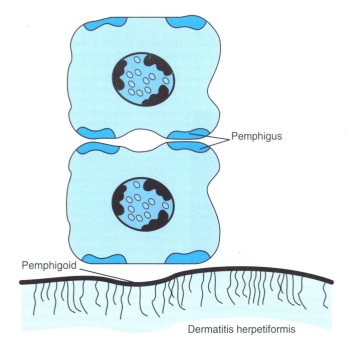

Connective tissue diseases

The group of connective tissue diseases or **collagenoses** comprises several disorders characterized by autoimmune phenomena taking place in mesenchymal tissues:

- **Systemic scleroderma** (Fig. 19.30) starts typically with fibrosis of the hands and the face with gradual progression and involvement of the lung, oesophagus and kidneys. Localized scleroderma (morphoea) is limited to a few sclerotic plaques or streaks in the skin.
- **Systemic lupus erythematosus** clinically shows a butterfly-like erythema with scaling on the cheeks, while discoid lupus erythematosus forms discrete scaly erythematous lesions. In the systemic form, arthritis, central nervous system involvement and renal insufficiency may follow.
- **Dermatomyositis** is often associated with internal malignancies. The skin of the face and the upper trunk shows a violaceous erythema, and the muscles of the shoulder girdle are weak and sore due to myositis.
- In **mixed connective tissue disease**, there are features of more than one of these disorders. Circulating autoantibodies to nuclear and cytoplasmic antigens are of diagnostic significance in connective tissue diseases, but are not necessarily causally related to the disease.

Vasculitis

There are two typical examples of vasculitis in the skin:

- **Allergic vasculitis** (Fig. 19.31) is an immune complex vasculitis often due to upper respiratory tract infection. Clinically, haemorrhagic papules occur particularly on the lower legs. Histology shows destruction of small dermal venules by numerous, often fragmented neutrophilic granulocytes and extravasated erythrocytes. Other organs (joints, bowel and kidney) may also be affected.
- **Polyarteritis nodosa** shows nodules often linearly arranged along arteries and occasional ulceration of the skin. The disease can be limited to the skin or can involve the skin in the course of generalized polyarteritis nodosa. In some cases, hepatitis B virus is the causative allergen. Vasculitis in general can also be a feature of other skin diseases as, for example, lupus erythematosus

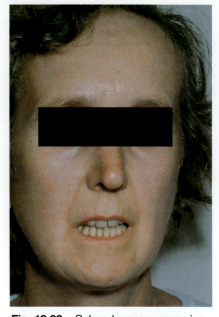

Fig. 19.30 Scleroderma: progressive scleroderma primarly affects hands, arms and face. The face shows narrowing of the mouth with radial furrows and a tightly stretched nasal skin. Lung and kidney involvement may occur after years.

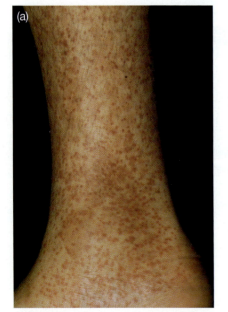
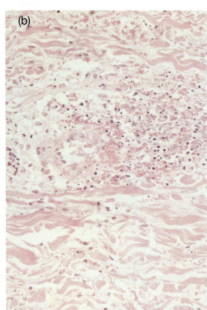
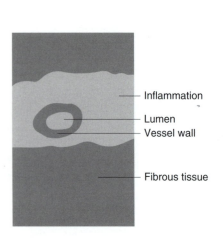

Inflammation
Lumen
Vessel wall

Fibrous tissue

Fig. 19.31 Allergic vasculitis: (a) slightly raised purpuric papules on the lower leg due to vasculitis of skin venules. (b, c) Histology shows a small vessel with necrotic vessel wall, infiltrated by neutrophils.

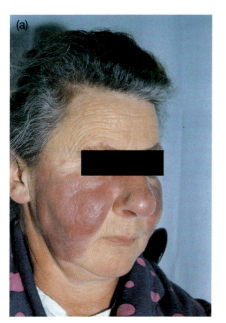
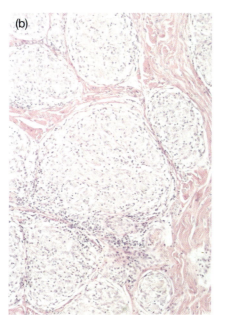
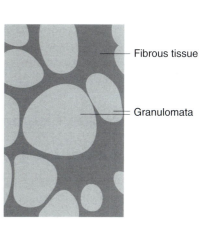

Fibrous tissue

Granulomata

Fig. 19.32 Cutaneous sarcoidosis: (a) bluish-red subcutaneous nodules and plaques in the face resembling perniones clinically. (b, c) Histology shows nodular infiltrates composed of epithelioid cells surrounded by a small rim of lymphocytes and collagen.

Granulomatous reactions

Granulomata often occur in infections with highly persistent micro-organisms. There are, however, examples of granuloma development without an evident infectious cause. **Granuloma annulare** presents with small, ring-like arranged, skin-coloured papules on the extremities. Histology shows a palisading granuloma with epithelioid cells arranged around centres of necrobiotic collagen. **Sarcoidosis** (Fig. 19.32) may show violaceous plaques and subcutaneous nodes in the skin, characterized by sharply circumscribed epithelioid and giant cell nodules surrounded by a sparse lymphocytic infiltrate. Sarcoidosis may be limited to the skin and may particularly involve old scars.

Pigmentary disorders

Vitiligo

Vitiligo is characterized by depigmentation in otherwise normal skin due to disappearance or impaired function of the melanocytes, probably caused by autoimmune phenomena. Sites most likely to be affected are the distal extremities and the regions around the orifices. The course is slowly progressive with incomplete remissions. Association with other autoimmune disorders (Hashimoto's thyroiditis, megaloblastic anaemia) may be found. As well as in vitiligo, depigmentation is often found following any type of skin inflammation (**postinflammatory depigmentation**). Additionally, hypopigmentation may involve an entire skin segment following Blaschko's lines.

Hyperpigmentation

Hyperpigmentation – due to increased melanin synthesis without an increase in the number of melanocytes – may be diffuse or circumscribed.

Diffuse hyperpigmentation may occur in Addison's disease. Circumscribed hyperpigmentation may also be postinflammatory. **Ephelides (freckles)** are other common examples of hyperpigmentation. *Café-au-lait* **macules** of several centimetres in diameter can be found in any individual. If there are more than six, they are usually associated with neurofibromatosis. As in hypopigmentation, segmental variants of hyperpigmentation exist.

Neoplastic skin diseases

Tumours of the epidermis

Seborrheic keratoses (basal cell papillomas) are benign proliferations of the epidermis and the papillary dermis in elderly people. The lesions are often hyperpigmented and characterized by tiny horn pearls. Chronic actinic damage of the skin may lead to **solar keratoses**: reddish, slightly scaling macules, histologically characterized by intraepithelial neoplasia with atypical nuclei and parakeratosis. **Bowen's disease** is synonymous with squamous cell carcinoma in situ of the skin, with grossly disturbed epidermal architecture, atypia and dyskeratosis.

Basal cell carcinoma is a locally destructive, but non-metastasizing tumour consisting of large, sharply circumscribed nests of keratinocytes sharing morphological features with basal cells. Clinically, a skin-coloured nodule, often centrally ulcerated, is evident (Fig. 19.33). In advanced cases, destruction of underlying bones may occur. **Fibrosing basal cell carcinoma** is a rare variant, which extends beyond the clinically visible margins and often recurs.

Invasive squamous cell carcinoma of the skin may arise from normal skin, actinic keratosis or Bowen's disease. It occurs particularly in sun-damaged skin in elderly people, grows slowly and produces occasionally metastatic deposits in the lymph nodes and rarely in inner organs (Fig. 19.34).

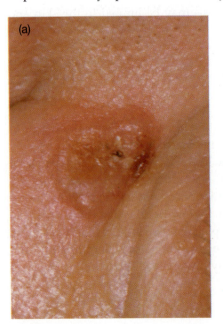
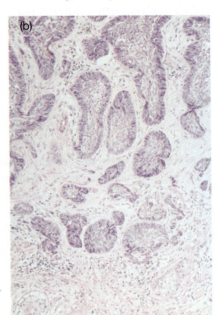
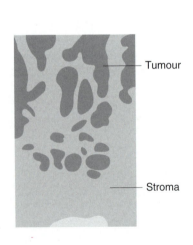

Tumour

Stroma

Fig. 19.33   Basal cell carcinoma: (a) there is a flat nodule with a depressed, ulcerated central portion and a rim of tiny, translucent papules at the periphery. (b, c) Histologically, there are nests of tumour cells with a basaloid appearance at the peripheral cells, embedded in a tumour-specific stroma with a loose collagenous network.

Fig. 19.34 Basal cell carcinoma versus squamous cell carcinoma. Main histological features: (a) basal cell carcinoma shows round nests of epithelial cells resembling basal cells of the epidermis; the nests are embedded in a specific, loose tumour stroma. (b) Squamous cell carcinoma shows irregular nests with central keratinization frankly invading the surrounding dermis.

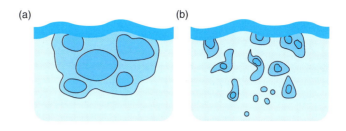

(a)   (b)

Melanocytic tumours

BENIGN MELANOCYTIC NAEVI

The **melanocytes** in the skin can give rise to benign naevi and to malignant melanoma. Acquired benign common naevi develop during the first two decades of life as brown macules, histologically characterized by the presence of nests of naevus cells at the dermoepidermal junction (**junctional naevus**) (Fig. 19.35). Subsequently, the lesion becomes dome-shaped and histology shows naevus cells at the junction and in the dermis (**compound junctional** and **intradermal naevus**) and still later the naevus becomes depigmented and fibrotic (**intradermal naevus**) with loss of the junctional component. In some patients, various numbers of so-called **dysplastic naevi** with larger size, uneven pigmentation and histologically evident atypia may occur. Patients with numerous dysplastic naevi, which is often inherited (**dysplastic naevus syndrome**), carry an increased risk of developing malignant melanoma anywhere on the skin. Uncommon variants of melanocytic naevi include: **congenital naevi** (often very large and hairy); **Spitz naevus**, which may be confused with malignant melanoma; and **blue naevus**, characterized by dendritic intradermal melanocytes.

MALIGNANT MELANOMA

Malignant melanoma may arise from giant congenital naevi, from common naevi, from dysplastic naevi or – most often – from normal skin.

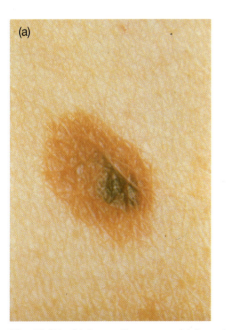

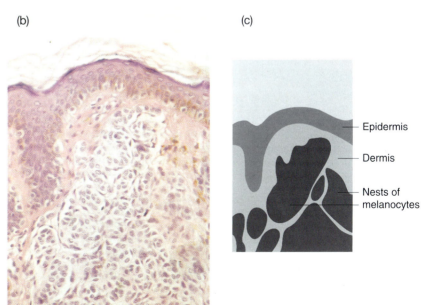

(a)   (b)   (c)

Epidermis

Dermis

Nests of melanocytes

Fig. 19.35 Melanocytic naevus: (a) there is a regularly but indistinctly outlined oval plaque, which is light brown in colour and appears more or less symmetrical. (b, c) Histologically, nests of evenly shaped naevus cells are present in the superficial dermis.

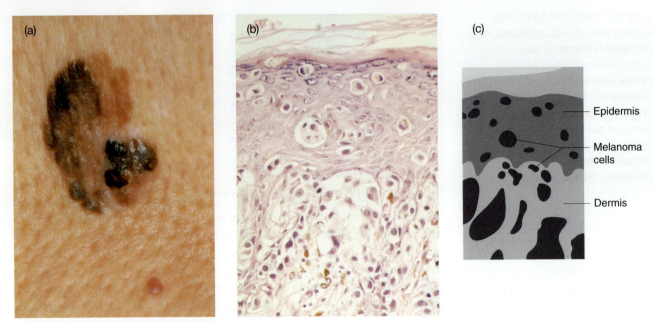

Fig. 19.36   Malignant melanoma: (a) there is an irregularly shaped, sharply demarcated plaque showing variation of colour ranging from light brown to deep black. Slight scaling is evident in the nodular portion on the lower right part of the lesion. (b, c) In contrast to benign naevi, malignant melanoma shows an abundance of highly atypical tumour cells, forming nests throughout the epidermis and also in the dermis.

Proliferation of melanoma cells starts at the dermoepidermal junction with single cells and nests of melanocytes moving upwards through the epidermis (**melanoma in situ**), clinically appearing as a black macule. Subsequently, melanoma cells scatter in the papillary dermis, but the lesion remains thin (**invasive melanoma, radial growth phase**) (Fig. 19.36). Later, proliferation and invasiveness increase and nodules are formed (**invasive melanoma, vertical growth phase**). The risk of metastatic spread increases with the maximum vertical tumour thickness (Fig. 19.37): lesions thinner than 0.75 mm are almost always cured by excision, whereas lesions thicker than 3 mm are highly likely to develop lymph node and visceral metastases.

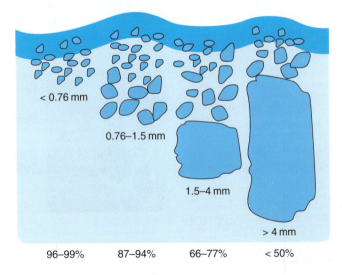

Fig. 19.37   Lesion thickness and prognosis in malignant melanoma (percentages denote 5-year survival rate).

Types of soft tissue tumour
- **Dermatofibroma** is a lenticular dermal nodule consisting of fibroblasts and coarse collagen bundles
- **Lipomas** present as soft subcutaneous tumours
- **Leiomyomas** present as grouped tender papules
- **Telangiectatic naevi** and **haemangiomas** may be confined to the skin or may be associated with other organ abnormalities
- **Neurofibromas** may appear as solitary, inconspicuous papules or can be multiple and disfiguring in neurofibromatosis

Malignant soft tissue tumours
- **Angiosarcoma** of the scalp is typically found in old patients
- **Classic Kaposi's sarcoma** is a slowly growing angiosarcoma usually starting on the lower extremities of elderly men
- **AIDS-related Kaposi's sarcoma**, in contrast, rapidly shows disseminated skin and mucous membrane lesions

---

CASE STUDY 19.8

A middle-aged woman presented with a brown to black, sharply circumscribed, irregularly outlined plaque on the lower leg. It had developed over 5 years. During the last few months, changes in colour (focal depigmentation, deep black areas, reddish inflammatory areas) and a black, dome-shaped papule within the lesion had occurred. A diagnosis of malignant melanoma was clinically suspected and histologically confirmed, with a maximum vertical tumour thickness of 3.5 mm. Four years later, lymph node metastases occurred, and another 3 years later the patient died of disseminated disease.

Soft tissue tumours

Soft tissue tumours mainly arise from fibroblasts, fat cells, muscle cells, endothelial cells and Schwann cells. Malignant tumours are rare.

Lymphomas and related disorders

Virtually all systemic lymphomas, leukaemia and histiocytoses can secondarily involve the skin. In contrast, **mycosis fungoides** is a typical example of a primary malignant lymphoma of the skin (Fig. 19.38). It starts with eczematoid patches, which become infiltrated plaques and finally give rise to rapidly growing dome-shaped tumours or to generalized erythroderma. Histologically, there is a dense dermal infiltrate of atypical T-helper lymphocytes (CD4+) with gyrate nuclei and a tendency to invade the epidermis. Systemic involvement and leukaemic spread may occur.

Diseases of the skin appendages

Hair

There may be hair shaft anomalies, increased hair growth and a decreased hair growth, with the last condition being the most common hair disorder. **Male pattern baldness** is an example of a diffuse, non-scarring alopecia. **Alopecia areata** is an autoimmunologically mediated hair loss in sharply circumscribed areas, where the follicles remain intact and regrowth is possible (**reversible alopecia**). Scarring alopecia may be due to a special type of folliculitis, lupus erythematosus or other inflammatory conditions. There is clinically evident loss of hair follicles and therefore the alopecia is irreversible.

Nails

Besides congenital abnormalities, nails may be affected by micro-organisms (dermatophytes, *Candida* spp., Gram-negative bacilli) or can show special types of dystrophy in inflammatory skin diseases (for example pits and onycholysis in psoriasis, longitudinal streaks in alopecia areata and chronic contact dermatitis).

Sebaceous glands

Sebaceous glands are particularly involved in acne vulgaris and rosacea as discussed above.

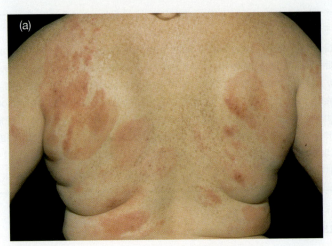

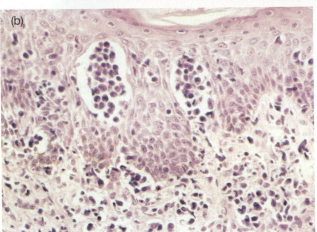

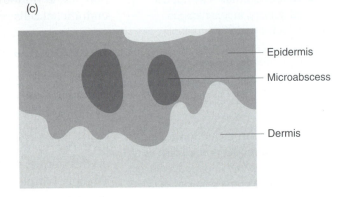

Fig. 19.38 Mycosis fungoides (cutaneous T-cell lymphoma): (a) there are confluent erythematous plaques on the back, some of the plaques showing a kidney shape. (b, c) Atypical lymphocytes with hyperchromatic and cleaved nuclei are scattered throughout the dermis and epidermis, forming intraepidermal microabscesses.

Sweat glands

Increased sweating in a humid atmosphere or in skin areas affected by inflammatory dermatosis may lead to **miliaria**, with numerous tiny vesicles at the orifices of the eccrine sweat glands. Abscesses of the apocrine sweat glands are common in the axillae and in the groins and may be an accompanying feature of severe acne.

The skin in systemic disease

Metabolic disorders

Diabetes mellitus is the most common example of a metabolic disorder affecting the skin, often secondarily due to neuropathy and angiopathy (Fig 19.39). Another example is **porphyria cutanea tarda**, in which a hereditary defect in porphyrin metabolism manifests itself in adult life with blister formation in sun-exposed areas and on slight traumata. Furthermore, many 'inborn errors of metabolism' show skin signs besides the prominent changes of inner organs.

Neoplastic disorders

In internal neoplasia, involvement of the skin can occur either by metastatic spread or by the development of paraneoplastic syndromes. **Acanthosis**

Fig. 19.39 Neurotrophic ulcers: this patient has diabetes. Owing to diabetic neuropathy he has become insensitive to pain. Prolonged pressure on the sole has led to a large callosity and finally to an ulcer with concomitant infection of the underlying bones.

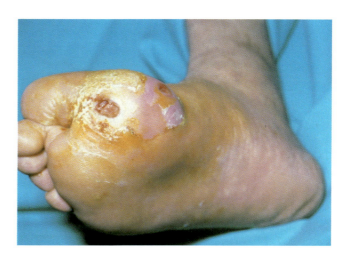

CASE STUDY 19.9

A 60-year-old patient presented with massive oedema and redness of the dorsum of the right foot, hyperkeratosis on the soles and a coin-sized ulcer on the weight-bearing area of the right foot. Furthermore, there were multiple yellowish to red papules on the buttocks and reddening and scaling in the perianal area. The patient had suffered from diabetes mellitus for a couple of years. The dermatological diagnoses were erysipelas of the right leg, a neurotrophic ulcer on the sole, multiple eruptive xanthomas on the buttocks accompanying rapid deterioration of blood glucose levels, and candida intertrigo in the perianal zone.

nigricans maligna is associated with gastrointestinal or bronchial tumours and shows clinically visible papillomatosis and hyperpigmentation in the flexures. Other potentially paraneoplastic syndromes are pruritus and pruritic exanthemas and severe manifestations of infectious skin diseases (such as generalized herpes zoster).

Psychological abnormalities

Psychological factors have some bearing on the course of particular skin diseases as, for example, atopic dermatitis. **Self-infliction** due to psychological disturbances may manifest itself by multiple ulcers, burns or abscesses, and may cause great diagnostic difficulties.

Chapter 20   Breast disease

> **Learning objectives**
>
> To appreciate and understand:
> - Effects of ageing and hormonal influences on breast tissue
> - Range of inflammatory disorders affecting the breast and benign mastopathy
> - Benign and malignant neoplastic conditions affecting the breast
> - Role of the pathologist in managing breast cancer and in screening for breast cancer

Normal anatomy and development

Breast development begins early in gestation; at week 6 the ectoderm buds into the underlying mesenchyme. These buds grow and branch and become canalized resulting in the system of ducts seen radiating from the nipple (Fig. 20.1). The distal end of the duct system gives rise to the **secretory unit** comprising the terminal duct with surrounding acini.

Before puberty the male and female breasts are similar with only few widely scattered rudimentary secretory units. The breasts enlarge in females at puberty, under the influence of oestrogen and progesterone. This is primarily due to an increase in the amount of adipose tissue but also results from a small increase in the number of secretory units which show distinct lobule formation as a result of the presence of more acini (Figs 20.2 and 20.3). Ducts and acini are lined by a double layer of epithelium: an inner secretory epithelial layer and an outer layer of myoepithelium. During pregnancy when oestrogen and progesterone levels increase further there is additional development of the mammary gland with a marked increase in the number of secretory units and the onset of secretory activity (Figs 20.4 and 20.5).

In postmenopausal women breast **involution** occurs. There is a reduction in the number of secretory units, often accompanied by a reduction in the amount of adipose tissue. Some of the ducts may show a microcystic change and contain inspissated secretions (Fig. 20.6).

Congenital abnormalities

Congenital abnormalities of the breast are rare. They include the absence of one or both breasts (**amazia**) or one or both nipples (**athelia**). Additional breasts (**polymastia**) or nipples (**polythelia**) may also occur along the milk line between the anterior axilla and the medial aspect of the thigh.

Fig. 20.1 An idealized illustration of the breast.

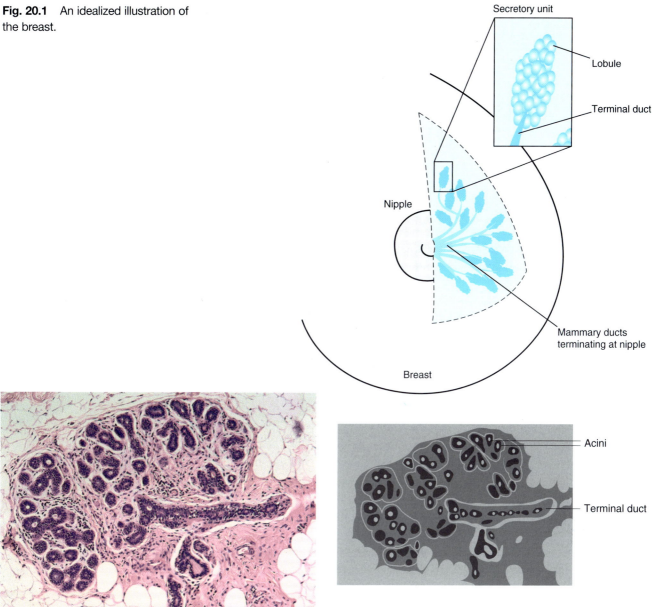

Fig. 20.2 The secretory unit of the breast (or terminal duct lobular unit) in non-pregnant women of reproductive age.

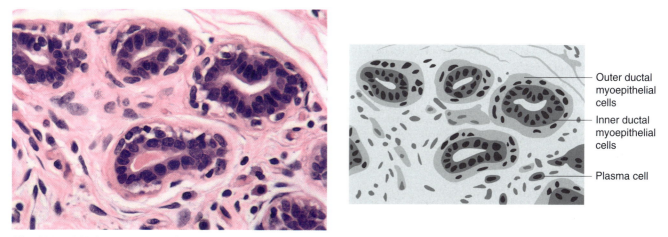

Fig. 20.3 A high-power view of secretory acini with the inner epithelial and outer layer of myoepithelial cells. Note the plasma cells in the surrounding loose intralobular (acinar) connective tissue.

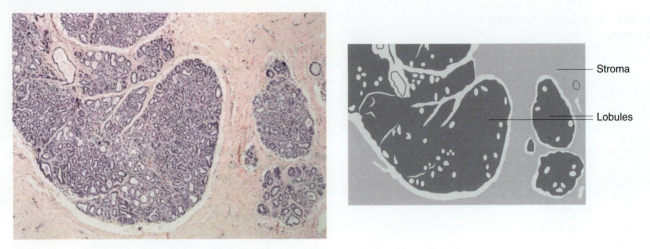

Fig. 20.4   A breast in late pregnancy. There is a marked increase in the number of lobules.

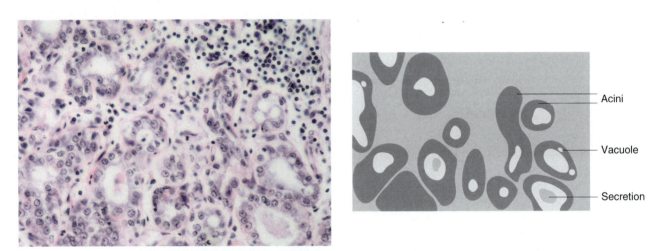

Fig. 20.5   A high-power view showing the inner layer of epithelium of the acini to be vacuolated and have a columnar appearance. A small amount of secretion is present in the lumen of some of the acini.

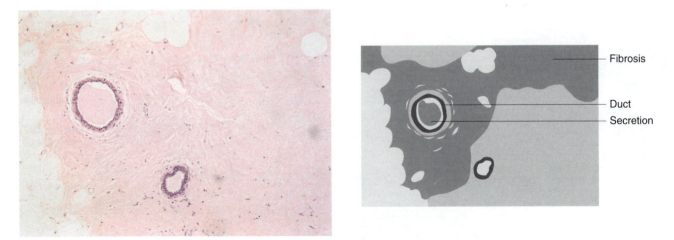

Fig. 20.6   Postmenopausal breast with fibrous replacement of adipose tissue, microcystic change and inspissated secretion in ducts.

Benign (non-neoplastic) conditions

Infective inflammatory disorders

ACUTE PYOGENIC MASTITIS

Acute mastitis is an inflammatory condition of the breast most often occurring during lactation. The clinical features are the same as acute inflammation occurring elsewhere in the body. Pyogenic bacteria, usually *Staphylococcus aureus*, gain entry via the ducts or when suckling causes an abrasion to the nipple. If not treated promptly, extensive abscess formation with subsequent scarring may occur.

CHRONIC INFECTIONS

Acute pyogenic mastitis which has been inadequately treated, or prolonged infection with bacteria of low virulence, may give rise to chronic infection. Sinus formation and scarring may be a long-term consequence of such an infection. True chronic infections of the breast are uncommon: tuberculosis may involve the breast by haematogenous, lymphatic or direct spread. Typical caseating granulomata are seen which may lead to sinus formation. **Actinomycosis**, **blastomycosis** and **coccidioidomycosis** are other rare granulomatous diseases of the breast.

Non-infective inflammatory disorders

MAMMARY DUCT ECTASIA

Ectasia, a condition of uncertain aetiology, is characterized by dilatation of the mammary ducts (Figs 20.7 and 20.8). It occurs primarily in premenopausal, multiparous women, although nulliparous women are occasionally affected. It is often asymptomatic, but may give rise to a firm, poorly defined mass or a browny cream, sometimes bloodstained, nipple discharge. Nipple retraction simulating a carcinoma may also occur. If a duct leaks, a prominent periductal chronic inflammatory cell infiltrate may develop. Large numbers of plasma cells may be present and this leads to the name plasma cell mastitis in the older literature. If a duct ruptures, a granulomatous reaction similar to that seen in fat necrosis may occur.

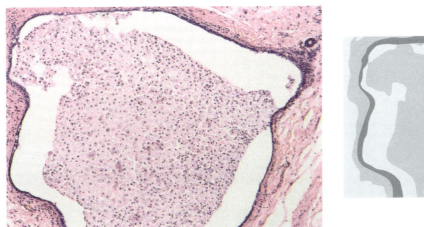
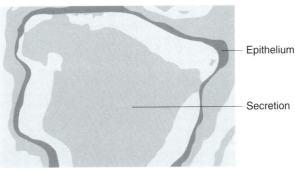

Epithelium

Secretion

Fig. 20.7 A dilated mammary duct lined by attenuated epithelium and containing secretion.

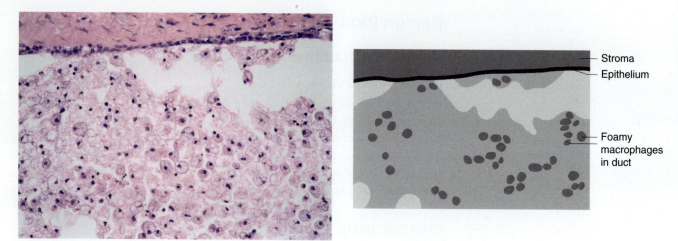

Fig. 20.8   Foamy macrophages present in the duct secretion. These can be found in the nipple discharge.

FAT NECROSIS

Fat necrosis is thought to occur following trauma to the adipose tissue of the breast, although a history of injury may only be obtained in about half the cases. Clinically the lesion presents as a hard lump which may simulate cancer particularly if there is retraction of the overlying skin. Trauma to the adipose cells results in necrosis with the release of lipids. The initial acute inflammatory infiltrate is rapidly superseded by a granulomatous reaction (Fig. 20.9).

SILICONE-INDUCED GRANULOMA

Silicone breast implants have been used for breast reconstruction following mastectomy and for breast augmentation. The bag of silicone becomes surrounded by a fibrous capsule and if small leaks occur these may elicit a granulomatous reaction (Fig. 20.10).

Benign mastopathy

The benign mastopathies are an important but poorly defined group of parenchymal changes that are seen commonly in the breasts of women of reproductive age. Each of these parenchymal changes (Fig. 20.11) may be

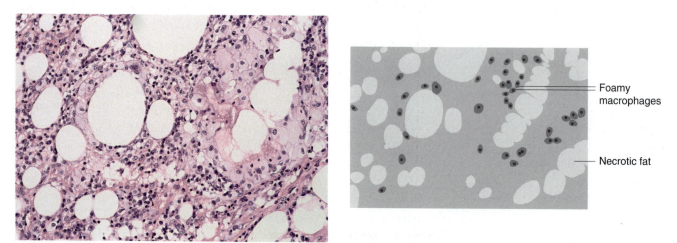

Fig. 20.9   Fat necrosis showing necrotic fat and foamy macrophages. Giant cells can often be found but are not easily seen in this photomicrograph. Note the acute and chronic inflammatory infiltrate in the background.

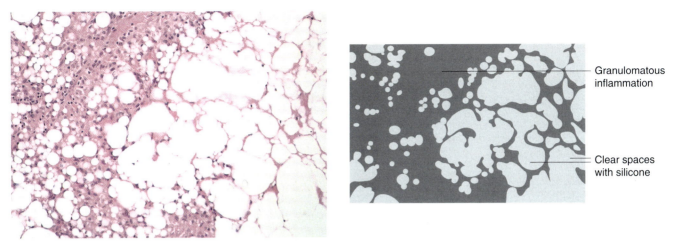

Fig. 20.10 Silicone-induced granuloma: histological appearances are similar to fat necrosis. Note the transparent fragments of silicone just visible in the clear spaces.

Fig. 20.11 The spectrum of benign mastopathy.

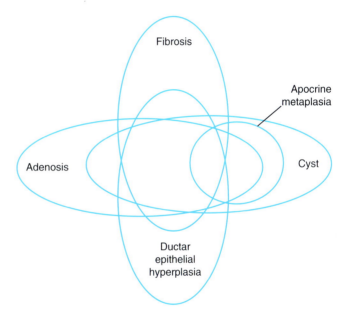

present in varying degrees, giving rise to a wide spectrum of disorders in the breast. This condition is so common that minor changes may be regarded as being within the limits of normality. In some women, however, the changes are more florid and can give rise to considerable morbidity with pain, cyst formation and breast lumpiness.

The terminology relating to this condition is confusing. Previously a number of different labels including fibrocystic disease, mammary dysplasia, cystic mastopathy and mastitis have been advocated. None is entirely satisfactory as they tend to emphasize only one or two of the disease components that may be present, and may even not reflect the changes observed. We therefore advocate the all-encompassing term **benign mastopathy** to cover the spectrum of changes observed.

AETIOLOGY AND SIGNIFICANCE

The aetiology of benign mastopathy is uncertain, but it is assumed that hormonal changes during reproductive years are important. This condition is important for two reasons. First the disease may present as a lump requiring to be distinguished from a carcinoma. Second, it is now recognized that if ductal epithelial hyperplasia is present this indicates an increased risk for the subsequent development of malignancy (Table 20.1).

Table 20.1   Risk factors for breast cancer

Increased risk	Risk multiplier	Decreased risk
First degree family history (mother/sister)	× 2–3[a]	
Early menarche	× 1.2	Late menarche
Late menopause	× 1.5	Early menopause or oophorectomy < 35 years
Late pregnancy	× 1.5	Early pregnancy
Nulliparity	> × 1.5	
Ductal epithelial hyperplasia	× 2	
Atypical ductal hyperplasia/ atypical lobular hyperplasia	× 5	
Ductal carcinoma in situ	× 10	
Radiation[b]		

[a] Approximate increase in risk compared with general population.
[b] Risk relates to exposure level. Exposure to diagnostic X-rays increases risk minimally.

COMPONENTS OF BENIGN MASTOPATHY

- **Cyst formation**: the cysts develop from the secretory unit and may be single or multiple. They may be microscopic or several centimetres in diameter and contain yellow or clear serous fluid (Figs 20.12 and 20.13). Macroscopically, intact cysts may have a blue, domed appearance. **Apocrine metaplasia** may occur in the epithelium lining the cyst (Fig. 20.14).
- **Fibrosis**: an increase in the dense interlobular connective tissue which extends into the lobules is often present. This may be quite extensive (see Fig. 20.12) or a subtle change often difficult to assess histologically.
- **Adenosis**: this is an increase in the number and size of lobules occurring outside pregnancy (Fig. 20.15). When this occurs in association with fibrosis it is termed **sclerosing adenosis** (Fig. 20.16).
- **Ductal epithelial hyperplasia**: this refers to a proliferation of the inner layer of epithelial cells lining the mammary ducts. Mild ductal

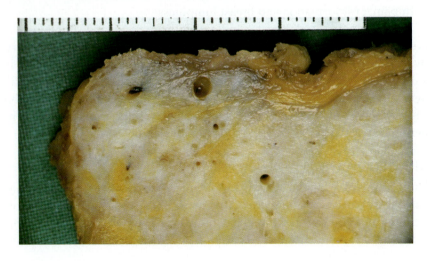

Fig. 20.12 Gross specimen of breast showing marked white fibrosis and a few small cysts.

epithelial hyperplasia refers to stratification of the ductal epithelium up to 3–4 cells thick (Fig. 20.17). Severe ductal epithelial hyperplasia occurs when the lumina are filled with cells (Fig. 20.18). Moderate ductal epithelial hyperplasia falls between the two. It is important that ductal epithelial hyperplasia is distinguished from ductal carcinoma in situ (see pp. 490–1).

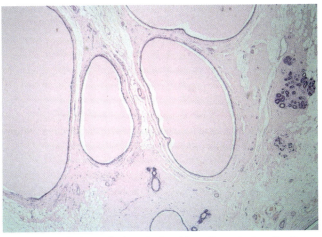
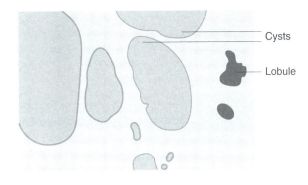

Fig. 20.13   Thin-walled cysts lined by attenuated epithelium.

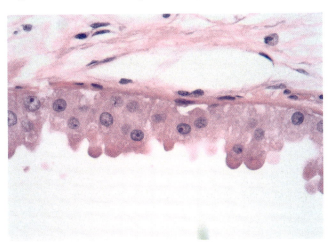
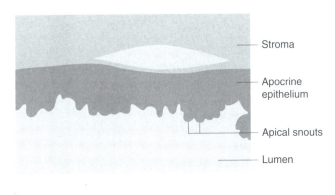

Fig. 20.14   Apocrine epithelium lining a breast cyst. The cells have abundant finely granular eosinophilic cytoplasm. Note the apical snouts releasing secretion into the lumen.

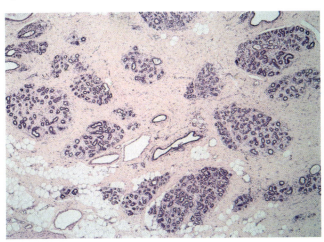
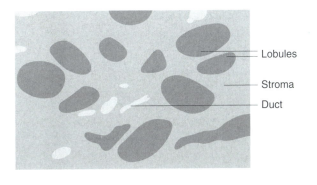

Fig. 20.15   Adenosis showing an increase in the number and size of breast lobules in a case of benign mastopathy

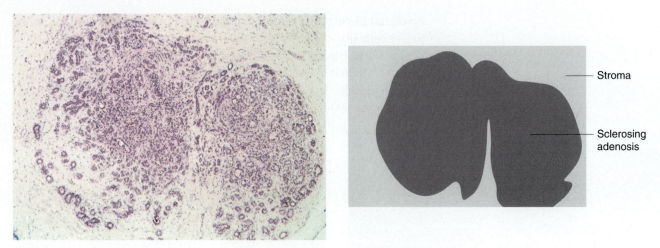

Fig. 20.16   Sclerosing adenosis: there is distortion of the individual acini by fibrous tissue resulting in a pseudoinfiltrative pattern which may be mistaken for carcinoma. However, the overall lobular architecture is preserved.

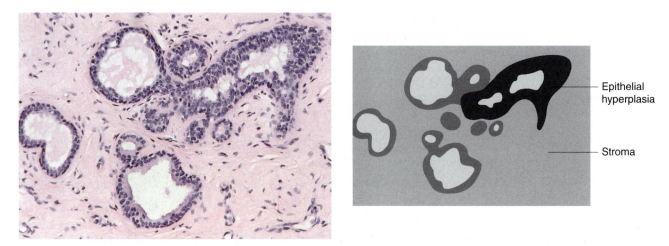

Fig. 20.17   Mild epithelial ductal hyperplasia (top right acinus) with heaping of cells up to 3–4 thick lining the lumen.

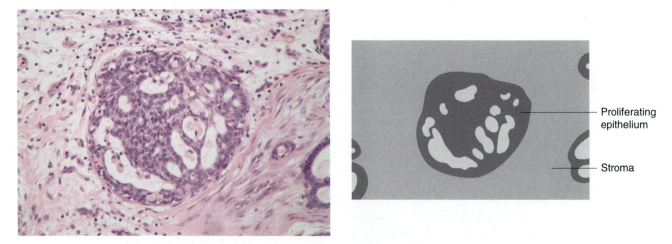

Fig. 20.18   Severe ductal epithelial hyperplasia: note the untidy, haphazard, overlapping arrangement of both lining epithelial and myoepithelial cells filling the lumen. Necrosis is characteristically absent. Immunohistochemistry would show that both epithelial and myoepithelial cells are involved in the proliferative process.

Rarely, a condition called **atypical ductal hyperplasia** is encountered in breast specimens. Here the epithelial proliferation exhibits some but not all of the histological features of ductal carcinoma in situ. The implication of this term is that it is a premalignant state which may eventually give rise to carcinoma. Indeed approximately 10% of women with a biopsy showing atypical ductal hyperplasia will develop carcinoma over 10 years.

Radial scar and complex sclerosing lesions

These rarely palpable, benign lesions cause stellate parenchymal distortion that mammographically (Fig. 20.19) can be indistinguishable from carcinoma. Both radial scar and complex sclerosing lesions have similar histological appearances (Figs 20.20 and 20.21), although the term radial scar is confined to lesions less than 10 mm in diameter.

Microglandular adenosis

Microglandular adenosis is a rare cause of a breast mass. There is a non-encapsulated proliferation of acini which spill out into the surrounding parenchyma. Myoepithelial cells are often absent; hence this condition may be mistaken for tubular carcinoma. However, the epithelial cells in microglandular adenosis lack the atypia (nuclear pleomorphism, disordered cellular architecture) of carcinoma cells.

Fig. 20.19 Mammogram showing stellate distortion of the breast tissue caused by a radial scar. The round blobs of calcification are benign. (Courtesy of Dr M. Creagh-Barry, Poole General Hospital.)

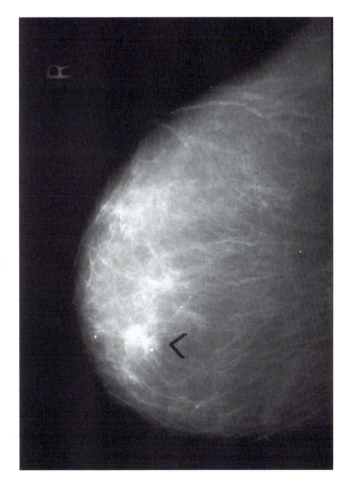

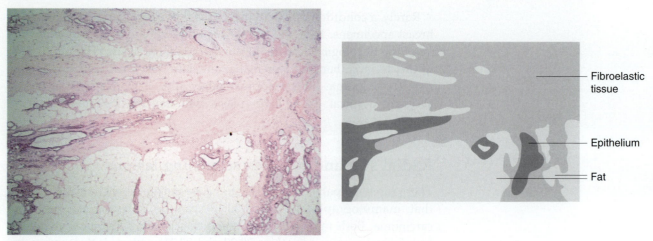

Fig. 20.20   Radial scar showing a central scarred area with radiating bands of fibroelastotic tissue. Ductal epithelial hyperplasia may be marked.

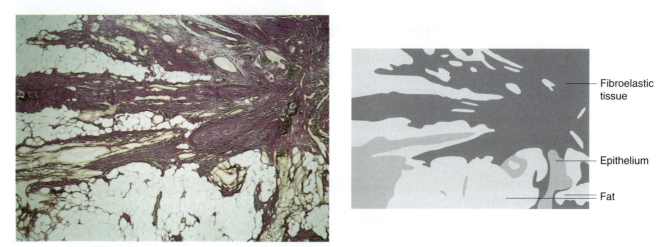

Fig. 20.21   Same specimen as Fig. 20.20 stained with an elastic stain showing marked deposition of elastin (black) in the stroma.

Neoplasms

Benign neoplasms

ADENOMA

Ductal adenomas are rare benign epithelial tumours and may develop anywhere in the breast. They present as a lump (usually less than 40 mm) consisting of well-demarcated, non-encapsulated acini in a fibrous stroma. Adenomas of the nipple also form a mass comprising densely packed duct structures but the epithelial component may have a papillary architecture. The acini in both these conditions usually have an outer myoepithelial layer.

PAPILLOMA

Papillomas are rare benign neoplasms occurring within mammary ducts of middle-aged women. They present with a nipple discharge which may be bloody. The lesions are usually 5–10 mm in diameter and consist of fibrovascular cores covered with a double layer of epithelium. Those located centrally near the nipple are usually single. The more peripherally located lesions may be multiple, can show epithelial atypia and are associated with an increased predisposition to mammary carcinoma.

FIBROADENOMA

Fibroadeoma is a relatively common cause of a mobile mass in the breast of a young premenopausal woman. Fibroadenomas are usually solitary and less than 50 mm, but may occasionally be large or multiple. Their status as a neoplasm is questionable as there is proliferation of both stroma and epithelium (Figs 20.22 and 20.23) and they tend to regress with age. They do not predispose to subsequent carcinoma although very rarely the epithelial component may exhibit changes of carcinoma in situ, like that of normal breast epithelium.

PHYLLODES TUMOUR

Phyllodes tumours are reminiscent of fibroadenomas consisting of both stromal and epithelial components. They are rare tumours affecting middle-aged and elderly women, forming a mass which can grow rapidly to greater than 50 mm. Grossly, the lesion may be encapsulated and small papillary structures may just be visible.

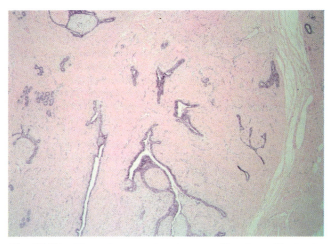
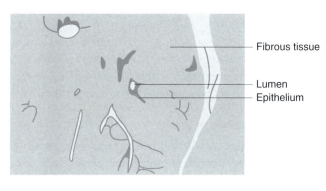

Fig. 20.22   Fibroadenoma showing a proliferation of both stroma and epithelium to form a well-circumscribed non-encapsulated mass.

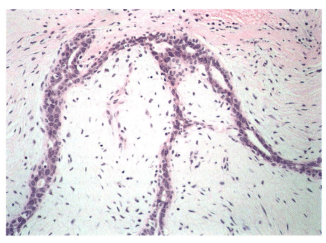
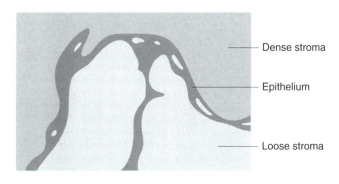

Fig. 20.23   The cellularity of the stroma in a fibroadenoma can vary considerably. Occasionally there is a florid proliferation of stroma resulting in compression, distortion and elongated ductal structures as seen here.

Microscopy shows a hypercellular stroma forming broad leaf-like structures projecting into clefts. The clefts and projections are lined by benign epithelial cells. The majority have a favourable outcome, although 10% of benign phyllodes tumours recur owing to incomplete excision. Malignant phyllodes tumours show stromal overgrowth relative to the epithelial component and a high stromal mitotic count. These malignant phyllodes tumours have a poor prognosis. The sarcomatous component metastasizes via the bloodstream, often to bone or lung. Lymph node involvement is rare.

Malignant neoplasia

CARCINOMA IN SITU

Carcinoma in situ is a term used to describe cytologically malignant epithelial cells which are still confined by their normal basement membrane. This term in many respects is a paradox, as the definition of carcinoma requires there to be a breach of the basement membrane by the malignant cells. Nevertheless, in the breast two forms of carcinoma in situ are recognized:

- **ductal** carcinoma in situ (DCIS)
- **lobular** carcinoma in situ (LCIS).

The former is more common than the latter, but our knowledge regarding the natural history and incidence of these conditions is limited. A postmortem study of young and middle-aged women dying from non-breast-related disease showed that 18% had in situ breast carcinomas (DCIS and LCIS). This suggests the premalignant phase of the disease is prolonged or that only some cases progress to invasive mammary carcinoma.

Ductal carcinoma in situ

DCIS is usually impalpable but can rarely present as a palpable solitary mass. It does, however, represent about 20% of mammographically detected malignancies. The malignant epithelial cells cause expansion of the mammary ducts but remain confined by the duct basement membrane. The disease is usually unicentric but can on occasion be extensive. Several different morphological subtypes of DCIS are recognized (Figs 20.24 and

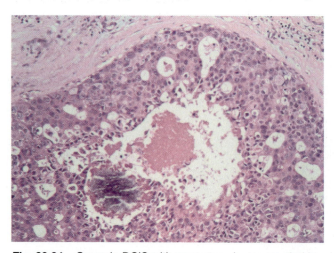
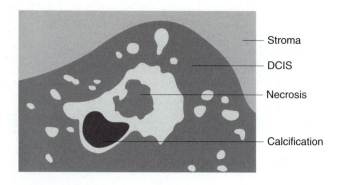

Stroma

DCIS

Necrosis

Calcification

Fig. 20.24   Comedo DCIS with mammary duct expanded by pleomorphic tumour cells exhibiting central necrosis. Note central granular calcification of necrotic debris.

remains stable, although substantial gains in the quality of life have been achieved. The exact aetiology of this disease remains to be established. Great advances in the pathogenesis of this disease at a molecular level have been made and the sequence of events involved in the development of breast carcinoma is beginning to unfold.

Research has shown abnormalities (such as breaks, deletions or point mutations) of chromosome 1, 3, 11, 13 and 17, but these are not recognized in every case of breast cancer. These genetic changes may account in part for the activation of oncogenes (for example *erb* B, *c-myc*, H-*ras*, *int2*), or the loss of tumour suppressor genes (retinoblastoma gene, *RB*) observed in many cases. Aberrant expression of these oncogenes leads to altered production of growth factors and their receptors (transforming growth factor-α and insulin-like growth factor, for example) and altered expression of nuclear proteins involved in cell cycle regulation such as p53.

There are a number of risk factors that predispose to the development of mammary carcinoma. These relate principally to reproductive and family history (see Table 20.1). Large breasts seem not to increase the risk of breast cancer, presumably because breast size is determined predominantly by the amount of adipose tissue. However, women with large breasts do tend to present with slightly larger tumours, as the tumours are more difficult to detect.

Presenting features

The incidence of breast cancer increases with increasing age and therefore is found most commonly in postmenopausal women. It is, however, not uncommon in women of reproductive age but is rare in women less than 25 years old. It commonly presents as a firm irregular lump. Tethering of the skin or to deeper fascial planes or pectoral muscles may be seen in advanced cases. Lymph nodes may be palpable if metastases have occurred. Up to 50% of tumours occur in the upper outer quadrant of the breast.

Types of invasive breast cancer

There are several different types of invasive mammary carcinoma which are classified histologically (Table 20.2). All probably start in the secretory unit as an area of ductal carcinoma in situ, although at the time of diagnosis this may not be evident as the invasive tumour may have overgrown the in situ component.

Fig. 20.29 Gross section of breast showing a firm mass with irregular crab-like extensions into the surrounding stroma. The lesion has a gritty 'unripe pear' texture on section. These appearances correspond to tumours with a high fibrous tissue content, such as invasive mammary carcinomas of no special histological type and lobular carcinomas.

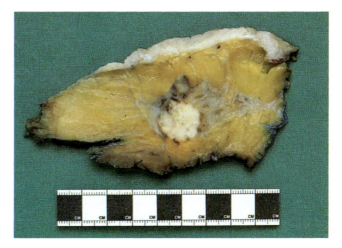

Table 20.2   Histological subtypes of invasive breast carcinoma presenting clinically

Infiltrating mammary carcinoma of no special histological type (Fig. 20.30)	80%
Lobular carcinoma (Fig. 20.31)	5%
Medullary carcinoma (Fig. 20.32)	2%
Tubular carcinoma	2%
Mucoid carcinoma (Fig. 20.33)	1%
Other	10%
In situ carcinomas	
Spindle/metaplastic carcinoma	
Apocrine	
Papillary	
Secretory	
Tubulolobular	
Adenocystic	
Metastatic tumours, e.g. gastric, lung	

The gross appearances depend predominantly on the amount of stromal fibrous tissue or mucin secretion rather than the epithelial (tumour) cell content. The majority are greater than 10 mm diameter by the time they are palpable and form hard irregular masses (see Fig. 20.29). A few tumours are soft and well demarcated and others may have a well-circumscribed glistening gelatinous cut surface due to extensive mucin production (**mucoid carcinoma**).

CASE STUDY 20.1

A 63-year-old women presented with a 6-week history of progressive thoracic back pain over 5 weeks. The pain was aggravated by movement and radiated around the lower chest towards her abdomen. Examination revealed a 50 mm firm irregular mass in the left breast with palpable axillary lymph nodes. There was no other significant past medical history. Urea electrolytes and liver function tests were normal. A chest radiograph revealed a lytic lesion with destruction of the tenth thoracic vertebra. An isotope bone scan showed no other lesions. Fine-needle aspirate of the breast mass revealed carcinoma cells. A diagnosis of metastatic mammary carcinoma was made. The woman was taken to theatre, the vertebral body decompressed and grafted with homologous bone. Histology confirmed the presence of a poorly differentiated mammary carcinoma of no special histological type. Postoperatively she was given tamoxifen and radiotherapy was given to the breast, axilla and spine. Five years later she presented with progressive continuous lower back pain. A full blood count showed a slight normochromic/normocytic anaemia and leukocytosis. Radiography of the lumber spine showed no apparent abnormality. A presumptive clinical diagnosis of metastatic mammary carcinoma was made. She was transferred to a terminal care ward where she died 3 weeks later. A postmortem examination was requested. This confirmed the presence of an invasive mammary carcinoma 35 mm in diameter in the left breast with lymph node involvement. Removal of the vertebral bodies showed no evidence of metastatic carcinoma either macroscopically or microscopically apart from histological foci in the tenth thoracic vertebrae. Examination of the renal system showed the right kidney to be swollen and congested with pus in the renal calyces. The postmortem examination showed death to be the result of acute pyelonephritis.

This case history shows that the clinical presumption of metastatic carcinoma in the absence of histological confirmation can be wrong and may on occasionally deny patients treatment of remedial conditions. (See section on death certification, Chapter 23.)

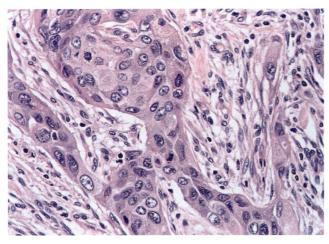
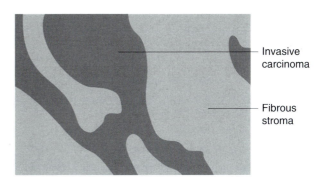

Invasive
carcinoma

Fibrous
stroma

Fig. 20.30   Invasive mammary carcinoma of no special histological type: the histological appearances vary considerably. In this view of a poorly differentiated carcinoma, atypical spheroidal epithelial cells infiltrate a fibrous stroma in sheets. There is a marked degree of cytological/nuclear pleomorphism and mitotic activity. Other tumours may show better formed acini (ducts/glands) and less pleomorphism or mitotic activity.

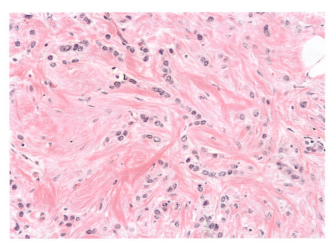
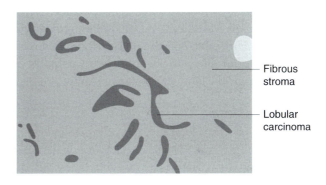

Fibrous
stroma

Lobular
carcinoma

Fig. 20.31   Infiltrating lobular carcinoma histologically consists of small uniform cells in a dense fibrous stroma, classically growing in single (Indian) file pattern as shown here. The malignant cells may also form concentric rings around established structures such as normal mammary ducts and vessels.

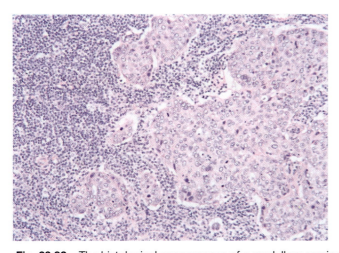
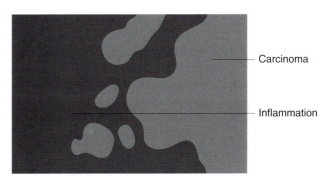

Carcinoma

Inflammation

Fig. 20.32   The histological appearances of a medullary carcinoma showing syncytial sheets of large pleomorphic epithelial cells with surrounding heavy lymphocytic infiltrate.

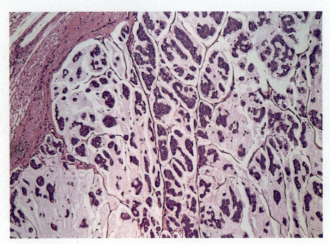
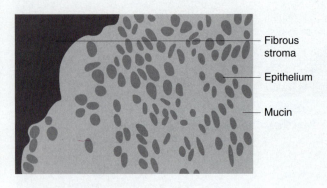

Fibrous stroma

Epithelium

Mucin

Fig. 20.33   A mucoid carcinoma with small groups of malignant epithelial cells in large pools of mucin.

Spread

Breast cancer is now regarded as a systemic disease, as patient outcome depends on the presence or absence of metastases at the time of diagnosis. Spread may occur locally by direct invasion of the chest wall or via lymphatics or the bloodstream. The axillary lymph nodes are more commonly involved than the internal mammary lymph nodes at the time of diagnosis. However, not all enlarged lymph nodes necessarily contain metastatic tumour; in up to 30% of cases of palpable axillary lymph nodes careful histological examination shows reactive changes only.

Prognostic factors

The rarer special histological types of breast cancer, such as mucoid and tubular carcinomas, are associated with an excellent prognosis. The outlook for the majority of breast cancer patients is less good and depends on the presence or absence of metastases at the time of diagnosis. This is, however, difficult to determine because micrometastases may remain occult for 20 years or more before becoming clinically evident. There are, however, a number of parameters (for example lymph node status, tumour grade and diameter – see Table 20.3) which can give a guide to likely patient survival, and these may be of value in deciding patient management. Tumour grade for infiltrating mammary carcinomas of no special histological type is determined by applying a score to the degree of nuclear pleomorphism, tubule formation and mitotic rate. Grade 1 tumours are well differentiated, grade 2 moderately differentiated and grade 3 poorly differentiated. Tumour oestrogen receptor status is also of prognostic value and provides a guide to treatment with hormonal therapy. Of all the different prognostic factors axillary lymph node status is the single most important factor. The more lymph nodes involved, the poorer the prognosis.

MANAGEMENT OPTIONS OF A WOMAN WITH A BREAST LUMP

For a woman to find a breast lump is a traumatic event. This needs to be handled with understanding and compassion by the clinician. Sometimes careful examination will, in fact, reveal no lump and the woman can be reassured. In others, the presence of a lump will be confirmed. As always, a complete history is important. Simple cysts can be treated by fine-needle aspiration. If a mass remains after draining, or the cyst fluid is blood-

---

The most common sites of spread of breast cancer
- Regional lymph nodes
- Bone
- Liver
- Lungs
- Brain

Table 20.3   Prognosis factors and survival rates

Prognosis factors	Proportion of patients surviving 5 years (%)
Axillary lymph node	
Histologically negative nodes	90
1 positive node	75
5 positive nodes	20
Tumour grade	
Grade 1	85
Grade 2	60
Grade 3	40
Tumour diameter	
< 20 mm	75
< 40 mm	60
< 60 mm	35

Hormone receptors and breast cancer

Breast carcinoma cells may (like normal mammary epithelial cells) contain oestrogen receptors. Activation of these receptors by oestrogen is thought to result in nuclear processing with the production of mRNAs responsible for progesterone receptors and growth factors. Oestrogen receptor-positive tumours have a better prognosis than oestrogen receptor-negative tumours, the receptor protein being a marker of tumour differentiation. Tamoxifen acts partly by an antioestrogen effect blocking oestrogen receptors. This relatively non-toxic drug has been shown to improve the survival of breast cancer patients, particularly those with oestrogen receptor-positive tumours. However, some patients with oestrogen receptor-negative tumours have also been found to benefit.

stained, further investigation is required. As a general rule all breast lumps should be investigated. The management of these cases can be assisted by fine-needle aspiration (Figs 20.34 and 20.35) and imaging techniques (mammography and ultrasonography). If the lesion is thought to be benign by clinical examination, cytology and imaging, the lump may be left and observed. If the findings are equivocal, there may be a lumpectomy. If the findings indicate a malignant tumour, the doctor and patient can jointly decide the best method of management before definitive treatment.

Mastectomy is performed less often today: there is an increasing tendency to treat early breast cancer by lumpectomy and radiotherapy accompanied

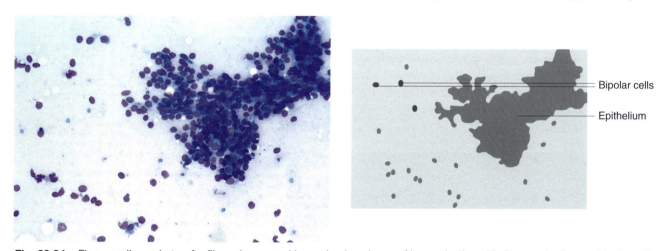

Fig. 20.34 Fine-needle aspirate of a fibroadenoma with a cohesive clump of hyperplastic epithelium and adjacent bipolar cells thought to be of myoepithelial origin (Giemsa stain).

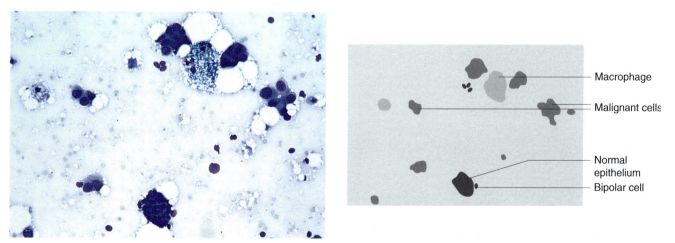

Fig. 20.35 Fine-needle aspirate of a breast carcinoma with discohesive pleomorphic carcinoma cells. Also present is a clump of normal breast epithelium and a foamy macrophage (Giemsa stain).

usually with axillary lymph node sampling. Recent studies have shown that survival is comparable for women treated with lumpectomy and radiotherapy as with mastectomy. **Early breast cancer** is a clinical term given to a tumour which is apparently operable without evidence of locally advanced disease (skin ulceration or systemic metastases, for example). Axillary lymph nodes may be palpable. The prognostic information derived from the histological examination of the tumour and lymph nodes allows planning of adjuvant therapy. This may include radiotherapy and/or chemotherapy. **Tamoxifen**, a well-tolerated antioestrogen, has also been shown to improve the survival of breast cancer patients, particularly postmenopausal women.

Differential diagnosis of breast lump
- Benign mastopathy
- Fat necrosis
- Fibroadenoma
- Carcinoma

Breast cancer screening

Several studies have shown that the smaller a breast tumour is when detected, the better the prognosis. It follows that, if it were possible to detect the tumour at a preclinical stage (when the lesion is impalpable), prognosis may be enhanced. Advances in radiology have now made this a practical proposition. Mammography can now be used to detect microcalcification (Fig. 20.36) or parenchymal changes associated with tumours. Thus in the late 1980s a breast-screening programme was instituted in the UK for women aged aged 50–64 years. Similar programmes in the USA and Sweden have shown that up to a 30% reduction in mortality over 5–8 years in women screened can be expected. Screening will not necessarily reduce mortality dramatically because, although the screening process in part detects lethal tumours sooner (**lead-time bias**), more non-lethal, slowly growing tumours will be detected during the same period (**length–time bias**). Furthermore there is the possibility that those patients most at risk do not participate in the programme (**selection bias**).

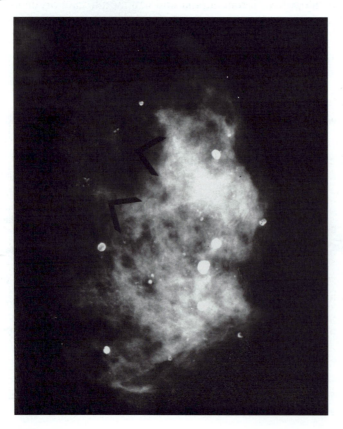

Fig. 20.36 Mammogram showing large rounded masses of benign calcification and areas of fine irregular microcalcification of a type associated with malignancy. (Courtesy of Dr M. Creagh-Barry, Poole General Hospital.)

In the UK the screening programme is run by a specialist team of radiologists, surgeons and pathologists. Women aged 50–64 years are called on a 3-yearly cycle for a mammogram. A small proportion (5–10%) of women require to be recalled due to an abnormality detected in the preliminary mammogram. Further assessment would include detailed clinical examination, and further mammography possibly with ultrasonography and fine-needle aspiration. Depending on the findings most women can be reassured. A few women (1% of total screened) following assessment may have a lesion suspicious of malignancy and require a biopsy. For impalpable lesions a radiologically guided wire may be inserted into the breast lesion immediately before the operation. This enables the surgeon to localize the area to be removed at surgery.

Approximately 50% of patients requiring a biopsy will be found to have a malignancy. The other patients will be found to have benign lesions, for example benign mastopathy, radial scars, involuted fibroadenomas, etc. The frequency of the different types of malignant lesions is different from those found in the symptomatic patients. There is an increased frequency of DCIS and well-differentiated invasive carcinomas, for example tubular carcinoma.

Other neoplasms

Other rare benign and malignant neoplasms of the breast occur. A few examples include fibroma, fibrosarcoma, angioma, angiosarcoma, lipoma and lymphoma.

The male breast

Benign mastopathy, fibroadenoma and carcinoma may occur in the male breast but are much less common than in women. Indeed, carcinoma in a male breast accounts for about 1% of all breast carcinomas. This is perhaps due to the smaller amount of duct epithelium present in male breasts capable of undergoing transformation.

Gynaecomastia

Gynaecomastia is the term given to the relatively common condition of male breast hypertrophy. This is a benign condition which may be unilateral or bilateral. It occurs as a result of raised oestrogen levels, for example, hormonal therapy in carcinoma of the prostate or in chronic liver failure where there is reduced breakdown of endogenous oestrogens. It may also be idiopathic in peripubertal boys. Some drugs with a steroid nucleus, such as digitalis or spironolactone, may also induce gynaecomastia. Histologically there is an increase in both the fibrous stroma and ducts. The ducts may also show some ductal epithelial hyperplasia.

Chapter 21   Lymphoid disease

Learning objectives

To appreciate and understand:
❏ Alterations in lymphoid system structure and function in disease
❏ Pathology of reactive changes in lymphoid tissues and the relationship to immune responses
❏ Major types of Hodgkin's and non-Hodgkin's lymphoma
❏ Relationship between 'lymphoma' and 'leukaemia'

The lymphoid system

The lymphoid system is composed of specific cells diffusely distributed and organized in recognizable organs throughout the body. The physiological functions of the system are concerned with immune defence and are dealt with in Chapter 6.

The constituent cells are predominantly bone marrow derived, but modified vascular endothelium and the specialized epithelia in the thymus and mucosa-associated lymphoid tissue, together with the fibroblasts responsible for the stromal framework, are also integral parts of the immune system.

The **central lymphoid tissues of bone marrow and thymus** are concerned with the production of **B-** and **T-cell lymphoid precursors** in their antigen-independent phase. The bone marrow is also responsible for the production of haemopoietic cells and monocyte precursors of the histiocyte/macrophage system.

The **peripheral lymphoid tissues** provide a home for the immunocompetent products of the bone marrow and thymus and are concerned with the response to antigenic stimulation. Many types of lymphoid cells are in constant recirculation in the blood and lymph, and hence physiological and neoplastic proliferation often involves both central and peripheral lymphoid tissues.

Understanding the structure and function of lymphoid tissue in some organs is incomplete. 'Skin-associated lymphoid tissue' and other secondary lymphoid tissues await better understanding in the future.

The changes that take place in lymphoid tissues in physiological responses and neoplastic proliferations involve all cell types to a greater or lesser degree and produce the recognizable functional and structural abnormalities which are the subject of this chapter.

The main lymphoid organs
■ Central/primary lymphoid tissue
  ● Bone marrow
  ● Thymus
■ Peripheral/secondary lymphoid tissue
  ● Lymph nodes
  ● Spleen
  ● Mucosa-associated lymphoid tissue (MALT)
  ● Skin-associated lymphoid tissue

The main cell types of lymphoid organs
● Lymphocytes of B- and T-cell types
● Tissue histiocytes and phagocytic macrophages
● Accessory cells including follicular dendritic cells and interdigitating dendritic cells
● Cells of the granulocyte series

Fig. 21.1 Normal haemopoiesis and lymphopoiesis. A large increase in cell numbers takes place at each stage.

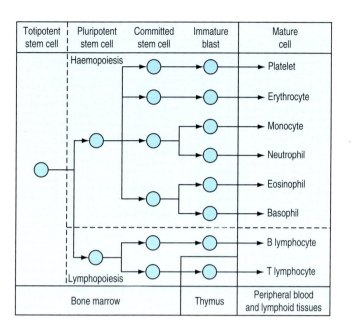

Totipotent stem cell	Pluripotent stem cell	Committed stem cell	Immature blast	Mature cell
	Haemopoiesis			Platelet
				Erythrocyte
				Monocyte
				Neutrophil
				Eosinophil
				Basophil
				B lymphocyte
	Lymphopoiesis			T lymphocyte
	Bone marrow		Thymus	Peripheral blood and lymphoid tissues

Normal structure and function

Bone marrow

In the adult, haemopoietically active bone marrow is largely confined to the axial skeleton and proximal femora (Fig. 21.1). In infants and young children, marrow in the long bones of the limbs is similarly active and may become functional again in adult life in conditions of reactive hyperplasia. In the fetus, liver and spleen are also major haemopoietic organs. In adult life, in cases of reactive hyperplasia and primary or secondary neoplasia of the bone marrow, haemopoiesis may take place in liver, spleen, lymph nodes and even soft tissues, where it is termed **extramedullary haemopoiesis**.

Production of mature circulating blood cells begins with a **totipotent stem cell** which gives rise to increasingly committed **progenitor cells** which finally become **mature cells** that enter the peripheral blood. B lymphocytes are derived from the bone marrow directly, whereas T lymphocytes require a period of maturation in the thymus. These antigenically independent lymphocytes subsequently enter peripheral lymphoid tissues where, on exposure to antigenic stimulation, they undergo further maturation.

Lymph nodes

Lymph nodes (Fig. 21.2) are the most intensively studied and the most biopsied part of the peripheral lymphoid system. Much of the nomenclature of normal and abnormal structure and function is based on nodal lymphoid tissue.

Resting lymph nodes are small, usually impalpable structures which are widely distributed but are concentrated in certain clinically important anatomical regions such as the neck, axilla, groin and retroperitoneum. When antigenically stimulated or involved by infection or malignancy, lymph nodes enlarge, sometimes massively, and become clinically

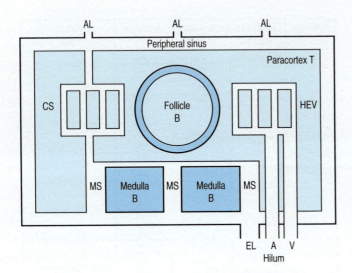

Fig. 21.2 Lymph node. AL, afferent lymphatic; EL, efferent lymphatic; A, artery; V, vein; HEV, high endothelial venules; CS, cortical sinus; MS, medullary sinus; B, B-cell area; T, T-cell area.

palpable. Enlargement may be localized, in which case the anatomical site may suggest the source of infection or primary malignancy, or generalized in which case additional aetiological factors must be considered.

The structure of the lymph node is fully developed only when exposed to antigenic stimulation and the conventional description of normal microanatomy refers to such a node.

The lymph node is bounded by a thin fibrous **capsule** which is penetrated on the cortical side by afferent lymphatics and at the hilum by an efferent lymphatic, artery and vein. From the capsule a network of fibrous **trabeculae** traverses the node, forming a fine mesh of collagen fibres which support the other parts of the node and play a role in the traffic of cells within the node.

The afferent lymphatics join the **peripheral sinus** which gives off numerous branches that divide to form the labyrinthine **cortical sinusoidal network** and then coalesce to form the **medullary sinuses** which drain into the efferent lymphatic. The sinuses are lined by specialized **sinus lining cells** which have both endothelial and phagocytic functions. These cells divide the sinusoidal compartment from the interstitial compartment and are responsible for regulating cell traffic, as well as the passage of antigens, antibodies and interleukins between the two compartments. Resident phagocytic macrophages within the sinuses play a major role in the filtering of micro-organisms and particulate matter from the lymph.

The nodal artery enters at the hilum and divides into arterioles and finally into a rich capillary network which extends throughout the node. The capillaries coalesce in the paracortex to form postcapillary venules known as **high endothelial venules** after their plump cuboidal endothelium. These join into larger venules and leave the node as the nodal vein. The vascular compartment is separated from the interstitium by endothelium. The specialized endothelium of the high endothelial venules regulates the traffic of lymphocytes between node and blood.

The interstitial compartment is divided into a superficial **cortex**, deeper **paracortex** and **medulla**. The immune response is the result of complex collaboration and hence the three distinct areas of the interstitium contain a mixture of cell types. However, the cortex is primarily concerned with the B-cell response while the paracortex is primarily a T-cell area. The medulla is the site of plasma cell reaction and antibody production.

The main compartments of a lymph node
■ Sinusoidal system
■ Arteriovenous system
■ Extravascular interstitium, which is further divided into:
  ● Cortex or lymphoid follicles
  ● Paracortex
  ● Medulla

The cortex is distributed as multiple discrete **primary** or **secondary follicles**. In unstimulated nodes the primary follicle is an inconspicuous structure composed of an aggregate of small lymphocytes. After antigenic stimulation, the secondary follicle becomes a prominent structure composed of a **germinal centre** surrounded by a thin **mantle zone** composed of small lymphocytes of various types. The germinal centre predominantly contains **centroblasts** and **centrocytes**, the former giving rise to the latter. **Phagocytic macrophages**, which are responsible for removing apoptotic cell debris, and **follicular dendritic cells**, which are responsible for presenting antigen to follicular B cells, are the accessory cells of the follicle.

The other B-cell area is found in the medulla, which is the main nodal site of plasma cell production. Under antigenic stimulation small lymphocytes transform into B immunoblasts which give rise to mature immunoglobulin-secreting plasma cells.

The paracortex lies between the follicles and contains the high endothelial venules. Under antigenic stimulation small T lymphocytes transform into T immunoblasts which in turn give rise to small immunocompetent T lymphocytes. Interdigitating reticulum cells are the major accessory cells of the paracortex. They are closely related to the Langerhans' cells of the skin and present antigen to T lymphocytes.

Mucosa-associated lymphoid tissue

Mucosa-associated lymphoid tissue (MALT) (Fig. 21.3) refers to the specialized lymphoid defences of mucosal tissues. The gastrointestinal tract has been most intensively studied and the **Peyer's patches** of the ileum provide the model for the system.

A large amount of lymphoid tissue is present in the gastrointestinal tract with the exception of the normal stomach. It is diffusely distributed throughout and organized into nodules in the ileum, appendix and distal

---

MALT tissues
- Gastrointestinal tract
- Salivary and lacrimal glands
- Respiratory tract
- Genitourinary tract

Fig. 21.3 Normal Peyer's patch. L, lymphatic; A, artery; V, vein; HEV, high endothelial venules; C, capillary network; B, B-cell area; T, T-cell area.

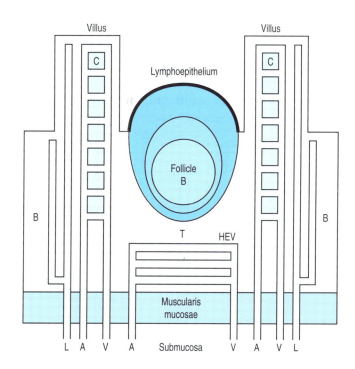

colon. The foremost function of this MALT is the defence of the body from the external environment, and lymphocytes consequently exist in intimate relationship with epithelium.

The normal Peyer's patch consists of a lymphoid follicle composed of a **germinal centre** and **mantle zone** similar to a lymph node but additionally has a well-developed **marginal zone**, similar to the white pulp of the spleen. The marginal zone is closely applied to the overlying specialized intestinal epithelium, termed **lymphoepithelium**, and **intraepithelial B lymphocytes** derived from the marginal zone are distributed within the lymphoepithelium. **Intraepithelial T lymphocytes** are distributed in the epithelium of the crypts and villi. The zone between the follicle and muscularis mucosae contains venules of high endothelial type and a mainly T-lymphocyte population, thus corresponding to the paracortex of the lymph node. The villi and the remainder of the lamina propria contain lymphatics and numerous plasma cells, thus corresponding to the medulla of the lymph node.

MALT operates as a linked system and immunity generated in one part of the system is shared with other organs by circulation of lymphoid cells capable of recognizing either the endothelium of the mucosal vessels by means of molecules termed vascular addressins or the epithelium by means of chemotactic factors. Antigen in the gut lumen is transported across the lymphoepithelium into the germinal centres of the Peyer's patch to generate dividing cells which enter the bloodstream via the mesenteric lymph nodes and thoracic duct. Maturation takes place, possibly in the spleen, and the activated lymphoid cells home to mucosal surfaces throughout the body where they develop into IgA-secreting plasma cells.

The spleen

The normal adult spleen weighs approximately 100–200 g and lies between the systemic and portal circulations. Lymph nodes filter lymph: the spleen filters blood and plays a physiological role in phagocytosis of effete red blood cells, micro-organisms and foreign materials (Fig. 21.4).

The splenic artery enters at the hilum and, accompanied by radicles of the splenic vein and lymphatics, branches widely, surrounded by a cuff of collagen. Arteries divide to form arterioles which are surrounded by lymphoid tissue known as the **white pulp**. The splenic capillaries divide

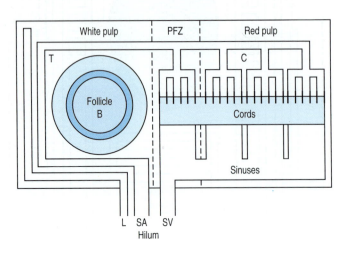

Fig. 21.4 Normal spleen. L, lymphatic; SA, splenic artery; SV, splenic vein; C, capillaries; PFZ, perifollicular zone; B, B-cell area; T, T-cell area.

within the **red pulp** and lose their endothelium to form highly specialized structures, the sheathed capillaries in which the endothelium is replaced by a sheath of phagocytic macrophages through which blood must pass en route to the sinuses. There is no direct connection with the sinuses and blood must traverse the connective tissues of the **splenic cords** before passing through slits in the sinusoidal basement membrane and the specialized sinusoidal endothelium which is related to the high endothelial venules of the lymph nodes. The sinuses coalesce to form the splenic vein which enters the portal circulation, thereby providing easy access to the liver for metabolic breakdown products and lymphocytes. Lymphatics arise in the T-lymphocyte area of the white pulp and accompany the splenic vessels to the hilum.

The **perifollicular zone** resembles the red pulp but has a more dilated sinusoidal network. It may be responsible for the slow circulation of approximately 10% of the splenic blood flow. The red pulp comprises 75% of the splenic volume, the perifollicular zone 10% and the white pulp the remainder.

The splenic lymphoid tissue is found in the white pulp where it is divided into a **periarteriolar T-cell predominant area**, corresponding to the paracortex of lymph nodes, and **B-cell predominant follicles**. The follicles have a germinal centre and mantle zone equivalent to lymph node follicles but additionally the mantle is surrounded by a **marginal zone** of medium-sized lymphocytes with abundant cytoplasm, related to cells found in ileal Peyer's patches. A less well defined but quantitatively equivalent population of B and T lymphocytes is distributed in the red pulp and perifollicular zone and may correspond to the medulla of lymph nodes.

Thymus

The thymus is composed of intimately related epithelial and lymphoid elements which collaborate principally in the maturation of T lymphocytes which have undergone partial maturation in the bone marrow (Fig. 21.5).

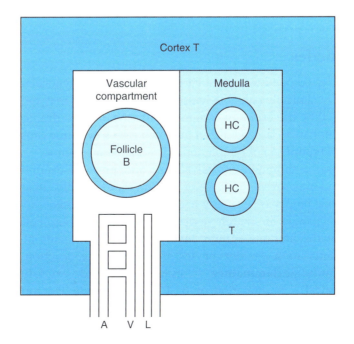

Fig. 21.5 Normal thymus. L, lymphatic; A, artery; V, vein; HC, Hassall's corpuscle; B, B-cell area; T, T-cell area.

Embryologically, the thymus is derived from the third and fourth pharyngeal pouches and contains derivatives of all three germ layers. The thymic primordia migrate caudally and fuse in the midline to occupy their final position in the anterior mediastinum.

Lymphocytes from the fetal liver and bone marrow colonize the organ which develops a **cortex** and **medulla**. Small medullary epithelial tubes differentiate into **Hassall's corpuscles**. The thymus enlarges until puberty after which time it involutes, persisting in an atrophic state into old age.

The thymus is composed of lobules divided into cortex and medulla. The cortex is composed of densely packed lymphocytes in a network of **thymic epithelial cells** whereas in the medulla lymphocytes are less numerous and epithelium more prominent. **Hassall's corpuscles** are found in the medulla and are made up of concentrically keratinized epithelium. The thymic vessels penetrate the capsule and are accompanied by connective tissue ensheathed by thymic epithelial cells, forming a functional vascular compartment.

In the thymus, in both cortex and medulla, T lymphocytes predominate and mature from a small population of **large subcapsular thymocytes**, derived from bone marrow derived **prothymocytes**, via medium-sized **cortical thymocytes** to **small medullary thymocytes**. In the vascular compartment B lymphocytes are found as **germinal centres** within the perivascular connective tissue in a medullary location. They are also found as **isolated perivascular B lymphocytes** in both cortex and medulla. A distinct population of activated B lymphocytes has been identified around Hassall's corpuscles. Other cell populations include **cortical macrophages**, **Langerhans' cells**, **neuroendocrine cells** and **germ cells**.

The thymus varies markedly in structure with age. The maximum weight occurs at puberty. Thereafter, germinal centres become less numerous and gradually both epithelial and lymphocytic components undergo involution until eventually the thymus is composed largely of fat with only a few remaining lymphoid aggregates.

Reactive changes

Lymph nodes

Lymph nodes respond to a wide variety of stimuli by **hyperplasia** which may result in clinically palpable **lymphadenopathy**. This may be localized, suggesting that the stimulus originated in the tissues drained by the afferent lymphatics, or generalized in which case a systemic cause may be suspected. **Hypoplasia** of lymph nodes is much less common.

In all cases a thorough clinical history and physical examination are essential and may reveal the cause of the lymphadenopathy. In some cases a lymph node biopsy is necessary to establish the diagnosis.

Reactive changes in lymph nodes invoke the complex collaborative response of the immune system, involving the constituents of all three compartments to a greater or lesser extent. The reaction may be predominantly **inflammatory** – hyperaemia and exudation – or **immunological** – proliferation of B, T and histiocyte/macrophage cell lines. In certain diseases particular reactions predominate, resulting in recognizable patterns which have diagnostic importance (Fig. 21.6).

Causes of lymphadenopathy
- Infection and infestation
- Connective tissue/autoimmune diseases
- Reaction to foreign material
- Reaction to drugs
- Immunodeficiency
- Primary neoplasia
- Metastatic neoplasms
- Idiopathic

Fig. 21.6 The different patterns of reaction in lymph nodes: (a) unstimulated lymph node; (b) sinus hyperplasia; (c) follicular and medullary hyperplasia; (d) paracortical hyperplasia; (e) granulomatous lymphadenopathy; (f) necrotizing lymphadenopathy. F, follicle; G, granuloma; N, necrosis.

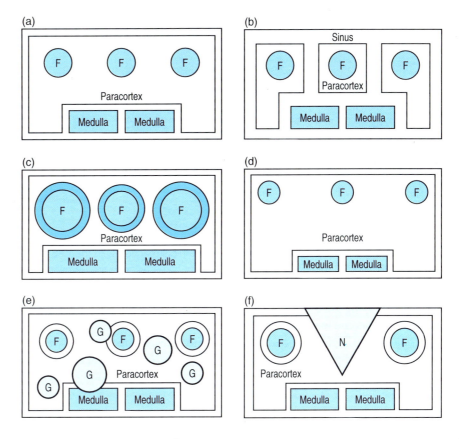

ACUTE LYMPHADENITIS

In lymph nodes draining sites of pyogenic infections and ulcerated lesion of the gut, inflammatory changes predominate – **acute lymphadenitis**. The sinuses are dilated and filled with protein-rich lymph, neutrophil granulocytes and macrophages. Nodal blood vessels are dilated. The inflammation may spill out into surrounding tissues and, particularly in the case of staphylococcal infection, the node may be destroyed, resulting in abscess formation.

FOLLICULAR HYPERPLASIA

As the B-cell immune response develops, primary follicles are converted to secondary follicles with active germinal centres. Although usually

Causes of follicular hyperplasia
- Bacterial infections
- Viral infections
- Rheumatoid arthritis

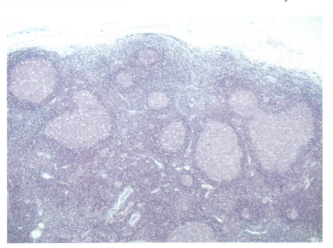

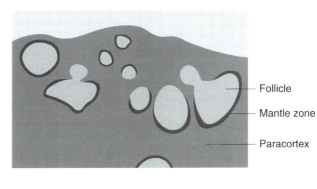

Follicle

Mantle zone

Paracortex

Fig. 21.7 Follicular hyperplasia: multiple follicles of different shapes and sizes are seen.

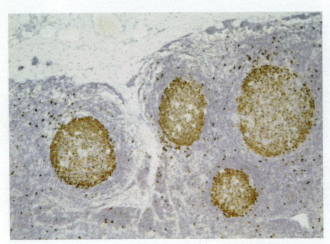
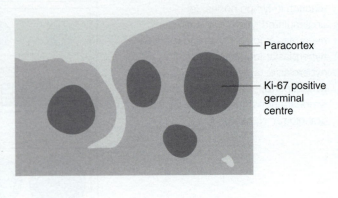

Paracortex

Ki-67 positive
germinal
centre

Fig. 21.8 Follicular hyperplasia: immunocytochemical reaction with the Ki-67 antibody directed against an antigen present in dividing cells, shows that most proliferative activity takes place in the germinal centre.

associated with medullary and paracortical reaction, the hyperplastic follicles may come to dominate the lymph node to such an extent that other components are overwhelmed (Figs 21.7 and 21.8). While in some cases the cause may be obvious, such as cervical lymphadenopathy accompanying acute bacterial tonsillitis, in others the exact cause may never be determined.

MEDULLARY HYPERPLASIA

Proliferation of plasma cells in the medullary cords usually accompanies follicular hyperplasia but in some cases of the B-cell response, plasma cells may dominate the node. The causes are the same as for follicular hyperplasia.

PARACORTICAL HYPERPLASIA

In certain conditions, the paracortex undergoes expansion at the expense of the other compartments. A characteristic diffuse proliferation of T immunoblasts, interdigitating dendritic cells and high endothelial venules distinguishes paracortical hyperplasia from follicular hyperplasia.

Dermatopathic lymphadenopathy occurs in chronic inflammatory skin diseases. The paracortex contains numerous interdigitating dendritic cells, possibly derived from cutaneous Langerhans' cells which have arrived from the inflamed skin via afferent lymphatics, together with macrophages containing lipid and melanin produced by the breakdown of epidermal cells.

SINUS HYPERPLASIA

Lymph nodes draining inflammatory and neoplastic lesions frequently undergo hyperplasia of the sinus lining cells which, together with resident histiocytes, fill and expand the sinuses (Fig. 21.9).

GRANULOMATOUS LYMPHADENOPATHY

The **histiocytic reaction** may result in the formation of granulomata which may be few in number and associated with other patterns of reaction or numerous enough to replace the whole lymph node. Multinucleate giant cells develop in many cases and necrosis may supervene. Later, healing by fibrosis with superimposed calcification may occur (Fig. 21.10).

Causes of paracortical hyperplasia
- Viral infections, particularly herpes group
- Drug hypersensitivity reactions, particularly anticonvulsants
- Dermatopathic lymphadenopathy

Causes of granulomata in lymph nodes
- Infections
  - Mycobacteria
  - Toxoplasmosis
  - Fungi
- Sarcoidosis
- Foreign body reaction
  - Inhaled/injected material
  - Prostheses
- Reaction to carcinoma

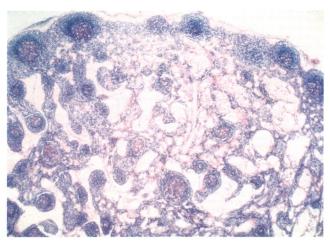

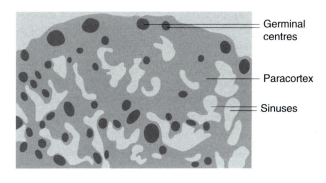

Germinal
centres

Paracortex

Sinuses

Fig. 21.9   Sinus hyperplasia: an abdominal lymph node showing expansion of the peripheral and cortical sinus network.

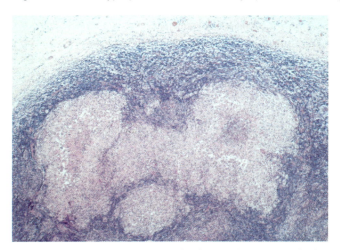

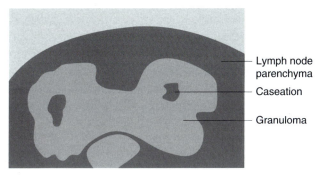

Lymph node
parenchyma

Caseation

Granuloma

Fig. 21.10   Granulomatous lymphadenopathy: a case of tuberculosis showing granulomata, some exhibiting caseous necrosis.

**Causes of necrotizing
lymphadenopathy**

■ Infections
  ● *Mycobacterium
    tuberculosis*
  ● Yersiniae
  ● Cat-scratch disease
  ● Lymphogranuloma
    venereum
■ Other causes
  ● Drug hypersensitivity
    reactions
  ● Systemic lupus
    erythematosus
  ● Idiopathic – Kikuchi's
    disease

NECROTIZING LYMPHADENOPATHY

In certain conditions, necrosis of parts of the lymph node associated with a histiocytic or neutrophilic reaction occurs.

IMMUNODEFICIENCY

Deficiency or suppression of lymph node function is less common than hyperplasia and is seldom a cause for biopsy. In **congenital combined immunodeficiency** and following radiotherapy there is pronounced hypoplasia of the lymphoid compartments of the nodes, leaving largely the vascular and connective tissue framework. When either B- or T-cell function is selectively deficient in **congenital immunodeficiency** or HIV infection, the corresponding zones of the node are hypoplastic. Immunodeficient patients are prone to infections, frequently due to unusual opportunistic organisms, and consequently the zones which retain function may undergo hyperplasia in response. Somewhat paradoxically, therefore, immunodeficient patients may present with lymph node enlargement in the early stages of the disease.

Immunosuppression following HIV infection and organ transplantation is associated with a high incidence of Epstein–Barr virus infection. Despite defective immune function, a vigorous B-cell reaction follows which may progress through **polyclonal** and **oligoclonal** stages to **monoclonal lymphoma**.

CASE STUDY 21.1

A 25-year-old man presented to his general practitioner complaining of headaches and malaise. Physical examination revealed a group of enlarged, firm lymph nodes in the left cervical region. The rest of the physical examination was normal. A full blood count revealed a mild leukocytosis. The clinical differential diagnosis was: lymphoma; metastatic carcinoma; or infection.

Metastatic carcinoma is unusual in younger age groups, and lymphoma – probably Hodgkin's disease – was considered to be most likely. A lymph node biopsy was performed to establish a diagnosis. Part of the node was submitted for histopathological analysis and part for microbiological culture. Microscopic examination of the node showed marked follicular hyperplasia with small clusters of histiocytes and poorly formed granulomata located in both cortex and paracortex (Fig. 21.11). Caseous necrosis of the granulomata was absent and only very occasional multinucleated giant cells were present. Culture of the node for bacterial infection was negative. The differential diagnosis of granulomatous lymphadenopathy in this patient was considered to be:

- tuberculosis
- sarcoidosis
- infectious mononucleosis
- toxoplasmosis

- syphilis
- brucellosis
- leishmaniasis.

Tuberculosis and sarcoidosis were excluded because the granulomata in these conditions are generally much larger, show caseous necrosis in the case of tuberculosis and are not associated with follicular hyperplasia. There was no history of exposure to syphilis, brucellosis or leishmaniasis, and toxoplasmosis was considered most likely on the basis of the microscopic appearances of the lymph node, with infectious mononucleosis a much less likely alternative.

Serological tests were compatible with past infection with Epstein–Barr virus but positive at higher titres for *Toxoplasma gondii*. The histopathological diagnosis of toxoplasmosis was thus confirmed. The patient had already begun to show symptomatic improvement and no treatment was considered necessary. The source of the infection was thought to be a recently acquired domestic cat, but ingestion of contaminated meat could not be excluded.

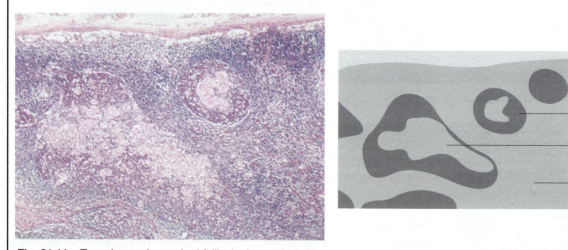

— Capsule

— Follicle

— Granuloma

— Paracortex

Fig. 21.11   Toxoplasmosis: marked follicular hyperplasia is accompanied by clusters of small, non-caseating granulomata.

Spleen

Enlargement of the spleen is usually a manifestation of systemic disease; primary splenic disease is rare. There are numerous causes of splenomegaly. However, unlike lymph nodes, the spleen is infrequently biopsied and the diagnosis is usually made by other investigations.

Enlargement of the spleen may result in increased destruction of blood cells within the expanded red pulp. The resulting syndrome of pancytopenia and compensatory bone marrow hyperplasia is termed **hypersplenism**. Atrophy or surgical removal results in failure of the spleen's role in red cell physiology. Red cells with characteristic abnormalities appear in the

Causes of deficient lymph node function
- Congenital defects of immunity
- Chemotherapy
- Radiotherapy
- HIV infection

Causes of splenomegaly

■ Infection and infestation
- ● Malaria
- ● Infectious mononucleosis
- ● Typhoid fever
- ● Tuberculosis
- ● Leishmaniasis, etc.

■ Sarcoidosis
■ Autoimmune/connective tissue diseases
■ Storage diseases
■ Amyloidosis
■ Congestion
■ Disorders of haemopoiesis
■ Lymphoma and leukaemia
■ Idiopathic

Causes of follicular hyperplasia in the spleen

- ● Bacterial infections
- ● Viral infections
- ● Rheumatoid arthritis
- ● Haemodialysis
- ● Autoimmune cytopenias

Causes of congestive splenomegaly

- ● Hepatic cirrhosis
- ● Hepatic veno-occlusive disease
- ● Portal vein thrombosis
- ● Congestive cardiac failure

Abnormalities of red blood cells with splenic destruction

- ● Congenital red cell disorders
- ● Haemoglobinopathies
- ● Autoimmune cytopenias
- ● Malaria

peripheral blood – this is known as **hyposplenism**. Patients are also prone to overwhelming infections, particularly by pneumococci. As with lymphadenopathy, the causes of splenomegaly may be considered in functional terms.

ACUTE SPLENITIS

During **acute septicaemic illnesses**, especially typhoid fever, lobar pneumonia and pyogenic bacterial infections, the spleen may enlarge to two or three times its normal size. There is marked congestion of the red pulp, infiltration of neutrophils, and phagocytosis of cell debris and bacteria by cordal macrophages. Staphylococcal septicaemia may lead to frank abscess formation.

FOLLICULAR HYPERPLASIA

Active germinal centres are normally present in children and adolescents. In adults, prominent follicular hyperplasia, frequently accompanied by plasmacytosis, may result in splenomegaly and hypersplenism.

DIFFUSE LYMPHOID HYPERPLASIA

Clinically apparent hyperplasia of the T-cell-predominant periarteriolar lymphoid tissue, corresponding to the paracortex in lymph nodes, is uncommon. However, it is an important feature of infectious mononucleosis where the proliferation of T cells, and numerous immunoblasts, extending into the red pulp is associated with spontaneous rupture of the spleen with consequent life-threatening haemorrhage.

CONGESTIVE SPLENOMEGALY

Splenic venous hypertension, transmitted back through dilated sinuses to the splenic cords, results in proliferation of cordal macrophages, followed by fibrosis. The consequent impediment to red cell circulation may result in hypersplenism. The spleen is typically firm and may become very large.

DISORDERS OF HAEMOPOIESIS

The spleen is largely responsible for the destruction of abnormal blood cells which accumulate in the congested cords, the sinuses being more or less empty in contrast to venous congestion. Both cordal macrophages and sinus lining cells are hyperplastic (Fig. 21.12).

In **myeloproliferative disorders** and destruction of the bone marrow, **extramedullary haemopoiesis** may occur in both cords and sinuses (Fig. 21.13).

GRANULOMATOUS SPLENOPATHY

There are numerous causes of **granuloma** formation in the spleen. Many are part of systemic disease and a few present with splenomegaly. The most important are disseminated infections with mycobacteria or fungi, and sarcoidosis (Fig. 21.14).

Diffuse proliferation of cordal macrophages also occurs as part of systemic disease. Splenomegaly and hypersplenism are typical in leishmaniasis, the viral haemophagocytic syndromes and inherited storage diseases.

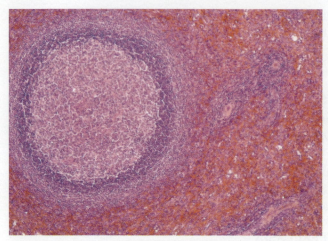

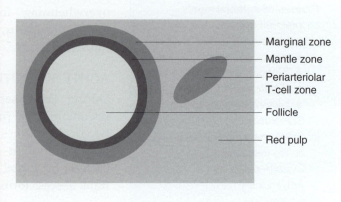

Marginal zone
Mantle zone
Periarteriolar T-cell zone
Follicle
Red pulp

Fig. 21.12   The spleen in hereditary spherocytosis: the lymphoid follicles are divided into a germinal centre, mantle zone and marginal zone. The periarteriolar T-cell zone is seen nearby. The splenic cords are congested with abnormal red cells while the sinuses are nearly empty.

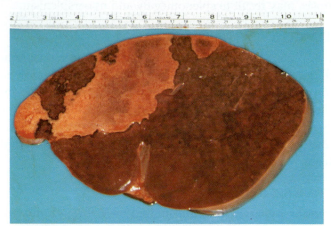

Fig. 21.13   The spleen in myelofibrosis: there is marked splenomegaly and large areas of necrosis.

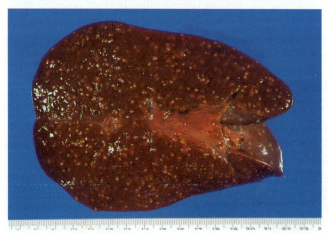

Fig. 21.14   The spleen in systemic candidiasis: multiple foci of candidal infection are seen throughout the spleen in a case of immunosuppression.

AMYLOIDOSIS

Deposition of amyloid proteins in the white or red pulp may result in pronounced splenomegaly. Hyposplenism may develop.

HYPOSPLENISM

Hyposplenism has been recorded in many diseases, often as a rare complication. In most the spleen is absent or reduced in size but in others it is enlarged.

Causes of hyposplenism
- Surgical removal
  - Following trauma
  - Therapeutic
  - Diagnostic
- Infarction
  - Sickle-cell disease
  - Thromboembolism
  - Vasculitis
  - Essential thrombocythaemia
- Coeliac disease
- Irradiation
- Amyloidosis
- Sarcoidosis

Thymus

A mass arising in the anterior mediastinum may be derived either from the thymus or local lymph nodes and biopsy is often required to establish the diagnosis.

True **corticomedullary hypoplasia** is rare and is associated with congenital immunodeficiency syndromes. **Corticomedullary hyperplasia** is also rare, but hyperplasia of the thymic follicles is more common.

FOLLICULAR HYPERPLASIA OF THE THYMUS

Follicular hyperplasia together with plasmacytosis occurs in a variety of diseases including rheumatoid arthritis, Graves' disease, Addison's disease and systemic lupus erythematosus. However, it assumes clinical importance in myasthenia gravis, in which some 75% of patients have some degree of follicular hyperplasia, many of the remainder having a **thymoma**. Patients with myasthenia gravis may benefit from thymectomy, but the relationship is poorly understood (Fig. 21.15).

CASTLEMAN'S DISEASE

This is a rare condition of unknown aetiology. Two-thirds of cases involve the mediastinum but other sites are affected. A large solitary mass is typical but multiple lesions may occur. The lymph node contains characteristic vessels surrounded by proliferating endothelial cells, hyaline material and concentric small lymphocytes. These structures are separated by thick-walled blood vessels or plasma cells. Patients may present only with a mass or with symptoms of fever, anaemia and polyclonal hypergamma-globulinaemia. The localized form may be cured by excision but the generalized form may progress rapidly with death due to intercurrent infection.

Neoplasia

Bone marrow, lymph nodes and extranodal lymphoid tissue

Primary neoplasia of the bone marrow may involve either the haemopoietic or lymphopoietic cell series. Primary neoplasia of the

---

Causes of an anterior mediastinal mass
- Thymic cysts
- Thymic hyperplasia
- Thymic neoplasms
- Castleman's disease
- Lymphomas

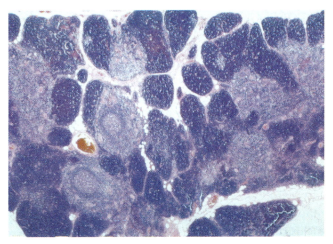
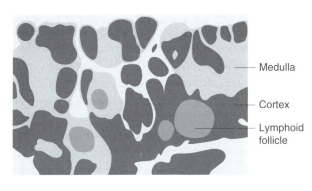

Medulla

Cortex

Lymphoid follicle

Fig. 21.15   The thymus in myasthenia gravis: the lymphoid follicules are hyperplastic and the thymic lobules, divided into the darker cortex and lighter medulla, are well seen.

peripheral lymphoid organs most commonly involves the lymphoid series; primary neoplasms of monocytic, histiocytic, accessory, granulocytic, vascular and connective tissue cells are rare. Metastatic neoplasms commonly involve bone marrow and lymph nodes and are a frequent discovery in biopsy specimens. Metastatic carcinomas are much commoner than sarcomas which preferentially metastasize to the viscera. Early metastases grow first within the peripheral sinus and then spread to replace the entire node (Fig. 21.16).

> **Primary neoplasia of the lymphoid system**
> ■ Hodgkin's disease
> ■ Non-Hodgkin's lymphoma
>   ● Lymphoid leukaemias
>   ● Nodal lymphomas
>   ● Extranodal lymphomas
> ■ Histiocytic neoplasia

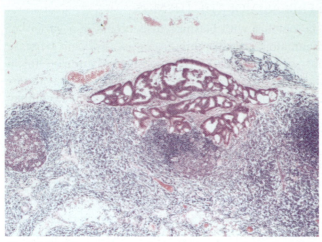
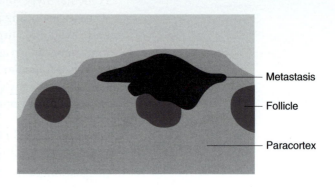

— Metastasis

— Follicle

— Paracortex

Fig. 21.16   Secondary carcinoma: an early metastasis growing within the peripheral sinus of a lymph node.

The lymphomas

Primary neoplasms of the lymphoid system might ideally be defined as neoplastic proliferations showing morphological and immunological resemblance to the cell population of origin. However, the cell of origin is not known in all cases and historical, morphological and anatomical criteria must still be used in current classification.

> **Characteristics of the lymphoid system**
> ● Lymphoid tissue is widely distributed but forms a linked system
> ● Lymphoid cells normally circulate in the blood and lymph
> ● Lymphoid cells proliferate and differentiate in response to immunological stimulation

COMPARISON WITH EPITHELIAL NEOPLASIA

Neoplastic proliferations of the lymphoid system differ from those of the solid organs in a number of respects. The usual concepts of differentiation and division into 'benign' and 'malignant' are difficult to apply to lymphoid neoplasia. Special criteria are therefore used, particularly for non-Hodgkin's lymphoma.

● **Grade**: non-Hodgkin's lymphomas are divided into low- and high-grade categories which have important biological, therapeutic and prognostic implications (Table 21.1). There are exceptions to these generalizations, and each lymphoma type has its own characteristics, but nevertheless the division into low and high grade has important implications for the choice of therapy.

● **Phase**: the nature of a lymphoma may change sometime after the initial diagnosis, similar to the chronic and acute phases described in myeloproliferative disorders. Just as small lymphoid cells may transform to large **'blast' cells** as part of the normal immune response, low-grade lymphomas may transform to **large cell 'blastic' forms**, sometimes as a terminal high-grade phase followed by rapid deterioration and death. The grade of a lymphoma may not therefore

Table 21.1   Comparison of low- and high-grade non-Hodgkin's lymphoma

	Low grade	High grade
Cell size	Mainly small	Large
Cell proliferation rate	Low	High
Growth rate	Slow	Fast
Stage at presentation		
Leukaemia	Often widespread	Often widespread
Nodal	Often widespread	Often localized
Extranodal	Often localized	Often localized
Visceral infiltration	Diffuse	Nodular[a]
Age at presentation	Older	Younger
Survival untreated	Medium to long	Short
Results of treatment	Slow progression	Killed or cured

remain constant during the whole of its natural history and occasionally different grades may coexist in different lymph nodes. Normal lymphoid cells circulate between bone marrow or thymus and the peripheral lymphoid tissues. Some lymphomas recapitulate this behaviour and are usually markedly leukaemic at presentation. In others only small numbers of cells usually enter the peripheral blood but a frankly leukaemic phase may supervene in most types of lymphoma.

- **Stage**: because lymphoid tissue is normally widely distributed, lymphomatous involvement of multiple sites, particularly central and peripheral lymphoid tissue, cannot be thought of as metastasis in the same light as epithelial neoplasia. This is particularly so for low-grade lymphomas in which involvement of bone marrow at presentation is common but survival is nevertheless prolonged. However, Hodgkin's disease and most high-grade lymphomas, which are often confined to one anatomical region at presentation, may later infiltrate the marrow and viscera in a tumorous fashion which resembles epithelial metastases in pattern and prognostic implications.

AETIOLOGY

In most types of lymphoma the aetiology is unknown. Epstein–Barr virus (EBV) is associated with Hodgkin's disease, Burkitt's lymphoma in African patients, and immunodeficient AIDS and post-transplant patients. EBV is a common virus and another factor must therefore be involved. The question remains mysterious with regard to Hodgkin's disease but the immunosuppression caused by endemic malaria, HIV infection and chemotherapy may be responsible in the other cases. Human T-cell lymphoma/leukaemia virus I (HTLV-I) has been implicated in T-cell lymphoproliferative disorders ranging from low-grade leukaemia to aggressive high-grade lymphomas in patients from Japan, Africa, the Caribbean and parts of the Americas. B-cell lymphomas of mucosa-associated lymphoid tissue have been related to reaction to gut flora, particularly chronic gastritis caused by infection with *Helicobacter pylori*, but the mechanism is uncertain.

Aetiological factors in lymphoma

- Viral infections
  - Epstein–Barr virus
  - Human T-cell lymphoma/leukaemia virus I
- Immune disorders
  - Inherited immunodeficiency
  - Human immunodeficiency virus infection
  - Transplant recipients
- Coeliac disease
- Connective tissue/autoimmune diseases
  - Rheumatoid arthritis
  - Sjögren's syndrome
  - Hashimoto's thyroiditis

INCIDENCE

In industrialized countries, lymphomas account for approximately 3% of all cancers. Non-Hodgkin's lymphomas as a group are twice as common as Hodgkin's disease. The geographical incidence of the various types of lymphoma varies from country to country but some regions have striking differences from the Western pattern. Asia has a low incidence of lymphomas in general, but Japan has a remarkably high incidence of T-cell lymphomas. Burkitt's lymphoma is so common in parts of tropical Africa that the incidence of non-Hodgkin's lymphomas rises to one-fifth of all cancers. HTLV-I lymphoma is prevalent in Japan and the Caribbean, and so-called 'immunoproliferative small intestinal disease' is common in the Middle East, causing it to be known as 'Mediterranean lymphoma'.

PRINCIPLES OF CLASSIFICATION

Hodgkin's disease represents some one-third of all lymphomas and is classified according to the mixture of the **reactive lymphoid cells** surrounding characteristic **Sternberg–Reed cells** and the development of fibrosis (Fig. 21.17a). The remainder are termed **non-Hodgkin's lymphomas**. They comprise some two-thirds of all lymphomas and are classified according to the grade of the proliferation, whether they arise from B or T cells and their resemblance to normal lymphoid cells (Fig. 21.17b).

HODGKIN'S DISEASE

Hodgkin's disease was the first lymphoma to be characterized, and the distinction from so-called non-Hodgkin's lymphomas remains clinically and pathologically important. It was long considered to be one disease, but there is growing evidence that two or possibly three different but related disorders may be involved. Furthermore, although most cases can be accurately defined, the boundaries between Hodgkin's disease and non-Hodgkin's lymphomas are not sharp – non-Hodgkin's lymphomas have been described to develop from Hodgkin's disease. Important differences in behaviour distinguish Hodgkin's disease from the non-Hodgkin's lymphomas (Table 21.2).

Clinical features

Hodgkin's disease may present at any age but has distinct peaks of incidence in early and late adult life. Like nodal non-Hodgkin's lymphomas, Hodgkin's disease most commonly presents with enlarged lymph nodes but a single node or group of nodes is usually involved – most commonly cervical and/or mediastinal. In the late stages, multiple nodes may become infiltrated but early generalized lymphadenopathy does not occur. Involved nodes are usually painless but may become painful after ingestion of alcoholic beverages. Systemic symptoms – malaise, fever, sweats, weight loss and pruritus – may be prominent.

Pathological features

An involved lymph node excised for biopsy is usually moderately firm in consistency and occasionally may be as large as 10 cm in diameter. On cross-sectioning, the freshly cut surface of the node resembles 'fish flesh'

Fig. 21.17 (a) Classification and percentage of each type for Hodgkin's disease. (b) Classification and percentage of each type for non-Hodgkin's lymphomas.

(a)

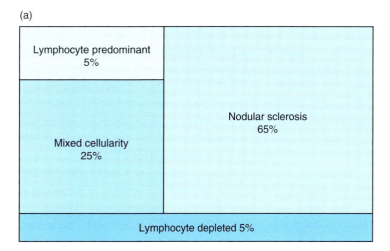

(b)

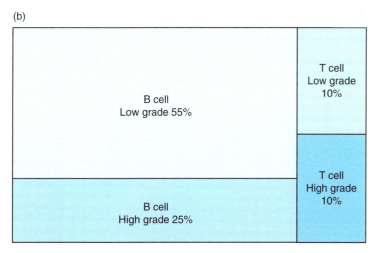

Table 21.2   Comparison of Hodgkin's disease and nodal non-Hodgkin's lymphoma

	Hodgkin's	Non-Hodgkin's
Age at presentation	Bimodal	Low grade: older High grade: younger
Constitutional symptoms	Common	Unusual
Stage at presentation	Often localized	Low grade: widespread High grade: localized
Pattern of spread	Predictable	Random
Visceral infiltration	Nodular	Low grade: diffuse High grade: nodular
Survival untreated	Short	Low grade: medium to long High grade: short
Results of treatment	Most cured	Low grade: slow progression High grade: killed or cured

and may be diffusely involved or sharply divided into nodules by firm fibrous bands in the nodular sclerosis subtype. This fibrosis may spread into adjacent tissues so that the nodes may be matted together. When located in the mediastinum, an infiltrating mass may result (Figs 21.18 and 21.19).

The hallmark of Hodgkin's disease is the presence of **Sternberg–Reed** and **Hodgkin's cells** in a mixed population of reactive cells including small lymphocytes, plasma cells, eosinophils and histiocytes. The Sternberg–Reed cell is a large lymphoid cell with abundant cytoplasm and a complex multilobated nucleus with multiple, very large nucleoli. The Hodgkin's cell is its mononuclear variant. The so-called classic Sternberg–Reed cell as seen in histological sections has two mirror image nuclei with central nucleoli, resembling an 'owl's eye'. These are always in the minority, other variants predominating (Fig. 21.20).

The Sternberg–Reed–Hodgkin cells of nodular lymphocyte predominant Hodgkin's disease are of B-cell origin. The origin of these cells in the other subtypes remains controversial. While generally considered to be neoplastic activated lymphoid cells, little conclusive evidence exists for their definitive identification as either B or T cells and even less for their relationship to any part of the normal lymphoid response.

In the absence of histogenetic information, Hodgkin's disease is classified according to the characteristics of the cell populations. The **Rye classification** is widely used (Table 21.3).

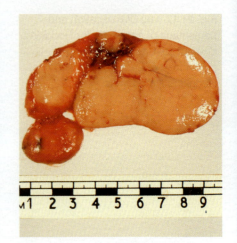

Fig. 21.18   Lymphoma: a case of mixed cellularity Hodgkin's disease showing the 'fish flesh' appearance typical of lymphomas.

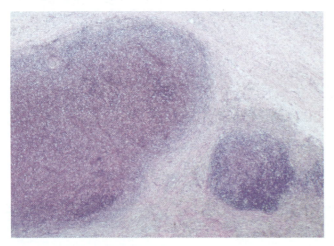

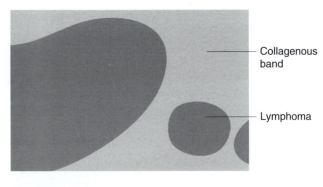

Collagenous band

Lymphoma

Fig. 21.19   Hodgkin's disease: nodular sclerosis subtype showing the lymphoma divided into nodules by thick collagenous bands.

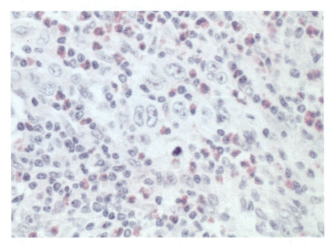

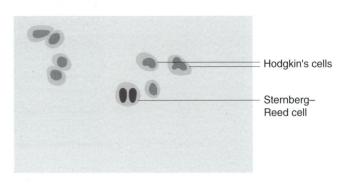

Hodgkin's cells

Sternberg–Reed cell

Fig. 21.20   Hodgkin's disease: a classic Sternberg–Reed cell with 'owl's eye' appearance in a background of Hodgkin's cells, small lymphoid cells and eosinophils.

Table 21.3   Rye classification

	Lymphocytes	SR cells	Other cells[a]	Fibrosis
Lymphocyte predominant	Numerous	Few	Mainly histiocytes	None
Mixed cellularity	Moderate	Moderate	Variable	Delicate
Lymphocyte depleted	Few	Numerous	Few	Diffuse
Nodular sclerosis	Variable	Variable	Variable	Dense, nodular

[a] Including plasma cells, eosinophils and histiocytes.
In addition, lymphocyte predominant is divided into nodular and diffuse subtypes. Nodular sclerosis is divided into grade I and grade II according to the proportion of the node occupied by pleomorphic Sternberg–Reed–Hodgkin cells, grade II cases having a worse prognosis.

Staging

Hodgkin's disease tends to spread predictably from the lymph node of origin to the next adjacent node and group of nodes. The spleen is involved in one-third of cases and in advanced cases, bone marrow, liver, lungs and other organs may be involved. The mode of dissemination of Hodgkin's disease is recognized in the Ann Arbor Staging System (Table 21.4).

Table 21.4   Ann Arbor Staging System

Stage I	A single lymph node region
Stage II	Two or more lymph node regions on the same side of the diaphragm
Stage III	Lymph node regions on both sides of the diaphragm
Stage IV	Visceral disease with or without lymph node involvement

To each main stage the following are appended:	
A	No constitutional symptoms
B	Fever, night sweats and/or weight loss

Prognosis

The prognosis of untreated Hodgkin's disease depends on the **subtype** as well as the **stage** at presentation. Lymphocyte-predominant and nodular sclerosis subtypes have the best prognosis, mixed cellularity is intermediate and lymphocyte depleted has the worst prognosis. The introduction of intensive therapy has meant that, although differences are maintained between subtypes, stage and age are now much more important. Long-term side effects of chemotherapy including acute myeloid leukaemia, other malignant neoplasms and pulmonary and cardiac complications of radiotherapy have come to assume increasing importance.

Some two-thirds of patients of all stages may now expect to be cured, the expectation approaching 100% for stage I disease.

NON-HODGKIN'S LYMPHOMAS

Non-Hodgkin's lymphomas (NHLs) are a diverse group of neoplastic disorders of the lymphoid system which may arise in central lymphoid tissue or peripherally in nodal or extranodal sites. Unlike Hodgkin's disease, much is known about the cell of origin of many NHLs although knowledge is still very incomplete. Rapid progress in the development of this understanding and of immunological techniques available in routine histopathological diagnosis has meant that older classifications have not stood the test of time and have had to be abandoned. Unfortunately several different classifications have developed as replacements and are still in current use. The classification developed in Kiel (Germany) is widely accepted in Europe, as well as being the most biologically and clinically sound, and will be used here (Table 21.5).

Table 21.5   Kiel classification, 1992 update

B cell	T cell
Low-grade malignant lymphomas	
Lymphocytic	Lymphocytic
Chronic lymphocytic leukaemia	Chronic lymphocytic leukaemia
Prolymphocytic leukaemia	Prolymphocytic leukaemia
Hairy cell leukaemia	
	Small cell cerebriform
	Mycosis fungoides, Sézary's syndrome
Lymphoplasmacytic/cytoid	Lymphoepithelioid
Plasmacytic	Angioimmunoblastic
Centroblastic–centrocytic	T-zone lymphoma
follicular ± diffuse	
diffuse	
Mantle cell	Pleomorphic, small cell
Monocytoid, including marginal zone cell	
High-grade malignant lymphomas	
Centroblastic	Pleomorphic, medium and large cell
Immunoblastic	Immunoblastic
Burkitt's lymphoma	
Large cell anaplastic	Large cell anaplastic
Lymphoblastic	Lymphoblastic
Rare types	Rare types

There are important differences in behaviour within the four main divisions, depending on whether the lymphomas are leukaemic, nodal or extranodal in type. Just as the normal immune response involves its separate parts acting together, some forms of lymphoma may involve more than one site, either at presentation or as the disease evolves.

The relationship of lymphomas to the normal lymphoid response

Many lymphomas retain features of the physiological lymphoid response to antigenic stimulation (Fig. 21.21). The neoplastic cells may closely resemble normal lymphoid cells in structure and function. Historically, it was proposed that the normal differentiation process might be arrested with consequent accumulation of cells at a certain point in the maturation

Fig. 21.21 The postulated relationship of lymphomas to the normal lymphoid response.

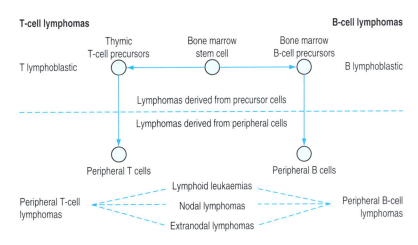

T-cell lymphomas   B-cell lymphomas

Thymic   Bone marrow   Bone marrow
T-cell precursors   stem cell   B-cell precursors

T lymphoblastic   B lymphoblastic

Lymphomas derived from precursor cells

Lymphomas derived from peripheral cells

Peripheral T cells   Peripheral B cells

Lymphoid leukaemias

Peripheral T-cell   Nodal lymphomas   Peripheral B-cell
lymphomas   lymphomas

Extranodal lymphomas

Clinical features of chronic lymphocytic leukaemia
- Older age group
- Abnormal lymphocytes in blood, bone marrow, lymph nodes, spleen, liver and tissues
- Late bone marrow failure
  - Anaemia
  - Thrombocytopenia
  - Haemorrhages
  - Infection
- Hypogammaglobulinaemia in 50% of cases
- Autoimmune haemolytic anaemia in 10% of cases
- Slowly progressive
- Rarely cured

Clinical features of acute lymphoblastic leukaemia
- Young age group
- Lymphoblasts in blood, bone marrow, thymus (T cell), lymph nodes, tonsils, spleen and tissues
- Early bone marrow failure
  - Anaemia
  - Thrombocytopenia
  - Haemorrhage
  - Infection
- Rapidly progressive
- May be cured by intensive therapy

pathway or a particular type of cell might be 'switched on', leading to proliferation of cells of that type.

Recent research into cell proliferation, differentiation and death has given support to these historical concepts and has shown that certain genetic mutations are associated with specific lymphoma types. It is now known that centroblastic–centrocytic lymphomas have a characteristic translocation of the *bcl2* gene on chromosome 18 to the immunoglobulin gene on chromosome 14 – the **t(14;18) translocation**. As a consequence, the bcl2 gene product is overexpressed resulting in reduction of apoptosis in the germinal centre. Phagocytic macrophages, responsible for removing apoptotic debris, disappear from the germinal centre and a population of affected follicle centre B cells accumulates, leading to the development of a lymphoma. A different mechanism has been demonstrated in mantle cell lymphoma. A **t(11;14) translocation** has been shown to shorten the cell cycle, thereby providing a competitive advantage for the affected cells and leading to the development of a lymphoma composed of cells resembling those normally found in the follicular mantle.

Molecular defects associated with other lymphoma types have also been described; however, the aetiological factors responsible for the abnormalities remain uncertain. In the future it may be possible to define characteristic genetic defects associated with each type of lymphoma and to develop new treatments based on this understanding.

Unfortunately, knowledge of the normal lymphoid response remains incomplete and it is consequently not possible to link all lymphomas to a physiological counterpart for classification purposes. This is particularly so for the peripheral T-cell lymphomas. Classification therefore remains partly descriptive rather than histogenetic.

LYMPHOID LEUKAEMIAS

Lymphocytic lymphomas

Lymphocytic lymphomas are usually of B-cell origin. Most are leukaemic at presentation and are termed **chronic lymphocytic leukaemia**. Bone marrow involvement is usually extensive, but a few cases are confined to lymph nodes. Most commonly the cells are small lymphocytes, resembling cells found in the blood and the follicular mantle, but occasionally **prolymphocytic (prolymphocytic leukaemia)** variants occur. **Hairy cell leukaemia** is derived from small B cells of unknown origin. The bone marrow and spleen are infiltrated but lymph node involvement is rare.

Lymphoblastic lymphomas

Lymphoblastic lymphomas may be of B- or T-cell type and are usually leukaemic at or soon after presentation, termed **acute lymphoblastic leukaemia**. T-cell lymphoblastic lymphoma involves the thymus primarily in most cases and has a poor prognosis. The cells are medium sized and derive from the precursor lymphoid cells of the bone marrow and thymus.

NODAL LYMPHOMAS

Most nodal lymphomas are of B-cell type and it is possible to relate the component neoplastic cells to physiological counterparts in the normal node. The normal physiology of the peripheral T-cell response is less well understood and the classification of nodal T-cell lymphomas is consequently less satisfactory (Fig. 21.22).

B-cell lymphomas of the lymphoid follicle

B-cell lymphomas of the lymphoid follicle derive from cells normally found in the follicular mantle or in the germinal centre.

Mantle cell lymphoma derives from a population of small lymphoid cells in the follicular mantle and may be leukaemic at presentation. The prognosis is considerably worse than other low-grade lymphomas.

Centroblastic–centrocytic lymphoma, often termed 'follicular lymphoma', is the neoplastic equivalent of the reactive follicle centre (Fig. 21.23). The commonest nodal NHL, accounting for some half of all cases, it is usually disseminated at presentation. However, behaviour is indolent. Treatment results in long remissions punctuated by recurrences. A late, high-grade **centroblastic phase** may supervene.

Lymphomas of the lymphoid follicle

■ **Low grade**
  ● Lymphocytic lymphoma
  ● Mantle cell lymphoma
  ● Centroblastic–centrocytic lymphoma

■ **High grade**
  ● Centroblastic lymphoma
  ● B-immunoblastic lymphoma
  ● Burkitt's lymphoma

Clinical features of centroblastic–centrocytic lymphoma
  ● Older age group
  ● Involved nodes are painless and enlarge slowly
  ● Bone marrow, spleen and liver often involved at presentation
  ● Terminal high-grade transformation common
  ● Generally slowly progressive

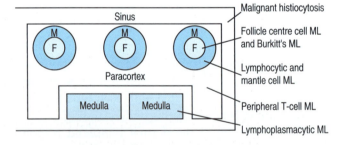

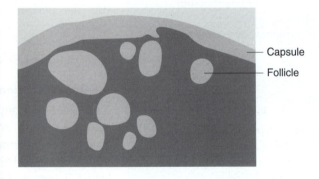

Fig. 21.22 The postulated relationship of peripheral non-Hodgkin's lymphomas to the compartments of the lymph node. ML, malignant lymphoma; M, follicular mantle; F, follicle centre.

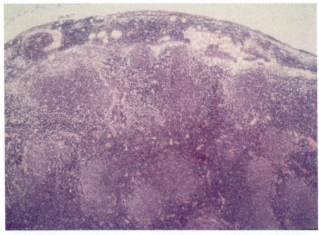

Fig. 21.23 Low-grade non-Hodgkin's lymphoma: centroblastic–centrocytic type showing persistent follicular architecture and infiltration of neoplastic lymphocytes through the capsule.

Fig. 21.24 High-grade non-Hodgkin's malignant lymphoma: centroblastic type showing large lymphoid cells, many in mitosis, and actively phagocytic macrophages similar to those found in the germinal centre.

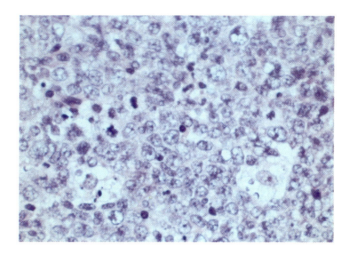

Centroblastic lymphoma may arise secondary to a pre-existing centroblastic–centrocytic lymphoma or as a primary high-grade lymphoma (Fig. 21.24).

Likewise, **B-immunoblastic lymphoma** may be primary or secondary to lymphocytic, lymphoplasmacytic, centroblastic–centrocytic or centroblastic lymphomas. A rapidly growing lymphoma, it carries the worst prognosis of all B-cell lymphomas.

B-cell lymphomas associated with paraproteinaemia

The following types of B-cell lymphoma associated with paraproteinaemia are recognized:

- lymphoplasmacytoid and lymphoplasmacytic lymphoma
- plasmacytic lymphoma and plasma cell myeloma.

Lymphoplasmacytoid, lymphoplasmacytic and plasmacytic lymphomas are the neoplastic equivalents of stages in the normal development of plasma cells from small memory lymphocytes. The lymphoplasmacytoid/ -cytic types are related to lymphocytic lymphoma but have varying degrees of plasma cell differentiation and are less often leukaemic. Secretion of monoclonal immunoglobulin results in paraproteinaemia in one-third of cases. IgM secretion produces a clinical hyperviscosity syndrome termed **Waldenström's macroglobulinaemia**.

Pure plasmacytic lymphoma confined to lymph nodes is mysteriously rare. Most pure plasma cell proliferations involve the bone marrow where they are termed **solitary plasmacytoma** or, much more commonly, **multiple** or **plasma cell myeloma**, after the destructive masses of plasma cells that form in the bone marrow. Plasma cell leukaemia is rare.

Lymphomas associated with viral infections

Endemic Burkitt's lymphoma is found in certain tropical countries with a high incidence of malaria, particularly Africa. Extranodal involvement of jaw, retroperitoneum and viscera predominates. **Non-endemic Burkitt's lymphoma** occurs in other parts of the world but the majority of cases do not contain Epstein–Barr virus. A nodal or abdominal visceral presentation is most common and some cases are leukaemic. The cell of origin remains uncertain but a pre-centroblastic germinal centre cell is proposed.

Clinical features of plasma cell myeloma

- Older age group
- Monoclonal immunoglobulin or light chains (Bence Jones protein) in blood
- Systemic amyloidosis in 10% of cases
- Lytic bone lesions and fractures common
- Renal failure common
- Slowly progressive

Lymphomas associated with viral infections

- **Epstein–Barr virus**
  - Burkitt's lymphoma
  - Lymphoma following HIV infection
  - Lymphoma following organ transplantation
- **Human T-cell lymphoma/leukaemia virus**
  - Pleomorphic, small, medium and large T cell

Lymphoma following **HIV infection and organ transplantation** is usually high-grade NHL of Burkitt or immunoblastic type. Epstein–Barr virus may be isolated from many cases. Extranodal presentation with a high incidence of central nervous system involvement is characteristic. The lymphoproliferative process appears to progress from polyclonal virus-induced hyperplasia through an oligoclonal phase to monoclonal lymphoma.

In areas where it is endemic, **HTLV-I infection** may, in some individuals, produce a chronic polyclonal proliferation of T cells which eventually becomes a monoclonal lymphoma. A chronic phase characterized by infiltration of bone marrow and skin by small pleomorphic lymphocytes may precede the development of an extremely aggressive high-grade lymphoma composed of medium to large pleomorphic T cells. A leukaemic phase, hypercalcaemia and hypogammaglobulinaemia are common.

Peripheral T-cell lymphomas

In Europe and North America, peripheral T-cell lymphomas are uncommon. The classification is at this time less satisfactory than for B-cell lymphomas, not assisted by the coexistence of different patterns and grades in different anatomical sites in the same patient. The more important nodal types are described above.

EXTRANODAL LYMPHOMAS

Lymphomas which arise in tissues other than bone marrow, thymus, lymph nodes and spleen are termed extranodal lymphomas and comprise some one-third of all lymphomas. Primary lymphomas have been described in almost every organ but those arising in the gastrointestinal tract and skin are the most common (Figs 21.25 and 21.26). Just as many nodal lymphomas have been shown to derive from stages in the immune response, recent research has in many cases demonstrated a relationship between extranodal lymphomas and the normal lymphoid tissue of the organ involved.

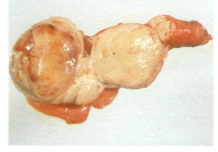

Fig. 21.25   Extranodal lymphoma of the testis; the 'fish flesh' appearance is maintained in the extranodal site.

B-cell lymphomas of MALT

B-cell lymphomas may arise in organs which normally have MALT but, in addition, the salivary glands and thyroid, which normally lack MALT, may

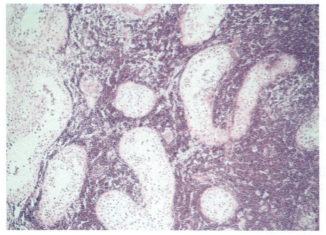

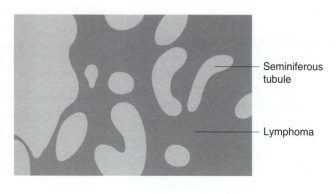

Seminiferous tubule

Lymphoma

Fig. 21.26   Extranodal lymphoma of the testis: the lymphoma infiltrates between the seminiferous tubules before destroying them.

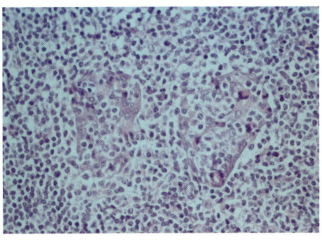

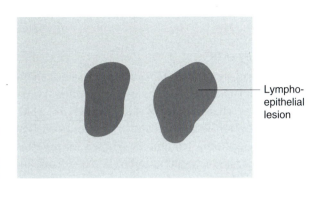

Lympho-epithelial lesion

Fig. 21.27   Lymphoma of the salivary gland: a lymphoma of MALT showing a typical lymphoepithelial lesion in which marginal zone lymphocytes infiltrate salivary epithelium.

Fig. 21.28   Extranodal lymphoma of the stomach: a high-grade non-Hodgkin's lymphoma resembling a carcinoma.

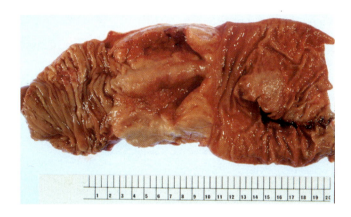

Pathological features of low-grade B-cell lymphomas of MALT

- Lymphoepithelial lesions
- Variable plasma cell differentiation
- Reactive lymphoid follicles
- Late dissemination

Primary lymphomas of the gastrointestinal tract

■ **B-cell lymphomas**
- Lymphomas of MALT
  - ○ low grade
  - ○ high grade
  - ○ immunoproliferative small intestinal disease
- Lymphomatous polyposis
- Burkitt's lymphoma
- Rare types

■ **T-cell lymphomas**
- Enteropathy-associated T-cell lymphoma
- Rare types

---

develop identical lymphomas following autoimmune inflammation in rheumatoid arthritis and Hashimoto's thyroiditis respectively. Lymphomas of MALT recapitulate many of the features of normal MALT including the intimate relationship of marginal zone lymphocytes and epithelium (Fig. 21.27). Most are low grade and late dissemination, preferentially to other MALT sites, conveys an excellent prognosis. Transformation to high-grade lymphoma occasionally occurs and is associated with a greatly worsened prognosis (Fig. 21.28).

A peculiar type of small intestinal lymphoma of MALT in which extreme plasma cell differentiation and secretion of IgA heavy chains occurs is termed **immunoproliferative small intestinal disease** or **Mediterranean lymphoma** in recognition of its high incidence in the Middle East.

Lymphomas of the gastrointestinal tract

Quantitatively, lymphomas of the gastrointestinal tract are the most important extranodal lymphomas. Secondary lymphomatous deposits are common.

Lymphomatous polyposis presents as multiple polyps throughout the gastrointestinal tract. It corresponds to nodal **mantle cell lymphoma** and has an aggressive course with rapid spread to peripheral lymphoid tissue.

Enteropathy-associated T-cell lymphoma may complicate coeliac disease. Perforation, haemorrhage and early dissemination convey a poor prognosis. The cell of origin is probably the intraepithelial T lymphocyte which is present in normal intestinal mucosa and increased in numbers in coeliac disease.

Lymphomas of skin

Skin lymphomas are of B- and T-cell types and are characterized by indolent behaviour with late dissemination and sometimes spontaneous regression. B-cell lymphomas share some of the features of MALT lymphomas, but epithelial infiltration is not a feature. Of the T-cell lymphomas, **small cell cerebriform lymphoma** (commonly known as **mycosis fungoides**) is best known. The lymphoma begins as infiltration of dermis and epidermis by small T lymphocytes of helper/inducer type with complex cerebriform nuclei. It may progress to a leukaemic phase with lymph node involvement (**Sézary's syndrome**) or eventually transform to a high-grade T-cell lymphoma.

Secondary infiltration of the skin by lymphoma and myeloid leukaemia is common and may be the presenting feature of these diseases.

HISTIOCYTIC NEOPLASIA

Neoplasia of the monocyte/histiocyte pathway is rare. Classification is according to differentiation (Table 21.6).

Details of the **monocytic leukaemias** and **Langerhans' cell histiocytosis** will be found elsewhere. Other histiocytic neoplasms are extremely rare.

Table 21.6   Classification of histiocytic neoplasia

Bone marrow monocytes	Monocytic leukaemias
Tissue and nodal histiocytes	Malignant histiocytosis
Accessory cells	Langerhans' cell histiocytosis
	Follicular dendritic and interdigitating dendritic cell sarcomas

Neoplasia of the spleen

Primary neoplasms confined to the spleen are rare. Most cases of neoplastic splenomegaly are due to secondary infiltration.

With the exception of hairy cell leukaemia, **low-grade NHLs** produce multiple nodules of similar size throughout the spleen while Hodgkin's disease and **high-grade NHLs** produce fewer but much larger nodules of varying size. Hairy cell leukaemia infiltrates the cords and sinuses in a diffuse fashion. In **chronic myeloproliferative disorders**, particularly myelofibrosis and chronic myelocytic leukaemia, the splenic red pulp is infiltrated by haemopoietic cells of erythroid, myeloid and megakaryocytic lineage, whereas in **acute myeloblastic leukaemia**, blast forms of myeloid lineage predominate. Metastases of carcinomas are seldom of clinical importance as they generally represent advanced disseminated disease. Malignant melanoma, breast and lung primaries are most common.

Hypersplenism may follow neoplastic infiltration of the spleen and spontaneous rupture may rarely occur.

Neoplasia of the thymus

Neoplasms presenting in the anterior mediastinum may arise primarily within the thymus or in adjacent lymph nodes with or without secondary

---

Clinical features of mycosis fungoides
- **Patch stage**: erythematous patches on trunk and extremities
- **Plaque stage**: elevated, itchy red/brown scaly plaques
- **Tumour stage**: rounded, ulcerated tumorous masses

Splenic neoplasia
- ■ Lymphomas
  - Hodgkin's disease
  - Low-grade non-Hodgkin's
    - ○ lymphocytic
    - ○ lymphoplasmacytic
    - ○ hairy cell leukaemia
    - ○ centroblastic–centrocytic
  - High-grade non-Hodgkin's
- ■ Myeloproliferative disorders
  - Myelofibrosis
  - Chronic myelocytic leukaemia
  - Acute myeloblastic leukaemia
- ■ Metastatic carcinoma

Superior vena cava syndrome
- Dilated veins of upper chest and neck
- Oedema and plethora of face and neck
- Oedema of conjunctiva and visual disturbances
- Headache

Paraneoplastic syndrome
'A non-metastatic manifestation of neoplasia caused by the production by the neoplasm of hormonal or other factors which affect the functions of other organs.'

Fig. 21.29 Thymoma: the gland is greatly enlarged and resembles a lymphoma because of the substantial reactive lymphoid population.

infiltration of the thymus. It is often impossible to distinguish between primary and secondary thymic involvement and anterior mediastinal neoplasms are therefore considered together.

Neoplasms of the anterior mediastinum may present with symptoms resulting from varying degrees of infiltration into mediastinal tissues including large vessels, airways, heart, lung and chest wall. Dyspnoea, the superior vena cava syndrome and pain in the chest, neck and arms are typical with aggressive types. Alternatively, a variety of paraneoplastic syndromes may be the first evidence of disease. Myasthenia gravis associated with thymoma is the best known.

THYMOMAS

Thymomas are derived from the thymic epithelium and recapitulate the association between epithelium and lymphoid tissues in the thymus. The neoplastic epithelial component is heavily infiltrated by T cells and cortical and medullary patterns are recognized. About a quarter of thymomas invade locally into the mediastinum and lung but very few metastasize to distant sites. Those with a cortical pattern have a worse prognosis than those of pure medullary type. The stage noted at time of resection provides a good indication of prognosis as cases confined to the gland at surgery tend not to recur (Figs 21.29 and 21.30).

Myasthenia gravis occurs in one-third of cases of thymoma. Hypogammaglobulinaemia, anaemias, polymyositis and Graves' disease are less common.

OTHER THYMIC NEOPLASMS
- **Thymic carcinomas** are aggressive malignant neoplasms of various types including squamous cell carcinoma and oat cell carcinoma.
- **Thymic carcinoids** resemble their counterparts in other organs. Metastases occur in three-quarters of cases and some are associated with ectopic ACTH production.
- **Germ cell neoplasms** are most commonly benign teratomas. Germinomas and other malignant germ cell tumours are rare and have a poor prognosis.
- **T-cell lymphoblastic lymphomas** may present with a thymic mass but frequently become leukaemic T-cell lymphoblastic leukaemia.
- **B-cell sclerosing lymphoma of the mediastinum** is a high-grade NHL

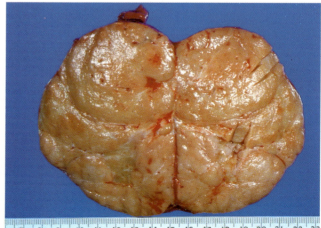

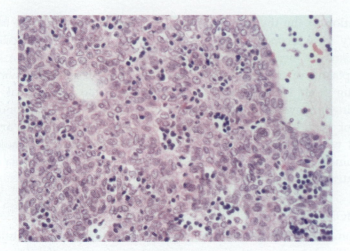

Fig. 21.30 Thymoma of cortical pattern: the solid thymic epithelium maintains its intimate relationship with small T cells.

in which large B cells are associated with dense fibrosis. The origin is thought to be the population of B cells which surrounds Hassall's corpuscles. Young women are most commonly affected and without intensive therapy the prognosis is poor (Fig. 21.31).

- **Nodular sclerosis Hodgkin's disease** commonly involves the anterior mediastinum, frequently with cervical lymph node involvement.

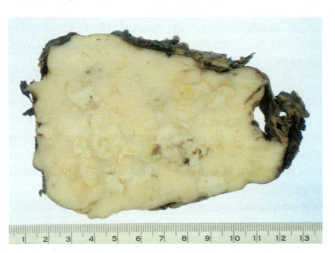

Fig. 21.31 Lymphoma of the thymus: 'High-grade sclerosing B-cell lymphoma' showing infiltrative border and areas of necrosis.

CASE STUDY 21.2

A 35-year-old woman presented to her general practitioner complaining of recent onset of headaches, visual disturbances and shortness of breath. Physical examination revealed dilatation of the veins of the neck and upper thorax, oedema of the face and conjunctivae and stridor on auscultation of the chest. The remainder of the physical examination was normal with no palpable lymphadenopathy. Urgent admission to hospital was arranged. Chest radiographs and computed tomography showed a solid mass filling the anterior mediastinum and infiltrating the superior vena cava, trachea and lung, The 'superior vena cava syndrome' is almost always caused by malignant neoplasia and the clinical differential diagnosis was:

- lymphoma
- thymoma
- thymic carcinoma
- malignant germ cell neoplasm
- carcinoma of the lung.

Lymphoma was considered most likely in view of the patient's age and lack of systemic symptoms. A needle biopsy was performed followed by irradiation to reduce the obstruction of airways and vessels. Microscopic examination of the biopsy showed a population of medium to large round cells, many in mitosis, a second population of small lymphocytes and strands of collagen (Fig. 21.32). A single Hassall's corpuscle was found, indicating that the neoplasm had originated within or invaded into the thymus. Hodgkin's disease could be excluded by the lack of Sternberg–Reed cells and the monomorphic nature of the neoplastic cells. The differential diagnosis was considered to be:

- lymphoma (B-cell sclerosing lymphoma of the mediastinum or T-cell lymphoblastic lymphoma)
- thymoma
- thymic carcinoma
- germinoma.

To clarify the nature of the neoplastic cells, immunocytochemical staining of the microscopic sections for B-cell, T-cell and epithelial differentiation was performed. The large neoplastic cells were positive for B-cell markers whereas the reactive small lymphocytes were shown to be T cells. Epithelial markers were negative except in Hassall's corpuscle.

The diagnosis of 'high-grade B-cell sclerosing lymphoma of the mediastinum' was made and the patient treated by irradiation of the mediastinum and systemic chemotherapy. The local symptoms responded rapidly and 3 years after diagnosis the patient remains in remission.

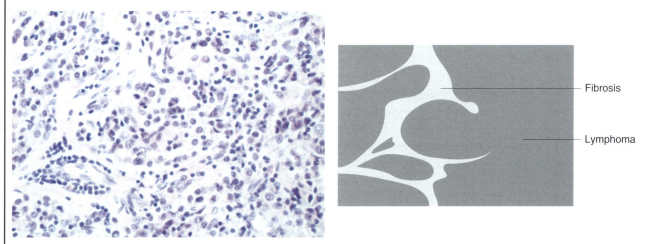

Fig. 21.32 Lymphoma of the thymus: 'high-grade sclerosing B-cell lymphoma' showing neoplastic large B cells, a background population of small non-neoplastic T cells and characteristic fibrosis.

Chapter 22   Bone, joint and soft tissue disease

Learning objectives

To appreciate and understand:
- ❏ Factors involved in maintaining bone structure and function
- ❏ Disturbances in homoeostasis resulting in metabolic bone diseases
- ❏ The clinical presentation of metastatic tumours in bone (common) and primary bone tumours (rare)
- ❏ Different types of arthritis
- ❏ Infections of the skeletal system and the importance of early diagnosis
- ❏ Presenting features and prognosis of soft tissue tumours

Bone: structure and function

Bone has several functions:

- It forms a rigid endoskeleton which supports the body and protects the viscera, and provides attachments for muscles.
- It has a major role in the metabolism of calcium and other minerals.
- It contains haemopoietic marrow, which in healthy adults is confined largely to the axial skeleton.

Bone consists of cells, organic matrix and mineral. **Osteoblasts** are mesenchymal cells which produce bone. **Osteoid**, a matrix rich in protein and mucopolysaccharides, is laid down and is subsequently mineralized to form bone. Some osteoblasts are incorporated into bone and become relatively inactive osteocytes which communicate with one another through cell processes that run through canaliculi within the bone. **Osteoclasts**, multinucleated cells of the macrophage/monocyte series, are responsible for resorption of bone. Through the action of carbonic anhydrase they produce a low pH and release lysosomal proteases, which together remove the bone matrix. In health there are complex interactions between osteoblasts and osteoclasts which allow coupling of bone formation and resorption so that bone mass is kept relatively constant. The major protein in bone is type I collagen; there are also many non-collagenous proteins. The mineral component is **hydroxyapatite**, a crystalline form of hydrated calcium phosphate. Mineralization is promoted by the enzyme **alkaline phosphatase**; this enzyme is also produced by the liver, but the serum levels of the bone isoenzyme provide a useful indicator of osteoblastic activity.

Bone exists in two forms, lamellar and woven. **Lamellar bone**, where collagen bundles are arranged in parallel arrays, is structurally strong and

Fig. 22.1 The structure of normal bone. This diagram shows a transverse section through a long bone.

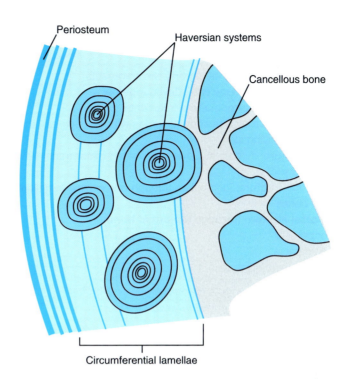

Periosteum

Haversian systems

Cancellous bone

Circumferential lamellae

forms the mature skeleton. The cortex of bones is composed of compact bone, arranged in concentric perivascular cylinders known as **haversian systems** or osteons which give the bone its strength; there are also subperiosteal and endosteal circumferential lamellae (Fig 22.1) on the outer and inner aspects of the cortex. The medullary cavity contains a meshwork of trabeculae of lamellar bone which separates the marrow spaces and forms **cancellous** (spongy) bone. When bone is laid down rapidly, during fetal growth or fracture healing or by bone-forming tumours, the collagen fibres are randomly arranged to form **woven bone**, which is weaker than lamellar bone.

Bone turnover

Bone is a metabolically active tissue; approximately 5% of the adult skeleton turns over each year. Bone formation is stimulated by mechanical loading during physical exercise and by growth hormone, androgens and somatomedins (insulin-like growth factors). Many factors, both systemic and local, control bone resorption. **Parathyroid hormone** and **vitamin D** both interact with receptors on osteoblasts which send a signal to neighbouring osteoclasts to initiate resorption. The physiological function of **calcitonin**, produced by the C cells of the thyroid, is unclear, but in pharmacological doses it inhibits bone resorption. Numerous substances influence local bone resorption; in inflammatory conditions, for example, these include prostaglandins and cytokines such as interleukin 1. After episodes of bone resorption, osteoblasts, stimulated by cytokines and growth factors released from the bone matrix, complete the bone turnover cycle.

Fractures and fracture healing

In health considerable force is required to break a normal bone, whereas abnormal bone may break after minimal trauma. There are several types of fracture, and many causes of pathological fracture (see box)

Fractures: types and causes
■ **Trauma to normal bone**
- **Simple fracture**: one break, giving two fragments
- **Impacted fracture**: bone ends driven together
- **Comminuted fracture**: multiple fragments
- **Compound fracture**: site communicates with exterior, e.g. through wound of overlying skin
- **Stress fracture**: incomplete, due to repeated minor trauma/overuse, e.g. runners
- **Greenstick fracture**: incomplete through one cortex, in children's pliable bones

■ **Pathological fracture (through abnormal bone)**
- Osteoporosis
- Osteomalacia
- Hyperparathyroidism
- Paget's disease
- Osteogenesis imperfecta
- Metastatic tumours in bone
- Primary bone tumours, both benign and malignant

As described in Chapter 6, healing of a fracture involves several processes:

- formation of callus
- repair of the fracture gap
- remodelling.

The force causing the fracture tears blood vessels, leading to haemorrhage between the bone ends and in the surrounding tissues, and also to death of bone around the fracture site. The periosteum reacts by proliferating and laying down **callus**, a bandage of reactive bone and cartilage which can be thought of as an attempt to immobilize the fracture site. A smaller amount of callus is also formed within the medullary cavity. Dead bone is resorbed from the fracture site and the fracture gap is filled by bone, under optimal conditions by direct ossification. Once continuity is restored the fracture callus is removed by the process of remodelling, which restores the bone contours to as near normal as possible. The process is more complete in children. Fracture healing may be delayed by local factors such as infection, vascular insufficiency and interposition of soft tissue at the fracture gap, and by systemic factors including malnutrition and steroid therapy (see box). Healing may be very slow (**delayed union**) or fail to occur (**non-union**), following which a false joint (**pseudarthrosis**) may form.

Factors delaying fracture healing
■ **Local**
- Inadequate immobilization
- Poor blood supply
- Infection
- Interposition of soft tissue
■ **General**
- Malnutrition, cachexia, uraemia
- Diabetes mellitus
- Steroid therapy

Generalized diseases of bone

The term 'metabolic bone disease' is applied to the group of acquired generalized skeletal disorders which are due to abnormalities of bone formation, mineralization or resorption. These include **osteoporosis**, **osteomalacia**, **hyperparathyroidism** and **renal osteodystrophy**.

Osteoporosis

In osteoporosis the bone mass is reduced below that required for its mechanical function. It is, however, of normal composition and is fully

Features of osteoporosis
- Mainly postmenopausal women
- Diminished bone mass
- Fractures of vertebrae, femur, radius
- Related to oestrogen lack

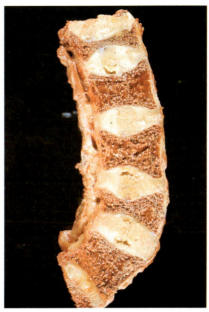

Fig. 22.2 Osteoporotic spine showing loss of height of the vertebral bodies with kyphosis.

mineralized. **Localized osteoporosis** occurs following immobilization, usually of a limb, and is a form of disuse atrophy. **Generalized osteoporosis** occurs typically in postmenopausal women (see box on p. 532) and is a major clinical and socioeconomic problem. After the menopause an acceleration of the normal age-related decrease in skeletal mass occurs, resulting in loss of bone, particularly in the cancellous bone of the vertebral bodies, ribs, pelvis and bone ends, where there is higher surface area and more rapid turnover. The cortices of long bones are also thinned. Severe osteoporosis results in crush fractures of the vertebral bodies leading to back pain and loss of height (Fig. 22.2), and to the common **fractures of the femoral neck** and **distal radius (Colles' fracture)**. Oestrogen deficiency is of major importance in the pathogenesis of postmenopausal osteoporosis, and early institution of hormone replacement therapy (HRT) can prevent or at least delay osteoporosis. Genetic factors, for example variations in the gene for the vitamin D receptor, are undoubtedly important. There are many other causes of osteoporosis (see box).

Osteomalacia and rickets

Osteomalacia ('soft bones') is due to reduced mineralization of newly formed bone matrix. The bones are soft, and may deform or fracture. In **rickets** in childhood, there is also growth disturbance and deformity, for example of the long bones, pelvis and skull.

Most cases of osteomalacia and rickets are caused by **vitamin D deficiency** (Fig. 22.3), particularly due to deficient intake and malabsorption. In osteomalacia a high proportion of the bone trabecular surface area is covered by an abnormally thick layer of osteoid. The bone is thus of reduced radiological density (**osteopenia**). Radiographs may show

Causes of osteoporosis

■ **Primary**
- Involutional age-related
- Postmenopausal oestrogen deficiency

■ **Secondary**
- Immobilization (local or general)
- Endocrine, e.g. Cushing's syndrome and steroid therapy
- Congenital, e.g. osteogenesis imperfecta
- Neoplastic, e.g. diffuse multiple myeloma or secondary carcinoma
- Gastrointestinal disease, e.g. malabsorption, liver disease

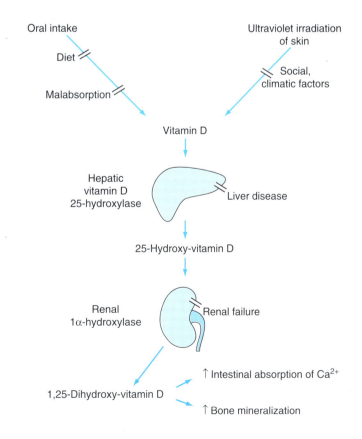

Fig. 22.3 Vitamin D metabolism and the principal causes of osteomalacia. The bars indicate how a pathway can be blocked.

pathological fractures. Transverse lucencies, known as **Looser's zones**, typically occur in long bones, pubic rami and scapulae, and are virtually pathognomonic of osteomalacia. In rickets, the epiphyseal plates are thickened and cupped due to failure of normal mineralization of cartilage and give rise to swollen wrists and knees; similar changes affect the chest wall, the rows of thickened costochondral junctions forming the so-called 'rickety rosary'.

Hyperparathyroidism

Hyperparathyroidism is classified as primary, secondary and tertiary (Table 22.1; see Chapter 18). Most patients with primary hyperparathyroidism do not develop bone disease; the 5–10% who do often complain of bone pain. The radiographs may show a generally abnormal bone texture with focal areas of lysis reflecting increased bone removal; subperiosteal cortical resorption, particularly of the phalanges, is typical. There may be generalized osteopenia. On microscopy there is increased osteoclastic activity, sometimes 'dissecting' the centre of bone trabeculae, and accompanied by marrow fibrosis and new bone formation. Occasionally large defects in the bone contain numerous osteoclasts, haemosiderin and fibrous tissue; these **'brown tumours'** may closely resemble giant cell tumour of bone, but respond to removal of the cause of the hyperparathyroidism.

Table 22.1   Types of hyperparathyroidism

Type	Cause	Serum calcium levels
Primary	80% parathyroid adenoma 15% hyperplasia 5% carcinoma	High
Secondary	Parathyroid hyperplasia, secondary to hypocalcaemia, e.g. renal failure	Low/normal
Tertiary	Autonomous nodule in parathyroid hyperplasia	High

Renal osteodystrophy

Patients with renal failure often develop generalized bone disease. The histological features (Fig. 22.4) are a combination of secondary hyperparathyroidism, which is present in 80–90% of patients, and osteomalacia, which is found in 20–40% and is due to reduced synthesis within the kidney of 1,25-dihydroxyvitamin D_3. In about one-third of patients there is increased bone density due to excessive woven bone formation; alternating bands of sclerotic and less dense bone in the vertebral column give an appearance known as a 'rugger jersey spine'.

Inherited conditions

OSTEOGENESIS IMPERFECTA (BRITTLE BONE DISEASE)

Patients with osteogenesis imperfecta are subject to repeated fractures and there is often skeletal deformity and short stature. The clinical features vary

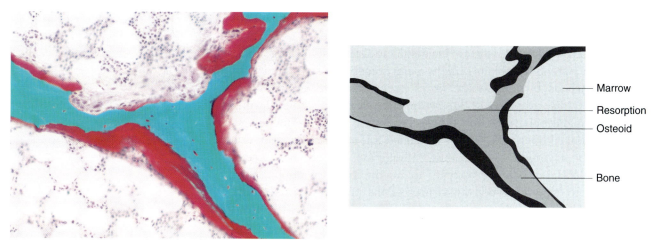

Fig. 22.4   Renal osteodystrophy. The features are a combination of osteomalacia and hyperparathyroidism. This undecalcified section shows a thickened layer of osteoid (red) on bone (green). A large area of resorption represents the increased turnover of hyperparathyroidism.

from mild forms with a moderately increased risk of fracture to severe cases which are lethal in the perinatal period. Osteogenesis imperfecta is due to mutations affecting the genes for type I collagen, the severity correlating with the extent of disruption of collagen synthesis and polymerization. Many patients have extraskeletal abnormalities, including blue sclerae (due to deficient scleral collagen), deafness and abnormal teeth (dentinogenesis imperfecta). Osteogenesis imperfecta must be excluded before multiple fractures in childhood are attributed to 'non-accidental injury'.

OSTEOPETROSIS (MARBLE BONE DISEASE)

Osteopetrosis is due to absence or malfunction of osteoclasts which results in failure of remodelling of the cartilaginous model of fetal bones. In severe cases the marrow cavity is greatly diminished, causing anaemia. Although the bones are of increased density, their structure is abnormal and they fracture readily. Narrowing of the exit foramina of the first or eighth cranial nerves may cause blindness or deafness. In severe cases bone marrow transplantation is indicated; normal osteoclasts derived from donor stem cells remodel the bones and the anaemia is relieved. Unfortunately, the cranial nerve palsies are usually irreversible.

ACHONDROPLASIA

Achondroplasia, which is the most common form of dwarfism, is due to a dominant gene with a high mutation rate. As a consequence most patients are new mutations and are born to normal parents. Failure of normal endochondral ossification at the epiphyseal plates leads to reduced bone growth. The clinical appearance is distinctive with very short limbs and a characteristic facial appearance. Neurological complications include spinal canal compression and hydrocephalus which may lead to death in infancy.

Other disorders of bone

Paget's disease of bone

One or many bones may be affected by Paget's disease, which is a disorder of bone turnover. The vertebrae, pelvis, skull and long bones are often affected. It is very common in elderly people of Anglo-Saxon stock (about 10% of those over 80 years), but rarer in other ethnic groups.

Paget's disease is frequently an incidental radiological finding; most symptomatic patients complain of bone pain, sometimes associated with deformity such as bowing of the limbs or enlargement of the head. Radiographs in the early stage of the disease show bone lysis often starting at one end of a long bone; with time there is progressive sclerosis due to new bone formation. Although the bone is thickened it is structurally weak due to the loss of haversian systems and pathological fracture may occur. Increased osteoclastic activity appears to be the primary abnormality, perhaps due to 'slow' infection by viruses of the paramyxovirus group. There is also increased bone formation, and the marrow spaces are filled with vascular fibrous tissue. Repeated cycles of bone resorption and formation lead to a characteristic 'mosaic' or 'jigsaw' pattern of cement lines in thickened bone trabeculae (Fig. 22.5). **Sarcomatous transformation** is an

> **Clinical features of Paget's disease**
> - Bone pain
> - Bowing or fracture
> - Deafness
> - Nerve or spinal cord compression
> - Sarcomatous transformation

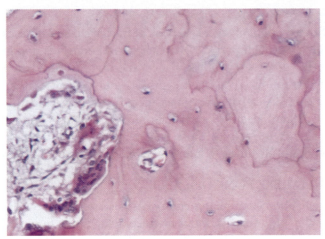
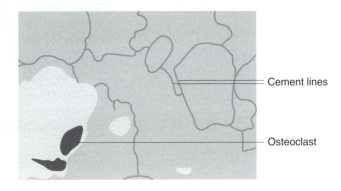

Cement lines

Osteoclast

Fig. 22.5 Paget's disease of bone. There are several large osteoclasts eroding bone. The 'mosaic' pattern of cement lines reflects previous episodes of irregular bone turnover.

uncommon but devastating complication of Paget's disease. Most tumours are **osteosarcomas** or **malignant fibrous histiocytomas** which metastasize early to the lungs; the prognosis of these high-grade tumours is poor. It is traditionally taught that increased blood flow through the skeleton in widespread Paget's disease causes high output cardiac failure; this is very rare in an otherwise healthy patient, but may be a contributory factor in patients with coexisting heart disease.

Fibrous dysplasia

Fibrous dysplasia is an abnormality of bone development which may affect one or several bones, typically the long bones, ribs and jaw. Most patients present in childhood or adolescence with swelling or pathological fracture; those with polyostotic disease in particular tend to develop progressive deformity, for example of the proximal femur (Fig. 22.6). The lesions of fibrous dysplasia consist of irregular trabeculae of woven bone likened to lobster claws, lying randomly in a fibroblastic stroma. **Albright's syndrome**, defined by polyostotic fibrous dysplasia, cutaneous pigmentation and endocrine abnormalities, especially precocious puberty, is commoner in girls.

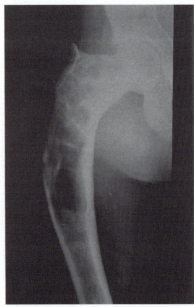

Fig. 22.6 Fibrous dysplasia. The bone is weak and a characteristic deformity of the femur develops.

Avascular necrosis (osteonecrosis)

Avascular necrosis is the death of bone due to interference with its blood supply, by definition in the absence of infection. There are many predisposing factors (see box).

Bone infarcts in the shaft of long bones are asymptomatic, but involvement of the subarticular bone – of the femoral head, for example (Fig. 22.7) – is often followed by collapse of the articular surface and secondary osteoarthritis.

Factors predisposing to avascular necrosis
- Trauma, e.g. fracture of the neck of femur or scaphoid; dislocation of hip
- Steroid therapy, e.g. in SLE, renal transplantation
- Alcoholism
- Dysbarism ('caisson disease') in divers and compressed air workers
- Sickle-cell disease
- Idiopathic

CASE STUDY 22.1

An elderly woman fell at home and was unable to walk. On admission a radiograph showed a subcapital fracture of the femoral neck with marked osteoporosis. The fracture was fixed using a pin and plate and she mobilized quickly. Some months later she developed pain in her hip and a total hip replacement was carried out. The femoral head showed avascular necrosis (see Fig. 22.7).

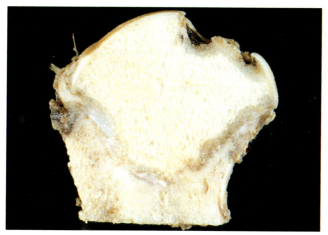

Fig. 22.7 Osteonecrosis of the femoral head, following a fracture. A large pale wedge-shaped area of necrosis is seen.

Bone tumours

Metastatic involvement of the skeleton is very common in patients with cancer; in contrast, with the exception of myeloma, a malignant tumour of plasma cells, primary bone tumours are rare. Only about 150 cases of the most common malignant bone tumour, osteosarcoma, are seen in the UK each year, but many patients are young and often require major surgery and aggressive chemotherapy. Because primary bone tumours are rare diagnosis is often delayed; bone pain or swelling merits early radiological investigation. A simplified classification of bone tumours is given in Table 22.2.

Metastatic tumours

Malignant tumours very commonly spread to bone, particularly to the vertebral column, ribs, flat bones of the limb girdles and the proximal ends of the humerus and femur – to sites usually occupied by haemopoietic marrow. Carcinomas of bronchus, breast, prostate, kidney and thyroid and, in children, neuroblastoma and rhabdomyosarcoma most commonly produce bone metastases. Many metastases are asymptomatic and are

Table 22.2   Classification of the common bone tumours

Metastatic tumours	Carcinoma, especially of bronchus, breast, prostate, kidney, thyroid (follicular) Neuroblastoma
Tumours of haemopoietic origin	Myeloma Lymphoma
Primary benign bone tumours	Osteoma Osteoid osteoma Osteoblastoma Osteochondroma Enchondroma Giant cell tumour
Primary malignant bone tumours	Osteosarcoma Chondrosarcoma Ewing's sarcoma Malignant fibrous histiocytoma/fibrosarcoma Chordoma

found only by radiography or isotope bone scans, or at postmortem examination. Metastases are usually osteolytic (Fig. 22.8); they cause bone pain and may lead to pathological fracture. Vertebral collapse often causes spinal cord compression and paraplegia which is usually irreversible if not treated within 48 hours. Metastatic carcinoma of prostate, and less commonly of breast, may stimulate much reactive bone formation producing radio-opaque 'sclerotic' metastases.

Multiple myeloma

Myeloma is a malignant proliferation of plasma cells which is usually confined to the bone marrow. Most patients are over 50 years of age, and may present with bone pain or pathological fracture, or with anaemia, renal impairment or hypercalcaemia. Overproduction of immunoglobulin chains by the tumour cells usually gives a monoclonal paraprotein found in the serum or in the urine (Bence Jones protein) and may cause a hyperviscosity syndrome. The ESR is normally very high.

The pathological features are of punched-out lytic lesions in the vertebrae, skull (Fig. 22.9), long and flat bones or of diffuse osteoporosis. Histology shows sheets of neoplastic plasma cells with varying degrees of differentiation. Myeloma varies in its aggressiveness, but many patients eventually die of their disease, often from renal failure or infection. Uncommonly, only a single skeletal deposit is present; patients with **solitary plasmacytomas** often develop multiple lesions within a few years.

Primary benign bone tumours

OSTEOID OSTEOMA

Osteoid osteoma (Fig. 22.10) is a small benign bone-forming tumour which usually occurs in the long bones of adolescents. Pain is typically worse at night and relieved by aspirin. The lesion is a small (<2 cm), intensely vascular tumour of osteoblasts forming bony trabeculae. On radiographs this nidus is radiolucent, but when located in the cortex is surrounded and

Features of metastatic tumours in bone
- Metastatic carcinoma to bone very common
- Lung, breast, prostate, kidney, thyroid commonest primaries
- Bone pain, pathological fracture, spinal cord compression

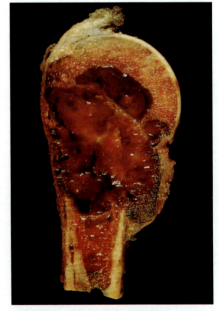

Fig. 22.8   Metastatic follicular carcinoma of thyroid. The humeral neck and head contain a large lytic deposit filled with soft haemorrhagic tumour. The patient had sustained a pathological fracture.

may be obscured by a thick layer of reactive bone; in these cases it can be well demonstrated by computed tomography. A histologically similar but larger lesion known as a **benign osteoblastoma** more commonly arises in the spine and may cause scoliosis or spinal cord compression; pain is less severe and there is less surrounding sclerosis. An osteoma is a well-defined mass of bone arising in the skull and nasal sinuses.

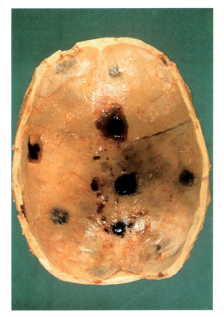

Fig. 22.9 Multiple myeloma. At autopsy the skull vault contains several large punched-out lytic lesions.

CASE STUDY 22.2

A girl of 16 presented with a mild scoliosis (lateral deviation) of the lumbar spine. She also complained of persistent pain, especially at night, and was taking numerous aspirins, which gave her relief. Plain radiography showed an area of sclerosis in the pedicle of the first lumbar vertebra, and increased uptake was noted at this level on isotope bone scan (Fig. 22.10a). The thickened bone was removed surgically and histological examination confirmed the preoperative diagnosis of an osteoid osteoma (Fig. 22.10b). Postoperatively the pain disappeared immediately and the patient's spine gradually straightened.

OSTEOCHONDROMA (OSTEOCARTILAGINOUS EXOSTOSIS)

Osteochondroma is a developmental abnormality which arises from a displaced piece of the epiphyseal growth plate. It consists of a cartilaginous cap on a bony stalk (Fig. 22.11a), attached to the metaphysis of long bones. Osteochondromas are usually painless lumps, although they can press on nerves or blood vessels. Multiple osteochondromas are found in **diaphyseal aclasis** (Fig. 22.11b), a disorder inherited as an autosomal dominant trait. Pain or resumption of growth in adult life should raise the suspicion of malignant change to chondrosarcoma; this is a rare event in solitary lesions and even in diaphyseal aclasis occurs in less than 1% of patients.

(a)

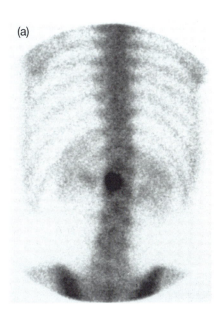

(b)

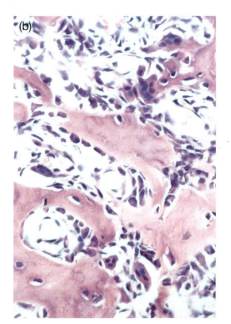

(c)

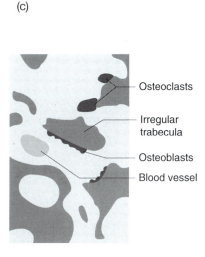

— Osteoclasts

— Irregular trabecula

— Osteoblasts

— Blood vessel

Fig. 22.10   Osteoid osteoma. An isotope bone scan (a) shows a focus of increased uptake over a tumour in the spine of a young girl. Histology (b, c) shows formation of irregular bony trabeculae by active osteoblasts. Osteoclastic resorption is also a feature.

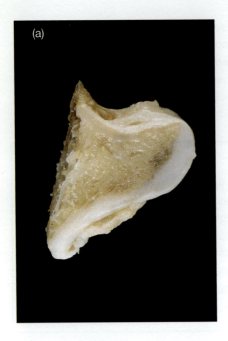

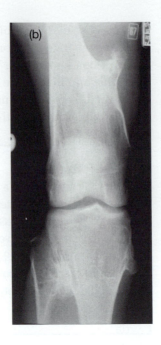

Fig. 22.11 An osteochondroma consists of a bony stalk and a cartilaginous cap (a). In diaphyseal aclasis (b), there are numerous exostoses and failure of remodelling of the metaphyses of the long bones.

ENCHONDROMAS

Enchondromas are lobulated masses of benign cartilage which arise within the medullary cavity. Well over half are found in the tubular bones of the hands and feet. Patients usually complain of swelling or suffer a pathological fracture. In **multiple enchondromas**, a disorder with no hereditary tendency, there may be a few or many enchondromas. If the lesions are often predominantly unilateral the condition is known as **Ollier's disease**. The risk of malignant change of solitary enchondromas is low, but about 25% of patients with multiple lesions, particularly those with lesions of the proximal limb bones and axial skeleton, develop chondrosarcoma.

GIANT CELL TUMOUR

Giant cell tumour arises in the epiphyses of long bones of young adults and consists of proliferating mononuclear tumour cells and numerous large osteoclastic giant cells (Fig. 22.12). Although the giant cells give the tumour its name, they are not themselves neoplastic. Giant cell tumours are locally aggressive tumours which may extend into soft tissue. Recurrence follows

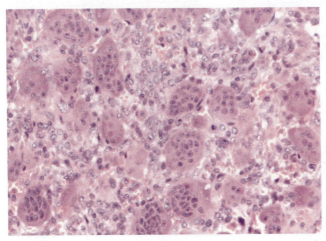

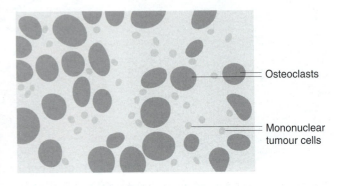

Osteoclasts

Mononuclear tumour cells

Fig. 22.12 Giant cell tumour of bone contains numerous osteoclasts and intervening mononuclear tumour cells.

curettage in 25% of patients and large lesions may require radical excision. Metastasis occurs in less than 5% of patients, most often due to sarcomatous transformation after radiotherapy.

Features of osteosarcoma

- Mainly adolescents
- 50% around knee
- Metaphyses of long bones
- Early pulmonary metastases
- Treat with chemotherapy and radiotherapy
- May complicate Paget's disease in elderly people

Primary malignant bone tumours

OSTEOSARCOMA

Osteosarcoma occurs mainly in adolescents and young adults, who usually complain of pain or swelling or develop a pathological fracture; in older patients a predisposing cause such as Paget's disease or previous irradiation is often found. Most osteosarcomas occur in the metaphysis of long bones (Fig. 22.13), over half around the knee. They are highly malignant tumours which destroy the cortex, extend into soft tissue and metastasize early by the bloodstream, mainly to the lungs. By definition, an osteosarcoma is a malignant tumour in which tumour cells form osteoid or bone. Bone may be present in large or tiny amounts giving densely sclerotic or entirely lytic tumours. Some tumours contain abundant malignant cartilage or fibrosarcomatous tissue. Osteosarcoma is usually treated by multiagent chemotherapy followed by surgery, and often by endoprosthetic replacement rather than amputation. Approximately 60% of patients survive 5 years, compared with 15–20% 25 years ago.

CASE STUDY 22.3

A girl of 12 presented with 6 months' history of pain in the knee. The radiograph showed a destructive lesion of the distal femur with a Codman's triangle of elevated periosteum (Fig. 22.13a). The biopsy showed a typical osteosarcoma (Fig. 22.13b). The patient received three courses of chemotherapy (doxorubicin and *cis*-platinum) after which the tumour was excised and a metallic prosthesis inserted. The resected specimen (Fig. 22.13c) showed that the soft tissue extension had shrunk, while microscopic examination showed no viable tumour indicating an excellent response to chemotherapy. The patient received three further courses of chemotherapy and remained well 3 years later.

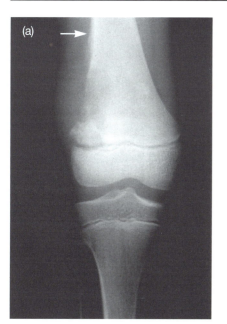
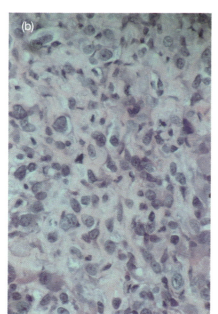
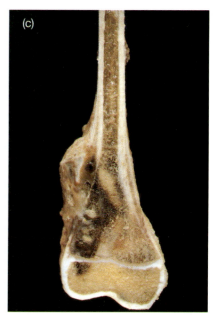

Fig. 22.13 Osteosarcoma. The radiograph (a) shows a destructive lesion within the metaphysis of the distal femur with cortical destruction, a soft tissue extension and a Codman's triangle due to elevation of the periosteum. On biopsy (b) pleomorphic tumour cells lay down a fine meshwork of osteoid. After chemotherapy the resection specimen (c) shows that the soft tissue extension has reduced in size, in keeping with a good response. Note that the tumour has spread through the growth plate into the epiphysis.

CHONDROSARCOMA

Chondrosarcoma differs greatly from osteosarcoma. It is usually a slowly growing tumour of middle-aged and elderly people, arising in the flat bones of the pelvic and shoulder girdles, and the proximal femur and humerus. Most chondrosarcomas develop in the medullary cavity, but some complicate osteochondromas, both solitary and in diaphyseal aclasis. In general, chondrosarcomas are of low-grade malignancy; they are locally aggressive but seldom metastasize. They are best treated by radical surgery, but their location in the axial skeleton makes complete curative excision difficult so that patients often die from slowly growing masses within the abdomen or thorax. Around 15% of chondrosarcomas are of high grade and metastasize to the lungs. Chondrosarcomas are usually resistant to cure by radiotherapy or chemotherapy.

EWING'S SARCOMA

Ewing's sarcoma is a highly malignant tumour occurring particularly in the diaphysis of long bones and in the flat bones of children and adolescents. The tumour consists of sheets of small round malignant cells; it extends through much of the medullary cavity, through the cortex and often forms a large soft tissue mass. There may be a layered 'onion skin' periosteal reaction. Some patients are unwell with fever, anaemia, elevated white cell count and raised ESR; these features may lead to an incorrect clinical diagnosis of osteomyelitis. The tumour metastasizes early to the lungs and bone marrow; treatment with chemotherapy combined with surgery enables half of the patients to survive 5 years. Recent evidence suggests that the tumour is of neuroectodermal origin; 90% of tumours show a characteristic **chromosomal translocation**, t(11;22)(q24;q12).

FIBROSARCOMA AND MALIGNANT FIBROUS HISTIOCYTOMA

Fibrosarcoma and malignant fibrous histiocytoma of bone occur mainly in adults and are destructive lesions which metastasize early by the bloodstream; about a quarter arise in Paget's disease or after irradiation. Histologically, they consist of spindle-shaped fibroblastic cells arranged in long fascicles (fibrosarcoma) or in radiating short bundles known as a storiform pattern (malignant fibrous histiocytoma). Separation of these two entities may be difficult for the pathologist and is of no practical importance.

Normal joint structure and function

Synovial joints (Fig. 22.14) allow a large range of movement, while synarthroses, such as those between the bones of the skull, allow very little movement.

The **articular cartilage** acts both as a smooth low friction surface and as a shock absorber; it contains chondrocytes, which synthesize collagen (mainly type II) and proteoglycan. The orientation of the collagen fibres is parallel to the joint surface in the superficial area, but is vertical in the deeper zone. Proteoglycan binds large amounts of water and, with collagen, forms a gel which resists compression. The **synovium** consists of a layer of synovial lining cells which lie on fibrous or adipose tissue. Synovial lining cells fall into two main categories: type A cells which are like macrophages, and type B cells which resemble fibroblasts. **Synovial**

Fig. 22.14   Structure of a synovial joint.

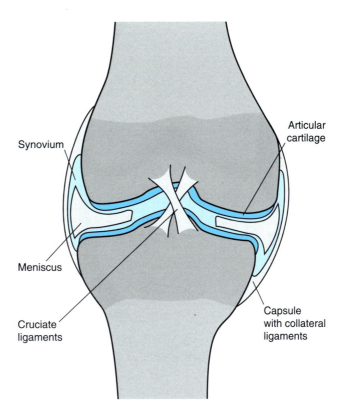

Synovium

Articular cartilage

Meniscus

Cruciate ligaments

Capsule with collateral ligaments

fluid is an ultrafiltrate of plasma to which hyaluronic acid is added by type B cells, thus increasing its viscosity. It acts as a lubricant between the articular surfaces and as nourishment to articular cartilage. Small numbers of mononuclear cells are present within the fluid in health, but the numbers increase greatly in arthritis.

Arthritis

Osteoarthritis

This degenerative disease particularly affects the weight-bearing joints (hips, knees, lumbar and cervical spine) and is common in elderly people. Patients complain of pain, stiffness and limitation of movement. The primary changes affect the articular cartilage: initially there is loss of proteoglycan, then the normally smooth surface becomes roughened, first with superficial flaking and then by deep vertical splits (**fibrillation**), following the orientation of the collagen fibres. As the full thickness of the cartilage is lost (Fig. 22.15), the exposed bone becomes thickened and polished (**eburnation**). Cysts may develop beneath the residual cartilage or exposed bone. At the periphery of the joint there is reactive proliferation of cartilage which undergoes ossification forming bony spurs of osteophytes, which if large may limit movement. The synovium may contain fragments of abraded bone and cartilage and a mild inflammatory infiltrate; these changes are secondary to cartilage damage.

In most cases there is no apparent cause for osteoarthritis; the pathogenesis of primary osteoarthritis is not well understood but genetic factors are important. In contrast the mechanisms are clear in a large number of disorders of joints which predispose to the development of secondary osteoarthritis (Table 22.3).

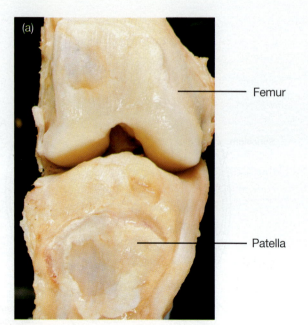

Femur

Patella

Fig. 22.15 Osteoarthritis of the patellofemoral joint (a). The articular cartilage is scored by linear grooves and is lost centrally with exposure of the underlying bone which becomes polished. On histology (b, c), the cartilage is progressively lost until bone is revealed.

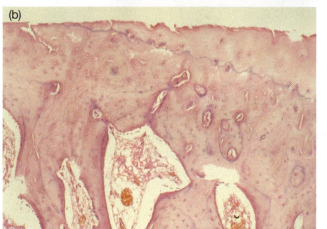

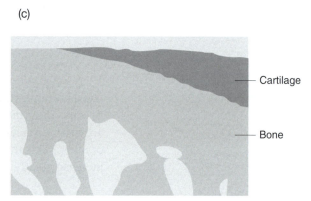

Cartilage

Bone

Table 22.3   Causes of secondary osteoarthritis

Previous joint damage	Rheumatoid arthritis
	Intra-articular fracture
	Osteonecrosis
	Previous septic arthritis
	Congenital dislocation of hip
	Slipped epiphysis
	Loose bodies
Abnormal stresses	Malaligned fracture
	Paget's disease
	Chronic overuse (?)
Metabolic	Gout
	Calcium pyrophosphate deposition
	Alkaptonuria
Neuropathies	Sensory neuropathy, e.g. diabetes
	Tabes dorsalis
	Syringomyelia

Neuropathic arthropathy (Charcot's joint) is a very severe form of osteoarthritis associated with insensitivity to pain or loss of proprioception.

Rheumatoid arthritis

Rheumatoid arthritis is a chronic relapsing remitting inflammatory disease which affects many systems, particularly the joints. Three-quarters of patients are female and although any age can be affected the peak lies between 30 and 45 years. Any synovial joint can be involved but the small joints of the hands and feet, the wrists, elbows, knees and shoulders are commonly affected. Cervical spine involvement with instability may lead to subluxation and spinal cord compression, a particular risk of general anaesthesia. The aetiology and pathogenesis of rheumatoid arthritis are discussed in Chapter 7 and in this section only the articular pathology will be described.

The principal abnormality is inflammation of the synovial lining of joints, tendons and bursae. The synovium (Fig. 22.16a, b) is hyperplastic and frondose and is infiltrated by large numbers of lymphocytes, plasma cells and, in active phases of the disease, neutrophils may be present. These changes account for the painful, stiff and swollen joints. The severe deformities which are often seen are due to secondary damage to the articular cartilage and joint structures. A layer of proliferating granulation tissue known as **pannus** grows over and erodes the articular cartilage from the synovial–cartilage junction (Fig. 22.16c). Similarly, the subchondral bone is removed by osteoclasts giving characteristic peripheral erosions. Destruction of tendons and joint capsule by granulation tissue contributes to the deformities seen in severe cases.

The pathological features of rheumatoid arthritis and osteoarthritis are compared in Fig. 22.17. The extra-articular manifestations of rheumatoid disease are summarized in the box on p. 546.

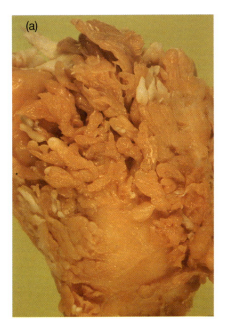

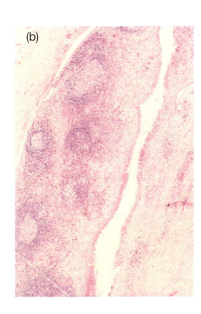

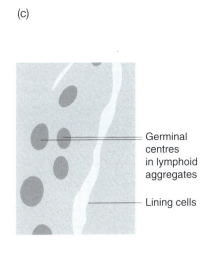

Germinal centres in lymphoid aggregates

Lining cells

Fig. 22.16   In rheumatoid arthritis the synovium (a) is hyperplastic and frondose, and brown stained due to accumulation of haemosiderin pigment. On histology (b, c) there is a chronic inflammatory infiltrate with lymphoid aggregates and germinal centres. The articular cartilage is eroded by vascular pannus (d, e).

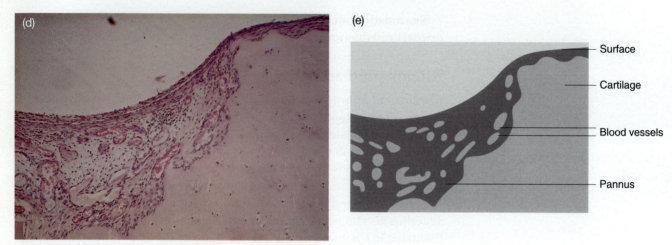

Fig. 22.16   contd

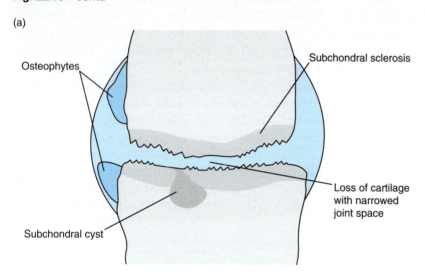

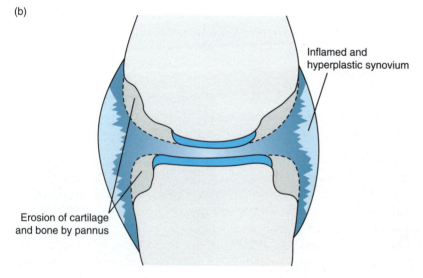

Fig. 22.17   A schematic comparison of (a) osteoarthritis and (b) rheumatoid arthritis.

Extra-articular manifestations of rheumatoid arthritis
- Anaemia
- Rheumatoid nodules
- Vasculitis
- Lymphadenopathy
- Sjögren's syndrome
- Felty's syndrome
- Pericarditis
- Pleurisy
- Pulmonary fibrosis
- Amyloidosis

Seronegative arthritis

The term seronegative arthritis refers to several forms of arthritis characterized by sacroiliac, spinal and peripheral joint involvement, in patients whose serum does not contain rheumatoid factors. The major types are **ankylosing spondylitis**, **psoriatic arthropathy**, reactive arthropathy (**Reiter's syndrome**) and the arthritis associated with ulcerative colitis and Crohn's disease.

The histocompatibility antigen HLA-B27 is expressed much more commonly in patients with these disorders than in the general population in whom the prevalence is around 5%.

ANKYLOSING SPONDYLITIS

Ankylosing spondylitis has a prevalence of 0.5–1% in developed countries, although in many individuals, particularly women, the symptoms are mild. Patients attending hospital are usually young men in their twenties who present with sacroiliac and lumbar pain and stiffness. A third or so will develop peripheral arthritis. In most patients the spondylitis does not progress, but in a minority spinal fusion results with formation of a rigid 'bamboo' spine. The association with HLA-B27 is particularly strong, over 90% of patients carrying the antigen.

Ankylosing spondylitis is characterized by inflammation at the site of insertion of ligaments into bone, which is followed by fibrosis and ossification. The peripheral joints show a synovitis similar to that found in rheumatoid arthritis. About a quarter of those patients with severe disease develop uveitis and a similar number develop aortitis, which may lead to aortic incompetence.

REITER'S SYNDROME (REACTIVE ARTHROPATHY)

Reiter's syndrome includes arthritis, conjunctivitis and urethritis, the last often due to infection by *Chlamydia* spp. or *Mycoplasma* spp. Some cases follow attacks of dysentery. The arthritis usually affects the large weight-bearing joints, and insertional tendonitis of the Achilles tendon is typical.

PSORIATIC ARTHROPATHY

About 5% of patients with psoriasis, usually those with nail involvement, develop a destructive arthritis of the distal interphalangeal and other joints. Sacroiliac and vertebral involvement are common.

Crystal arthropathy

GOUT

Patients with hyperuricaemia are at risk of developing arthritis due to deposition of urate crystals within the joints.

- **'Primary' hyperuricaemia** is due to poorly understood abnormalities of purine catabolism, in most cases as a result of decreased excretion rather than over-production of uric acid. The disease typically affects middle-aged men and there is often a family history.
- **'Secondary' hyperuricaemia** occurs in patients with malignant disease, in whom uric acid production is raised due to increased cell breakdown (particularly following chemotherapy), or in those taking drugs, such as thiazide diuretics, which interfere with renal excretion of urate.

The arthritis of gout may be acute or chronic. Acute gout typically involves the metatarsophalangeal joint of the big toe which is red, swollen and exquisitely painful, but other joints may be affected. Examination of aspirated joint fluid shows needle-shaped crystals free and within neutrophil polymorphs. The symptoms are rapidly relieved by anti-

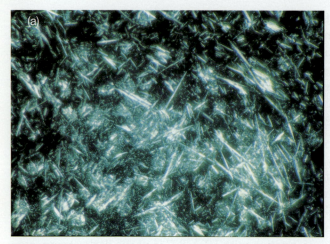
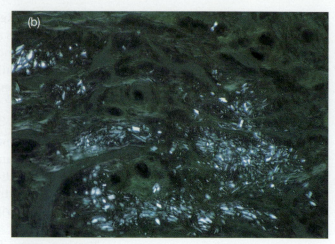

Fig. 22.18   The needle-shaped crystals of gout (a) contrast with the rhomboid crystals of calcium pyrophosphate disease (b).

inflammatory drugs. In **chronic tophaceous gout** chalky deposits of urate crystals (Fig. 22.18a) are found in articular cartilage which undergoes secondary degenerative change. Deposits are also seen in fibrous tissue and fibrocartilage, for example, the menisci and the pinna of the ear. The uricosuric drug **allopurinol** lowers the serum urate level.

CALCIUM PYROPHOSPHATE DEPOSITION DISEASE (PYROPHOSPHATE ARTHROPATHY, PSEUDOGOUT)

Deposition of calcium pyrophosphate crystals within joints (**chondrocalcinosis**) is common in elderly people and can also lead to acute or chronic arthritis. Typically the knees are involved. During acute attacks (**pseudogout**) rhomboid crystals can be detected within polymorphs on polarizing microscopy of joint fluid. Chronic deposition within the menisci, articular cartilage, synovium (Fig. 22.18b) and other articular structures gives a typical radiographic appearance. Although many patients are asymptomatic, chronic deposition of pyrophosphate is strongly linked with osteoarthritis. The precise relationship is not clear: although it may be simply coincidental, it seems more likely that pyrophosphate deposits cause or aggravate some cases of osteoarthritis. Pyrophosphate arthropathy is sometimes familial, and may be associated with hyperparathyroidism and haemochromatosis; these possibilities should be investigated in younger patients.

Bone and joint infections

Over the past 50 years the incidence of infections of the skeletal system has declined in developed countries, and the prognosis has improved with antibacterial therapy. In developing countries, infection remains a major cause of morbidity.

PYOGENIC INFECTIONS

Infection by pyogenic bacteria may follow direct inoculation into bone, following a compound fracture or surgery, but in most cases spread to bone is haematogenous, often from a trivial lesion such as a boil. **Haematogenous acute osteomyelitis** typically occurs in children; the causal organism is usually *Staphylococcus aureus* (Fig. 22.19), although other

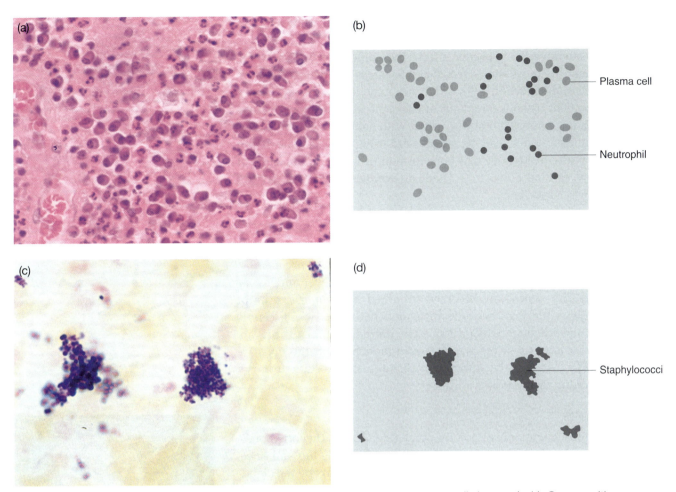

Fig. 22.19 In osteomyelitis a mixed inflammatory infiltrate of neutrophils and plasma cells is seen (a, b). Gram-positive staphylococci (c, d) are the commonest cause.

Complications of acute osteomyelitis
- Septicaemia
- Septic arthritis
- Growth disturbance
- Chronic osteomyelitis

bacteria may be responsible. Patients with sickle-cell anaemia, for example, are at risk of developing **salmonella osteitis**. Infection tends to localize in the dilated sinusoids of the metaphysis of long bones, where the resulting acute inflammatory reaction leads to vascular thrombosis causing local necrosis of bone. Radiographs may be misleadingly normal at this stage, when the infection can often be aborted by antibiotic therapy. If the infection is not treated early, pus tracks in the medullary canal and through the cortex and elevates the periosteum which lays down a shell of new bone (**involucrum**). If the penetrating arteries thrombose, much or all of the shaft of the bone may become necrotic, forming a **sequestrum** which may remain as a haven for organisms and a source for recurrent episodes of inflammation.

Before antibiotic therapy a quarter of patients died of acute osteomyelitis, usually from septicaemia. Other complications include **septic arthritis**, which may follow spread of infection to adjacent joints, particularly those such as the hip and shoulder where the metaphysis lies within the joint capsule. Damage to the epiphyseal plate often leads to growth disturbance, usually retardation, but occasionally overgrowth due to increased blood supply.

Chronic osteomyelitis may supervene with recurrent acute exacerbations and with chronically inflamed discharging sinuses. Squamous carcinoma may, on occasion, develop in these after many years.

Patients with long-standing chronic osteomyelitis are at risk of developing amyloidosis.

Subacute osteomyelitis typically affects the spine; the bodies of the lumbar vertebrae are most often affected and *S. aureus* is the most common organism, although infection with coliforms may follow genitourinary surgery. The patient usually complains of backache; the infection destroys bone and adjacent intervertebral disc, often with some vertebral collapse which may uncommonly lead to spinal cord compression. The lesion usually heals with considerable new bone formation. Localized infection of the metaphysis of long bones may result in **Brodie's abscesses**, cavities surrounded by sclerotic bone.

SEPTIC ARTHRITIS

Septic arthritis may follow a penetrating wound to the joint, direct spread from acute osteomyelitis or haematogenous spread. *S. aureus* is most commonly responsible and the onset is abrupt with high fever and a very painful joint. The synovium becomes inflamed and unless prompt treatment is given the joint becomes distended with pus, which causes destruction of the articular cartilage. Patients with rheumatoid arthritis are at particular risk from superimposed sepsis. In these patients the signs are less apparent and it may be difficult to distinguish infection from an exacerbation of the rheumatoid arthritis.

TUBERCULOSIS

Tuberculosis most commonly affects the spine (Fig. 22. 20), the long bones, where there is often involvement of adjacent joints such as hip and knee, and the tubular bones of the hands (**dactylitis**). Spread occurs by the bloodstream, usually from pulmonary disease. **Spinal tuberculosis** (Pott's disease) may lead to disc destruction, vertebral collapse and paraplegia. Infection sometimes tracks along tissue planes, for example within the sheath of the psoas muscle to form a **psoas abscess** presenting in the groin. In tuberculous arthritis the infection involves the subchondral bone; the articular cartilage is detached and destruction of the joint results.

OTHER INFECTIONS

Bacterial infection of the bones or joints was formerly common in **syphilis**. Arthritis may complicate **gonorrhoea** and **brucellosis**. In **Lyme disease**, a zoonosis is caused by the spirochaete *Borrelia burgdorferi* which is transmitted to humans by deer ticks; a destructive arthritis may be seen. Transient arthralgia is a feature of many common viral illnesses.

Pathology of joint replacement

About 50 000 hip replacements – the most common joint replaced – are performed each year in the UK, usually for osteoarthritis and rheumatoid arthritis; the aim is to restore mobility and relieve pain. Most prostheses for large joints are made of high molecular weight polyethylene and inert metallic alloys. The components are fixed to the bone by acrylic cement or by promoting ingrowth of fibrous tissue or bone into irregularities on the surface of the prostheses (non-cemented prostheses). Prostheses often loosen within 5–10 years, particularly in younger, heavier and more active patients; in general artificial hips last better than knees, because of the

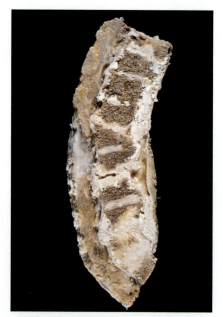

Fig. 22.20   In tuberculosis of the spine the infection starts close to the intervertebral disc, and may extend to involve the adjacent vertebrae.

increased stability of the ball and socket joint. Loosening results from resorption of bone around the prosthesis; in the minority of cases this is due to infection, but the incidence of sepsis has been greatly reduced by improved surgical technique. In most patients it appears that micro-movement between prosthesis and bone stimulates bone resorption. Wear particles of metal, polyethylene and acrylic cement cause a macrophage and foreign body giant cell response which also induces bone resorption and loosening. A vicious circle results with increasing bone loss; revision surgery, with insertion of a further prosthesis, is often required.

Soft tissue tumours

Benign soft tissue tumours, such as **lipomas**, **schwannomas** and **neurofibromas**, are fairly common. Most are small, superficially located and give few problems other than cosmetic ones.

In contrast, **soft tissue sarcomas** are uncommon, with an incidence of 20 cases per million of population per year. They are often large, deeply situated, usually within the limbs or retroperitoneum, and often present late. They cause considerable mortality and may require mutilating surgery including amputation. Soft tissue sarcomas form a heterogeneous group with very large numbers of histological types – a small number of important tumours are described in Table 22.4. In general soft tissue sarcomas form well-defined masses (Fig. 22.21), but the impression that

Prognostic factors in soft tissue sarcomas
- Size
- Site
- Grade
  - Extent of necrosis
  - Mitotic rate

Table 22.4   Some common soft tissue tumours

Tumour	Peak age	Common site	Comments
Benign			
Lipoma	40–60	Superficial, trunk and proximal limbs	Very common
Schwannoma	20–50	Head, neck, flexor aspect of limbs	Arise from nerves; usually solitary
Neurofibroma	20–40	Cutaneous nerves or large trunks	Usually single; multiple in neurofibromatosis
Leiomyoma	30–50	Cutaneous, genital, veins	Sometimes painful
Haemangioma	0–15	Head and neck	'Strawberry naevus' or 'port wine stain'
Malignant			
Liposarcoma	40–70	Retroperitoneum, deep in limbs	Variable grade and prognosis
Malignant fibrous histiocytoma	40–70	Retroperitoneum, deep in limbs	High grade
Leiomyosarcoma	50–70	Retroperitoneum, limbs	Varying grade
Rhabdomyosarcoma	5–15	Genitourinary, head and neck, limbs	Highly malignant
Synovial sarcoma	15–40	Limbs, near but not in joints	Misnomer: not of synovial origin

A large number of types of soft tissue tumours exist, and many are very rare. This table is therefore an oversimplification.

they are encapsulated is erroneous because tumour cells infiltrate the surrounding tissue. If the surgeon 'shells out' the tumour, local recurrence is very likely; the tumour should therefore be removed with a margin of normal tissue. It is desirable to identify the exact histological type of a sarcoma, but this may be difficult even with special stains and electron microscopy. In most cases the precise diagnosis is of less help in determining prognosis than a number of other factors. The anatomical site is important; tumours of the retroperitoneum and head and neck have a poorer outcome than those of the limbs, probably because of the difficulty in complete surgical removal. The risk of local recurrence depends largely on completeness of excision, and therefore on the site and on the skill of the surgeon. The histological grade, which is best estimated by the mitotic activity and extent of necrosis, and the size of the tumour are the best indicators of the risk of metastases.

Tumour-like lesions

FIBROMATOSES

The term fibromatoses is used to describe a number of benign but infiltrative proliferations of fibroblasts (or, more correctly, myofibroblasts); these are divided into superficial and deep groups.

Superficial fibromatoses

Palmar fibromatosis (Dupuytren's contracture) is a very common superficial fibromatosis of the palmar aponeurosis, within which nodules of fibroblasts form and in time are converted into bands of dense fibrous tissue. These cause clawing of the ring and little fingers. The condition is often bilateral. Similar lesions occur in the foot (**plantar fibromatosis**) and, rarely, in the penis (**Peyronie's disease**).

Deep fibromatoses

Deeply placed **musculoaponeurotic fibromatoses** may involve the muscles of the abdominal wall, thigh, shoulder, pelvis or retroperitoneum. These are more serious since they commonly recur repeatedly and, although they do not metastasize, they may cause the patient's death through involvement of vital structures.

PSEUDOSARCOMATOUS LESIONS

The importance of pseudosarcomatous lesions is that they may be overdiagnosed as sarcomas, with unnecessarily radical treatment.

Nodular fasciitis

Nodular fasciitis is a small superficial nodule found on the limbs or trunk, but especially on the forearm. It is so rapidly growing that it is often thought clinically to be a malignant tumour; the histological appearances can be equally alarming in that there are numerous mitotic figures, but these are normal in type. The condition is reactive and is entirely benign.

Myositis ossificans

Myositis ossificans is another fast-growing soft tissue swelling which resembles a sarcoma. It occurs mainly in adolescents and young adults and often, but not always, follows trauma. It tends to occur in the deep muscles

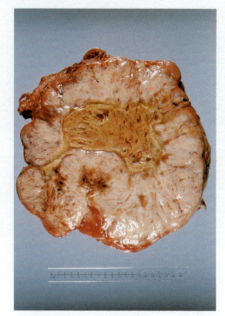

Fig. 22.21 A large soft tissue sarcoma with central necrosis. The tumour appears well defined and has been 'shelled out'. Where possible, these tumours should be excised with a margin of normal tissue.

of the thigh and buttock. It also is completely benign and matures into a well-formed mass of bone within 6 weeks or so.

Miscellaneous orthopaedic conditions

Back pain

Back pain is one of the most common complaints encountered by general practitioners, as 80% of the population suffer from it at some time in their lives. Most patients recover within 3 months, but the outlook for those whose pain lasts for over 6 months is poor, many becoming unable to work. Excluding those with infection, tumour, osteoporotic collapse or arthritis, the cause of the pain is often uncertain; it appears that most 'bad backs' are due to soft tissue rather than bony injury. Some of the commoner conditions giving rise to back pain are discussed briefly below.

PROLAPSED INTERVERTEBRAL DISC

The normal disc is situated between the vertebral bodies. It consists of a fibrous outer layer, the **annulus fibrosus**, and an inner mucinous core, the **nucleus pulposus**. Acute strain on the back, caused for instance by lifting excessive weights, may tear or stretch the annulus, allowing the nucleus to herniate posterolaterally and impinge directly on one of the dorsal roots, causing referred pain. Most patients are between 25 and 50. Although symptoms generally settle with a short period of bed rest and analgesia followed by physiotherapy, surgery is sometimes required for persistent neurological deficit.

SPONDYLOSIS

Vertebral spondylosis, a degenerative condition essentially similar to osteoarthritis, may affect the vertebral bodies or facet joints and is a common cause of cervical or lumbar back pain, often with radiation down the arms or legs.

SPONDYLOLISTHESIS

In spondylolisthesis, a condition seen in around 5% of the population, one vertebral body slips forward on the vertebral body below. It typically occurs at the lumbosacral level or between the fifth and fourth lumbar vertebrae. The condition may be due to congenital instability of the lumbosacral joints, trauma or degenerative changes. Patients usually complain of back pain and and may have sciatica. Spasm of the hamstrings may be striking. Neurological signs are uncommon.

Disorders of menisci

The menisci are demilunes of fibrocartilage which lie between the femoral condyles and tibial plateaux. Tears of the menisci are seen in two groups. Young patients often sustain a 'bucket-handle' tear during sport, usually due to a twisting injury on a flexed knee. The menisci of older patients may degenerate and split without a specific episode of trauma. The torn meniscus may cause locking of the joint, or give pain and joint effusion.

Not uncommonly the lateral meniscus undergoes myxoid degeneration with the formation of a meniscal cyst, palpable over the joint line.

Disorder of the tendons

Abnormalities are seen in both tendons and their surrounding synovial sheath. **Rupture of the Achilles tendon** typically occurs suddenly and dramatically during exercise in middle-aged individuals, usually at the site of degenerative changes. Surgical repair is often required. The tendons of the quadriceps and the long head of biceps may also rupture, usually due to degenerative changes in elderly patients.

Inflammation of the tendon sheaths (**tenosynovitis**) is often a feature of rheumatoid disease (see above). 'Irritative' tenosynovitis may follow overuse, particularly unaccustomed repetitive movements, and usually settles with rest. Bacterial infection is uncommon, but typically affects the flexor tendons of the forearm and hand.

Stenosing tenosynovitis, a fibrous thickening of the tendon sheath, may result in 'trigger finger'. In this, a nodular thickening of the tendon can only pass through the tendon sheath with difficulty, resulting in 'locking' of the finger in the flexed position.

Ganglia

A ganglion is a fibrous walled cyst containing mucoid material which typically occurs around the wrist. The pathogenesis of these very common lesions is uncertain, but is thought to be due to myxoid degeneration of periarticular soft tissue. They almost always recur after being hit by a heavy book, traditionally the family bible, and are better treated by excision.

Bursitis

A bursa is a cystic structure with a synovial lining, usually lying between a bony prominence and a tendon, and acting to reduce friction. Inflammation may follow excessive pressure or movement (as in prepatellar bursitis, housemaid's knee), although bacterial infection is sometimes seen. Bursitis may be a feature of rheumatoid arthritis.

Conclusion

Diseases of the musculoskeletal system are among the most common disorders seen in medical practice. In young patients, sports injuries and back pain interfere with the quality of life and have major economic consequences. The effects of osteoporosis and arthritis are particularly important in middle-aged and elderly people, and involvement of the skeleton is common in patients with cancer.

Chapter 23   Pathology in practice

Learning objectives

To appreciate and understand:

❏ How pathologists contribute to the management of disease and the technology available to do this

❏ Indications for frozen section diagnosis and cytology

❏ How to fill in a death certificate and order a postmortem examination

This book has introduced you to the pathological processes involved in the development of disease. Armed with this knowledge, you have the basis for an understanding of the many different branches of medicine. Most textbooks of pathology do not give the student an insight into the function of the pathology department and pathologist in the modern hospital. Ideally, a student would spend time in a pathology department to see the pathologist's importance to patient care, but with the increasing pressure from other subjects on the medical curriculum, few undergraduates are able to do this. That is the reason for including this chapter.

In the hospital setting the pathologist has several vital roles to play. The primary function is to report the findings in tissue removed from the living body (**biopsy**). This is probably the single most important investigation a patient undergoes. Examination of the biopsy by the pathologist allows a diagnosis to be obtained that assists in determining the future management of the patient. With the increasing complexity of medicine, pathologists are being more directly involved in patient care. Often a team approach with radiologists, surgeons and oncologists is required to arrive at the correct treatment for each patient.

Diagnostic methods available to the pathologist

- Light microscopy
- Electron microscopy
- Immunohistochemistry
- Cytology

Light microscopy

The core of diagnostic work is performed on tissue sections examined by light microscopy. Tissue is preserved in a fixative (usually formalin) and representative samples are subsequently embedded in paraffin wax. From the paraffin wax blocks 5 µm thick sections are cut and stained with **haematoxylin and eosin (H&E)** – a process that has not changed in over a century. Haematoxylin is a natural compound extracted from the heartwood of a tree (logwood) grown mainly in the West Indies. Eosin is a synthetic xanthine-based dye. The method of embedding tissue in paraffin wax requires a minimum processing period of about 4 hours. Most laboratories with a heavy workload prefer overnight processing, for logistic reasons.

Indications for frozen section
- Establish diagnosis: for instance, in a breast lump a diagnosis of malignancy would determine the nature of the operation
- Confirm the nature of tissue identified, for example parathyroid tissue during parathyroid surgery
- Confirm adequate excision of a malignant tumour by histological examination of excision lines
- Confirm that the tissue removed is diseased and suitable for diagnostic purposes. For example, an extensively necrotic tumour consists mainly of debris with only a small portion of recognizable tumour – for diagnostic purposes it is important to obtain viable tissue.

In some cases it is necessary to obtain a diagnosis more quickly. This is usually confined to intraoperative surgical events in which the diagnosis will have an immediate impact on patient management. The frozen section technique involves freezing a small piece of tissue in liquid nitrogen, from which 5 μm thick sections are then cut and stained. This is a particularly difficult procedure; however, skilled medical laboratory scientific officers can achieve a section quality approaching that obtained by conventional paraffin processing. The pathologist must exercise considerable care when interpreting frozen sections, as benign lesions may mimic malignant lesions and vice versa, more readily than in paraffin sections. The accuracy of frozen section diagnosis when compared with subsequent paraffin sections is approximately 98%. Diagnostic errors do occur, but the false-positive diagnosis of malignancy should be less than 1%.

Electron microscopy

In the 1950s electron microscopy became available and soon established itself as an important tool to assist the pathologist in solving particular diagnostic problems. A beam of electrons is passed through ultrathin tissue sections. The resulting images are magnified and focused by a column of electromagnetic lenses. The use of electrons allows higher magnifications (5000–500 000 ×) and higher resolution than that obtained by light microscopy, thus allowing detailed investigation of tissue ultrastructure. Electron microscopy cannot in general distinguish between benign and malignant tumours.

Uses of electron microscopy
- Classification of poorly differentiated tumours, for example identification of ultrastructural features of differentiation not visable by light microscopy, such as melanosomes in an amelanotic melanoma
- Renal biopsies, for example. identification of site of distribution of immune complexes important in the classification of glomerulonephritis
- Identification of tissue deposits, viruses, amyloid and inorganic materials, including asbestos

Immunohistochemistry

In the 1970s, with the advent of monoclonal antibodies, immunochemistry superseded many of the functions of electron microscopy. Polyclonal or antigen-specific monoclonal antibodies can be produced which are directed at specific antigens. These can thus detect signs of differentiation at a molecular rather than ultrastructural level. These antibodies can be applied to tissues and, having bound to a specific antigen, the antibody can be localized by a second monoclonal antibody directed against the first (Fig. 23.1). This second antibody is labelled with a tracer (either a fluorescent marker or an enzyme which will cause a chemical to precipitate out on the section).

Uses of monoclonal antibodies
- Classification of tumours: demonstration of antigenic determinants related to differentiation
- Classification of renal disease: demonstration of different types of immune complexes in glomeruli
- Identification of scanty (easily overlooked) tumour cells or organisms in tissue sections

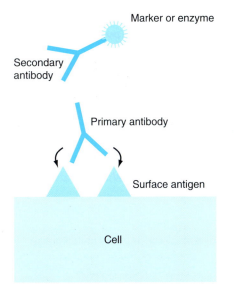

Fig. 23.1 Immunocytochemistry uses the reaction between a primary antibody and antigen to locate markers of cells types or cell products, within tissues. The primary antibody may be labelled directly or detected by a further (secondary) antibody as shown.

Uses of cytology
- Confirmation of malignancy in suspected cases, for example:
  - Sputum in patients with haemoptysis
  - Urine in patients with haematuria
  - Pleural effusions
  - Tissue masses, such as breast lumps
- Screening
  - Screening of the general population for cervical carcinoma
  - Urine from people at high risk of bladder carcinoma, for example workers in the dye industry
- Follow-up of patients with previous malignancy
  - Urine in patients with treated transitional cell carcinoma of the bladder or cervical smears in treated cases of cervical intraepithelial neoplasia

Examples of monoclonal antibodies directed against specific targets are given in Table 23.1. Immunochemistry can also be applied to cytology specimens.

Table 23.1   Examples of monoclonal antibodies available

Monoclonal antibodies	Target
Vimentin	General mesenchymal marker
Epithelial membrane antigen	Epithelial marker
Desmin	Muscle cells
Melanoma antigens	Melanocytes
Leukocyte common antigen	Lymphoid cells
Neurofilament	Neural cells

Cytology

The role of cytology and in particular fine-needle aspiration cytology has expanded in recent years. The technique involves obtaining a sample of cells which are then smeared or centrifuged on to a slide, stained and examined microscopically. Cells may be obtained from scraping mucosal surfaces (e.g. cervical smears) or by applying a vacuum to a standard venepuncture syringe and needle inserted through the skin into the tissue required to be examined.

The procedure has significant advantages over formal biopsies in that cytology is quick and relatively painless, rarely requiring anaesthesia. The process is technically simple, safe and may be performed virtually anywhere (on wards or at the patient's home, for example).

The skills involved in the interpretation of cytological preparations are similar to those used in light microscopy: smears are assessed for the types of cell present, nuclear/cytoplasmic ratio, and nuclear/cytological pleomorphism. Obviously, in cytological preparations it is not possible to assess tissue architecture. Hence one cannot comment on the presence or absence of stromal invasion, making it difficult to distinguish between in situ and invasive carcinomas.

In general the diagnostic specificity of cytology is less than that for histology. Frequently one can only state if a lesion is benign or malignant and indicate a possible diagnosis. This is nevertheless of value as it helps decide patient management.

Postmortem examinations

People who watch too much television may well believe that pathologists spend most of their time carrying out postmortem examinations and playing detective. It may come as a surprise that for most pathologists postmortem examinations comprise only a small proportion of their workload: indeed, many pathologists do not perform them. In the UK and many other countries deaths occurring in suspicious circumstances (such as murders) have postmortem examinations performed by specially trained forensic pathologists.

While perhaps being the least glamorous aspect of a pathologist's work, postmortem examinations do have an important place in the practice of medicine. They can play a central role in modern medicine being a definitive method of quality control and audit. The results provide accurate mortality data for research and public health planning.

Despite this, in developed countries there is a worrying decline in autopsy rates, and the reasons for this are unclear. It is possible that clinicians perceive advances in medical technology, and hence in their diagnostic skills, are making the postmortem examination an antiquated investigation. However, repeated postmortem studies over the decades have shown that the concordance between antemortem (clinical) and postmortem diagnoses remains little changed at around 75%. Indeed, these studies have shown that in about 10% of cases if the postmortem diagnosis had been known prior to death it would have significantly altered patient management! Cynics would argue that because of this, fear of litigation could account in part for the decline in postmortem examinations. There are also the perceived economic costs at a time when resource management and clinical budgeting are being introduced: perhaps the benefits to health care are not immediately apparent.

Another possible cause is the possible reluctance of doctors to request an examination which might lead to further distress of bereaved relatives. Doctors are rarely counselled on dealing with bereaved relatives, but if the situation is handled sensitively, relatives rarely refuse consent for a postmortem examination when requested. Furthermore, many relatives find it of value to know the findings. It should be noted that with careful technique it is difficult to recognize that a postmortem examination has been performed when the body is viewed afterwards by relatives.

Death certification

Following death, it is important that a death certificate is completed to allow disposal of the body. When the cause of death is known and 'natural'

Indications for postmortem examination
- Confirm/determine cause of death
- Investigation of suspicious/unexplained deaths (medicolegal deaths)
- Research
- Investigation of environmental/work-related deaths
- Evaluation of new methods of treatment
- Assistance in the Identification of new diseases, such as Legionnaires' disease
- Teaching
- (Tissue for transplantation)

Types of death to be reported to the Coroner, Procurator Fiscal or State Official
This list is not exhaustive and may vary in different countries
- Uncertainty about cause of death
- Illegal (non-spontaneous) abortions
- Accidents (including industrial); time interval immaterial
- Anaesthetic deaths (including local anaesthetics)
  - during operation
  - considered clinically due to anaesthetic
  - postoperative within 24 hours or cases in which the patient has not regained consciousness
- Death at or taken ill at work (not all deaths at work require referral)
- Blood transfusion
- Drugs (therapeutic or drugs of addiction)
- Electroconvulsive therapy
- Poisoning (including food poisoning)
- Prisoner (including police custody)
- Violence (unnatural deaths)
- Relative unhappy about the standard of medical care
- Persons in receipt of an occupational pension
- Suspected occupationally induced disease

MED A 000000
21

BIRTHS AND DEATHS REGISTRATION ACT 1953
(Form prescribed by the Registration of Births and Deaths Regulations 1987)

MEDICAL CERTIFICATE OF CAUSE OF DEATH

For use only by a Registered Medical Practitioner WHO HAS BEEN IN ATTENDANCE during the deceased's last illness.
and to be delivered by him forthwith to the Registrar of Births and Deaths.

Registrar to enter
No. of Death entry

Name of the deceased...

Date of death as stated to me...day of...Age as stated to me.........................

Place of death..

Last seen alive by me...day of...

1 The certified cause of death takes account of information obtained from post-mortem.
2 Information from post-mortem may be available later.
3 Post-mortem not being held.
4 I have reported this death to the Coroner for further action.
[See overleaf]

Please ring appropriate digit(s) and letter

a Seen after death by me.
b Seen after death by another medical practitioner but not by me.
c Not seen after death by a medical practitioner.

CAUSE OF DEATH

The condition thought to be the 'Underlying Cause of Death' should appear in the lowest completed line of Part 1.

CANCELLED

These particulars not to be entered in death register

Appropriate interval between onset and death

I(a) Disease or condition directly leading to death†.............. **BRONCHOPNEUMONIA**

(b) Other disease or condition, if any, leading to I(a)............. **SQUAMOUS CARCINOMA OF LUNG**

(c) Other disease or condition, if any, Leading to I(b)............. **SMOKING**

II Other significant conditions CONTRIBUTING TO THE DEATH but.............. **RHEUMATOID DISEASE** not related to the disease or condition causing it..........

The death might have been due to or contributed to by the employment followed at some time by the deceased.

Please tick where applicable

†*This does not mean the mode of dying, such as heart failure, asphyxia, asthenia, etc: it means the disease, injury, or complication which caused death.*

I hereby certify that I was in medical attendance during the above named deceased's last illness, and that the particulars and cause of death above written are true to the best of my knowledge and belief.

Signature ....

Residence...

Qualifications as registered .... by General Medical Council

Date.................................

For deaths in hospital: Please give the name of the consultant responsible for the above-named as a patient...

Fig. 23.2 Cause of death certificate used in the UK, partially completed. (The design of the Medical Certificate of Cause of Death is Crown Copyright and is reproduced with permission of the Controller of HMSO.)

the medical practitioner may complete the certificate. If the cause of death is unclear, or there are any suspicious (unnatural) circumstances, the deaths are reported to the Coroner (in England and Wales – Procurator Fiscal in Scotland or State Official in other countries). These judicial officers have statutory powers which enable further inquiry and if necessary an inquest to be held to determine the exact cause of death. This may include ordering a postmortem examination which does not require the relatives' consent.

Mortality statistics are published regularly by governmental bodies. This information is derived primarily from death certificates. Unfortunately this information is not completely reliable. As noted above, studies have shown that clinical diagnoses may be incorrect when compared with postmortem data. Secondly, an incorrect diagnosis may be mistakenly entered on the death certificate – this is surprisingly common. An example of an English death certificate is given in Fig. 23.2.

Research

Pathologists have an important role in the advancement of medicine. They are ideally placed to study diseases with the aim of providing new methods of treatment or health prevention. This may involve the documentation and publication, in the form of case reports, of new diseases or unrecognized features of known diseases. Pathologists may also be part of a research team with surgeons or other clinicians studying the efficacy and adverse effects of new forms of treatment. The most glamorous area of research currently attracting research money is molecular biology. Histopathological laboratories are ideally situated to apply the techniques and methods originally devised in biochemical laboratories, to the extensive range of pathological material they receive. The application of these sophisticated molecular techniques does, however, require dedicated facilities and personnel. Consequently, they are usually found in association with universities or research institutes. Nevertheless major advances are rarely the result of sudden breakthroughs. It is a well-known saying that the way forward in science is the result of 99% perspiration and 1% inspiration. Science advances slowly in small steps with the meticulous study of clearly identified problems. All types of research, whether practical or theoretical, are equally important in contributing to this process.

Management

One of the major challenges in medicine today is the balancing of health care demand with the ever-increasing cost of medical treatment against limited funding. To achieve this, doctors are being encouraged to undertake a new role as managers with greater emphasis being placed on the quality of health care delivered and cost effectiveness. For many doctors this new role is occupying a substantial part of their time as they practise their new skills in resource management (including budgeting) and personnel skills. Besides managing their own departments, pathologists are ideally suited by their insight and interaction with other clinical specialties to participate actively in total hospital management.

Medical audit

To determine whether resources are being utilized effectively, great emphasis is placed on the role of audit. This is defined as the systematic, critical analysis of medical care (methods of diagnosis and treatment) with comparison of defined standards in order to improve the quality of patient care. A simple example of audit in pathology would be the examination of the time interval between receipt of a specimen and the issuing of a report. An efficient turnaround is important as patients awaiting diagnosis may

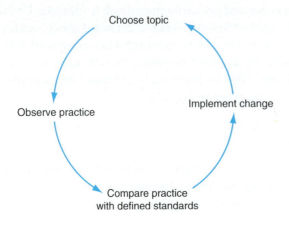

Fig. 23.3   The audit cycle.

unnecessarily occupy hospital beds which is costly. The important part of audit is to complete the feedback cycle (Fig. 23.3); if requisite standards are not met changes are implemented.

Teaching

Pathologists have an important role in the education and continuing education of surgeons, physicians and other health care workers in the causes and effects of disease and their prevention. Pathologists are also responsible for the training of future pathologists. The teaching of undergraduates can occupy a substantial part of the pathologist's time and tends to occur mainly in medical schools. The core material is usually taught in lectures supplemented by postmortem demonstrations, tutorials and problem-solving exercises. Recent advances in technology, including the innovative use of computers and video, should make the learning process more exciting.

Conclusion

As can be seen from this chapter, the pathologist has several roles to play. The responsibilities of particular pathologists may differ appreciably, depending on the institution at which they work. In universities there is a greater tendency for specialization, with individuals responsible for key areas such as renal pathology, soft tissue pathology, administration or teaching. In contrast, in a district general hospital there are rarely sufficient staff to develop highly specialized fields and a pathologist will have a wider range of responsibility covering many areas.

The future for pathology is exciting. Major advances in molecular biology are beginning to unravel the steps involved in the development of cancer. In time this will lead to the specific therapies directed against individual tumours. It is up to pathologists to embrace these developing technologies, and doing so will propel them into the forefront of modern medicine.

Further reading

General texts

Cotran RS, Kumar V, Robins SL. *Robin's Pathologic Basis of Disease*, 5th edn. Philadelphia: WB Saunders, 1994.

Ghadially FN. *Ultrastructural Pathology of the Cell and Matrix*, 3rd edn. London: Butterworths, 1988.

McGee JO'D, Isaacson PG, Wright NA (eds). *Oxford Textbook of Pathology*. Oxford: Oxford University Press, 1992.

McSween RNM, Whaley K (eds). *Muir's Textbook of Pathology*, 14th edn. London: Hodder & Stoughton, 1995.

Medawar P. *Advice to a Young Scientist*. New York: Harper & Row, 1979.

Parums DV. *Essential Clinical Pathology*. Oxford: Blackwell Science, 1996.

Report of the Joint Working Party of the Royal Colleges of Pathologists, Royal College of Physicians of London and Royal College of Surgeons of England. *The Autopsy and Audit*, 1991.

Underwood JCE. *Introduction to Biopsy Interpretation and Surgical Pathology*, 2nd edn. Berlin: Springer-Verlag, 1987.

Walter JB. *Walter & Israel's General Pathology*. Edinburgh: Churchill Livingstone, 1995.

Related disciplines

Molecular biology and genetics

Alberts B, Bray D, Lewis J, Raff M, Roberts K, Watson JD. *Molecular Biology of the Cell*, 3rd edn. New York: Garland, 1994.

Franks LM, Teich NM. *Introduction to the Cellular and Molecular Biology of Cancer*. Oxford: Oxford University Press, 1991.

Leder P, Clayton DA, Rubinstein E. *Introduction to Molecular Medicine*. New York: Scientific American Inc., 1994.

Rothwell NV. *Understanding Genetics: A Molecular Approach*. New York: Wiley-Liss, 1993.

Trent RJ. *Molecular Medicine: An Introductory Text for Students*. Edinburgh: Churchill Livingstone, 1993.

Weatherall DJ. *The New Genetics and Clinical Practice*. Oxford: Oxford University Press, 1991.

Immunology

Janeway CA, Travers P. *Immunobiology: The Immune System in Health and Disease*, 2nd edn. London and New York: Current Biology/Churchill Livingstone/Garland, 1996.

Reeves WG. *Lecture Notes on Immunology*. Oxford: Blackwell Scientific, 1996.

Roitt I. *Essential Immunology*, 8th edn. Oxford: Blackwell Scientific, 1994.

Roitt IM, Brostoff J, Male DK (eds). *Immunology*, 4th edn. London: Gower Medical, 1995.

Haematology

Campbell-Hughes NC. *Lecture Notes on Haematology*. Oxford: Blackwell Scientific, 1996.

Haematological Pathology. Edinburgh: Churchill Livingstone, 1995.

Hoffbrand AV, Pettit JE. *Essential Haematology*. Oxford: Blackwell Scientific, 1993.

Cytopathology

Gray W. *Diagnostic Cytopathology*. Edinburgh: Churchill Livingstone, 1995.

Kocjan GIL. *Grubb's Colour Atlas of Diagnostic Cytopathology*. Edinburgh: Churchill Livingstone, 1996.

McKee GT. *Diagnostic Cytopathology*. St Louis, MO: Mosby, 1996.

Pathology of individual systems

Cardiovascular disease

Davies MJ. *Colour Atlas of Cardiovascular Pathology*. Oxford: Oxford University Press, 1986.

Julian DG, Camm AJ, Fox KM, Hall RJC, Poole-Wilson PA. *Diseases of the Heart*, 2nd edn. Philadelphia: WB Saunders, 1996.

Respiratory disease

Craighead JE. *Pathology of Human Environmental and Occupational Disease*. St Louis, MO: Mosby, 1995.

McDowell E, Beals TF. *Biopsy Pathology of the Bronchi*. London: Chapman & Hall, 1986.

Sheppard M. *Practical Pulmonary Pathology*. London: Arnold, 1995.

Oral pathology

Cawson RA, Eveson JW. *Oral Pathology and Diagnosis*. London: Heinemann Medical, 1987.

Cawson RA, Odell EW. *Colour Guide. Oral Pathology*. Edinburgh: Churchill Livingstone, 1993.

Marsh P, Martin M. *Oral Microbiology*, 3rd edn. London: Chapman & Hall, 1992.

Odell E, Morgan P. *Biopsy Pathology of Oral Tissues*. London: Chapman & Hall, 1996.

Pindborg JJ. *Oral Cancer and Precancer*. Bristol: Wright, 1980.

Shear M. *Cysts of the Oral Regions*, 3rd edn. Bristol: Wright, 1982.

Soames JV, Southam JC. *Oral Pathology*, 2nd edn. Oxford: Oxford University Press, 1993.

Gastrointestinal disease

Day DW, Dixon MF. *Biopsy Pathology of the Oesophagus, Stomach and Duodenum*, 2nd edn. London: Chapman & Hall, 1996.

Morson BC, Dawson IMP, Day DW, Jass JR, Price AB, Williams GT. *Gastrointestinal Pathology*, 3rd edn. Oxford: Blackwell Scientific, 1990.

Owen DA, Kelly JK. *Atlas of Gastrointestinal Pathology*. Philadelphia: WB Saunders, 1994.

Talbot IC, Price AB. *Biopsy Pathology in Colorectal Disease*. London: Chapman & Hall, 1987.

Liver, pancreas and gallbladder

Cruickshank AH. *Pathology of the Pancreas*. New York: Springer-Verlag, 1995.

Go VLW, DeMagno EP, Gardner JD et al. (eds). *The Pancreas: Biology, Pathobiology and Disease*. New York: Raven Press, 1993.

MacSween RNM, Anthony PP, Scheuer PJ (eds). *Pathology of the Liver*, 2nd edn. Edinburgh: Churchill Livingstone, 1987.

Patrick RS, McGee JO. *Biopsy Pathology of the Liver*, 2nd edn. London: Chapman & Hall, 1988.

Scheuer PJ. *Liver Biopsy Interpretation*. Philadelphia: WB Saunders, 1994.

Sherlock S. *Disease of the Liver and Biliary System*, 9th edn. Oxford: Blackwell Scientific 1992.

Renal and urinary disease

Brenner BM, Rector FC (eds). *The Kidney*, 4th edn. Philadelphia: WB Saunders, 1991.

Hepinstall RH (ed.). *Pathology of the Kidney*. Boston: Little, Brown, 1992.

Tisher CC, Brenner BM (eds). *Renal Pathology with Clinical and Functional Correlations*, 2nd edn. Philadelphia: JB Lippincott, 1994.

Young RH (ed.). *Pathology of the Urinary Bladder*. New York: Churchill Livingstone, 1989.

Male genital pathology

Ansell ID. *Atlas of Male Reproductive Pathology*. Lancaster: MTP Press, 1985.

Bostwick DG, Dundore PA. *Biopsy Pathology of the Prostate*. London: Chapman & Hall, 1996.

Peterson RO. *Urologic Pathology*, 2nd edn. Philadelphia: JB Lippincott, 1992.

Gynaecological pathology

Coleman DC, Evans DMD. *Biopsy Pathology and Cytology of the Cervix*, 2nd edn. London: Chapman & Hall, 1996.

Fox H (ed.). *Hains and Taylor's Obstetrical and Gynaecological Pathology*. Edinburgh: Churchill Livingstone, 1987.

Fox H, Buckley CH. *Biopsy Pathology of the Endometrium*. London: Chapman & Hall, 1989.

Kraus FT, Damjanov I, Kaufman N (eds). *Pathology of Reproductive Failure*. Baltimore, MD: Williams & Wilkins, 1991.

Naeye RL. *Disorders of the Placenta, Fetus and Neonate: Diagnosis and Clinical Significance*. St Louis, MO: Mosby, 1992.

Paediatric pathology

DeSa D. *Pathology of Nonatal Intensive Care*. London: Chapman & Hall, 1994.

Gray ES. *Paediatric Surgical Pathology*. Edinburgh: Churchill Livingstone, 1995.

Keeling JW. *Fetal Pathology*. Edinburgh: Churchill Livingstone, 1994.

Parham DM. *Pediatric Neoplasia*. Philadelphia: Lippincott Raven, 1996.

Potter EL. *Potter's Pathology of the Fetus and the Infant*. St Louis, MO: Mosby Yearbook, 1996.

Wigglesworth J, Singer DB (eds). *Textbook of Fetal and Perinatal Pathology*. Oxford: Blackwell Scientific, 1991.

Neurological and eye disease

Adams JH, Graham DI. *Introduction to Neuropathology*, 2nd edn. Edinburgh: Churchill Livingstone, 1994.

Esiri MM, Oppenheimer DR. *Diagnostic Neuropathology*. Oxford: Blackwell Scientific, 1989.

Lee WR. *Ophthalmic Histopathology*. London: Springer-Verlag, 1991.

Poirier J, Gray F, Escourelle R. *Manual of Basic Neuropathology*. Philadelphia: WB Saunders, 1990.

Richardson EP. *Pathology of the Peripheral Nerve*. Philadelphia: WB Saunders, 1995.

Swash M, Schwartz M. *Biopsy Pathology of the Muscle*. London: Chapman & Hall, 1991.

Weller RO. *Colour Atlas of Neuropathology*. Oxford: Oxford University Press, 1984.

Weller RO. *Nervous System, Muscle and Eyes. Systemic Pathology*, 3rd edn, Vol 4. Edinburgh: Churchill Livingstone, 1990.

Endocrine disease

Kovacs K, Asa S. *Functional Endocrine Pathology*. Oxford: Blackwell Scientific, 1990.

Ljungberg O. *Biopsy Pathology of the Thyroid and Parathyroid*. London: Chapman & Hall, 1992.

Symmers W. *The Endocrine System*. Edinburgh: Churchill Livingstone, 1996.

Skin disease

Hunter JAA, Savin JA, Dahl MV. *Clinical Dermatology*. Oxford: Blackwell Scientific, 1989.

Kirkham N. *Biopsy Pathology of the Skin*. London: Chapman & Hall, 1991.

Mooi W-J, Krausz T. *Biopsy Pathology of Melanocytic Disorders*. London: Chapman & Hall, 1992.

Morse SA. *Atlas of Sexually-transmitted Disease*. Philadelphia: JB Lippincott, 1990.

Breast disorders

Hughes LE, Marvel RE, Webster DJT. *Benign Disorders and Diseases of the Breast: Concepts and Clinical Management*. London: Baillière Tindall, 1989.

Sloane J. *Biopsy Pathology of the Breast*. London: Chapman & Hall, 1985.

Trott P. *Breast Cytopathology*. London: Chapman & Hall, 1996.

Lymphoid disease

Henry K, Symmers W (eds). *Thymus, Lymph Nodes, Spleen and Lymphatics. Systemic Pathology*, 3rd edn, Vol 7. Edinburgh: Churchill Livingstone, 1992.

Isaacson PG, Norton AJ. *Extranodal Lymphomas*. Edinburgh: Churchill Livingstone, 1994.

Lennert K, Feller AC. *Histopathology of Non-Hodgkin's Lymphomas*, 2nd edn. Berlin: Springer-Verlag, 1992.

Stansfeld AG, d'Ardenne AJ (eds). *Lymph Node Biopsy Interpretation*, 2nd edn. Edinburgh: Churchill Livingstone, 1992.

Bone and soft tissue diseases

Bullough PG. *Bullough and Vigorita's Atlas of Orthopaedic Pathology*. St Louis, MO: Mosby-Wolfe, 1996.

Fletcher C. *Diagnostic Histopathology of Tumours*. Edinburgh: Churchill Livingstone, 1995.

Milgram JW. *Radiologic and Histologic Pathology of Nontumorous Diseases of Bones and Joints*. Northbrook: Northbrook Publishing, 1990.

Index

Metastatic sites (*contd*)
  lympoid tissue 514
  preferred 86
  spleen 526
Metazoal infections
  colon 271
  gastric 262
Methotrexate 17, 66, 110
Methyldopa 285, 430
Metoclopramide 430
Metropathia haemorrhagica 355
MHC *see* Major histocompatibility complex
Michaelis–Gutman bodies 323, 327, 333
Micro-organisms
  in dental plaque formation 228
  inhaled 216
  transmission 4
Microabscesses 296
Microadenoma 431
Microaneurysms, retina 423
Microangiopathic haemolytic anaemia 176
Microcalcification, breast tumours 498
Microcephaly, prenatal diagnosis 36
Microglandular adenosis 487
Microglandular hyperplasia, cervix 347
Microglial cells 60, 116, 396
Microglobulins 116
Micrognathia 303
Microinfarcts, retina 423
Micronodular cirrhosis 290
Microsatellite polymorphism 28
Microsporidiosis, immunosuppressed patients
    262
Mid-brain acqueduct stenosis 375
Mikulicz's disease and syndrome 244
Milia, sweat glands 476
Miliary tuberculosis *see* Tuberculosis
Milker's nodule 460
Mineralocorticoids 55
Minimal change disease 306–7, 311
Mis-sense mutation 22
Miscarriage *see* Abortion
Missile injury 399
Mites *see* Arthropods
Mitochondria 19, 34, 288
Mitochondrial cytopathy 417
Mitogen-activated protein kinases 64
Mitomycin C 17, 110
Mitosis 9, 19–20, 80, 110, 140
Mitosis (maturation) promoting factor 62
Mitral valves 181, 186, 187, 189
    stenosis 188, 218, 219
Molluscum contagiosum 460
Monoclonal antibodies 111, 112, 556–7
Monocyte chemotactic protein 1 (MCP-1) 120
Monocytic leukaemia 526
Monocytoid lymphoma 520
Mononeuritis multiplex 419
Mononeuropathy 419
Mononuclear infiltrates 216
Mononuclear phagocyte system 123
Mononucleosis, infectious 237–8, 511
Monosomy X *see* Turner's syndrome
Morphoea 470
Mortality data, accurate 558, 559
Mosaic, genetic 24
Mosquitoes 209
Motor neuron disease 408, 409, 417, 418
Moulds, inhaled 216
Mucin 248
Mucinous tumours
  colorectal 275
  ovary 362, 363
  pancreas 300
Mucocele
  gallbladder 298
  salivary 232, 244
Mucoepidermoid carcinoma 221
Mucoid carcinoma 494, 496
Mucolipidoses 36

Mucopolysaccharides 359, 434, 530
Mucopolysaccharidoses 36, 41
Mucor sp. 207, 208
Mucosa
  alimentary tract 248
  bronchial 194
  hypertrophy 255
  large bowel, prolapse 270
  nasal passages 192–3
  oesophageal 249, 250
  oral 234
Mucosa-associated lymphoid tissue (MALT)
  lymphoma 224, 275, 441, 516, 525
  normal structure and function 500, 503–4
Mucous membranes, in epidermolysis 456
Mucus, hypersecretion 255
Müllerian ducts 343
Müllerian tumour, malignant mixed 357
Multi-point linkage analysis 35
Multidrug resistance 110
Multiple endocrine neoplasia (MEN) syndromes
    95, 427, 432, 439–40, 441, 446, 447, 450
Multiple myeloma 128, 318, 523, 533, 538, 539
Multiple sclerosis 58, 408–10
Multiple systems degeneration 408
Mumps virus (paramyxovirus) infections
  and diabetes mellitus 448
  and germ cell tumours 334
  oral involvement 230, 237
  and pancreatitis 299
  and viral encephalitis 404
  and viral meningitis 404
  and viral orchitis 333
Muscle atrophy 68
Muscle cramps 433
Muscular dystrophies 33, 36, 41, 414–16
Muscularis propria, alimentary tract 248
Musculoaponeurotic fibromatoses 552
Musculoskeletal disorders, congenital 368,
    376–7
Mushroom worker's lung 216
Mutagens 22, 24, 99
Mutation 22–3
Mutation reversal 43
Myasthenia gravis 418–19, 513, 527
Myasthenia gravis-like syndrome *see*
    Eaton–Lambert syndrome
Myb and myc oncoproteins 93
Myc oncogene, and lung tumours 224
Mycetomas 208
Mycid reactions 464
Mycobacterial infections
  and Crohn's disease 263
  drug resistant 150
  and granuloma formation 126, 198
  in HIV/AIDS 146, 147–8, 149
  and lymph node granuloma 508
  and meningitis 388
  and necrotizing lymphadenopathy 509
  recurrent 390
  secondary gut involvement 261
  skin 461–2
  splenic candidiasis 512
  superantigens 158
  therapy 134
Mycobacterium avium 146, 147–8, 149, 150, 154
Mycobacterium avium-intercellulare 206
Mycobacterium bovis 152
Mycobacterium kansasii 206
Mycobacterium leprae 151
Mycobacterium marinum 462
Mycobacterium paratuberculosis 263
Mycobacterium tuberculosis 73, 148, 150, 151, 198,
    261, 388, 462, 509
Mycobacterium ulcerans 462
Mycoplasma infection
  and ARDS 218
  and HIV/AIDS 208
  in Reiter's syndrome 547
  salpingitis 360

Mycoplasma pneumoniae, community-acquired 209
Mycosis fungoides 475, 476, 520, 526
Myelin 58, 60
Myelofibrosis, spleen 512
Myeloid neoplasms *see* Leukaemia
Myelolipoma 446
Myeloma 76, 538
  see also Multiple myeloma
Myeloma kidney 318
Myelomeningocele 374
Myeloproliferative disorders, spleen 526
Myocardial damage 147
Myocardial infarction
  and atheroma 4
  and cerebral infarction 401
  clinical features 178–81
  coagulation necrosis 73
  complications 181
  in ischaemic heart disease 176
  and thrombosis 170
Myocardial infiltrations or depositions 184–5
Myocarditis 182–3, 205, 462
Myoglobin, and acute tubular necrosis 312
Myometrium, tumours 359–60
Myopathies
  alcoholic 417
  congenital 417
  inflammatory 416–17
  and mitochondrial genes 33–4
  muscular dystrophies 414–16
  penicillamine 417
  peripheral 306
  viral 416
Myoproliferative disorders 511
Myositis ossificans 552–3
Myotonic dystrophy 22, 36, 416
Myxoedema 417, 427, 436, 437
  see also Hypothyrodism
Myxoedema madness 434
Myxoid mitral degeneration 188

N-*myc*, overexpression 94
Naevus, melanocytic 473
Naevus flammeus or telangiectaticus 457
Nails 451
  disease 475
  dystrophy 456, 475
  fungal infection 462, 463, 475
  in psoriatic arthropathy 547
Nares 192
Nasal cavity, endometriosis 358
Nasal mucosa, chronic inflammation 122–7
Nasal passages 192–4
Nasal polyp, allergic 131
Nasal tumours 193–4
Nasolabial cyst 232
Nasopalatine duct (incisive canal) cyst 232
Nasopharyngeal carcinoma 106, 194
Natural killer (NK) cells 50, 70, 86, 107
Nausea and vomiting 306, 398, 430
NEC *see* Necrotizing enterocolitis
Neck
  oedema 194
  stiffness 398, 403, 405
Necrosis 71–3, 119
  endometrial 357
  and inflammation 114
  in liver failure 280
  in malignant tumours 79
Necrotizing enterocolitis (NEC) 262, 383, 385–6
Needle biopsy 88, 302, 331, 332, 529
Neisseria sp., in dental plaque 230
Neisseria gonorrhoeae 327, 345, 346, 360
Neisseria infection
  cervical 346
  chronic prostatitis 327
  meningitis 388, 389, 404
  salpingitis 360
  vaginal 345